Graham Roberts.

September 2008

Cambridge studies in Biological and Evolutionary Anthropology 53

Technique and Application in Dental Anthropology

Bringing together a variety of today's most accomplished dental researchers, *Technique and Application in Dental Anthropology* covers a range of topics germane to the study of human and other primate teeth. The chapters encompass work on both individuals and samples, ranging from prehistoric through recent times. The focus throughout the book is the methodology required for the study of modern dental anthropology, comprising the most up-to-date scientific methods in use today – ranging from simple observation to advanced computer-based analyses – which can be utilized by the reader in their own dental research. Originating from the twentieth anniversary meeting of the Dental Anthropology Association, this is a valuable reference source for advanced undergraduate and graduate students, academic researchers, and professionals in the social and life sciences, as well as clinicians.

JOEL D. IRISH is a Professor in the Department of Anthropology at the University of Alaska Fairbanks.

GREG C. NELSON is an Adjunct Assistant Professor in the Department of Anthropology at the University of Oregon.

Cambridge Studies in Biological and Evolutionary Anthropology

Series editors

Also available in the series

39 *Methods in Human Growth Research* Roland C. Hauspie, Noel Cameron & Luciano Molinari (eds.) 0 521 82050 2
40 *Shaping Primate Evolution* Fred Anapol, Rebecca L. German & Nina G. Jablonski (eds.) 0 521 81107 4
41 *Macaque Societies – A Model for the Study of Social Organization* Bernard Thierry, Mewa Singh & Werner Kaumanns (eds.) 0 521 81847 8
42 *Simulating Human Origins and Evolution* Ken Wessen 0 521 84399 5
43 *Bioarchaeology of Southeast Asia* Marc Oxenham & Nancy Tayles (eds.) 0 521 82580 6
44 *Seasonality in Primates* Diane K. Brockman & Carel P. van Schaik (eds.) 0 521 82069 3
45 *Human Biology of Afro-Caribbean Populations* Lorena Madrigal 0 521 81931 8
46 *Primate and Human Evolution* Susan Cachel 0 521 82942 9
47 *The First Boat People* Steve Webb 0 521 85656 6
48 *Feeding Ecology in Apes and Other Primates* Gottfried Hohmann, Martha Robbins & Christophe Boesch (eds.) 0 521 85837 2
49 *Measuring Stress in Humans: A Practical Guide for the Field* Gillian Ice & Gary James (eds.) 0 521 84479 7
50 *The Bioarchaeology of Children: Perspectives from Biological and Forensic Anthropology* Mary Lewis 0 521 83602 6
51 *Monkeys of the Taï Forest* W. Scott McGraw, Klaus Zuberühler & Ronald Noë (eds.) 0 521 81633 5
52 *Health Change in the Asia-Pacific Region: Biocultural and Epidemiological Approaches* Ryutaro Ohtsuka & Stanley J. Ulijaszek (eds.) 978 0 521 83792 7

Technique and Application in Dental Anthropology

Edited by

Joel D. Irish
University of Alaska, Fairbanks

Greg C. Nelson
University of Oregon

CAMBRIDGE
UNIVERSITY PRESS

CAMBRIDGE UNIVERSITY PRESS
Cambridge, New York, Melbourne, Madrid, Cape Town, Singapore, São Paulo

Cambridge University Press
The Edinburgh Building, Cambridge CB2 8RU, UK

Published in the United States of America by Cambridge University Press, New York

www.cambridge.org
Information on this title: www.cambridge.org/9780521870610

First published 2008

Printed in the United Kingdom at the University Press, Cambridge

A catalogue record for this publication is available from the British Library

ISBN 978-0-521-87061-0 hardback

Contents

Section III: Applied life and population history

Section IV: Forefront of technique

Contributors

Kalpana Agrawal
Department of Anatomy
Laboratory Block
Faculty of Medicine Building
21 Sassoon Road
Hong Kong

Sarah K. Amugongo
Department of Integrative Biology
University of California
3060 Valley Life Sciences Building
Berkeley
California 94720
USA

KaiYang Ang
Department of Biological Sciences
National University of Singapore
14 Science Drive 4
Singapore 117543
Republic of Singapore

Shara E. Bailey
Department of Anthropology
New York University
25 Waverly Place
New York
New York 10003
USA

Luca Bondioli
Museo Nazionale Preistorico Etnografico "Luigi Pigorini"
Sezione di Antropologia

P. le G. Marconi 14
00144 Rome
Italy

Jonathan M. Bunn
Old Main 330
Department of Anthropology
University of Arkansas
Fayetteville
Arkansas 72701
USA

M. Christopher Dean
Evolutionary Anatomy Unit
Department of Anatomy and Developmental Biology
University College London
London WC1E 6BT
UK

Charles M. FitzGerald
Department of Anthropology
McMaster University
Hamilton
Ontario
Canada L8S 4L9

Debbie Guatelli-Steinberg
Department of Anthropology
244 Lord Hall
124 West 17th Avenue
The Ohio State University
Columbus
Ohio 43210
USA

Edward F. Harris
Department of Orthodontics
College of Dentistry
The Health Science Center
University of Tennessee

Memphis
Tennessee 38163
USA

Brian Hemphill
Department of Sociology/Anthropology
California State University Bakersfield
9001 Stockdale Highway
Bakersfield
California 93311
USA

Simon Hillson
Institute of Archaeology
University College London
31–34 Gordon Square
London WC1H 0PY
UK

Leslea J. Hlusko
Department of Integrative Biology
University of California
3060 Valley Life Sciences Building
Berkeley
California 94720
USA

Louise T. Humphrey
Palaeontology Department
Natural History Museum
Cromwell Road
London SW7 5BD
UK

Joel D. Irish
Department of Anthropology
University of Alaska Fairbanks
Fairbanks
Alaska 99775
USA

Teresa E. Jeffries
Department of Mineralogy
The Natural History Museum
Cromwell Road
London SW7 5BD
UK

Helen M. Liversidge
Centre for Oral Growth and Development (Paediatric Dentistry)
Institute of Dentistry
Queen Mary's School of Medicine & Dentistry
Turner Street
Whitechapel
London E1 2AD
UK

Peter W. Lucas
Department of Anthropology
George Washington University
2110 G St NW
Washington
DC 20052
USA

John R. Lukacs
Department of Anthropology
University of Oregon
Eugene
Oregon 97403
USA

Roberto Macchiarelli
Laboratoire de Géobiologie
Biochronologie et Paléontologie Humaine
UMR 6046 CNRS
Université de Poitiers
40 av. du Recteur Pineau
86022 Poitiers Cedex
France

Michael C. Mahaney
Southwest National Primate Research Center
Southwest Foundation for Biomedical Research
PO Box 760549
San Antonio
Texas 78245
USA

Arnaud Mazurier
Etudes Recherches Matériaux
Dép. Géosciences
40 av. du Recteur Pineau
86022 Poitiers Cedex
France

Greg C. Nelson
Department of Anthropology
University of Oregon
Eugene
Oregon 97403
USA

Oliver T. Rizk
Department of Integrative Biology
University of California
3060 Valley Life Sciences Building
Berkeley
California 94720
USA

Christopher W. Schmidt
Department of Anthropology
University of Indianapolis
1400 E. Hanna Ave.
Indianapolis
Indiana 46227
USA

Gary T. Schwartz
Institute of Human Origins and School of Human Evolution and Social Change
PO Box 872402

Arizona State University
Tempe
Arizona 85287
USA

G. Richard Scott
Department of Anthropology/096
University of Nevada Reno
Reno
Nevada 89557
USA

Jessica R. Scott
Old Main 330
Department of Anthropology
University of Arkansas
Fayetteville
Arkansas 72701
USA

Robert S. Scott
Old Main 330
Department of Anthropology
University of Arkansas
Fayetteville
Arkansas 72701
USA

Zhongquan Sui
Department of Botany
University of Hong Kong
Pokfulam Road
Hong Kong

Hugh T. W. Tan
Department of Biological Sciences
National University of Singapore
14 Science Drive 4
Singapore 117543
Republic of Singapore

Mark Teaford
Center for Functional Anatomy and Evolution
Johns Hopkins University School of Medicine
725 North Wolfe St.
Baltimore
Maryland 21205
USA

Linda M. Thompson
Department of Anthropology
University of Oregon
Eugene
Oregon 97403
USA

Christy G. Turner II
School of Human Evolution and Social Change
PO Box 872402
Arizona State University
Tempe
Arizona 85287
USA

Peter S. Ungar
Old Main 330
Department of Anthropology
University of Arkansas
Fayetteville
Arkansas 72701
USA

Acknowledgments

We wish to acknowledge the expertise and efforts of the various authors who contributed chapters, and thank them for sticking with us throughout the long duration of this project – from conception to conclusion; without them this book would not have been possible, or at least it would have been considerably shorter! Thomas Moore and several anonymous reviewers of our original book proposal offered useful advice on how to improve the final product's organization and expand upon its content. Heather Edgar, Tammy Greene, Diane Hawkey, Brian Hemphill, Bob Pastor, and several article reviewers provided valuable guidance during compilation of the volume. We are grateful to our editor at Cambridge University Press (CUP), Dr. Dominic Lewis, and appreciate the hard work of the CUP support and production staff.

Finally, JDI thanks Christy G. Turner II, who fostered an already "budding" interest in teeth and dental anthropology, and his parents, Lloyd and Violet Irish, and wife, Carol, for their guidance and support. GCN thanks his wife Charissa for her love and support and daughters Sarah, Greta, and Laura for putting up with a dad who was always looking at their teeth. On the professional side GCN thanks three primary mentors (alpha order) Clark Howell, John Lukacs, and Tim White.

Section I
Context

1 *Introduction*

JOEL D. IRISH AND GREG C. NELSON

1.1 Introduction

Introductory chapters in edited biological anthropology volumes often follow a stock, six-part formula: (1) explain why a component/ability/process of the human/non-human primate body/skeleton is of consequence, and can tell us so much about the origins/adaptation/affinities/health of an individual or population, (2) characterize the sub-field that studies said component/ability/process, (3) sing the myriad praises, and/or mention several shortcomings of that sub-field, (4) present an historical overview, (5) summarize the contributed chapters and relate how they tie in with parts 1–4, and (6) provide a vision of the sub-field's future direction(s). Such predictability may explain why many readers skip the Introduction, and head straight for the "meat" (i.e., the substantive chapters) of such books. For that reason we will leave out much of this standard material, with the exception of the chapter summaries, and primarily recount the genesis of the present volume; summaries are still presented to acknowledge the many talented contributors who made this volume possible, and to highlight and link together their diverse and, in some cases, cutting-edge dental research under a common, unifying theme, i.e., methodology.

In brief, it is unnecessary to expound on the qualities of the body/skeleton component covered in this volume – the dentition, or the sub-field of study used – dental anthropology, and/or, for that matter, the merits of such study (e.g., enamel is hard and preserves well, enamel does not remodel, the interaction between teeth and environment, the high genetic component in expression, teeth evolve slowly, both living and dead subjects can be directly compared, etc.); these issues were all previously detailed in innumerable books, including: Brothwell's (1963) *Dental Anthropology*, Kelley and Larsen's (1991) *Advances in Dental Anthropology*, and many others (e.g., Alt *et al.*, 1998; Dahlberg, 1971; Harris, 1977; Hillson, 1986, 1996; Jordan *et al.*, 1992; Kieser, 1990; Nichol, 1990; Scott, 1973; Scott and Turner, 1997). Indeed, it is precisely because of the

Technique and Application in Dental Anthropology ed. Joel D. Irish and Greg C. Nelson
Published by Cambridge University Press.

many useful attributes of teeth, and their study, that so many dental publications exist.

With regard to the history of dental anthropology, most of these same publications contain pertinent information (see Dahlberg, 1991), whereas others focus on the subject, especially concerning early accomplishments in the sub-field (e.g., Scott, 1997). Moreover, Richard Scott and Christy Turner contributed an updated history of dental study, concentrating on the twentieth century, to this volume (Chapter 2); thus, again, there is no need to provide such an overview here in the Introduction.

Lastly, as practicing dental anthropologists we, the editors, do have our respective visions regarding where the sub-field stands, and where it is headed. But why take our word for it? A principal goal of this volume is to illustrate the current and future direction(s) of dental anthropology in the subsequent chapters (a.k.a., the "meat").

1.2 Origins of the present volume

The creation of an edited volume was set in motion at the 2004 Dental Anthropology Association (DAA) meeting in Tampa, Florida; a question arose concerning what to do about the DAA's 20th anniversary meeting that was to be held the following year in Milwaukee, Wisconsin. The DAA is an international organization whose yearly gatherings are held in conjunction with those of the American Association of Physical Anthropologists (AAPA); additional details are provided in Chapter 2. Regarding the question, it was decided that a dental anthropology symposium should be organized. Past DAA president, John Lukacs, suggested that it cover the "state of the science" in the sub-field. That is, what established approaches are being used and what may be on the horizon? We supported the idea and set about organizing a symposium for 2005 that, fittingly, was entitled "Dental Anthropology 20 Years After: The State of the Science." The abstract in the 2005 AAPA meeting issue describes the symposium's intent:

> Commemorating the 20th anniversary meeting of the Dental Anthropology Association, this symposium highlights recent research in the sub-field that is illuminating issues of fundamental anthropological importance. Using both established and innovative new methodological and technological approaches, scholars with interests ranging from the micro- to macroscopic levels of structure and expression present their latest findings on dental genetics, histology, growth and development, pathology, and morphometrics across a broad range of living and

> fossil human and non-human primate taxa. Thus, unlike many symposia that focus on specific topics and/or regions, the unifying theme here is diversity. The intent is to assess the current state of the sub-field, emphasize its insights into diverse anthropological questions, and explore its potential future directions. (Irish and Nelson, 2005, p25)

Thirteen papers by 20 authors and co-authors were presented. A discussion led by John Lukacs and DAA past-president, Edward Harris, followed. At least a dozen or so additional researchers could have easily been added to the program if time allowed. In any event, the symposium succeeded in its stated goals and was well received. As such, it was decided that the next logical step was to publish and disseminate the papers.

1.3 Content, links, and objectives

All lead and most co-authors in the symposium, many of whom are renowned researchers in their respective areas of study, contributed to the present volume. Most subjects covered here are either unchanged or represent substantial expansions relative to the original material. To address the obligatory exclusion of some important context and research in the symposium, and based on the advice of the anonymous reviewers of our book proposal, several additional chapters (2, 3, 7, 12, and 17) were solicited.

Although the subsequent 17 chapters do highlight sub-field diversity (i.e., the original stated intent), they are linked together here by an overarching theme that stresses methodology, to warrant use of the phrase "technique and application" in the title. Specifically, they comprise a range of methods – from basic observation and recording, to advanced computer-based imaging and analysis. The result is a cross section of modern dental study. Although many pertinent books have been published since *Advances in Dental Anthropology*, a truly comprehensive survey of methods – many of which can be readily employed by the reader – is not among them; the present volume is intended as a follow-up to that 1991 compendium. It can provide a useful reference for advanced undergraduate students, graduate students, and professionals in the social and life sciences, as well as interested dental clinicians. It should also be useful as a contemporary reader in courses covering human and other primate teeth; as it now stands, many instructors supplement their main text by placing assorted current journal articles and book chapters on library reserve for their students.

To provide a framework for the various topics, this volume is divided into four parts or sections: (1) Context, (2) Applications in Assessing Population Health, (3) Applied Life and Population History, and (4) Forefront of Technique. The focus and sequence of these sections also serve to take us from where we are at present, to where we are headed as a sub-field of biological anthropology.

The first section includes this Introduction, the aforementioned history by Scott and Turner, and a review of statistical applications in dental anthropology by Edward Harris (Chapter 3). As Harris relates in his introduction, "[i]t may seem odd to have a chapter on statistics in a book discussing advances in dental anthropology." However, a thorough understanding of how to apply and interpret the results of statistical methods is, today, a necessity in almost all areas of dental research. Thus, his chapter provides additional "context" for the remainder of the volume.

The second section contains five chapters that address various aspects of population health at the micro- through macroscopic levels of analysis. First, in Chapter 4, Debbie Guatelli-Steinberg explores the use of perikymata (i.e., enamel growth layers evident on sides of crowns) within hypoplastic defects to estimate duration of growth disruptions in recent and fossil human teeth. Her comparisons indicate that mean stress periods in a sample of Alaskan Inupiaq were greater than in Neandertals; a comparable finding was noted for *Australopithecus* versus *Paranthropus*. Second, using laser ablation inductively coupled plasma mass spectrometry, Louise Humphrey, Teresa Jeffries, and Christopher Dean (Chapter 5) evaluate lead and zinc distributions in human deciduous tooth enamel. Their findings, that both elements vary in concentration throughout the crown (e.g. high at the enamel surface), have implications for reconstructing early life history from elemental studies of teeth. Third, in Chapter 6, Simon Hillson covers the most important and pervasive of all dental diseases: caries. He discusses the etiology and diachronic variation of caries, from prehistoric through recent times and, in the process, provides background for the two subsequent section chapters. Fourth, John Lukacs and Linda Thompson (Chapter 7) conduct a global survey of published caries data, and conclude that there is a difference in prevalence by sex throughout much of human prehistory. In contrast to standard anthropological explanations of sex differences that focus on culture and behavior, they propose that differences in caries susceptibility by sex are due to differing life history events, particularly those surrounding women's reproductive biology. Lastly, Brian Hemphill (Chapter 8) closes out this section by introducing a new quantitative approach that links the examinations of dental pathology prevalence with dental pathology pervasiveness. An analysis of individuals at the site of Tepe Hissar, Iran revealed that, depending upon individual gender and status, an increase in wealth did not necessarily lead to a corresponding improvement in dental health.

The volume's third section is comprised of six contributions relating to life and population histories. Gary Schwartz and Christopher Dean (Chapter 9) start things off by focusing on dental growth and development in non-human primates. Using examples from a sub-fossil lemur (*Megaladapis edwardsi*) and living great ape (*Gorilla gorilla*), they show how construction of a bar chart illustrating dental chronology (initiation, duration, and completion of the dentition) can complement and clarify life history inferences derived from other means. This growth and development theme is carried over into the study of humans by Helen Liversidge in Chapter 10. She describes ways to measure dental growth and maturation, presents various methods to estimate age from these references, compares the methods, and finally provides some useful insight and recommendations. Peter Ungar and Jonathan Bunn (Chapter 11) next demonstrate the use of a computer-based approach, i.e., dental topographic analysis, to interpret primate dental functional morphology. Beyond summarizing this novel approach, they present findings on diet in two Old World monkey species through a comparative study of variation in occlusal slope and relief at given attrition stages.

Like the three preceding chapters, Christopher Schmidt's contribution (Chapter 12) addresses dental development, age, and idiosyncratic features. In this case, however, these and other dental indicators (along with additional evidence) are discussed in the context of helping forensic dental anthropologists, together with forensic dentists, to identify accident and crime scene victims. Moving from identifying individuals to estimating relatedness among populations, Shara Bailey (Chapter 13) compares the teeth of Neandertals and modern humans to determine if observed morphological differences are typical of sub-specific or closely related specific taxa. To help gauge the level of these differences, comparisons are made with *Pan* – a sister taxon of *Homo*. Lastly, Chapter 14, by Oliver Rizk, Sarah Amugongo, Michael Mahaney, and Leslea Hlusko, provides something of a bridge to the rest of the volume. Beginning with an overview of prior dental heritability research, it relates how dental variation (a major component of the preceding chapters) is influenced by genetic factors, and how future quantitative genetics research will help us to better understand the evolution of our primate relatives and ancestors.

The fourth and final section, as its title indicates, highlights the forefront of dental technique. This is not to say that the preceding chapters do not; as noted, they entail such topics as high-tech recording and computer-based applications, a new quantitative approach, and future directions in genetics, among others. And, of course, "cutting-edge" techniques do not necessarily have to be "high-tech" (e.g., see FitzGerald and Hillson (below)). However, Chapter 15 certainly is. In their exploration of incision, Kalpana Agrawal, KaiYang Ang, Zhongquan Sui, Hugh Tan, and Peter Lucas go beyond traditional bite mechanics to explore how the fracture mechanics of food may affect tooth shape. Noting that spatulate-shaped incisors of primates are rare in other mammals, they report that such teeth are well adapted for two things: peeling fruit and stripping leaves – both of which involve more than simple biting. On the other hand, Charles Fitzgerald and Simon Hillson (Chapter 16) simply, but inventively, update an old low-tech method, i.e., dental measurements, while reviewing their analysis of human dental reduction since the Pleistocene. Rather than mesiodistal and buccolingual crown diameters, that are susceptible to even slight attrition, they record less vulnerable cervical diameters using specially designed calipers.

Still, what good is a section on cutting-edge dental research without the inclusion of at least some truly ground-breaking methodology? In Chapter 17, Peter Ungar, Robert Scott, Jessica Scott, and Mark Teaford describe dental microwear texture analysis, and use it in the study of eight anthropoid taxa. This new imaging technique provides a fast, objective alternative to standard SEM microwear analyses, and provides much more information on diet and tooth use. The final contribution (Chapter 18) by Roberto Macchiarelli, Luca Bondioli, and Arnaud Mazurier involves actual "space-age" technology. Using monochromatic high photon flux-based μCT analyses on a variety of extinct hominoids and hominids, they were able to obtain high-resolution images of internal dental structures; this new approach, though currently beyond the reach of many dental researchers, provides a potential glimpse of the future, in that it yields useful data without resorting to traditional, destructive thin-sectioning of teeth.

1.4 Conclusion

This introduction has, we hope, whetted your appetite for what follows. The 17 chapters comprising the "meat" of *Technique and Application in Dental Anthropology* provide an excellent snapshot of "the state of the science" as the first decade of the twenty-first century winds down. In putting this volume together, we strived to include both established and up-and-coming researchers to present as broad a representation of sub-field methodology as space allowed. Therefore, it should contain at least a few valuable nuggets for every reader, whether student, professional, or clinician. After all, because of the many aforementioned attributes of teeth, along with their ubiquity in the fossil record, most individuals with an interest in human/non-human primate origins/adaptation/affinities/health are *de facto* dental anthropologists. Since, as we all know and are forever repeating, "teeth are the hardest substance in the body," they are terrific little time capsules that retain numerous, pertinent data. As we continue to refine, develop, and apply dental anthropology techniques, our ability to retrieve these data will only increase – so that the next 20 years will, undoubtedly, be even more productive than the last 20.

References

Alt, K. W., Rösing, F. W., and Teschler-Nicola, M., eds. (1998). *Dental Anthropology: Fundamentals, Limits, and Prospects*. New York: Springer.

Brothwell, D., ed. (1963). *Dental Anthropology*. New York: Pergamon Press.

Dahlberg, A. A., ed. (1971). *Dental Morphology and Evolution*. Chicago: The University of Chicago Press.

Dahlberg, A. A. (1991). Historical perspective of dental anthropology. In *Advances in Dental Anthropology*, ed. M. A. Kelley and C. S. Larsen. New York: Wiley-Liss, pp. 7–11.

Harris, E. F. (1977). Anthropologic and genetic aspects of the dentition of Solomon Islanders, Melanesia. Ph.D. Dissertation, Arizona State University.

Hillson, S. (1986). *Teeth*. Cambridge: Cambridge University Press.

Hillson, S. (1996). *Dental Anthropology*. Cambridge: Cambridge University Press.

Irish, J. D. and Nelson, G. C. (2005). Session 9. Dental anthropology 20 years after: the state of the science. *American Journal of Physical Anthropology*, **Supplement 40**, 25–6.

Jordan, R. E., Abrams, L., and Kraus, B. S. (1992). *Kraus' Dental Anatomy and Occlusion*. St. Louis: Mosby Year Book.

Kelley, M. A. and Larsen, C. S. eds. (1991). *Advances in Dental Anthropology*. New York: Wiley-Liss.

Kieser, J. A. (1990). *Human Adult Odontometrics*. Cambridge: Cambridge University Press.

Nichol, C. R. (1990). Dental genetics and biological relationships of the Pima Indians of Arizona. Ph.D. Dissertation, Arizona State University.

Scott, G. R. (1973). Dental morphology: a genetic study of American white families and variation in living southwest Indians. Ph.D. Dissertation, Arizona State University.

Scott, G. R. (1997). Dental anthropology. In *History of Physical Anthropology. Volume 1, A-L.*, ed. F. Spencer. New York: Garland Publishing, pp. 334–340.

Scott, G. R. and Turner, C. G. II. (1997). *The Anthropology of Modern Human Teeth: Dental Morphology and its Variation in Recent Human Populations*. Cambridge: Cambridge University Press.

2 *History of dental anthropology*

G. RICHARD SCOTT AND CHRISTY G. TURNER II

2.1 Introduction

In 1991, Albert A. Dahlberg wrote "Historical perspective of dental anthropology" for the volume *Advances in Dental Anthropology* (Kelley and Larsen, 1991). A few years later, the senior author (Scott, 1997) wrote an historical paper on "Dental anthropology" for Frank Spencer's 1997 edited volume on the *History of Physical Anthropology*. Dahlberg was both a dentist and a pioneer in the field of dental anthropology. Because of those two abiding interests, his historical treatment focused as much on developments in oral biology as on the history of dental anthropology per se. Scott, a physical anthropologist, dealt with the early history of dental research, but the overall focus of his article revolved around the manner in which teeth have been used in anthropological research. Given the recency of these two articles, we do not want to simply reiterate points already made. Moreover, in no way is this general contribution comparable to articles on the history of dental anthropology in circumscribed geographic areas, such as those written for Australia (Brown, 1992, 1998) and Hungary (Kósa, 1993). We applaud these efforts and encourage other workers to document the history of the field in their country or region.

Our goal is to focus broadly on the growth of dental anthropology during the twentieth century and comment on potential directions in the twenty-first century. Specifically, this chapter addresses: (1) how scholars have used teeth to address and resolve anthropological problems, (2) recent developments in the field, including the founding of the Dental Anthropology Association, the growth of dental anthropology in Russia and China, and the spate of new dental books published during the past 15 years, (3) the development and significance of standardization in the field, (4) a survey showing how physical anthropologists teach dental anthropology directly, or incorporate its methods and principles into closely allied courses in osteology, bioarchaeology, human biology, primate anatomy, and paleoanthropology, and (5) recent and projected trends in dental anthropology.

Technique and Application in Dental Anthropology ed. Joel D. Irish and Greg C. Nelson
Published by Cambridge University Press.

2.2 How teeth have been used to further the aims of anthropological inquiry

The role of the physical anthropologist is to describe biological variation and explain it in terms of adaptation, evolution, and history. As teeth are under strong genetic control and are also the only hard part of the skeleton directly exposed to the environment, this variation takes different forms (Scott and Turner, 1988). Genetic information is sought in the size, shape, and morphology of teeth, along with numerical deviations away from a species' dental formula. Some variation is environmental in origin, such as the crown wear produced by normal food mastication; wear may also be of cultural origin, in that it is not induced by chewing, but is a byproduct of intentional and unintentional cultural practices that leave an imprint on the teeth (Milner and Larsen, 1991). Because teeth develop along a strongly programmed developmental path, environmental stressors are inferred by micro- and macrostructural defects in the enamel and dentine.

If dental anthropologists are concerned with genetic and environmental variation provided by teeth, who are the objects of study? *Homo sapiens*, or recent and modern humans, are the primary focus of dental anthropologists. However, dental anthropologists also study fossil ancestors back to the point of hominid origins and beyond – to fossil and living primates. Species studied outside this order, while interesting as animal models for stress, asymmetry, development, inheritance, and the like, are not considered part of dental anthropology per se, as the problems addressed are biological rather than anthropological in nature. Perhaps this is an artificial distinction, but boundaries have to be drawn somewhere or the entire field of oral biology would have to be reviewed – a daunting task. In discussing historical foundations for research on recent humans, fossil hominids, and non-human primates, each section is divided roughly by research before and after 1950, about the time physical anthropologists started thinking in terms of the modern evolutionary synthesis.

2.2.1 Research on recent humans (living, skeletal)

In pre-Darwinian times, the nascent field of physical anthropology focused on human racial variation and classification. Teeth played almost no role in these early discussions, as workers focused on externally visible characteristics like skin, hair, and eye color, hair and nose form, stature, etc. By the end of the nineteenth century, with but few exceptions (e.g., P. Broca and crown wear, W. H. Flower and tooth crown size, L. H. Mummery and oral pathology), teeth had yet to enter anthropological consciousness in any significant way (Scott, 1997).

In the early twentieth century, scholars began to pay attention to teeth as an additional system that could provide insights into human variation. Most of the emphasis was on human skeletal remains because techniques for making impressions of the living were limited. Aleš Hrdlička, who had access to an enormous sample of Native American skeletal remains at the Smithsonian Institution, was among the first to note interesting dental morphological distinctions between major human groups. In particular, Hrdlička (1911, 1920) noted that American Indians were distinguished from other human populations by the development of pronounced marginal ridges on the lingual surface of the upper incisors (i.e., shoveling). W. K. Gregory (1922), in his opus *The Origin and Evolution of the Human Dentition*, also noted morphological attributes of recent humans, but he did not feel that inter-group variation was pronounced or significant.

Although Hrdlička authored many books, he never wrote one devoted entirely to teeth. That task was left to other pioneers in the field, including T. D. Campbell (1925) in Australia and J. C. M. Shaw (1931) in South Africa. These workers studied the size, morphology, number, wear, and pathology of Australian aboriginals and South African black populations, respectively. Given the paucity of comparative data, their books were largely descriptive in nature. To complement these early dental monographs, other significant contributions during this period include R. W. Leigh's (1925) analysis of oral pathology under varied environmental conditions, W. M. Krogman's (1927) paper on anthropological aspects of human teeth, C. Nelson's (1938) study of the Pecos Pueblo population, and M. S. Goldstein's (1948) work on the teeth of Texas Indian crania. Other key contributions at this time were Percy Butler's (1937, 1939) (Figure 2.1) articles on the field effect in the mammalian dentition. One of the most influential papers in the history of dental anthropology, A. A. Dahlberg's (1945) "The changing dentition of man," applied Butler's concept of dental fields to human teeth, forever changing the manner in which anthropologists would analyze metric, morphologic, and numeric variation in the dentition.

P. O. Pedersen's (1949) (Figure 2.2) *The East Greenland Eskimo Dentition*, with its extensive set of observations on Inuit teeth and a bibliography citing articles in a diverse array of languages, ushered in a new age for dental anthropology. At this same time, following key theoretical developments that led to the modern evolutionary synthesis, anthropologists started paying more heed to genetics and process, and less to typology and classification. G. W. Lasker's (1950) paper "Genetic analysis of racial traits of the teeth" set the stage for new ways of thinking about the inheritance and utility of dental morphological variation. In the late 1940s, Dahlberg (1951) initiated a major dental casting project among the Pima Indians of Arizona. After modest beginnings with plaster casts made from wax bite impressions, Al and Thelma Dahlberg went on to collect

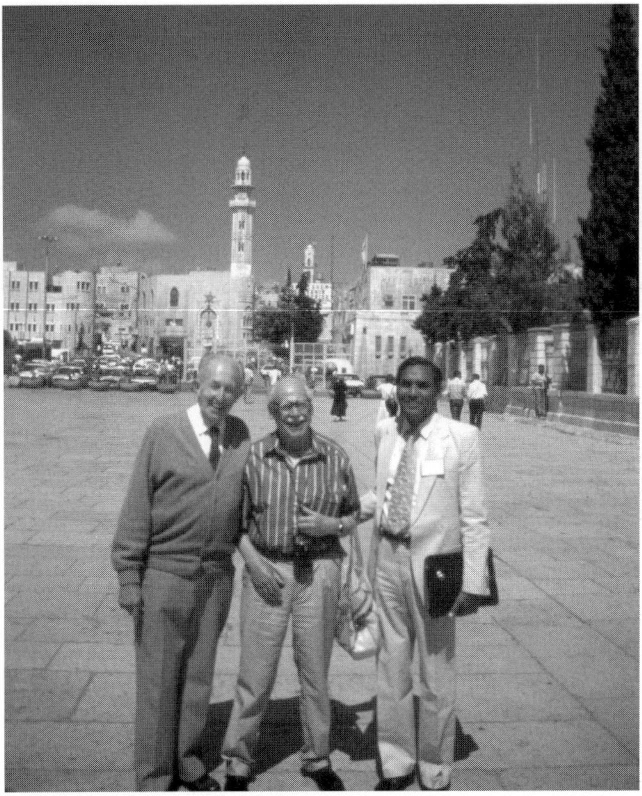

Figure 2.1 Albert A. Dahlberg, Percy Butler and V. R. Reddy at 8th International Symposium on Dental Morphology, Jerusalem, Israel, 1989.

over 8000 Pima Indian casts (many in families, many individuals replicated for growth and development studies). From this foundation, Dahlberg was able to build up some of the first characterizations of the extant American Indian dentition.

The 1950s saw a flurry of activity in the anthropological uses of teeth. C. F. A. Moorrees (1957) published *The Aleut Dentition*, which covered all facets of dental anthropology, from size, morphology, and number to pathology and oral tori. T. Murphy (1959a, 1959b) developed new standards for scoring tooth crown wear based on the pattern of dentine exposure, a scheme that provided far more information on wear than the Broca scale of the late nineteenth century. Lasker (1957) discussed the potential uses of dental morphology in the interpretation of forensic remains, while Bertram Kraus (1951, 1957; Kraus and Jordan, 1965; Kraus *et al.*, 1959) conducted pioneering work in dental genetics and ontogeny.

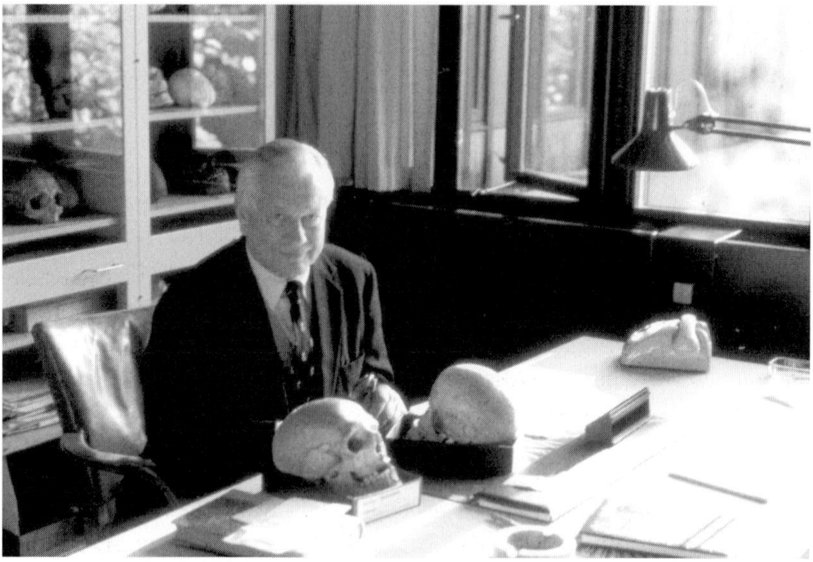

Figure 2.2 P. O. Pedersen at the Panum Institue, University of Copenhagen, 1986.

S. M. Garn, along with his colleagues at the Fels Institute, began publishing dozens of articles that focused on dental variation, development, and interactions between variables.

Although the term "dental anthropology" had been used earlier, one of the crystallizing events of the field was the publication of *Dental Anthropology*, edited by Don R. Brothwell (1963). This work emanated from the Symposia of the Society for the Study of Human Biology. A perusal of the contents is telling. Of 15 contributions, 3 dealt with primate teeth, 1 with fossil hominid teeth, and 11 with recent human populations. That balance approximates the overall focus of dental research during the middle of the twentieth century.

Following the publication of *Dental Anthropology*, the field greatly expanded in terms of practitioners and publications. From 1963 to the present, hundreds of articles and dissertations have dealt with various aspects of the human dentition. Topical trends include an ever increasing emphasis on methodologically standardized studies of tooth crown and root morphology and dimensions, increased interest in oral health concerns, especially the negative impacts of agriculture, and a greatly expanded interest in the study of developmental stress as measured by growth defects, in particular linear enamel hypoplasia. The International Symposium of Dental Morphology, which first met in 1965, would meet on a regular basis across the next four decades, leaving in its wake a number of significant edited volumes that highlighted current research in dental ontogeny, genetics, and variation (Butler and Joysey, 1978; Dahlberg, 1971; Kurten, 1982; Mayhall and Heikkinen, 1999; Moggi-Cecchi, 1995; Pedersen *et al.*, 1967; Radlanski and Renz, 1995; Russell *et al.*, 1988; Smith and Tchernov, 1992; Zadzinska, 2005).

2.2.2 Research on fossil hominids

As teeth are extremely hard and durable, it is not surprising that they make up a significant portion of the fossil record. This is certainly as true for hominid fossils as for any other tooth-bearing lineage. What is perhaps more surprising is that, until recently, hominid fossil teeth did not receive their just due. Of course, the Piltdown skull and dentition were examined by early twentieth-century scholars and many, who had no close familiarity with teeth, were duped into thinking this specimen was an early hominid. Even Hrdlička (1923, p. 216) was fooled, noting "The Piltdown teeth . . . are already human or close to human." Gerrit Miller (1915, 1918) pointed out the pronounced incongruity of the skull and jaw, observing that the former was clearly human while the latter was in all likelihood a chimpanzee. At this time, many scholars thought Miller's arguments were convincing although the British establishment, led by Sir Arthur Keith, Grafton Elliot Smith, and W. P. Pycraft, refused to accept any interpretation that did not associate the cranium with the mandible. Although Piltdown remained in the pantheon of hominid fossils until 1953, Miller was vindicated when the find was exposed as a hoax by K. Oakley and J. S. Wiener (Weiner, 1955; Weiner and Oakley, 1954).

Although the first half of the twentieth century saw a number of papers on the jaws and teeth of the South African Australopithecines and European Neanderthals, the only major treatise on fossil hominids was Franz Weidenreich's (1937) *The Dentition of* Sinanthropus pekinensis. For fossil and living hominoids, W. K. Gregory and M. Hellman (1926) wrote "The Dentition of *Dryopithecus* and the Origin of Man," wherein they compared the dentitions of fossil apes, living primates, and modern humans. Hrdlička (1924) also weighed in on comparisons of fossil hominid and primate dentitions. However, there remained a paucity of literature on fossil hominid teeth during the early twentieth century, possibly attributable to the small number of workers in hominid paleontology, and the greater difficulties in transportation – making access to collections difficult. After 1950, studies of fossil hominid teeth slowly accelerated with each new find. By 1956 there were enough Australopithecine fossils for J. T. Robinson to pen a monograph on *The Dentition of the Australopithecinae*. Shortly thereafter, P. V. Tobias (1967) provided a detailed description of the dentition of *Australopithecus (Zinjanthropus) boisei*.

During the middle of the twentieth century, there was no deficiency of studies on hominid fossil teeth. However, such studies usually provided detailed descriptive data on the fissures, pits, fossae, sulci, ridges, cingular manifestations, root grooves, and radicals of the crowns and roots of individual fossils. The problem was often the lack of context and standards. While this was true of studies that focused on morphology and shape, it was not true of odontometrics. Authors who made significant contributions in this area include C. L. Brace (1967; Brace and Mahler, 1971), D. W. Frayer (1978) and M. Wolpoff (1971), who focused on metric trends in hominid dental evolution from the Australopithecines to modern *Homo sapiens* of the Mesolithic. C. E. Oxnard (1987) also applied multivariate morphometric analysis to tooth size variables of living apes, fossil primates, and Australopithecines to evaluate the evolution of sex dimorphism in hominid and primate evolution. For the most part, authors have concentrated on buccolingual and mesiodistal diameters, but at least for these variables, extensive comparative data were available to help workers evaluate differences and trends in tooth size and size sequence polymorphisms.

Standardized morphological observations on robust Australopithecines and early *Homo* were carried out by B. Wood and his colleagues in the 1980s (Wood and Abbott, 1983; Wood and Engleman, 1988, Wood and Uytterschaut, 1987, Wood *et al.*, 1983, 1988). Now that representative samples of fossils were available, it was possible to characterize different taxa in terms of the frequencies of specific traits, a great improvement over the older strategy of individual fossil descriptions. Bermúdez de Castro (1986, 1988, 1993; Bermúdez de Castro and Nicolás, 1995; Bermúdez de Castro *et al.*, 1993, 1999, 2001) has played a significant role in describing the size and morphology of Middle Pleistocene hominids from Spain. Although Neanderthals have long been known for their taurodont molars, shoveled incisors, and pronounced incisor basal cingula (Adloff, 1907), detailed descriptions of their morphology are only now starting to appear (see Bailey, 2002, 2004; Bailey and Hublin, 2006; Bailey and Lynch, 2005; Irish, 1998).

2.2.3 *Research on non-human primates*

Recently, there has been an upsurge in research on the dentition of non-human primates. Early in the twentieth century, a few workers published data on primate teeth (see Adloff, 1908; Gregory, 1916; Gregory and Hellman, 1926; Hrdlička, 1923), but their attention was devoted primarily to size and morphology. A. Schultz (1935), noting the undue emphasis on size and morphology, presented valuable data on eruption and decay in non-human primate teeth. Later, LeGros Clark (1960) provided a detailed description of the morphology and

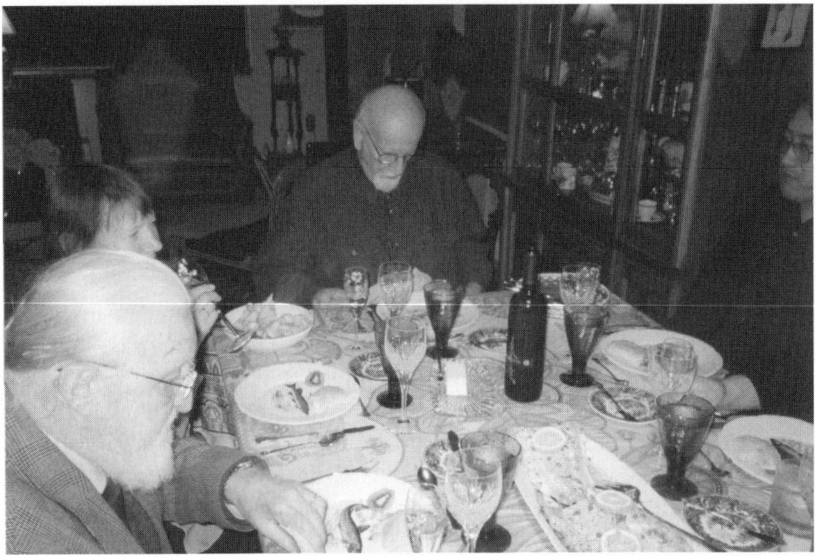

Figure 2.3 Dinner gathering at the home outside of Seattle, Washington, belonging to Daris R. Swindler (center) and wife Kathy, attended by C. Loring Brace (left) and others following the multiple scientist examination of the Kennewick Man skeletal remains.

numerical variation in non-human primate dentitions in his classic text *The Antecedents of Man*.

Recently, D. Swindler (Figure 2.3) has provided two excellent monographs on non-human primate teeth, the first being the *Dentition of Living Primates* published in 1976. Swindler (2002) updated this important volume and retitled it *Primate Dentition: An Introduction to the Teeth of Non-human Primates*. These volumes cover dozens of primate species, with illustrations, descriptions of dietary behavior, eruption sequences, crown morphology, and tables of summarized data on MD and BL dimensions, with descriptive statistics based on small samples, and not simply individual primates.

Over the past 25 years, many researchers, including M. C. Dean, R. A. Eaglen, R. Kay, W. G. Kinzey, D. Guatelli-Steinberg, J. Lukacs, J. Sirianni, A. Rosenberger, and others, have developed new insights into the variation and development of primate teeth. These authors address issues across a range of topics, including tooth comb formation in prosimians, developmental rates, growth disturbances, enamel thickness, canine honing, microwear analysis, and the interaction of crown morphology and dietary behavior. With the basic foundation laid for the size, shape, and morphology of non-human primate teeth, more problem-oriented research is now possible on tooth form, function, and evolution.

2.3 Recent developments in the field

Since 1991, there have been at least three broadly influential developments in the field: (1) the Dental Anthropology Association, founded in 1986, enlarged the size of its small *Newsletter*, changed the name to *Dental Anthropology*, and adopted the standards and styles of a professional journal, all carried out under the editorship by Alice M. (Sue) Haeussler, (2) English translations were made for the large and largely unread body of dental anthropology studies written in Russian, and a dental anthropology research program was initiated in the People's Republic of China, and (3) the publication of several books designed to be used as textbooks, as well as scientific references, in dental anthropology. There are, of course, many other advances since 1991, including increased course offerings in dental anthropology in a number of universities and colleges, continued publication of the assembled papers for the International Dental Morphology meetings, development of new methods, descriptions of new fossil dentitions, and new syntheses on human and non-human dental variation, among other subjects.

2.3.1 Dental Anthropology Association

In 1985, a small group of dental anthropologists went out for dinner during the American Association of Physical Anthropologists (AAPA) meeting in Knoxville, TN. After some discussion, they identified more than 160 anthropologists and dentists with an interest in dental anthropology. Given the number of scholars in the field and a worldwide interest in the subject, these individuals formed a Dental Anthropology Group (DAG). At the next annual meeting of the AAPA (April, 1986), held in Albuquerque, New Mexico, the Dental Anthropology Association was founded by M. Y. İşcan and 41 other signatories (İşcan, 1989).

The Dental Anthropology Association began publishing the *Dental Anthropology Newsletter* in 1986, the same year the organization was founded. The first issue had only three pages while the second had nine, including the constitution and by-laws. Although the association and its published organ, the *Dental Anthropology Newsletter*, started out modestly, it would see extensive growth over the next 20 years. In 1989, S. R. Loth, Florida Atlantic University, became *DAN* Editor. In 1990, the task was taken over by A. M. (Sue) Haeussler at Arizona State University. Year by year during the course of her 12 year editorship, the newsletter increased in page length and quality with each new issue. Haeussler also initiated a Board-approved name change by dropping "newsletter" from the cover in 2000, because the Association's publication had grown far beyond a simple newsletter. Moreover, scientific articles submitted for publication received peer reviews under her editorship, which in essence made *Dental Anthropology* a professional journal. Her last issue was published in 2002, in conjunction with the present editor, E. F. Harris, University of Tennessee. Staying with Haeussler's efforts to continuously improve the publication, Editor Harris initiated an on-line distribution of the journal in 2006 in PDF format with high quality color illustrations.

In addition to the three yearly issues of *Dental Anthropology*, the organization, along with other specialty organizations, holds its annual meetings with the American Association of Physical Anthropologists. At these meetings there are both verbal and poster presentations, and the awarding of prizes for outstanding student papers. Appropriately, the student prize for the DAA is named after Albert A. Dahlberg, a true pioneer in the field of dental anthropology. From its humble beginnings in 1986, the association now has well over 250 members with a good mix of representatives from every continent.

2.3.2 Dental anthropology in Russia and China

Dental anthropology was pioneered in the Russian Federation (formerly the USSR) by A. A. Zoubov, Russian Academy of Sciences, Institute of Ethnography, Moscow. For over 40 years, Zoubov and his many graduate students and colleagues have collected wax bite dental impressions from thousands of primary school children throughout the old USSR. In hundreds of articles and books, they have reported the analyses of crown morphology following the Dahlberg standards, as well as using a uniquely Russian system of molar groove patterning of the occlusal surface that Zoubov (1977) calls odontoglyphics. The odontoglyphic method works best with unworn teeth. Hence, Zoubov and his students have focused traditionally on dental variation in children under 15 years of age.

The very large amount of Russian dental morphological information is not only largely unknown and unused by dental anthropologists who do not read Russian, but much of this literature is very difficult to obtain outside of Russia. Few American libraries subscribe to the relevant Russian journals, and dental anthropology symposia volumes printed in Russia almost never find their way

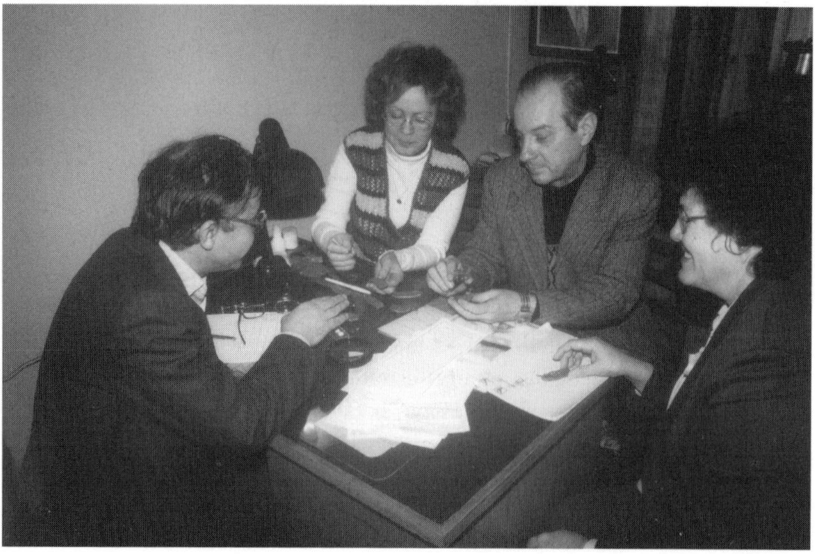

Figure 2.4 Alexander A. Zoubov (second from right) and Natalia Haldeyeva (center) with doctoral students and Jacqueline A. Turner (right), Institute of Ethnography, Russian Academy of Sciences, Moscow (CGT 2-11-87:15).

outside of the Russian Federation. Unlike archaeology and ethnology, there are only a few physical anthropological studies that have utilized the Russian literature (but see Scott and Turner, 1997, who included the extensive data sets of Zoubov and Haldeyeva (1979) (Figure 2.4) in their worldwide synthesis of crown-trait frequencies). General reviews of Russian physical anthropology, including dental anthropology, were prepared by Turner (1987a, 1987b). A major work that concentrated on dental morphological variation in Russia, the Caucasus, and Central Asia was written by Haeussler (1996).

While dental anthropology has many contributors in Russia, eastern and southern Asia, and the Pacific basin, including a number of internationally acclaimed scholars, only recently has major dental anthropology research begun in China. This activity is led by Liu Wu (1992), Institute of Vertebrate Paleontology and Paleoanthropology, and his associates. Wu and Xianglong (1995) provide a brief description of the morphology of Chinese Neolithic samples and fossil hominids, and discuss research directions in dental anthropology. Major goals of an ever-expanding dental research program include delineating the relationship between Chinese and neighboring populations in east Asia, studying temporal trends and microevolution in China since the late Pleistocene, and providing a dental-based interpretation of the origins of modern Chinese populations.

2.3.3 Recent books on dental anthropology

Since 1991, a number of significant books that cover key aspects of dental anthropology have been published. These volumes include J. Kieser's (1991) *Human Adult Odontometrics*, M. Kelley and C. Larsen's (1991) *Advances in Dental Anthropology*, S. Hillson's (1996) *Dental Anthropology*, G. R. Scott and C. G. Turner's (1997) *The Anthropology of Modern Human Teeth*, J. R. Lukacs' (1998) *Human Dental Development, Morphology, and Pathology*, and P. W. Lucas' (2004) *Dental Functional Morphology*. Dental anthropology courses taught in the 1970s had to rely on dental anatomy texts, edited volumes (e.g., Dahlberg, 1971), or monographs that focused on a specific geographic region (e.g., Moorrees, 1957). Thanks largely to Cambridge University Press, new syntheses of crown size, morphology, and function have provided university professors with a variety of texts for dental anthropology courses at the advanced undergraduate and graduate levels.

2.4 History of standardized dental reference plaques

While dental morphology has long been used as an aid in the classification of vertebrates, especially mammals (see Keil, 1966; Owen, 1840–45; Peyer, 1968), its use in defining sub-groups or races within a species has largely been limited to anthropology. Because dental and other biological differences between groups within a species are smaller than differences between species, a function of time and evolution, there is an inherent need for greater precision in trait identification. One can hardly go wrong differentiating a narwhal tusk from the tusk of an elephant, or the incisor of a fresh water beaver from that of a sea otter. Although the variation in human dental morphology is much less than these two typological examples, it is not so great that experienced workers are often unable to identify a human tooth from anywhere in the world. While a single tooth can be identified as human, it is generally held that a "racial" identification cannot be made from a single tooth because races or intra-species groups are defined on a populational basis, and characterizing populations requires the use of several individuals and several traits.

Early "standards" employed to classify within-trait variation were based on textual or conceptual descriptions, such as the four class ranking used by Hrdlička (1920) for upper incisor shoveling: none, trace, semi, and shovel-shaped. He could see that shoveling might be present or absent, but he also observed that intermediate grades might occur within any human group. Nevertheless, workers continued to describe dental and other traits on a present or absent basis for many years after this classic paper. It was not until A. A.

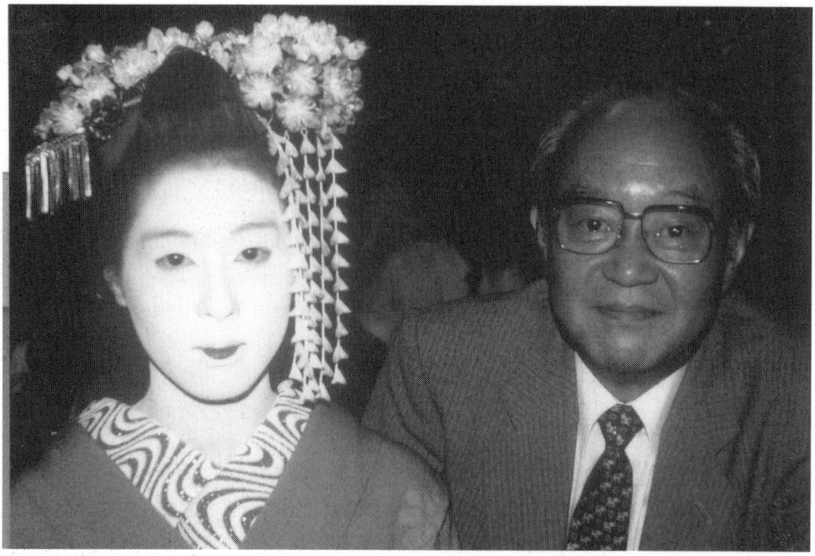

Figure 2.5 Kazuro Hanihara and entertainment, following a conference he organized at the International Research Center for Japanese Studies, Kyoto, Japan (CGT 9-26-90:22).

Dahlberg began producing his plaster reference plaques for dental variation after World War II that ranked scales were developed for several other dental traits, including Carabelli's trait, the protostylid, and the hypocone, among others. The value of these reference plaques was immense, not only in identifying the intermediate conditions, but they also reduced intra- and inter-observer error.

Ranked scale traits of the dentition are the sort that are difficult to measure in a metrical fashion due to minimal or variable landmarks, unlike many osteological traits such as head length and breadth. As such, dental traits like these are often referred to as non-metric traits. Non-metric traits can be present or absent, and when present they exhibit various degrees of expression from trace to pronounced in size. In theory, this variation of expression is thought to be due to a threshold effect in a polygenic system. By this we mean that the more alleles and chromosomal loci that are involved in determining a trait's presence, the stronger will be its expression, and the more common will the trait be in a given population (Scott and Turner 1997). Hence precision of observations followed the development of the Dahlberg reference plaques at the Zoller Dental Laboratory of the University of Chicago. Dahlberg's plaques on permanent crown traits also inspired another pioneer in dental anthropology, Kazuro Hanihara (Figure 2.5), to develop comparable standards for primary teeth.

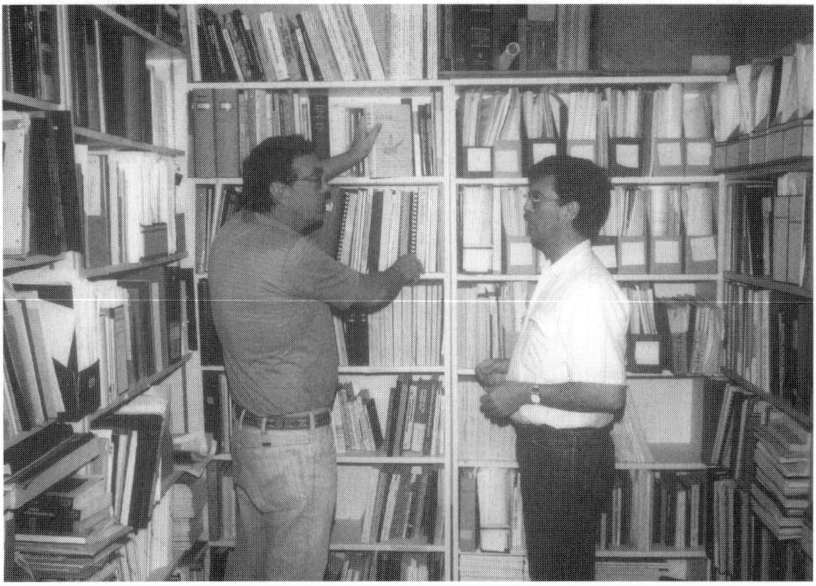

Figure 2.6 The authors Christy G. Turner II (left) and G. Richard Scott (right), Department of Anthropology, Arizona State University, Tempe (KDT 1–88:14).

Following a brief period of study with Dahlberg in 1962 at his University of Chicago laboratory, the junior author set out to study the dentition of Arctic peoples for his Ph.D. dissertation, with an emphasis on the Aleuts of Alaska. In addition to the Aleut skeletons he excavated on Umnak Island, he also visited several museums that possessed large collections of Arctic human remains, most derived from archaeological excavations. Because the Dahlberg plaques markedly enhance an observer's precision in classifying intra-trait variation, Turner (1967) was able to demonstrate small but meaningful differences between eastern and western Aleut dental characteristics. These differences, coupled with those based on an intermediate island grouping, revealed that clines existed in trait frequencies. Clines were then considered to be hallmarks of natural selection, but because the human occupation of the Aleutian Islands was post-glacial, and throughout the 1000-mile long chain, the islands were effectively identical as far as teeth were concerned. Hence, the plaques made possible a strong inference that clines are not necessarily produced solely by natural selection. Other evolutionary processes, alone or in combination, could also give rise to clinal variation.

In light of the theoretical significance derived by the use of the Dahlberg plaques, and knowing that several other traits could usefully be added to the Dahlberg list, Turner, assisted by his students (especially G. R. Scott) (Figure 2.6), began a long-term project to develop ranked-scale plaques for additional traits, starting with lower molar cusps 6 and 7. It was decided that, wherever possible, at least five grades of occurrence and one of absence would be defined on the basis of the multiregional collection of human teeth and casts in the Arizona State University collections assembled by Turner and D. H. Morris. Experimentation quickly showed that intra- and inter-observer error increased with the addition of more intermediate classes. Importantly, the large dental collection was carefully searched for examples of trait expression that had minimal expression, assuming that minimal expression was at or near the observable morphogenetic threshold. An effort was made to develop a minimum of one new standard plaque each year.

By 1990, a method of standardized observations had evolved that was called the Arizona State University Dental Anthropology System, in short, ASUDAS. Turner *et al.* published rules for use of the ASUDAS in 1991. While use of the reference plaques is relatively easy, not all are equally so (Nichol and Turner 1986), and the rules provided in Turner *et al.* (1991) should be read and followed carefully, even by experienced observers. Inter-observer error should be minimized in comparative studies, particularly those like the above-mentioned Aleut microevolution study, or those involving affinity assessment in NAGPRA investigations.

Researchers in at least 36 countries are using the Arizona State University standard reference plaques. Table 2.1 shows where sets of these plaques have been sent on request, and the number of individuals who have made these requests since 1985. More than half of the requests have come from workers in the USA. Presumably these requests are related to the large number of skeletal studies that have resulted from NAGPRA legal requirements to determine affiliation of prehistoric skeletal assemblages in museums and institutions in the US. Table 2.1 suggests that the ASUDAS standards are being used widely, if not on a global scale. Most conspicuously absent are nations in the Middle East, Central Asia, most of Africa, and parts of South America. Plaque requests were filled before 1985, but the records are incomplete. It is doubtful if requests were made from any more than a few workers in these unrepresented regions.

2.5 Course work in dental anthropology

Our Spring, 2006 survey of the Dental Anthropology Association membership, submitted to about 250 individuals, asked which members taught courses in dental anthropology, and which of a list of 20 topics were covered in their courses. Altogether, 30 topics were identified. About 10 % of the membership replied, which is probably representative since many members are either

Table 2.1 *Distribution of ASU DAS reference plaques*[a] *(n = 242)*

County	Sets	Percent	Country	Sets	Percent
Argentina	2	0.8	Ireland	2	0.8
Australia	3	1.2	Italy	5	2.1
Austria	1	0.4	Japan	4	1.6
Brazil	1	0.4	Jordan	1	0.4
Canada	14	5.8	Mexico	1	0.4
Chile	1	0.4	Mongolia	1	0.4
China	2	0.8	Netherlands	1	0.4
Croatia	2	0.8	Northern Ireland	1	0.4
Czech Republic	1	0.4	New Zealand	1	0.4
Denmark	1	0.4	Poland	1	0.4
England	10	4.1	Portugal	4	1.6
Finland	2	0.8	Russia	3	1.2
France	4	1.6	Scotland	1	0.4
Germany	1	0.4	South Africa	3	1.2
Greece	2	0.8	Spain	7	2.9
Guatemala	1	0.4	Thailand	1	0.4
Hungary	1	0.4	Taiwan	1	0.4
Indonesia	1	0.4	United States	154	63.6

[a] Sets distributed mainly from 1983 to 2006; sets distributed in the 1970s and early 1980s were incomplete because plaques were being developed – these are not included in this listing.

students, dental professionals outside of anthropology, or physical anthropologists who instruct primarily osteology or some other specialization within physical anthropology. Our survey assumed that most professionals who identified themselves as full or part-time dental anthropologists within and outside of the US were members of the Dental Anthropology Association; thus, it would be largely redundant to survey other associations, especially the larger and broader American Association of Physical Anthropologists, or various large organizations that deal mainly with clinical dentistry. Responses outside of the US came from 10 members.

Table 2.2 lists the course content responses to our survey. Thirty "topics" or course elements were identified, the lowest seven of which were solicited with the category of "other" in the itemized listing on the questionnaire. Since evolution is the major theoretical paradigm in biological anthropology, and is embedded in most courses, we felt no need to ask about a topic such as method and theory, which is commonly a separate graduate level archaeological or cultural anthropological course in many anthropology departments.

Fifty percent or more of the courses represented in Table 2.2 included instruction in dental anatomy, dental morphology, non-metric morphology, human

Table 2.2 *Dental anthropology course content*

Topical area included in course	No. courses[a] (total = 26)	Percent
Dental anatomy	23	88.5
Dental morphology	23	88.5
Non-metric morphology	20	76.9
Human population variation	18	69.2
Human dental evolution	16	61.5
Oral pathology	15	57.7
Mid-term and final exams	15	57.7
Lab practical quiz	14	53.8
Fossil hominid dentition	13	50.0
Primate dentition	12	46.1
Vertebrate dental evolution	12	46.1
Genetics	11	42.3
Dental embryology	11	42.3
Laboratory research project	10	38.5
Comparative vertebrate	10	38.5
Dental impressing	9	34.6
Statistics	7	25.9
Wear, behavior, modification	6	23.1
Graduate reading section	5	19.2
X-ray techniques	4	15.4
Dental anthropology history	4	15.4
Odontometry	4	15.4
Teeth in population history	3	11.5
Dental histology	3	11.5
Forensic dentistry	2	7.7
Developmental timing	2	7.7
Tooth function	2	3.8
Paleopathology	1	3.8
Oral biology	1	3.8
Clinical odontometry	1	3.8

[a] Seventeen (65.4 %) of 26 reported courses had the term "dental anthropology" in their title, either alone or with other designations.

population variation, human dental evolution, oral pathology, and fossil hominid dentition. Of the other topics that were taught in less than 50 % of the courses, primate dentition, genetics, dental embryology, and vertebrate dental evolution were the most frequently reviewed. No course was concerned with all of the topics in Table 2.2. As for number of topics per course, the mean was 10, and the range was 3 to 19. The lower number of topics was covered in courses without dental anthropology in their title. These values suggest that, on average, about one week of instruction was given per topic. Institutionally, most respondents taught on a semester basis, usually 15 weeks of instruction. Where textbooks were required, Hillson's (1996) *Dental Anthropology* was most frequently mentioned, followed by Scott and Turner's (1997) *The Anthropology of Modern Human Teeth.*

Table 2.2 suggests that dental anthropology courses emphasize dental anatomy, non-metric morphology, and human dental evolution. Oral pathology was emphasized slightly more than fossil hominid dentition despite the strong emphasis on human dental evolution, but the difference is hardly significant. Courses that have a more clinical orientation are those based in dental schools, or in liberal arts colleges where dental anthropology is to some degree a service course for undergraduate pre-dental or health science majors. Generally speaking, dental anthropology is a specialized domain of anthropology departments, and it is oriented mainly at undergraduate students (only 20 % had a graduate reading section). As far as we know, there were no courses devoted to dental anthropology before 1950, although pioneers in physical anthropology such as A. Hrdlička, and later workers such as S. M. Garn, and A. A. Dahlberg, concentrated their teaching and research on topics that are commonly dealt with today in dental anthropology courses. While dental anthropology is a freestanding specialty within physical anthropology, it has its strongest links with teaching and research in human osteology, forensic anthropology, bioarchaeology, and paleoanthropology.

2.6 Trends in dental anthropological research

Walker (1997) provides a useful review of the quantity and topical nature of dental anthropological research between 1966 and 1996 – an era that witnessed a veritable explosion of the sub-field. Searching Medline, he found that 3 % of the total dental literature was devoted to dental anthropology, a significant increase from earlier periods. From 1966 to 1975, the number of dental articles in the *American Journal of Physical Anthropology (AJPA)* increased from 8.4 % to about 20 % of total content. This finding is in accord with our analysis of decadal volumes of *AJPA*. Although there was a lull in dental publications in the 1930 volume, the frequency of dental articles in every other volume ranged from 8.0 % to 19.4 %, with a mean of around 11 %. We found, as did Walker, that there was distinct rise in *AJPA* dental content from 1970 to 1990. Surprisingly though, the 2000 volume witnessed a drop-off to about 6.5 %, attributable to some extent to the much greater number of articles on mtDNA and primates. Of course, there are other outlets for dental anthropological research, so it is too early to tell if 2000 is an aberration.

Although the total number of papers on modern and recent populations still exceeds those that focus on hominid fossils or non-human primates, we found the same trend that Walker (1997) reports – to wit, there has been a dramatic increase in the number of dental papers that focus on fossil hominids. Although such studies do not ignore tooth size and morphology, there has been an increased emphasis on growth and development and also developmental disturbances (i.e., hypoplasia).

It is difficult to assess the impact of repatriation on dental anthropological studies. Many of the samples being repatriated from the Smithsonian Institution have been subjected to intense study of all attributes of bones and teeth, including tooth size, morphology, pathology, crown wear, etc. However, there may be some lag in the publication of such materials. To compensate for the loss of research materials in the United States, some American scholars are turning to problems in other parts of the world where skeletal collections are numerous and often little studied.

Projecting into the future, there will never be a paucity of research materials for the dental anthropologist, whether they are from living humans, archaeological remains, fossil hominids, or non-human primates. On the theoretical front, we anticipate great strides will be made in the next few decades on understanding the development of teeth as meristic structures. It is well established that the size of one tooth is not independent of the size of other teeth but, instead, there is some form of component structure in the dentition. Understanding the genetics of these components is the next step. This includes a greater understanding of the role of homeobox genes in dental development (see Weiss, 1990). At some point in the twenty-first century, human genome research should contribute key insights to studies of dental ontogeny. To complement the enhanced understanding of gene/tooth interaction, technological advances applied to the observation and quantification of tooth size, shape, morphology, and pathology will revolutionize future studies.

Despite the growth of dental anthropology over the past 100 years, there is still much work to do. For example, measurements on skulls (craniometrics) are far more readily available for world populations than measurements on teeth (odontometrics). While some areas of the world are well known in terms of dental morphological variation (see the New World [Turner, 1985], Africa [Irish, 1993], India [Hawkey, 2002]), other regions have not been fully fleshed out for complete sets of crown and root trait frequencies (e.g., parts of Europe, the Middle East, central Asia). This fact became apparent when we synthesized morphological data on a worldwide scale (Scott and Turner, 1997). The study of tooth crown wear remains a promising avenue of research for inferences on diet and dietary behavior, but standards have to be refined and applied more uniformly to enhance comparative studies. A fascinating area for the dental anthropologist is the systematic treatment of cultural wear, that is, patterned wear reflecting behaviors other than normal food mastication. Although the subject has been reviewed in some depth (see Milner and Larsen, 1991), observations often remain focused on the individual rather than the sample. Based on recent articles and abstracts, the one area of dental anthropology that is receiving a great deal of attention today is the study of growth disturbances. Using scanning electron microscopy, detailed studies of perikymata development are adding depth and nuance to an area where observations of linear enamel hypoplasia were based traditionally on visual inspection, with or without the use of hand-held lenses. With an ever-expanding number of researchers focusing on human, fossil hominid, and non-human primate dentitions, we anticipate that the twenty-first century will see exponential growth and revolutionary developments in the field of dental anthropology – trends reflected by the broad range of topics and methods employed in the subsequent chapters.

References

Adloff, P. (1907). Die Zähne des Homo Primigenius von Krapina. *Anatomischer Anzeiger*, **31**, 273–82.

Adloff, P. (1908). *Das Gebiss des Menschen und der Anthropomorphen*. Berlin: Julius Springer.

Bailey, S. E. (2002). Neanderthal Dental Morphology: Implications for Modern Human Origins. Ph.D. Dissertation, Arizona State University.

Bailey, S. E. (2004). A morphometric analysis of maxillary molar crowns of Middle-Late Pleistocene hominins. *Journal of Human Evolution*, **47**, 183–98.

Bailey, S. E. and Hublin, J.-J. (2006). Dental remains from the Grotte du Renne at Arcy-sur-Cure (Yonne). *Journal of Human Evolution*, **50**, 485–508.

Bailey, S. E. and Lynch, J. M. (2005). Diagnostic differences in mandibular P4 shape between Neandertals and anatomically modern humans. *American Journal of Physical Anthropology*, **126**, 268–77.

Bermúdez de Castro, J. M. (1986). Dental remains from Atapuerca (Spain) I. Metrics. *Journal of Human Evolution*, **15**, 265–87.

Bermúdez de Castro, J. M. (1988). Dental remains from Atapuerca/Ibeas (Spain). II. Morphology. *Journal of Human Evolution*, **17**, 279–304.

Bermúdez de Castro, J. M. (1993). The Atapuerca dental remains. New evidence (1987–1991 excavations) and interpretations. *Journal of Human Evolution*, **24**, 339–71.

Bermúdez de Castro, J. M. and Nicolás, M. E. (1995). Posterior dental size reduction in hominids: the Atapuerca evidence. *American Journal of Physical Anthropology*, **96**, 335–56.

Bermúdez de Castro, J. M., Durand, A. I., and Ipiña, S. L. (1993). Sexual dimorphism in the human dental sample from the SH site (Sierra de Atapuerca, Spain): a statistical approach. *Journal of Human Evolution*, **24**, 43–56.

Bermúdez de Castro, J. M., Rosas, A., and Nicolás, M. E. (1999). Dental remains from Atapuerca-TD6 (Gran Dolina site, Burgos, Spain). *Journal of Human Evolution*, **37**, 523–66.

Bermúdez de Castro, J. M., Sarmiento, S., Cunha, E., Rosas, A. and Bastir, M. (2001). Dental size variation in the Atapuerca-SH Middle Pleistocene hominids. *Journal of Human Evolution*, **41**, 195–209.

Brace, C. L. (1967). Environment, tooth form, and size in the Pleistocene. *Journal of Dental Research*, **46**, 809–16.

Brace, C. L. and Mahler, P. E. (1971). Post-Pleistocene changes in the human dentition. *American Journal of Physical Anthropology*, **34**, 191–203.

Brothwell, D. R., ed. (1963). *Dental Anthropology*. New York: Pergamon Press.

Brown, T. (1992). Dental anthropology in south Australia. *Dental Anthropology Newsletter*, **6**, 1–3.

Brown, T. (1998). A century of dental anthropology in South Australia. In *Human Dental Development, Morphology, and Pathology*, ed. J. R. Lukacs. Eugene: University of Oregon Anthropological Papers, No. 54, pp. 421–441.

Butler, P. M. (1937). Studies of the mammalian dentition. I. The teeth of *Centetes ecaudatus* and its allies. *Proceedings of the Zoological Society of London* B, **107**, 103–132.

Butler, P. M. (1939). Studies of the mammalian dentition. Differentiation of the post-canine dentition. *Proceedings of the Zoological Society of London* B, **109**, 1–36.

Butler, P. M. and Joysey, K. A., eds. (1978). *Development, Function and Evolution of Teeth*. New York: Academic Press.

Campbell, T. D. (1925). *The Dentition and Palate of the Australian Aboriginal*. Adelaide: Hassell Press.

Clark, W. E. L. (1960). *The Antecedents of Man*. Chicago: Quadrangle Books.

Dahlberg, A. A. (1945). The changing dentition of man. *Journal of the American Dental Association*, **32**, 676–90.

Dahlberg, A. A. (1951). The dentition of the American Indian. In *The Physical Anthropology of the American Indian*, ed. W. S. Laughlin, New York: The Viking Fund, pp. 138–76.

Dahlberg, A. A., ed. (1971). *Dental Morphology and Evolution*. Chicago: University of Chicago Press.

Dahlberg, A. A. (1991). Historical perspective of dental anthropology. In *Advances in Dental Anthropology*, ed. M. A. Kelly & C. S. Larsen, pp. 7–11. New York: Wiley-Liss.

Frayer, D. W. (1978). *Evolution of the Dentition in Upper Paleolithic and Mesolithic Europe*. Lawrence, KS: University of Kansas Publications in Anthropology, Number 10.

Goldstein, M. S. (1948). Dentition of Indian crania from Texas. *American Journal of Physical Anthropology*, **6**, 63–84.

Gregory, W. K. (1916). Studies on the evolution of the primates, parts 1 and 2. *Bulletin of the American Museum of Natural History*, **35**, 239–355.

Gregory, W. K. (1922). *The Origin and Evolution of the Human Dentition*. Baltimore: Williams and Wilkins.

Gregory, W. K. and Hellman, M. (1926). The dentition of *Dryopithecus* and the origin of man. *American Museum of Natural History Anthropological Papers*, **28**, 1–117.
Haeussler, A. M. F. (1996). Dental anthropology of Russia, Ukraine, Georgia, Central Asia: evaluation of five hypotheses for Paleo-Indian Origins. Ph.D. Dissertation, Arizona State University.
Hawkey, D. (2002). *The Peopling of South Asia: Evidence for the Affinities and Microevolution of Prehistoric Populations of India and Sri Lanka.* Spolia Zeylanica: Bulletin of the National Museum of Sri Lanka, Volume 39.
Hillson, S. (1996). *Dental Anthropology*. Cambridge: Cambridge University Press.
Hrdlička, A. (1911). Human dentition and teeth from the evolutionary and racial standpoint. *Dominion Dental Journal*, **23**, 403–17.
Hrdlička, A. (1920). Shovel-shaped teeth. *American Journal of Physical Anthropology*, **3**, 429–65.
Hrdlička, A. (1923). Variations in the dimensions of the lower molars in man and anthropoid apes. *American Journal of Physical Anthropology*, **6**, 423–38.
Hrdlička, A. (1924). New data on the teeth of early man and certain European fossil apes. *American Journal of Physical Anthropology*, **7**, 109–137.
Irish, J. D. (1993). Biological Affinities of Late Pleistocene Through Modern African Aboriginal Populations: The Dental Evidence. Ph.D. Dissertation, Arizona State University.
Irish, J. D. (1998). Ancestral dental traits in recent Sub-Saharan Africans and the origins of modern humans. *Journal of Human Evolution*, **34**, 81–98.
İşcan, M. Y. (1989). The emergence of dental anthropology. *American Journal of Physical Anthropology*, **78**, 1.
Keil, A. (1966). *Grundzüge der Odontologie*. Berlin: Gebrüder Borntraeger.
Kelley, M. A. and Larsen, C. S., eds. (1991). *Advances in Dental Anthropology*. New York: Wiley-Liss.
Kieser, J. A. (1991). *Human Adult Odontometrics: The Study of Variation in Adult Tooth Size*. Cambridge Studies in Biological and Evolutionary Anthropology (No. 4). Cambridge: Cambridge University Press.
Kósa, F. (1993). Directions in dental anthropological research in Hungary, with historical retrospect. *Dental Anthropology Newsletter*, **7**, 1–10.
Kraus, B. S. (1951). Carabelli's anomaly of the maxillary molar teeth. *American Journal of Human Genetics*, **3**, 348–55.
Kraus, B. S. (1957). The genetics of the human dentition. *Journal of Forensic Sciences*, **2**, 419–27.
Kraus, B. S. and Jordan, R. E. (1965). *The Human Dentition Before Birth.* Philadelphia: Lea and Febiger.
Kraus, B. S., Wise, W. J., and Frei, R. H. (1959). Heredity and the craniofacial complex. *American Journal of Orthodontics*, **45**, 172–217.
Krogman, W. M. (1927). Anthropological aspects of the human teeth and dentition. *Journal of Dental Research*, **7**, 1–108.
Kurtén, B., ed. (1982). *Teeth: Form, Function, and Evolution*. New York: Columbia University Press.
Lasker, G. W. (1950). Genetic analysis of racial traits of the teeth. *Cold Spring Harbor Symposia on Quantitative Biology*, **15**, 191–203.

Lasker, G. W. (1957). Racial traits in the human teeth. *Journal of Forensic Sciences*, **2**, 401–19.
Leigh, R. W. (1925). Dental pathology of Indian tribes of varied environmental and food conditions. *American Journal of Physical Anthropology*, **8**, 179–99.
Lucas, P. W. (2004). *Dental Functional Morphology: How Teeth Work*. Cambridge: Cambridge University Press.
Lukacs, J. R., ed. (1998). *Human Dental Development, Morphology, and Pathology: A Tribute to Albert A. Dahlberg*. Eugene: University of Oregon Anthropological Papers, No. 54.
Mayhall, J. T. and Heikkinen, T., eds. (1999). *Dental Morphology 1998: Proceedings of the 11th International Symposium on Dental Morphology*. Oulu: Oulu University Press.
Miller, G. S., Jr. (1915). The jaw of the Piltdown man. *Smithsonian Miscellaneous Collection*, **65**, 1–31.
Miller, G. S., Jr. (1918). The Piltdown jaw. *American Journal of Physical Anthropology*, **1**, 1–32.
Milner, G. R. and Larsen, C. S. (1991). Teeth as artifacts of human behavior: intentional mutilation and accidental modification. In *Advances in Dental Anthropology*, ed. M. A. Kelly and C. S. Larsen. New York: Wiley-Liss, pp. 357–78.
Moggi-Cecchi, J., ed. (1995). *Aspects of Dental Biology: Paleontology, Anthropology, and Evolution*. Cortona: International Institute for the Study of Man.
Moorrees, C. F. A. (1957). *The Aleut Dentition*. Cambridge: Harvard University Press.
Murphy, T. (1959a). The changing pattern of dentine exposure in human tooth attrition. *American Journal of Physical Anthropology*, **17**, 167–78.
Murphy, T. (1959b). Gradients of dentine exposure in human molar attrition. *American Journal of Physical Anthropology*, **17**, 179–86.
Nelson, C. T. (1938). The teeth of the Indians of Pecos Pueblo. *American Journal of Physical Anthropology*, **23**, 261–93.
Nichol, C. R. and Turner, C. G., II (1986). Intra- and inter-observer concordance in classifying dental morphology. *American Journal of Physical Anthropology*, **59**, 299–315.
Owen, R. (1840–45). *Odontography or a Treatise on the Comparative Anatomy of the Teeth*. London: Bände.
Oxnard, C. E. (1987). *Fossils, Teeth and Sex: New Perspectives on Human Evolution*. Seattle: University of Washington Press.
Pedersen, P. O. (1949). The East Greenland Eskimo dentition. *Meddelelser om Grønland*, **142**, 1–244.
Pedersen, P. O., Dahlberg, A. A., and Alexandersen, V., eds. (1967). Proceedings of the International Symposium on Dental Morphology. *Journal of Dental Research*, **46 (suppl. to no. 5)**, 769–992.
Peyer, B. (1968). *Comparative Odontology*. Chicago: University of Chicago Press.
Radlanski, R. J. and Renz, H., eds. (1995). *Proceedings of the 10th International Symposium on Dental Morphology*. Berlin: Christine and Michael Brünne GbR.
Robinson, J. T. (1956). *The Dentition of the Australopithecinae*. Pretoria: Transvaal Museum Memoir 9.

Russell, D. F., Santoro, J. P., and Sigogneau-Russell, D., eds. (1988). *Teeth Revisited: Proceedings of the VIIth International Symposium on Dental Morphology*. Paris: Mémoires du Muséum National D'Histoire Naturelle, Series C, Tome 53.

Schultz, A. H. (1935). Eruption and decay of the permanent teeth in primates. *American Journal of Physical Anthropology*, **19**, 489–581.

Scott, G. R. (1997). Dental anthropology. In *History of Physical Anthropology, Volume 1, A-L.*, ed. F. Spencer. New York: Garland Publishing, pp. 334–340.

Scott, G. R. and Turner, C. G., II. (1988). Dental anthropology. *Annual Review of Anthropology*, **17**, 99–126.

Scott, G. R. and Turner, C. G., II. (1997). *The Anthropology of Modern Human Teeth: Dental Morphology and its Variation in Recent Human Populations*. University of Cambridge Press, Cambridge.

Shaw, J. C. M. (1931). *The Teeth, the Bony Palate, and the Mandible in the Bantu Races of South Africa*. London: Bale and Danielsson.

Smith, P. and Tchernov, E., eds. (1992). *Structure, Function and Evolution of Teeth*. London: Freund Publishing House Ltd.

Spencer, F., ed. (1997). *History of Physical Anthropology.* Two volumes. New York: Garland Publishing.

Swindler, D. R. (1976). *Dentition of Living Primates*. London: Academic Press.

Swindler, D. R. (2002). *Primate Dentition: An Introduction to the Teeth of Non-Human Primates*. Cambridge: Cambridge University Press.

Tobias, P. V. (1967). *Olduvai Gorge: The Cranium and Maxillary Dentition of Australopithecus (Zinjanthropus) boisei*. Cambridge: Cambridge University Press.

Turner, C. G., II (1967). *The Dentition of Arctic Peoples*. Ph.D. dissertation, University of Wisconsin, Madison. Published (1991), Garland Publishing, Inc., New York.

Turner, C. G., II (1985). Dental evidence for the peopling of the Americas. *National Geographic Research Reports*, **19**, 573–96.

Turner, C. G., II (1987a). Physical anthropology in the USSR today. Part I. *Quarterly Review of Archaeology*, **8**, 11–14

Turner, C. G., II (1987b). Physical anthropology in the USSR today. Part II. *Quarterly Review of Archaeology*, **8**, 4–6.

Turner, C. G., II, Nichol, C. R., and Scott, G. R. (1991). Scoring procedures for key morphological traits of the permanent dentition: the Arizona State University dental anthropology system. In *Advances in Dental Anthropology*, ed. M. A. Kelley and C. S. Larsen. New York: Wiley-Liss, pp. 13–31.

Walker, P. L. (1997). Trends in dental anthropological research. *Dental Anthropology Newsletter*, **11**, 1–2.

Weidenreich, F. (1937). The dentition of *Sinanthropus pekinensis*: a comparative odontography of the hominids. *Paleontologica Sinica, New Series D*, Whole series **101**, 1–180.

Weiner, J. S. (1955). *The Piltdown Forgery*. London: Oxford University Press.

Weiner, J. S. and Oakley, K. P. (1954). The Piltdown fraud: available evidence reviewed. *American Journal of Physical Anthropology*, **12**, 1–8.

Weiss, K. M. (1990). Duplication with variation: metameric logic in evolution from genes to morphology. *Yearbook of Physical Anthropology*, **33**, 1–23.

Wolpoff, M. H. (1971). *Metric Trends in Hominid Dental Evolution*. Cleveland: Case Western Reserve University Press.

Wood, B. A. and Abbott, S. A. (1983). Analysis of the dental morphology of Plio-Pleistocene hominids. I. Mandibular molars: crown area measurements and morphological traits. *Journal of Anatomy*, **136**, 197–219.

Wood, B. A. and Engleman, C. A. (1988). Analysis of the dental morphology of Plio-Pleistocene hominids. V. Maxillary postcanine tooth morphology. *Journal of Anatomy*, **161**, 1–35.

Wood, B. A. and Uytterschaut, H. (1987). Analysis of the dental morphology of Plio-Pleistocene hominids. III. Mandibular premolar crowns. *Journal of Anatomy*, **154**, 121–56.

Wood, B. A., Abbott, S. A., and Graham, S. H. (1983). Analysis of the dental morphology of Plio-Pleistocene hominids. II. Mandibular molars – study of cusp areas, fissure pattern and cross sectional shape of the crown. *Journal of Anatomy*, **137**, 287–314.

Wood, B. A., Abbott, S. A., and Uytterschaut, H. (1988). Analysis of the dental morphology of Plio-Pleistocene hominids. IV. Mandibular postcanine root morphology. *Journal of Anatomy*, **156**, 107–39.

Wu, L. (1992). Dental anthropology in China. *Dental Anthropology Newsletter*, **7**, 2–3.

Wu, L. and Xianglong, Z. (1995). Preliminary impression of current dental anthropology research in China. *Dental Anthropology Newsletter*, **9**, 1–5.

Zadzinska, E., ed. (2005). *Current Trends in Dental Morphology Research*. Lodz: University of Lodz Press.

Zoubov, A. A. (1977). Odontoglyphics: the laws of variation of the human molar crown relief. In *Orofacial Growth and Development*, ed. A. A. Dahlberg and T. M. Graber. The Hague: Mouton Publishers, pp. 269–282.

Zoubov, A. A. and Haldeyeva, N. (1979). *Ethnic Odontology of the USSR*. Moscow: Nauka [in Russian].

3 *Statistical applications in dental anthropology*

EDWARD F. HARRIS

3.1 Introduction

Statistical methods have become a mainstay in physical anthropology – and a working knowledge of statistics is as necessary in dental anthropology as in any other aspect of the field. It may seem odd to have a chapter on statistics in a book discussing advances in dental anthropology. Statistics are tools – they are means of investigating questions – not ends in themselves, and they should not drive or limit the research. Also, there are no "dental" statistics; we are dealing with the same descriptive and inferential methods used in other areas of physical anthropology and in biology generally. On the other hand, access to and familiarity with statistical methods are two essentially separate issues that have molded, and continue to influence, the development of dental anthropology, as demonstrated elsewhere in this volume.

NB

This is not the first effort at characterizing the use of statistics in dental anthropology, and I will mention just a few key precedents. Going back a good ways, Wilder (1920) provided a rudimentary introduction to descriptive statistics in his manual on anthropometry; however, this was readily surpassed by Rudolf Martin's (1928) classic three-volume work "Lehrbuch der Anthropology," that has a 49-page chapter on statistical methods. Martin's review was meant for all physical anthropology, with no specific mention of teeth in this chapter. The mean and measures of dispersion were described, along with the two-sample (group comparison) t-test, and Karl Pearson's correlation coefficient. Common to reviews in that pre-calculator era, graphical and tabular methods were described that facilitate hand calculation (see, comparably, Croxton and Cowden, 1939). Later, Denys Goose (1963) authored a chapter on dental measurements in the historically important symposium that resulted in the volume entitled "Dental Anthropology," edited by Don R. Brothwell (1963). However, his review mostly describes crown measurements rather than statistical approaches. Additional examples are presented below.

Technique and Application in Dental Anthropology ed. Joel D. Irish and Greg C. Nelson
Published by Cambridge University Press.

The present chapter is not intended as a primer. The field of biological statistics (biometry) has become far too broad, too detailed, and is expanding too rapidly to make any synopsis possible. Instead, several key points in the origins and applications of statistics in dental anthropology are presented, with an emphasis on continuous data. For readers interested in additional methodological details and the chronological development of biometry, there has been an approximate lineage of popular texts over the past century. One suggested set of selections would be: Pearl (1940), the many editions of Yule and Kendall (e.g. 1950) and Fisher (e.g. 1954), Snedecor (1948), Steel and Torrie (1960), Sokal and Rohlf (1995), and Zar (1999). This list represents a highly selected and biased sequence, but does point out the agricultural and animal-husbandry roots of biometry.

3.2 Quantifying teeth

3.2.1 Beginnings

There is a long tradition of measuring teeth and jaws in anthropology (see references in de Terra, 1905; Gregory and Hellman, 1926; and Selmer-Olsen, 1949). This interest in quantification meshes with physical anthropologists' expertise in anthropometry and osteometry, but a good deal of impetus derived from dentists who took an interest in size variations. The renowned American dentist G. V. Black published tooth size "standards" in his small text "Descriptive Anatomy of the Human Teeth," with the first edition in 1897, and these values have been broadly cited and reprinted (including typographic errors, see Moss and Chase, 1966) throughout the twentieth century (Ash, 1984). It is apparent that T. D. Campbell borrowed from Black in his choice of what tooth dimensions to measure and how to display the statistics. This is predictable since Campbell was trained as a dentist and, indeed, wrote his classic odontography "Dentition and Palate of the Australian Aboriginal" (1925) in partial fulfillment of his dental degree. In turn, J. C. Middleton Shaw, author of the landmark odontography "The Teeth, The Bony Palate and the Mandible in Bantu Races of South Africa," (1931) also was a dentist, and he too paralleled Black's choice of what to measure and how to table the summary statistics.

The problem has not been the unavailability of tooth dimensions, but how to analyze them to address anthropological questions. De Terra's (1905) formative solutions were to compare the range of tooth sizes and, also, to see whether crown shape (plotting crown length by breadth) would distinguish among contemporary human groups. A group's range seldom is distinctive, though, because it is a measure of dispersion rather than central tendency and, because it relies on just two values, it is easily distorted by outliers (and the range often depends on sample size). Crown length–breadth comparisons also proved of little use in separating human groups because of the considerable sameness within the human species. This occurs in part because of the positive inter-correlations between dimensions and among tooth types (e.g. Moorrees and Chadha, 1962; Moorrees and Reed, 1964; Ono, 1960).

For much of the twentieth century, dental anthropologists persisted in hoping that the amassment of crown-size data would provide insights into inter-group variation. Moorrees' study of the Aleuts (1957) is a case in point. He carefully tabled the comparative data from the literature (which were meager then). Despite considerable scrutiny, Moorrees could come to few conclusions: (1) men have larger crown diameters than women on average, (2) average tooth sizes and sample variances in humans reflect the morphogenetic field concepts developed by Butler (1939) and applied to humans by Dahlberg (1945), and (3) contemporary European groups are typified by selective size reduction of the maxillary lateral incisors. As for using tooth dimensions to distinguish among human groups, Moorrees was disheartened, concluding that, "odontometry is of limited value in population studies" (1957, p. 100).

Over time, the earlier interest in using dental metrics (or other data) to classify humans into "groups" as an end in itself has waned (Washburn, 1951), and the method of tabling groups' mean tooth sizes and "looking" for patterns has been replaced with multivariate methods (e.g. Reyment, 1991; Slice, 2005; Sneath and Sokal, 1973). Moorrees' vague dismissal of size (in favor of morphology) is quite similar to the short shrift given to metrics by Lasker and Lee (1957, p. 403) who concluded that, "one can say that, in general, there are large-toothed and small-toothed races." In fairness, rather little data on dental metrics had been published at that time.

3.2.2 Expanding horizons

When Goose (1963) reviewed the kinds of tooth measurements made by anthropologists, his "list" consisted just of maximum mesiodistal and buccolingual crown diameters, plus the crown module (MD+BL/2) and crown index (BL/MD × 100). These few measures were about the only ones that were obvious when using sliding calipers. This was a technical limitation; indeed, sliding calipers were a valuable triumph over prior methods (Conneally *et al.*, 1968; Garn *et al.*, 1967a).

Morphological traits are geometrically complex, generally three-dimensional configurations. Quantifying size, let alone shape, is difficult, but there have been some creative forays in this direction. Corruccini (1978, 1979) used the insightful approach of measuring the size of cusps defined as the chord between their marginal grooves. The contention was that crown size is a composite of the constituent cusps and that cusp size may provide more fundamental measures of the tooth's genetic information. Recent work seems to substantiate this assumption (Townsend *et al.*, 2003). Similarly, Biggerstaff, in a flurry of publications (e.g. 1969a, 1969b, 1975), pursued the study of crown components (basal cusp areas, inter-cusp distances) measured from occlusal photographs. Biggerstaff's efforts were precocious given the labor-intensive methods then required, but the key issue is the collection of continuous, metric data that are amenable to parametric statistical analysis and model building. Technology has increased rapidly: Hartman (1989) devised a coordinate analysis applied to the molars of hominoid taxa; his study also describes multivariate methods for evaluating size and shape differences among groups; similar work has led to the current search for quantitative trait loci in the dentition (e.g. Leamy *et al.*, 2005; Shimizu *et al.*, 2004; Workman *et al.*, 2002).

Other creative efforts were employed by Wood and collaborators (e.g. Suwa *et al.*, 1995), who used a planimeter to measure basal cusp areas from occlusal photographs of individual teeth. A planimeter is a clever analog device that, when the periphery of an area of any form is manually scribed, will generate the form's two-dimensional area (Dinh and Harris, 2005; Macho and Moggi-Cecchi, 1992). Advancements now permit distances and areas to be measured in relatively easy computer-assisted fashions (e.g., Kanazawa *et al.*, 1983; Kondo and Townsend, 2006). These methods yield novel ratio-scale data; statistically, this means that ordinal-scale data as supplied by visually distinguishable (anthroposcopic) grades can be replaced with continuous-scale measurements that may more accurately reflect the biological nature of the size–shape variation (Bailey, 2004; Harris and Dinh, 2006; Hlusko *et al.*, 2004).

Aas (1979) used depth of the lingual fossa as a proxy for the degree of lingual incisor shoveling. This approach is not sensitive to the form of the marginal ridges (that produce the trait), and depth measurements can be affected by lingual tubercles (Turner *et al.*, 1991), but, valuably, this approach converts what would otherwise be ordinal-grade frequencies (e.g. Hrdlicka, 1920) into continuous data that are more amenable to statistical treatment.

Researchers have explored the collection of volumetric data. One approach uses moiré contourography (Mayhall and Kanazawa, 1989; Mayhall and Kageyama, 1997) which, to date, has been informative but labor-intensive. Dentistry is, on the other hand, on the cusp of benefiting from major advances in computed tomography (e.g. Davis and Wong, 1996; Nakajima *et al.*, 2005) that will routinely provide operator-selected planar data as well as tissue-specific areas and volumes.

3.3 Testing distributions and technical errors

Long ago, Francis Galton (1883) suggested that, "The object of statistical science is to discover methods of condensing information concerning large groups of allied facts into brief and compendious expressions suitable for discussion." This aspect of statistics would now be termed "descriptive statistics." Statisticians talk about moments of a distribution, and it is informative to test these for a given dataset to: (1) confirm that the data meet expectations (Tukey, 1977) but, equally importantly, (2) check for biological and/or cultural reasons why a distribution departs from normality. The first moment of a distribution of measurements has a trivial solution: it is always zero. The variance – the most common measure of dispersion – is the second central moment. Statistical packages make it effortless to assess sample skewness (g_1, asymmetry, third moment) and kurtosis (g_2, peakedness, fourth moment). There are higher moments (described in physics books), but they have no obvious biological interpretation.

Unfortunately, nothing that is complex enough to be interesting can be measured without error. Measurement "error" combines issues of precision and accuracy. Accuracy is how close an obtained value is to its true value (Sokal and Rohlf, 1995). Errors can be viewed primarily as technical issues. Calipers with just 1 mm increments are less accurate than those with electronic readouts to 0.001 mm. CAT scans (computed axial tomography) with 1 mm "slices" (pixels or voxels) have less accuracy (resolution) than those at 0.5 mm or thinner. Precision, in contrast, is the closeness of repeated measurements of the same quantity. This has to do with the consistency (measurement style) within and between observers. Sokal and Rohlf (1995, p. 13) note that, "Unless there is bias in a measuring instrument, precision will lead to accuracy. We therefore mainly need be concerned with the former." Regardless of what is being measured, there is no substitute for practice, familiarity, and experience (Kieser *et al.*, 1990; Utermohle and Zegura, 1982).

Statistically, the issue is to confirm that measurement errors are: (1) random rather than systematic, and (2) appreciably smaller than the inter-group differences claimed to be of biological importance. These are separate issues, but they commonly are confused and confounded. Both depend on having repeated measurements on the same specimens so within-operator measures of variability can be assessed.

Systematic errors are easy to visualize. Suppose you measured the teeth of sample A, then, while traveling to the next museum to measure the teeth of sample B, you drop your only pair of calipers (really hard!). Later you're elated to discover that teeth of group B are 0.47 mm bigger than those of group A – thus confirming your hypothesis. This silly, but plausible, example of a systematic bias can only be detected with duplicate measurements of the same specimens.[1] Subtler examples are more common than this contrived one (Utermohle and Zegura, 1982), especially when comparing between observers. For a single observer, systematic errors may diminish as the person becomes more consistent with experience, or they may increase due to fatigue.

Systematic biases can be tested with paired t-tests or, more generally, repeated-measures analysis of variance. Either approach tests whether the sample means are equal or, more specifically, that the mean difference of the paired measurements does not differ from zero. A paired t-test matches each specimen's first and second measurement, so the difference is tested as a function of the standard error of the mean difference. This measure of variability is always smaller than the more common group-comparison t-test (or factorial ANOVA), so it is more efficient – more likely to discover a difference if one actually exists. In other words, a paired t-test is less likely to produce a type II statistical error (i.e. acceptance of a false null hypothesis).

The related issue is how big is the "random" component of intra-observer repeatability error? Kieser (Kieser *et al.*,1990; Kieser and Groeneveld, 1991) describes some insightful tests of the levels of within- and among-observer variability for human odontometrics. An obvious test might be to calculate the correlation coefficient between the two sets of data, but this is misleading because a correlation coefficient produces a false sense of security because the coefficient always tends toward 1.0, unless the paired data are extremely discordant. Also, the correlation offers no sense of the extent of the discrepancies; a correlation coefficient measures the strength of association between two variables, not the agreement between them, and the test of significance is irrelevant as to how closely paired measurements agree (Bland and Altman, 1996a, 1996c, 1999). Parenthetically, the same criticism holds when the "accuracy" of a method of estimating age is correlated with actual age at death (reviewed by Rösing and Kvaal, 1998).

Gunnar Dahlberg, the statistician and geneticist (not the dental anthropologist Albert Dahlberg), developed a simple means of expressing the average discrepancy between repeated measurements (Dahlberg, 1940). This measure of precision has come to be labeled the Dahlberg statistic:

$$d = \sqrt{\frac{\sum_{i=1}^{n} (X_{1i} - X_{2i})}{2n}}, \tag{3.1}$$

where X_{1i} and X_{2i} are the first and second measurements of specimen *i*. The unit of measurement does not cancel out, so *d* is expressed as the average difference due to measurement imprecision. The denominator is $2n$, where *n* is the number of specimens (Knapp, 1992).

Table 3.1 *Repeated mesiodistal measurements (mm) on 30 maxillary right central incisors*

Pair	Lab 1	Lab 2	Difference	Difference Squared
1	8.3	8.2	0.1	0.01
2	8.1	8.2	−0.1	0.01
3	8.4	8.5	−0.1	0.01
4	9.1	8.9	0.2	0.04
5	8.3	8.2	0.1	0.01
6	8.4	8.2	0.2	0.04
7	7.4	7.7	−0.3	0.09
8	8.0	7.8	0.2	0.04
9	8.2	8.3	−0.1	0.01
10	8.6	8.6	0.0	0.00
11	7.3	7.6	−0.3	0.09
12	7.7	7.6	0.1	0.01
13	8.6	8.7	−0.1	0.01
14	9.4	9.3	0.1	0.01
15	9.2	9.1	0.1	0.01
16	9.2	9.2	0.0	0.00
17	9.1	9.1	0.0	0.00
18	8.4	8.3	0.1	0.01
19	8.2	8.5	−0.3	0.09
20	7.7	8.0	−0.3	0.09
21	8.0	7.9	0.1	0.01
22	8.0	8.0	0.0	0.00
23	8.1	7.9	0.2	0.04
24	8.0	8.0	0.0	0.00
25	8.5	8.5	0.0	0.00
26	8.7	8.1	0.6	0.36
27	8.6	8.0	0.6	0.36
28	8.6	8.7	−0.1	0.01
29	8.7	8.6	0.1	0.01
30	8.6	8.5	0.1	0.01

Dahlberg's statistic can easily be computed within any spreadsheet program, though Bland and Altman (1996c) suggest using a one-way ANOVA, which yields identical results. The ANOVA method points up the fact that there can be more than just two repetitions of data collection (see Winer *et al.*, 1991, for an in-depth discussion of repeatability analysis using ANOVA.) Beware, though, that any systematic difference between trials will inflate the estimate of typical error (Hopkins, 2000). One also needs to be assured that repeatability errors are independent of size (Bland and Altman, 1986, 1996a, 1996b, 1996c, 1999).[2]

Table 3.1 lists the mesiodistal crown diameters from 30 adults, each measured by two observers several years apart using different calipers. The Dahlberg

Table 3.2 *ANOVA for the data in Table 3.1*

Source	df	Sum of Squares	Mean Square
Subjects	29	13.494	0.465
Residual	30	0.690	0.023

statistic is 0.152 mm, which is the average difference due to technical error. The same result is obtained from ANOVA where the two measurements for each tooth are nested within subject, so "subjects" in Table 3.2 is the inter-individual variation and "residual" is the within-individual variation due to measurement differences (that could be termed here labs nested within subjects). The square root of the residual mean square – frequently termed "root mean square" – is $\sqrt{0.023} = 0.152$, which is the Dahlberg statistic and, synonymously, the within-subject deviation and the TEM (technical error of measurement).

This approach is presented in some detail because variations introduced by technical errors often are overlooked – which is potentially risky – and also because the same concept can be used with different data to estimate a variable's fluctuating asymmetry (FA). FA is a measure of size differences between left–right pairs of homologous structures (Bailit *et al.*, 1970; Van Valen, 1962). Comparing the size differences between homologous paired structures (i.e. the body's ability to produce the same phenotype twice) is comparable to assessing the imprecision between a researcher's ability to measure the same structures twice. Utermohle and Zegura (1982) and Utermohle *et al.* (1983) review 11 methods of assessing repeatability error.

3.4 Phenetic distance

3.4.1 Quantitative frequencies

Physical anthropologists encounter peoples distributed across time and space – indeed, they search them out. How can we assess how "close" groups are one to another based on some set of dental variables? This is a facet of the broad topic of numerical taxonomy (e.g. Lestrel, 2000; Slice, 2005; Sneath and Sokal, 1973), and reconstructing phylogenetics, even within a species, is of interest because all biological groups have an evolutionary history.

Constandse-Westermann (1972) has a thorough, but now dated, review of the plethora of formulae devised to estimate biological dissimilarity among groups. Without bogging down in the finer points, the issue is to develop a numerical value that reflects the phenetic distance between a pair of groups based on a suite of measurements. There are two impediments here, how to optimize the: (1) formula that produces the measure of distance, and (2) battery of variables measured. Sokal and Sneath (1963), Sneath and Sokal (1973), and others address the actual underpinnings of the selection procedures here.

In terms of an actual formula, we can begin rather midstream in the historical development of methods by viewing Penrose's size coefficient (1954) in order to develop some discussion points:

$$C_Q^2 = \frac{\left(\sum_{i=1}^{m}(\bar{X}_{ij} - \bar{X}_{ik})\right)^2}{m^2}. \tag{3.2}$$

This equation requires only the sample means for the *m* variables in groups *j* and *k*. If the means were identical in the two samples ${C^2}_Q$ would be zero, and the larger its value, the less similar the groups are judged to be. Statistically, this simple-to-calculate equation has various shortcomings. What if there are missing data, so that some averages are based on more specimens than others? What if the sample variances differ among variables? Should not, say, a 5 mm difference between two means with small sample variances count for more than the same difference for a variable with large variances? What if the variables are inter-correlated? Correlated variables share redundant information – and most tooth size dimensions are positively inter-correlated (Harris and Bailit, 1988; Moorrees and Reed, 1964). Penrose's formula (${C^2}_Q$) accounts for none of these potentially important issues. There also is no way to assess whether a ${C^2}_Q$ value is significant statistically, though this is not an important issue (Smith, 1972).

Of note, each of these shortcomings of the Penrose (and similar) distance formulas had been solved much earlier by Mahalanobis (1936) with his generalized distance statistic (D^2). Even today, D^2 persists as the gold standard for continuous variables. D^2 standardizes the means and variances of all variables and eliminates intertrait correlations (Cooley and Lohnes, 1971).

The strong attraction of a simpler formula, such as Karl Pearson's CRL (coefficient of racial likeness) and Penrose's distance, size and shape (above), is their ease of calculation (Pearson, 1926, 1928). In contrast, calculating D^2 by hand is formidable, though most statistical packages now have programs that make detailed analyses using D^2 effortless – though each program differs in terms of the nature of the statistics that can be output.

The D^2 statistic is not a panacea. It requires complete data sets, which can be a particular problem with odontometrics because tooth dimensions can be missing for any number of reasons (unerupted, avulsed, broken, worn, carious, filled, and so on). If missing data are limited, programs are available in larger statistical packages to estimate missing values using multivariate equations based on the variables that are available for that case (see Prossinger, 1998). The injudicious "populating" of data with many missing cells can, of course, substantively increase inter-trait associations and diminish sample variance because of how the missing values are predicted. Also, the covariance structure at the heart of the analysis is based on all of the individuals in all of the groups, so if groups subsequently are added or deleted, the whole analysis needs to be recalculated. This is not true when using simple formulae that do not develop the variance–covariance data structure.

O'Rourke and Crawford (1980) used D^2 to quantify the phenetic relationships among four contemporary population samples in Mexico. Harris and Bailit (1987) used D^2 to evaluate the phenetic relationships among 12 groups living in island Melanesia. Used as a measure of biological distance, all variables are used in order to estimate the overall extents of dissimilarity (Sneath and Sokal, 1973). This contrasts with the stepwise approach, where the intent is to maximize discrimination among groups using just those variables that actually distinguish significantly among groups. It is, of course, useful to know which variables contribute to which group dissimilarities, and this information comes from the standardized discriminant coefficients that show each variable's unique contribution to each canonical axis. Blackith and Reyment (1971) and Reyment (1991), among others, review various other approaches to investigating which variables contribute to which patterns of group differences.

Numerous alternatives to D^2 have been applied to dental data, particularly methods that use sample means so sample size can vary due to missing data (though this carries risks). The statistical approach that has gotten much recent attention was developed by Relethford and Blangero (1990; also see Relethford, 1991, 1994, 2002). Their statistic (termed F_{ST}) is comparatively complex, but the concept is this: each trait's contribution to F_{ST} is determined by the difference of means between a pair of groups, but this difference is reduced for: (1) traits based on small sample sizes, and/or (2) traits with low heritability (h^2) estimates, and/or (3) inter-correlated traits.

Hanihara and Ishida (2005) have applied F_{ST} to tooth-crown dimensions to assess contemporary patterns of odontometric variation. Hanihara and Ishida's study is noteworthy because of their global assessment (72 samples) and the finding from the F_{ST} analysis that most human variation resides within groups rather than among them, which agrees with results from other biological systems (e.g. Lewontin, 1972; Relethford, 2002). Hanihara and Ishida's paper also shows that much insight can be gained from multivariate methods that do not calculate phenetic distances, but, instead, array the groups on canonical axes derived from principal components from the battery of measured variables.

3.4.2 *Trait frequencies*

Evidence suggests that morphological dental traits, such as molar cusp size and depth of incisor shoveling, are expressed as quasi-continuous polygenic traits (e.g. Falconer, 1967; Grüneberg, 1952), though little work actually has been done to test this assumption for tooth traits in humans (e.g. Harris and Bailit, 1980; Townsend *et al.*, 1990). This model of inheritance fits many sample distributions, where a trait in an individual is absent or present and, when present, can range from small to large (Scott, 1977, 1980), which supports the development of ordinal-grade anthroposcopic scales to record trait expression (see, notably, Turner *et al.*, 1991).

Problems arise in attempts to use these ordinal-scale data in phenetic studies, and problems are exacerbated because of historically poor decisions. Dental anthropologists have been enamored with the use of C. A. B. Smith's mean measure of divergence (MMD) (e.g. Grewal, 1962; Sjøvold, 1973), which was not developed to be a measure of phenetic distance and, along with a profusion of misunderstandings by successive researchers, it seems that published results in this area are effectively uninterpretable and, at best, extremely suspect. Overviews of the development of MMD are provided in Sjøvold (1973, 1977) and Harris and Sjøvold (2004). There fundamentally are two problems. One, numerous errors have crept in to how the MMD is calculated, and this problem is pernicious since virtually no author is at all specific how the statistic was calculated. Secondly, the statistic is not amenable to the morphological data collected: data are collected using ordinal grades, but most of this information is discarded because MMD only accepts dichotomous data. There currently is no solution to this problem because of mathematical constraints. Bedrick *et al.* (2000) published a generalized distance formula that can incorporate both continuous and discrete data, but, in fact, it too requires that the ordinal data be dichotomized. Loss of information by developing "cut-points" to partition ordinal data into single frequencies discards important biological information; of equal note, the researcher can manipulate the cut-points to bias the results in different directions.

3.5 Group discrimination

Dental anthropologists often deal in one way or another with the forensic-demographic issues of sex, race,[3] and age identification. These are patently statistical issues because, dentally, there is considerable overlap in tooth size and form between the sexes, among races, and across ages (e.g. Harris, 2003). The statistical issue often is how to maximize the likelihood of correctly assigning a specimen to a group, *and*, in the process, gaining insight into how (and, ultimately, why) the variables differ among the groups. The question often can be addressed with discriminant analysis, which was introduced to physical anthropology by the polymath Jan Bronowski using dental examples (Bronowski and Long, 1951, 1952, 1953).

Discriminant analysis (DA) warrants discussion because it has several applications, all of which are relevant to dental anthropology. DA can be used to develop multivariate (canonical) formulae that maximally separate two or more groups.[4] This is valuable for sex discrimination (e.g. De Vito and Saunders, 1990; Ditch and Rose, 1972; Owsley and Webb, 1983). Once dental metrics have been collected from known males and females in a biological population, then DA can derive the set of weighted variables that maximally distinguish between the sexes (reviewed by Teschler-Nicola and Prossinger, 1998). Inspection of the canonical axis is, in itself, informative as to what variables optimally separate the groups (and why). The logical next step is to use the derived formula to determine the most likely group affiliation of unknown specimens (Bronowski and Long, 1953), where "group" can be sex, population, species, or other categorical affiliation. The use of logistic regression analysis has, however, supplanted DA in some applications (e.g. Pregibon, 1981; Tabachnich and Fidell, 2001) because it carries fewer assumptions and can be used with combinations of categorical and continuous variables (e.g. Edgar, 2005; Lease and Sciulli, 2005). A third application is to use MDA to calculate phenetic distances (i.e. Mahalanobis' D^2) among groups as discussed in a prior section. These other two applications are briefly reviewed below.

3.5.1 Sexual dimorphism

Men tend to have larger teeth than women (e.g. Garn *et al.*, 1967b; Sciulli *et al.*, 1977; Teschler-Nicola and Prossinger, 1998), but there is considerable overlap in their distributions because humans are not particularly dimorphic (Figure 3.1). This modest dimorphism precludes definitive separation of the sexes in archeological or forensic contexts (Rehg and Leigh, 1999) because there is so much overlap, even when analyzed multivariately. Other primates (Kelley, 1995a, 1995b), notably the cercopithecidae (Swindler, 1976, 2002), possess far greater male–female differences in tooth size. Crown size differences are applicable in forensic and osteological contexts because they can help ascertain a specimen's sex (e.g. Brown and Townsend, 1979; Lund and Mornstad, 1999; Sherfudhin *et al.*, 1996) – notably so in sub-adults where secondary sexual characteristics are not yet developed – and this is a prime application

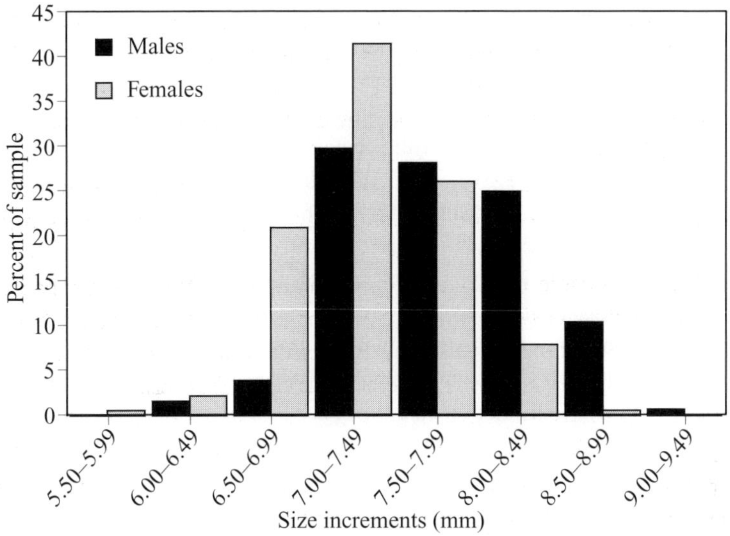

Figure 3.1 Sexual dimorphism in crown size is subtle in humans. The size distribution of males is shifted to the right compared to females, but there is almost complete overlap even for this, the buccolingual dimension of the mandibular canines, which typically is the most dimorphic crown dimension in humans. Statistically, males are 6.1% larger than females in this sample, which is highly significant statistically (F = 59.0 with 1 and 298 df), but of little help for sex determination. (Data from Harris and Burris, 2003.)

for multivariate discriminant functions analysis (Cooley and Lohnes, 1971). Alt *et al.* (1998) show how tooth dimensions at the crown–root junction (see Hillson *et al.*, 2005) are more sexually dimorphic than crown dimensions and, so, are more useful for multivariate sex assignment.

3.5.2 Group assignment

DA can assign an unknown individual to one of a known set of groups. This is the basis of Bronowski and Long's (1952) classic illustration of DA. They measured four variables on the primary canines of contemporary "apes" (an aggregate of chimps, gorillas, and orangs), then evaluated how each of eight Australopithecine specimens compared multivariately to this ape reference group. They subsequently calculated D^2 distances for the eight specimens to a sample of contemporary humans. These separate calculations were inefficient, but they made the point that the Australopithecine specimens were multidimensionally quite different from apes and closer to the human sample. Being substantially closer to modern humans does not confirm anything phylogenetically because the Australopithecine specimens could be even more similar to another untested taxonomic group. The example does illustrate the concept and methodology (see, for example, Klecka, 1980, for fuller details).

Kieser and Groeneveld (1989) tested the allocation of individuals to one of three contemporary groups (South African blacks and whites, and South American Indians) using 28 MD and BL crown diameters (omitting M3s). Conventional allocation with the jackknife procedure correctly assigned 65 to 80 % of the individuals back to their correct group (correct assignment, of course, assumes one knows that an unknown specimen is from one of the known groups). They went on to show, however, that these conventional percentages carry no information as to the degree of confidence (i.e. no probability of correct assignment). Using Campbell's (1980, 1984) method of predictive allocation, only about 10 to 50 % of these same individuals were correctly allocated to their group with statistical confidence, and numerous subjects were "highly atypical of the populations from which they were drawn. This casts a gloomy light on the usefulness of odontometric data in the allocation of fossil or forensic specimens" (Kieser and Groeneveld, 1989, p. 335).

3.6 Age estimation

3.6.1 Ratio-scale data

There are numerous biological parameters tied to a person's progress toward maturity and/or senescence (Rösing and Kvaal, 1998). Gustafson (1950, 1966) and Johanson (1971), among others, review the earlier literature, showing that attrition, diminution of the pulp chamber, cementum apposition, and root transparency all increase in an age-progressive fashion, though rates differ among phenomena as well as race, sex, and culture. Maples and several others (e.g. Lucy and Pollard, 1995; Lucy *et al.*, 1996; Maples, 1978; Maples and Rice, 1979) suggest statistically appropriate methods of handling multiple variables.

The age changes do not have to be the degenerative changes seen in adulthood. It is useful in some circles to assess a child's height age or weight age (e.g. Peterson and Chen, 1990; Tanner, 1976) to monitor children's growth. Liversidge *et al.* (1993) suggest that age estimation can be obtained by measuring formative tooth length and estimating a child's age at death from predictive equations developed by regressing formative tooth length on age. Liversidge and coworkers provide predictive equations for the primary, and some permanent teeth. The method shows promise of providing finer age estimation than using ordinally spaced morphological grades. Liversidge and Molleson (1999a, 1999b) show that the method can be applied to radiographs of the teeth, so extracted elements are unnecessary.

Regression analysis is the statistical method appropriate for predicting age (independent variable) from some biological variable when the data are measured on a continuous scale. For example, in youths, the pulp chamber in a tooth's crown is large, containing blood vessels and nerves. One of the pulp's functions is to form dentin, which it does along the inner walls of the chamber throughout life (Bhaskar, 1980). Consequently, pulp dimensions diminish progressively with age. Chambers may even become obliterated in older ages by this process. If starting conditions were uniform enough among people and the rate of deposition were uniform enough across time, a person's age could be predicted with useful accuracy.

Using data from Woods *et al.* (1990), the correlation coefficient ($r = -0.58$) between age and the mesiodistal width of the maxillary central incisor pulp chamber is negative and highly significant statistically, so there is a solid association here, but r^2 (the coefficient of determination) is just 0.34, indicating that only about one third of the variation in pulp width is accounted for by variation in age. The linear regression of pulp width on age is significant; correlation and regression ask different questions of the same data, so the P-values of their tests are identical. The equation is:

$$\text{Age} = 56.39 - 11.17\ (\text{Pulp Width}). \tag{3.3}$$

This relationship is shown in Figure 3.2, and there is progressive diminution of width with age. But, note the specimens with wholly occluded pulp chambers at zero along the Y-axis. Perhaps a curvilinear relationship would fit these data better than a straight line. The regression equation for a second order polynomial is $Y = a + b_1X + b_2X^2$, and this model fits better; a straight line has an associated r^2 of 0.34 and this increases to 0.37 (a small but statistically significant increase) for a curvilinear relationship that accounts for the steeper rate of secondary dentin deposition in older ages (Table 3.3). Critically, the statistical output shows that the first- and second-order terms are both significant, so there is justification in using the more complex model:

$$\text{Age} = 51.74 - 9.43\ (\text{Pulp Width}) + 2.36\ (\text{Pulp Width})^2. \tag{3.4}$$

If we tried a third-order polynomial to see whether a sharper curve would fit the data better, the term is not significant ($p = 0.68$), so we need to settle on Equation 3.4. On the other hand, this is a good example where we could improve the homogeneity of the sample and, thereby, improve the precision of the age estimates by developing formulae specific to race and sex, assess whether the person has missing teeth adjacent to the central incisor that promote

Table 3.3 *Results of regressing maxillary central incisor pulp width on chronological age*

Term	Estimate	SEM	t-test	*P*-value
Linear Model				
Intercept	56.39	2.21	25.48	<0.0001
Pulp width	−11.17	1.15	−9.70	<0.0001
Quadratic Model				
Intercept	51.74	3.19	16.22	<0.0001
Pulp width	−9.43	1.43	−6.58	<0.0001
Pulp width^2	2.36	1.17	2.01	0.0461

"jiggling" and trauma to the incisor, and account for other extraneous sources of variation.

Occlusal attrition is another example of a dental condition that is age-progressive, especially in non-westernized peoples experiencing a coarser diet; various detailed scoring systems have been devised to assess the extent of wear (e.g. Murphy, 1959a, 1959b; Smith, 1984). Richards and Brown (1981) and Molnar *et al.* (1983) developed a computer-assisted measuring system, documenting that the worn area (exposed dentin) of a molar's occlusal surface increases in a predictive fashion with advancing age. It would seem that a curvilinear regression model would best fit the data since extensive wear will involve all of the occlusal surface after cusps are abraded away, causing the extent of involvement to stabilize at 100 %. Differences in slopes (regression of wear on age) could, usefully, suggest differences between sexes or among dietary regimens as well as data for biomechanical studies.

3.6.2 Ordinal-scale data

Various age-dependent dental changes lend themselves to quantitative measurement (e.g. reduction in MD tooth crown size with attrition; Brook *et al.*, 2006), but others involve morphological changes that are easy to see, but hard to measure on a ratio scale. The use of logistic regression analysis blurs this distinction (e.g. Hosmer and Lemeshow, 2000). Some developmental processes can be thought of as "events." For example, a tooth either has erupted into the oral cavity or it has not yet (Liversidge, 2003). A primary tooth either is in the oral cavity or it has been exfoliated (Moorrees *et al.*, 1963). A permanent tooth crown has formed in its bony crypt, but it has not yet initiated root mineralization (Anderson *et al.*, 1976). These are examples of discrete events;

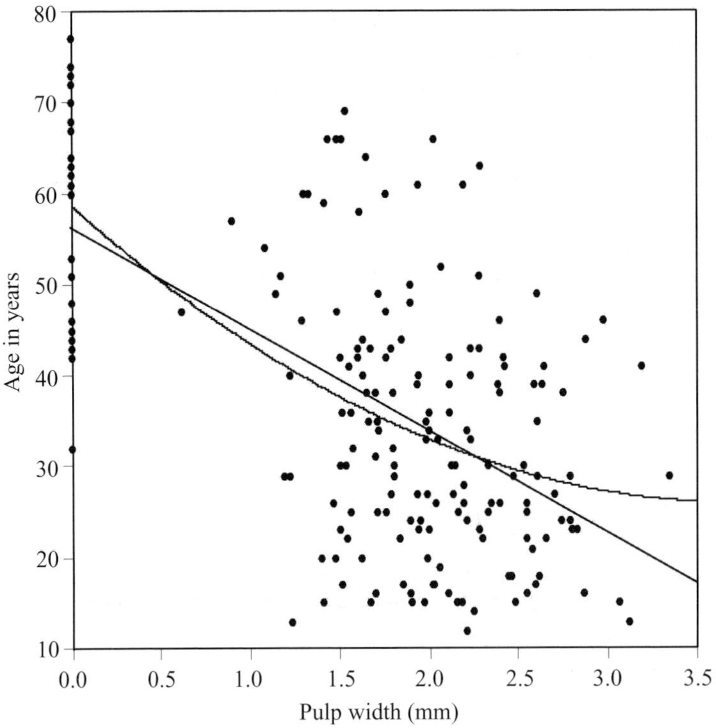

Figure 3.2 Bivariate plot between age at examination (on the abscissa, independent variable) and maximum mediolateral width of the pulp chamber in maxillary central incisors (on the ordinate, dependent variable). Note the several cases of occluded pulp chambers along the *X*-axis at zero. American blacks and whites and males and females are pooled here to simplify presentation. (Data from Woods *et al.*, 1990.)

each maturational event either has occurred or it has not. Because a person's genotype fairly closely governs the tempo of tooth maturation (Merwin and Harris, 1998; Pelsmaeker *et al.*, 1997), the normative age at which an event occurs (within a race and sex) can be known with some accuracy. This is the basis for physiological age assessment, such as that using hand–wrist bone development (Greulich and Pyle, 1959; Tanner *et al.*, 1975), tooth eruption (Liversidge, 2003), or tooth mineralization (Demirjian *et al.*, 1973; Demirjian and Goldstein, 1976; Moorrees *et al.*, 1963). It merits emphasizing that the intent in each instance is to estimate the age at *onset* (i.e. age of *attainment*) of the event.

If an event is normally distributed across time, any of several statistical methods that use cumulative distribution functions will yield concordant results (Hayes and Mantel, 1958; Heidman, 1986; Smith, 1991). For example, we may want to determine the average age at which the mandibular first molar completes crown formation, or the average age at which the maxillary primary second molar exfoliates. Familiar methods are probit analysis (Haavikko, 1970; Jaswal, 1983; Moorrees *et al.*, 1963; Moorrees and Kent, 1981), survival analysis (Holman and Jones, 1998, 2003; Leroy *et al.*, 2003), and logistic regression analysis (Diamanti and Townsend, 2003; Magnusson, 1982; Psoter *et al.*, 2003).

Smith (1991) is one of the few to appreciate that, for demographic and forensic purposes, a different statistic may be more appropriate, namely the "average" age of a person at a stage (e.g. Anderson *et al.*, 1976; Harris and McKee, 1990). In archeological cases, for example, a tooth's emergence and mineralization status can be assessed, but not when or how long previously these developmental events occurred (Konigsberg and Holman, 1999).

3.7 Additional considerations

3.7.1 The special case of factor analysis

Factor analytic techniques consist of a spectrum of multivariate approaches aimed at discovering the underlying, latent structure among variables. The types of factor analysis vary depending on the assumptions placed on the data (Gorsuch, 1983; Harman, 1976).

Common factor analysis (CFA) can serve several different purposes. One is as a data-reduction technique, and, because several variables contribute to a factor's score, the factors tend to be more informative than conventional univariate data (e.g. Corruccini, 1983; Harris and Smith, 1982; Townsend and Brown, 1979). For example, tooth dimensions often are inter-correlated because they have a common etiology (e.g. Jernvall and Thesleff, 2000; Kettunen and Thesleff, 1998; Potter *et al.*, 1968, 1976; Weiss, 1990). CFA is an efficient way of re-expressing the shared variance in fewer, canonical dimensions. Tooth dimensions lend themselves to factor analysis because they are numerous (e.g. Hillson *et al.*, 2005) and obviously covary in size within individuals (e.g. Moorrees and Reed, 1964). An obvious inference is that tooth "size" is an overarching factor that affects the developing size of all teeth within an individual, even though the teeth form at different times and in different places and take on various morphologies (Potter and Nance, 1976; Potter *et al.*, 1968, 1976). Biologically, these inter-correlations mean that the information of the various tooth dimensions is repetitive, so the number of dimensions measured exceeds the number of underlying axes of genetic and/or developmental control (Plikus *et al.*, 2005). Statistically, the inter-correlations mean that the information from the original

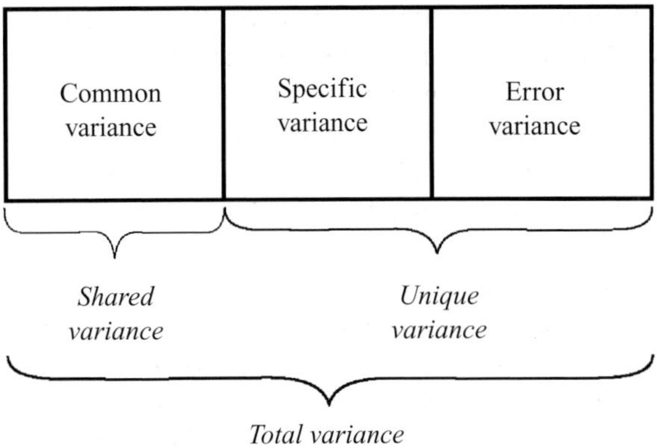

Figure 3.3 Common factor analysis (CFA) assumes that a variable's variance is the aggregate of three components, namely (1) common variance shared with other measured variables, (2) variance specific to that variable, and (3) error variance (mostly due to technical errors). CFA analyzes just the common variance (hence the name). PCA, in contrast, simply treats the total variance. The goal with CFA is to use the common variance to extract the underlying (latent) axes of variation that explain why the variables are inter-correlated, generally depending on an hypothesis. With PCA, the goal is to extract the maximum variance in the original variables using the fewest composite (canonical) variables, which are the principal components.

measurement battery can be expressed in terms of far fewer linear combinations of optimally weighted composite variables (canonical axes).

CFA is valuable for investigating the latent structure of a data set. The use of latent factors has been pursued more extensively in areas such as psychology and quantitative genetics (e.g. Kelloway, 1998; Neale and Cardon, 1992) than in anthropology. Usefully, factor analysis can be applied both as an exploratory tool – to discover the regularity and order in phenomena, and as a confirmatory tool – to verify hypotheses (e.g. Harman, 1976).

3.7.2 Principal components analysis

Several researchers have examined the structure of correlations among tooth crown diameters in humans (Harris and Bailit, 1988; Lombardi, 1975; Potter *et al.*, 1968; Townsend, 1976; Townsend and Brown, 1979, 1981) and non-human primates (e.g. Henderson, 1975; Henderson and Greene, 1975; Kanazawa *et al.*, 1989). Scrutiny suggests that most of these studies actually relied on principal components analysis (PCA). While the terminology between common factor analysis and PCA is considerably confused and overlapping among authors, there is an important difference in concepts (Figure 3.3). PCA is a technique for data reduction; it assumes that *all* of the observed variation can be re-expressed as fewer linear combinations of the original variables. PCA produces determinate variables that express all of the original data on a few composite axes. Factor analysis, in contrast, involves a testable model concerning that the latent structure is based on just the common variance. Factors are latent (underlying, not directly measurable) variables that are indeterminate. Unfortunately, this important distinction often is blurred in practice because both methods reduce the original variables to fewer canonical axes based on inter-trait correlations, and they can produce quite similar results. Moreover, statistical programs often can perform CFA or PCA depending on which options are selected (or fail to be selected). But, factor analysis assumes that there is an underlying causal structure. With tooth-size data, there would be, for example, the assumption of a "size" determining factor that affects all dimensions to some degree, thus driving the observed positive, statistical inter-correlations (e.g. Harris and Bailit, 1988; Potter and Nance, 1976; Potter *et al.*, 1968, 1976).

Applications in anthropology almost always use R-mode analysis, where subjects are rows and variables are columns, so the factors are composites of the variables. The matrix can be transposed, though, to produce Q-mode analysis, where the subjects are clustered rather than the variables. This is a useful alternative to conventional cluster analysis (e.g. Sneath and Sokal, 1973) where individuals sharing similar dimensions cluster together – and the goal is to evaluate *why*.

3.7.3 Bilateral asymmetry

The causes of bilateral asymmetry – differences between homologous left–right structures – have long been of interest to dental anthropologists (e.g. Adams and Niswander, 1967; Bailit *et al.*, 1970; Kieser *et al.*, 1986). One motivating reason is the numerous paired dental elements (10 deciduous and up to 16 pairs of permanent teeth), and, since various measurements can be made on each tooth type, there can be lots of dental variables to analyze. The underpinning assumption is that genetic information on the two sides of the body is identical, so differences are due to developmental and/or environmental signals that perturb the left and right phenotypes from being the same. There are various sorts of left–right asymmetry (Auffray *et al.*, 1999; Van Valen, 1962), but most work has focused on fluctuating asymmetry, where the magnitude of left–right differences in proportional to the stress experienced during development (Polak, 2003).

Various methods of analysis have been proposed (e.g. Palmer, 1994; Palmer and Strobeck, 2003), but the optimal method is that of Van Dongen *et al.* (1999)

who describe the use of a restricted maximum likelihood mixed regression model. In keeping with Palmer and Strobeck, these authors promote double determinations of all measurements; otherwise technical noise (measurement error) cannot be separated from FA (Greene, 1984; Smith *et al.*, 1982). Van Dongen's method provides statistical tests that address six issues, namely whether: (1) FA, corrected for DA and TEM, is significant statistically, (2) FA differs among samples, (3) FA differs among traits, (4) DA is discernible statistically, (5) there is heterogeneity (interaction) between samples and variables, (6) there is heterogeneity among samples.

The usefulness of tooth crowns for studies of asymmetry is considerable. Unlike bones (and tooth roots; Bishara *et al.*, 1999; Wittwer-Backofen *et al.*, 2004), crowns do not change in size after formation, except by degradative processes (wear, fillings, caries, dissolution, abfraction), so people of any age in a sample can, in theory, be pooled to enhance sample size. Teeth also form at different ages, thus reflecting a person's health at different intervals of life, though this is confounded by the distal teeth in a morphogenetic field being more labile to stressors as well as intrinsically more variable.

3.8 Conclusion

As noted at the outset, statistics are tools, not ends in themselves. This synoptic review addresses just a few statistical issues commonly encountered in the dental anthropological literature. Space limitations – given the breadth of "biometry" – prevent any in-depth review, but the intent has been to highlight some issues common to many applications. I have spent perhaps too much time reviewing measurement *techniques* rather than statistical tests, but the one informs the other. Less often is the dental anthropologist in possession of a statistical technique that demands exposition. Instead, awareness of the statistical possibilities ought to direct the data analysis and, ideally, enhance interpretation and the understanding of causation.

References

Aas, I. H. (1979). The depth of the lingual fossa in permanent maxillary incisors of Norwegian Lapps. *American Journal of Physical Anthropology*, **51**, 417–19.

Adams, M. S. and Niswander, J. D. (1967). Developmental "noise" and a congenital malformation. *Genetics Research*, **10**, 313–17.

Alt, K. W., Riemensperger, B., Vach, W., and Krekeler, G. (1998). Tooth root length and tooth neck diameter as indicators in sex determination of human teeth. *Anthropologischer Anzeiger* **56**, 131–44 [in German].

Anderson, D. L., Thompson, G. W., and Popovich, F. (1976). Age of attainment of mineralization stages of the permanent dentition. *Journal of Forensic Science*, **21**, 191–200.

Ash, M. M. (1984). *Wheeler's Dental Anatomy, Physiology, and Occlusion.* Philadelphia: W. B. Saunders Company.

Auffray, J-C., Debat, V., and Alibert, P. (1999). Shape asymmetry and developmental stability. In *On Growth and Form: Spatio-Temporal Pattern Formation in Biology*, ed. M. A. J. Chaplain, G. D. Singh, and J. C. McLachlan. Chichester: John Wiley & Sons Ltd. pp. 309–324.

Bailey, S. E. (2004). A morphometric analysis of maxillary molar crowns of Middle-Late Pleistocene hominins. *Journal of Human Evolution*, **47**, 183–98.

Bailit, H. L., Workman, P. L., Niswander, J. D., and MacLean, C. J. (1970). Dental asymmetry as an indicator of genetic and environmental conditions in human populations. *Human Biology*, **42**, 626–38.

Bedrick, E. J., Lapidus, J., and Powell, J. F. (2000). Estimating the Mahalanobis distance from mixed continuous and discrete data. *Biometrics*, **56**, 394–401.

Bhaskar, S. N. (1980). *Orban's Oral Histology and Embryology*, 9th edn. St Louis: CV Mosby Company.

Biggerstaff, R. H. (1969a). The basal area of posterior tooth crown components: the assessment of within tooth variations of premolars and molars. *American Journal of Physical Anthropology*, **31**, 163–70.

Biggerstaff, R. H. (1969b). Electronic methods for the analysis of the human post-canine dentition. *American Journal of Physical Anthropology*, **31**, 235–42.

Biggerstaff, R. H. (1975). Cusp size, sexual dimorphism, and heritability of cusp size in twins. *American Journal of Physical Anthropology*, **42**, 127–40.

Bishara, S. E., Vonwald, L., and Jakobsen, J. R. (1999). Changes in root length from early to mid-adulthood: resorption or apposition? *American Journal of Orthodontics and Dentofacial Orthopedics*, **115**, 563–8.

Black, G. V. (1897). *Descriptive Anatomy of the Human Teeth.* Philadelphia: S. S. White Dental Manufacturing Company.

Blackith, R. E. and Reyment, R. A. (1971). *Multivariate Morphometrics.* New York: Academic Press.

Bland, J. M. and Altman, D. G. (1986). Statistical methods for assessing the difference between two methods of measurement. *Lancet*, **1**, 307–10.

Bland, J. M. and Altman, D. G. (1996a). Statistical notes: measurement error and correlation coefficients. *British Medical Journal*, **313**, 41–2.

Bland, J. M. and Altman, D. G. (1996b). Statistical notes: measurement error proportional to the mean. *British Medical Journal*, **313**, 106.

Bland, J. M. and Altman, D. G. (1996c). Statistical notes: measurement error. *British Medical Journal*, **313**, 744.

Bland, J. M. and Altman, D. G. (1999). Measuring agreement in method comparison studies. *Statistical Methods in Medical Research*, **8**, 135–60.

Bronowski, J. and Long, W. M. (1951). Statistical methods in anthropology. *Nature*, **168**, 794.

Bronowski, J. and Long, W. M. (1952). Statistics of discrimination in anthropology. *American Journal of Physical Anthropology*, **10**, 385–94.

Bronowski, J. and Long, W. M. (1953). The Australopithecine milk canines. *Nature*, **172**, 251.

Brook, A. H., Underhill, C., Foo, L. K., and Hector, M. (2006). Approximal attrition and permanent tooth crown size in a Romano-British population. *Dental Anthropology*, **19**, 23–8.

Brothwell, D. R., editor. (1963). *Dental Anthropology*. New York: Oxford.

Brown, T. and Townsend, G. C. (1979). Sex determination by single and multiple tooth measurements. *Occasional Papers in Human Biology*, **1**, 1–16.

Butler, P. M. (1939). Studies of the mammalian dentition: differentiation of the post-canine dentition. *Proceedings of the Zoological Society of London*, **109**, 1–36.

Campbell, N. A. (1980). Robust procedures in multivariate analysis. *Applied Statistics*, **29**, 231–7.

Campbell, N. A. (1984). Some aspects of allocation and discrimination. In *Multivariate Statistical Methods in Physical Anthropology: A Review of Recent Advances and Current Developments*, ed. G. N. Van Vark and W. W. Howells. Boston: D. Reidel Publishing Company, pp. 177–92.

Campbell, T. D. (1925). *Dentition and Palate of the Australian Aboriginal*. Adelaide: Hassell Press.

Conneally, P. M., Merritt, A. D., Quinn, B. E., and Potter, R. H. (1968). Semi-automatic digital printing caliper for tooth measurement. *Journal of Dental Research*, **47**, 51.

Constandse-Westermann, T. S. (1972). *Coefficients of Biological Distance*. The Netherlands: Oosterhout N. B.

Cooley, W. W., and Lohnes, P. R. (1971). *Multivariate data analysis*. New York: John Wiley & Sons, Inc.

Corruccini, R. S. (1978). Crown component variation in hominoid upper first premolars. *Archives of Oral Biology*, **23**, 491–4.

Corruccini, R. S. (1979). Molar cusp-size variability in relation to odontogenesis in hominoid primates. *Archives of Oral Biology*, **24**, 633–4.

Corruccini, R. S. (1983). Principal components for allometric analysis. *American Journal of Physical Anthropology*, **60**, 451–3.

Croxton, F. E. and Cowden, D. J. (1939). *Applied General Statistics*. New York: Prentice-Hall, Inc.

Dahlberg, A. A. (1945). The changing dentition of man. *Journal of the American Dental Association*, **32**, 676–90.

Dahlberg, G. (1940). *Statistical Methods for Medical and Biological Students*. London: George Allen & Unwin, Ltd.

Davis, G. R. and Wong, F. S. (1996). X-ray microtomography of bones and teeth. *Physiological Measurement*, **17**, 121–46.

Demirjian, A., Goldstein, H., and Tanner, J. M. (1973). A new system of dental age assessment. *Human Biology*, **45**, 211–27.

Demirjian, A. and Goldstein, H. (1976). New systems for dental maturity based on seven and four teeth. *Annals of Human Biology*, **3**, 411–21.

de Terra, M. (1905). *Beitrage zu einer Odontographie den Menschenrassen*. Berlin: Berlinishche Verlagsanstalt.

De Vito, C. and Saunders, S. R. (1990). A discriminant function analysis of deciduous teeth to determine sex. *Journal of Forensics*, **35**, 845–58.

Diamanti, J. and Townsend, G. C. (2003). New standards for permanent tooth emergence in Australian children. *Australian Dental Journal*, **48**, 39–42.

Dinh, D. P. and Harris, E. F. (2005). A study of cusp base areas in the maxillary permanent molars of American Whites. *Dental Anthropology*, **18**, 22–9.

Ditch, L. E. and Rose, J. C. (1972). A multivariate dental sexing technique. *American Journal of Physical Anthropology*, **37**, 61–4.

Edgar, H. J. (2005). Prediction of race using characteristics of dental morphology. *Journal of Forensic Science*, **50**, 269–73.

Falconer, D. S. (1967). The inheritance of liability to diseases with variable age of onset, with particular reference to diabetes mellitus. *Annals of Human Genetics*, **31**, 1–20.

Fisher, R. A. (1954). *Statistics for Research Workers*, 12th edn. Edinburgh: Oliver and Boyd.

Galton, F. (1883). *Inquiries into Human Faculty and its Development*. London: Macmillan.

Garn, S. M., Helmrich, R. H., and Lewis, A. B. (1967a). Transducer caliper with readout capability for odontometry. *Journal of Dental Research*, **46**, 306.

Garn, S. M., Lewis, A. B., Swindler, D. R., and Kerewsky, R. S. (1967b). Genetic control of sexual dimorphism in tooth size. *Journal of Dental Research*, **46**, 963–72.

Goose, D. H. (1963). Dental measurement: an assessment of its value in anthropological studies. In: *Dental Anthropology*, ed. D. R. Brothwell. New York: Pergamon Press, pp. 125–48.

Gorsuch, R. (1983). *Factor Analysis*, 2nd edn. Hillsdale: Lawrence Erlbaum Publishers.

Greene, D. L. (1984). Fluctuating dental asymmetry and measurement error. *American Journal of Physical Anthropology*, **65**, 283–9.

Gregory, W. K. and Hellman, M. (1926). The dentition of Dryopithecus and the origin of man. *Anthropological Papers of the Museum of Natural History*, **28**, 1–122.

Greulich, W. W. and Pyle, S. I. (1959). *Radiographic Atlas of Skeletal Development of the Hand and Wrist,* 2nd edn. Stanford: Stanford University Press.

Grewal, M. S. (1962). The rate of genetic divergence in the C57BL strain of mice. *Genetical Research*, **3**, 226–37.

Grüneberg, H. (1952). Genetical studies on the skeleton of the mouse. IV. Quasi-continuous variations. *Journal of Genetics*, **51**, 95–114.

Gustafson, G. (1950). Age determination on teeth. *Journal of the American Dental Association*, **41**, 45–54.

Gustafson, G. (1966). *Forensic Odontology*. New York: American Elsevier Publishing Company.

Haavikko, K. (1970). The formation and the alveolar and clinical eruption of the permanent teeth: an orthopantomographic study. *Suomen Hammaslaakariseuran Toimituksia*, **66**, 103–70.

Hanihara, T. and Ishida, H. (2005). Metric dental variation of major human populations. *American Journal of Physical Anthropology*, **128**, 287–98.

Harman, H. H. (1976). *Modern Factor Analysis*, 3rd edn. Chicago: University of Chicago Press.

Harris, E. F. (2003). Where's the variance? Variance components in tooth sizes of the permanent dentition. *Dental Anthropology*, **16**, 84–94.

Harris, E. F. and Bailit, H. L. (1980). The metaconule: a morphologic and familial analysis of a molar cusp in humans. *American Journal of Physical Anthropology*, **53**, 349–58.

Harris, E. F. and Bailit, H. L. (1987). Odontometric comparisons among Solomon Islanders and other Oceanic peoples. In *The Solomon Islands Project: A Long Term Study of Health, Human Biology and Culture Change*, ed. J. S. Friedlaender. Oxford: Oxford University Press, pp. 215–64.

Harris, E. F. and Bailit, H. L. (1988). A principal components analysis of human odontometrics. *American Journal of Physical Anthropology*, **75**, 87–99.

Harris, E. F. and Burris, B. G. (2003). Contemporary permanent tooth dimensions, with comparisons to G. V. Black's data. *Journal of the Tennessee Dental Association*, **83**, 25–9.

Harris, E. F. and Dinh, D. P. (2006). Intercusp relationships of the maxillary permanent first and second molars in American Whites. *American Journal of Physical Anthropology*, in press.

Harris, E. F. and McKee, J. H. (1990). Tooth mineralization standards for blacks and whites from the middle southern United States. *Journal of Forensic Science*, **35**, 859–72.

Harris, E. F. and Sjøvold, T. (2004). Calculation of Smith's Mean Measure of Divergence for intergroup comparisons using nonmetric data. *Dental Anthropology*, **17**, 83–93.

Harris, E. F. and Smith, R. J. (1982). Occlusion and arch size in families: a principal components analysis. *Angle Orthodontist*, **52**, 135–43.

Hartman, S. E. (1989). Stereophotogrammetric analysis of occlusal morphology of extant hominoid molars: phenetics and function. *American Journal of Physical Anthropology*, **80**, 145–66.

Hayes, R. L. and Mantel, N. (1958). Procedures for computing the mean age of eruption of human teeth. *Journal of Dental Research*, **37**, 938–47.

Heidmann, J. (1986). Comparison of different methods for estimating human tooth-eruption time on one set of Danish national data. *Archives of Oral Biology*, **31**, 815–17.

Henderson, A. M. (1975). *Dental Field Theory: An Application to Primate Dental Evolution*. Ph.D. dissertation, University of Colorado, Boulder.

Henderson, A. M. and Greene, D. L. (1975). Dental field theory: an application to primate evolution. *Journal of Dental Research*, **54**, 344–50.

Hillson, S., FitzGerald, C., and Flinn, H. (2005). Alternative dental measurements: proposals and relationships with other measurements. *American Journal of Physical Anthropology*, **126**, 413–26.

Hlusko, L. J., Maas, M. L., and Mahaney, M. C. (2004). Statistical genetics of molar cusp patterning in pedigreed baboons: implications for primate dental development and evolution. *Journal of Experimental Zoology, Part B, Molecular and Developmental Evolution*, **302**, 268–83.

Holman, D. J. and Jones, R. E. (1998). Longitudinal analysis of deciduous tooth emergence: II. Parametric survival analysis in Bangladeshi, Guatemalan, Japanese, and Javanese children. *American Journal of Physical Anthropology*, **105**, 209–30.

Holman, D. J. and Jones, R. E. (2003). Longitudinal analysis of deciduous tooth emergence: III. Sexual dimorphism in Bangladeshi, Guatemalan, Japanese, and Javanese children. *American Journal of Physical Anthropology*, **122**, 269–78.

Hopkins, W. G. (2000). Measures of reliability in sports medicine and science. *Sports Medicine*, **30**, 1–15.

Hosmer, D. W. and Lemeshow, S. (2000). *Applied Logistic Regression*, 2nd edn. Hoboken: John Wiley & Sons, Inc.

Hrdlicka, A. (1920). Shovel-shaped teeth. *American Journal of Physical Anthropology*, **3**, 429–65.

Jaswal, S. (1983). Age and sequence of permanent-tooth emergence among Khasis. *American Journal of Physical Anthropology*, **62**, 177–86.

Jernvall, J. and Thesleff, I. (2000). Reiterative signaling and patterning during mammalian tooth morphogenesis. *Mechanisms of Development*, **92**, 19–29.

Johanson, G. (1971). Age determination from human teeth. *Odontologisk Revy*, **22** (suppl 22), 1–126.

Kanazawa, E., Sekikawa, M., Kamiakito, Y., and Ozaki, T. (1989). Metrical study on teeth and mandible in *Macaca fuscata fuscata. 2.* Principal component analysis. *Nichidai Koko Kagaku* **15**, 138–44 [in Japanese].

Kanazawa, E., Sekikawa, M., and Ozaki, T. (1983). Three-dimensional measurements of the occlusal surface of upper first molars in a modern Japanese population. *Acta Anatomica* (Basel), **116**, 90–96.

Kelley, J. (1995a). Sexual dimorphism in canine shape among extant great apes. *American Journal of Physical Anthropology*, **96**, 365–89.

Kelley, J. (1995b). Sex determination in Miocene catarrhine primates. *American Journal of Physical Anthropology*, **96**, 391–417.

Kelloway, E. K. (1998). *Using LISREL for Structural Equation Modeling: A Researcher's Guide*. London: SAGE Publications.

Kettunen, P. and Thesleff, I. (1998). Expression and function of FGFs-4, -8, and -9 suggest functional redundancy and repetitive use as epithelial signals during tooth morphogenesis. *Developmental Dynanmics*, **211**, 256–68.

Kieser, J. A. and Groeneveld, H. T. (1989). Allocation and discrimination based on human odontometric data. *American Journal of Physical Anthropology*, **79**, 331–8.

Kieser, J. A. and Groeneveld, H. T. (1991). The reliability of human odontometric data. *Journal of the Dental Association of South Africa*, **46**, 267–70.

Kieser J. A., Groeneveld H. T., McKee J., and Cameron N. (1990). Measurement error in human dental mensuration. *Annals of Human Biology*, **17**, 523–8.

Kieser, J. A., Groeneveld, H. T., and Preston, C. B. (1986). Fluctuating dental asymmetry as a measure of odontogenic canalization in man. *American Journal of Physical Anthropology*, **71**, 437–44.

Klecka, W. R. (1980). *Discriminant Analysis*. Beverly Hills: Sage.

Knapp, T. R. (1992). Technical error of measurement: a methodological critique. *American Journal of Physical Anthropology*, **87**, 235–6.

Kondo, S., and Townsend, G. C. (2006). Associations between Carabelli trait and cusp areas in human permanent maxillary first molars. *American Journal of Physical Anthropology*, **129**, 196–203.

Konigsberg, L. and Holman, D. (1999). Estimation of age at death from dental emergence and implications for studies of prehistoric somatic growth. In *Human Growth in the Past: Studies from Bones and Teeth*, ed. R. D. Hoppa and C. M. FitzGerald. Cambridge: Cambridge University Press, pp. 264–89.

Lasker, G. W. and Lee, M. M. C. (1957). Racial traits in the human dentition. *Journal of Forensic Science*, **2**, 401–19.

Leamy, L. J., Workman, M. S., Routman, E. J., and Cheverud, J. M. (2005). An epistatic genetic basis for fluctuating asymmetry of tooth size and shape in mice. *Heredity*, **94**, 316–25.

Lease, L. R. and Sciulli, P. W. (2005). Brief communication: discrimination between European-American and African-American children based on deciduous dental metrics and morphology. *American Journal of Physical Anthropology*, **126**, 56–60.

Leroy, R., Bogaerts, K., Lesaffre, E., and Declerck, D. (2003). The emergence of permanent teeth in Flemish children. *Community Dentistry and Oral Epidemiology*, **31**, 30–9.

Lestrel, P. E. (2000). *Morphometrics for the Life Sciences*. New Jersey: World Scientific.

Lewontin, R. C. (1972). The apportionment of human diversity. In *Evolutionary Biology*, Vol. 6, ed. T. Dobzhansky, T. Hecht, and W. C. Steere, pp. 381–398.

Liversidge, H. M. (2003). Variation in modern human dental development. In *Patterns of Growth and Development in the Genus Homo*, ed. J. L. Thompson, G. E. Krovitz, and A. J. Nelson. Cambridge: Cambridge University Press, pp. 73–113.

Liversidge, H. M., Dean, M. C., and Molleson, T. I. (1993). Increasing human tooth length between birth and 5.4 years. *American Journal of Physical Anthropology*, **90**, 307–13.

Liversidge, H. M. and Molleson, T. I. (1999a). Deciduous tooth size and morphogenetic fields in children from Christ Church, Spitalfields. *Archives of Oral Biology*, **44**, 7–13.

Liversidge, H. M., and Molleson, T. I. (1999b). Developing permanent tooth length as an estimate of age. *Journal of Forensic Science*, **44**, 917–920.

Lombardi, A. V. (1975). A factor analysis of morphogenetic fields in the human dentition. *American Journal of Physical Anthropology*, **42**, 99–104.

Lucy, D. and Pollard, A. M. (1995). Further comments on the estimation of error associated with the Gustafson dental age estimation method. *Journal of Forensic Science*, **40**, 222–7.

Lucy, D., Aykroyd, R. G., Pollard, A. M., and Solheim, T. (1996). A Bayesian approach to adult human age estimation from dental observations by Johanson's age changes. *Journal of Forensic Science*, **41**, 189–94.

Lund, H. and Mornstad, H. (1999). Gender determination by odontometrics in a Swedish population. *Journal of Forensic Odontostomatology*, **17**, 30–4.

Macho, G. A. and Moggi-Cecchi, J. (1992). Reduction of maxillary molars in *Homo sapiens sapiens*: a different perspective. *American Journal of Physical Anthropology*, **87**, 151–60.

Magnusson, T. E. (1982). Emergence of primary teeth and onset of dental stages in Icelandic children. *Community Dentistry and Oral Epidemiology*, **10**, 91–7.

Mahalanobis, P. C. (1936). On the generalized distance in statistics. *Proceeding of the National Institute of Science in India*, **2**, 49–55.

Maples, W. R. (1978). An improved technique using dental histology for estimation of adult age. *Journal of Forensic Science*, **23**, 764–70.

Maples, W. R. and Rice, P. M. (1979). Some difficulties in the Gustafson dental age estimations. *Journal of Forensic Science*, **24**, 168–72.

Martin, R. (1928). *Lehrbuch der Anthropologie in Systematischer Darstellung*. 3 Vols. Jena: Gustav Fischer.

Mayhall, J. T. and Kageyama, I. (1997). A new, three-dimensional method for determining tooth wear. *American Journal of Physical Anthropology*, **103**, 463–9.

Mayhall, J. T. and Kanazawa, E. (1989). Three-dimensional analysis of the maxillary first molar crowns of Canadian Inuit. *American Journal of Physical Anthropology*, **78**, 73–8.

Merwin, D. R. and Harris, E. F. (1998). Sibling similarities in the tempo of human tooth mineralization. *Archives of Oral Biology*, **43**, 205–10.

Molnar, S., McKee, J. K., and Molnar, I. (1983). Measurements of tooth wear among Australian aborigines: I. Serial loss of the enamel crown. *American Journal of Physical Anthropology*, **61**, 51–65.

Moorrees, C. F. A. (1957). *The Aleut Dentition: A Correlative Study of Dental Characteristics in an Eskimoid People*. Cambridge: Harvard University Press.

Moorrees, C. F. A. and Chadha, J. M. (1962). Crown diameters of corresponding tooth groups in the deciduous and permanent dentition. *Journal of Dental Research*, **41**, 466–70.

Moorrees, C. F. A., Fanning, E. A., and Hunt, E. E., Jr. (1963). Age variation of formation stages for ten permanent teeth. *Journal of Dental Research*, **42**, 1490–502.

Moorrees, C. F. A. and Kent, R. L., Jr. (1981). Interrelations in the timing of root formation and tooth emergence. *Proceedings of the Finnish Dental Society*, **77**, 113–17.

Moorrees, C. F. A. and Reed, R. B. (1964). Correlations among crown diameters of human teeth. *Archives of Oral Biology*, **9**, 685–97.

Moss, M. L. and Chase, P. S. (1966). Morphology of Liberian Negro deciduous teeth. I. Odontometry. *American Journal of Physical Anthropology*, **24**, 215–29.

Murphy, T. (1959a). The changing pattern of dentine exposure in human tooth attrition. *American Journal of Physical Anthropology*, **17**, 167–78.

Murphy, T. (1959b). Gradients of dentine exposure in human molar tooth attrition. *American Journal of Physical Anthropology*, **17**, 179–86.

Nakajima, A., Sameshima, G. T., Arai, Y., Homme, Y., Shimizu, N., and Dougherty, H., Sr. (2005). Two- and three-dimensional orthodontic imaging using limited cone beam-computed tomography. *Angle Orthodontist*, **75**, 895–903.

Neale, M. C. and Cardon, L. R. (1992). *Methodology for Genetic Studies of Twins and Families*. Dordrecht: Kluwer Academic Publishers.
Ono, H. (1960). Mesiodistal diameters of primary and permanent teeth and their correlation in the arch. *Kokubyo Gakkai Zasshi*, **27**, 221–34.
O'Rourke, D. H. and Crawford, M. H. (1980). Odontometric differentiation of transplanted Mexican Indian populations: Cuanalan and Saltillo. *American Journal of Physical Anthropology*, **52**, 421–34.
Owsley, D. W. and Webb, R. S. (1983). Misclassification probability of dental discrimination functions for sex determination. *Journal of Forensic Science*, **28**, 181–5.
Palmer, A. R. (1994). Fluctuating asymmetry analyses: a primer. In: *Developmental Instability: Its Origins and Evolutionary Implications*, ed. T. A. Markow. Dordrecht: Kluwer Academic Publishers, pp. 335–64.
Palmer, A. R. and Strobeck, C. (2003). Fluctuating asymmetry analyses revisited. In *Developmental Instability: Causes and Consequences*, ed. M. Polak. Oxford: Oxford University Press, pp. 279–319.
Pearl, R. (1940). *Introduction to Medical Biometry and Statistics*, 3rd edn. Philadelphia: W. B. Saunders Company.
Pearson, K. (1926). On the coefficient of racial likeness. *Biometrika* **18**(1), 105–17.
Pearson, K. (1928). Note on the standardization of method of using the coefficient of racial likeness. *Biometrika*, **20**, 376–9.
Pelsmaekers, B., Loos, R., Carels, C., Derom, C., and Vlietinck, R. (1997). The genetic contribution to dental maturation. *Journal of Dental Research*, **76**, 1337–40.
Penrose, L. S. (1953–1954). Distance, size and shape. *Annals of Eugenics*, **19**, 337–43.
Peterson, K. E. and Chen, L. C. (1990). Defining undernutrition for public health purposes in the United States. *Journal of Nutrition*, **120**, 933–42.
Plikus, M. V., Zeichner-David, M., Mayer, J. A. *et al.* (2005). Morphoregulation of teeth: modulating the number, size, shape and differentiation by tuning Bmp activity. *Evolutionary Development*, **7**, 440–57.
Polak, M. (2003). *Developmental Instability: Causes and Consequences*. Oxford: Oxford University Press.
Potter, R. H. and Nance, W. E. (1976). A twin study of dental dimension. I. Discordance, asymmetry and mirror imagery. *American Journal of Physical Anthropology*, **44**, 391–6.
Potter, R. H., Yu, P-L., Dahlberg, A. A., Merritt, A. D., and Conneally, P. M. (1968). Genetic structure of tooth size factors in size factors in Pima Indian families. *American Journal of Human Genetics*, **20**, 89–100.
Potter, R. H., Yu, P-L., Nance, W. E., and Davis, W. B. (1976). A twin study of dental dimension. II. independent genetic determinants. *American Journal of Physical Anthropology*, **44**, 397–412.
Pregibon, D. (1981). Logistic regression diagnostics. *Annals of Statistics*, **9**, 705–24.
Prossinger, H. (1998). The reconstruction of missing tooth dimensions as a prerequisite for sex determination. In *Dental Anthropology: Fundamentals, Limits, and Prospects*, ed. K. W. Alt, F. W. Rösing, and M. Teschler-Nicola. Vienna: Springer, pp. 501–518.

Psoter, W. J., Morse, D. E., Pendrys, D. G., Zhang, H., and Mayne, S. T. (2003). Median ages of eruption of the primary teeth in white and Hispanic children from Arizona. *Pediatric Dentistry*, **25**, 257–61.

Rehg, J. A. and Leigh, S. R. (1999). Estimating sexual dimorphism and size differences in the fossil record: a test of methods. *American Journal of Physical Anthropology*, **110**, 95–104.

Relethford, J. H. (1991). Genetic drift and anthropometric variation in Ireland. *Human Biology*, **63**, 155–65.

Relethford, J. H. (1994). Craniometric variation among modern human populations. *American Journal of Physical Anthropology*, **95**, 53–62.

Relethford, J. H. (2002). Apportionment of global human genetic diversity based on craniometrics and skin color. *American Journal of Physical Anthropology*, **118**, 393–8.

Relethford, J. H. and Blangero, J. (1990). Detection of differential gene flow from patterns of quantitative variation. *Human Biology*, **62**, 5–25.

Reyment, R. A. (1991). *Multidimensional Paleobiology*. Oxford: Pergamon Press.

Richards, L. C. and Brown, T. (1981). Dental attrition and degenerative arthritis of the temporomandibular joint. *Archaeologica Oceania*, **16**, 94–8.

Rösing, F. W. and Kvaal, S. I. (1998). Dental age in adults – a review of estimation methods. In *Dental Anthropology: Fundamentals, Limits, and Prospects*, ed. K. W. Alt, F. W. Rösing, and M. Teschler-Nicola. Wien: Springer, pp. 443–68.

Sciulli, P. W., Williams, J. A., and Gugelchuk, G. M. (1977). Canine size: an aid in sexing prehistoric Amerindians. *Journal of Dental Research*, **56**, 1424.

Scott, G. R. (1977). Classification, sex dimorphism, association, and population variation of the canine distal accessory ridge. *Human Biology*, **49**, 453–69.

Scott, G. R. (1980). Population variation of Carabelli's trait. *Human Biology*, **52**, 63–78.

Selmer-Olson, R. (1949). *An Odontometrical Study of the Norwegian Lapps*. Oslo: I Kommisjon hos Jacob Dybwad.

Shaw, J. C. M. (1931). *The Teeth, the Bony Palate and the Mandible in Bantu Races of South Africa*. London: John Bales, Sons and Danielsson, Ltd.

Sherfudhin, H., Abdullah, M. A., and Khan, N. (1996). A cross-sectional study of canine dimorphism in establishing sex identity: comparison of two statistical methods. *Journal of Oral Rehabilitation*, **23**, 627–31.

Shimizu, T., Oikawa, H., Han, J., Kurose, E., and Maeda, T. (2004). Genetic analysis of crown size in the first molars using SMXA recombinant inbred mouse strains. *Journal of Dental Research*, **83**, 45–9.

Sjøvold, T. (1973). The occurrence of minor non-metrical variants in the skeleton and their quantitative treatment for population comparisons. *Homo*, **24**, 204–33.

Sjøvold, T. (1977). Non-metrical divergence between skeletal populations. *Ossa*, **4**, suppl. 1.

Slice, D. E., editor. (2005). *Modern Morphometrics in Physical Anthropology*. New York: Kluwer Academics.

Smith, B. H. (1984). Patterns of molar wear in hunger-gatherers and agriculturalists. *American Journal of Physical Anthropology*, **63**, 39–56.

Smith, B. H. (1991). Standards of human tooth formation and dental age assessment. In *Advances in Dental Anthropology*, ed. M. A. Kelley and C. S. Larsen. New York: Wiley-Liss, pp. 143–168.

Smith, B. H., Garn, S. M., and Cole, P. E. (1982). Problems of sampling and inference in the study of fluctuating dental asymmetry. *American Journal of Physical Anthropology*, **58**, 281–9.

Smith, C. A. B. (1972). Coefficients of biological distance. *Annals of Human Genetics*, **36**, 241–45.

Sneath, P. H. A. and Sokal, R. R. (1973). *Numerical Taxonomy: The Principles and Practice of Numerical Classification*. San Francisco: W. H. Freeman and Company.

Snedecor, G. W. (1948). *Statistical Methods*, 4th edn. Ames, Iowa: Collegiate Press.

Sokal, R. R. and Rohlf, F. J. (1995). *Biometry: The Principles and Practice of Statistics in Biological Research*, 3rd edn. San Francisco: W. H. Freeman and Company.

Sokal, R. R. and Sneath, P. H. A. (1963). *Principles of Numerical Taxonomy*. San Francisco: W. H. Freeman and Company.

Steel, R. G. D. and Torrie, J. H. (1960). *Principles and Procedures of Statistics, with Special Reference to the Biological Sciences*. New York: McGraw-Hill Book Company, Inc.

Suwa, G., Wood, B. A., and White, T. D. (1995). Further analysis of mandibular molar crown and cusp areas in Pliocene and early Pleistocene hominids. *American Journal of Physical Anthropology*, **93**, 407–26.

Swindler, D. R. (1976). *Dentition of Living Primates*. New York: Academic Press.

Swindler, D. R. (2002). *Primate Dentition: An Introduction to the Teeth of Non-Human Primates*. Cambridge: Cambridge University Press.

Tabachnick, B. G. and Fidell, L. S. (2001). *Using Multivariate Statistics*. Boston: Allyn and Bacon.

Tanner, J. M., Whitehouse, R. H., Marshall, W. A., Healy, M. J. R., and Goldstein, H. (1975). *Assessment of Skeletal Maturity and Prediction of Adult Height (TW2 Method)*. London: Academic Press.

Tanner, J. M. (1976). Growth as a monitor of nutritional status. *Proceedings of the Nutritional Society*, **35**, 315–22.

Teschler-Nicola, M. and Prossinger, H. (1998). Sex determination using tooth dimensions. In *Dental Anthropology: Fundamentals, Limits, and Prospects*, ed. K. W. Alt, F. W. Rösing, and M. Teschler-Nicola. Vienna: Springer, pp. 479–500.

Townsend, G. C. (1976). *Tooth Size Variability in Australian Aboriginals: A Descriptive and Genetic Study*. Ph.D. dissertation, University of Adelaide, South Australia.

Townsend, G. C. and Brown, T. (1979). Family studies of tooth size factors in the permanent dentition. *American Journal of Physical Anthropology*, **50**, 183–90.

Townsend, G. C. and Brown, T. (1981). Morphogenetic fields within the dentition. *Australian Orthodontics Journal*, **7**, 3–12.

Townsend, G. C., Richards, L., and Hughes, T. (2003). Molar intercuspal dimensions: genetic input to phenotypic variation. *Journal of Dental Research*, **82**, 350–5.

Townsend, G. C., Yamada, H., and Smith, P. (1990). Expression of the entoconulid (sixth cusp) on mandibular molar teeth of an Australian aboriginal population. *American Journal of Physical Anthropology*, **82**, 267–74.

Tukey, J. W. (1977). *Exploratory Data Analysis*. Reading, Mass: Addision-Wesley.

Turner, C. G. II, Nichol, C. R., and Scott, G. R. (1991). Scoring procedures for key morphological traits of the permanent dentition: the Arizona State University dental anthropology system. In *Advances in Dental Anthropology*, ed. M. A. Kelley and C. S. Larsen. New York: Wiley-Liss, pp. 13–31.

Utermohle, C. J. and Zegura, S. L. (1982). Intra- and interobserver error in craniometry: a cautionary tale. *American Journal of Physical Anthropology*, **57**, 303–10.

Utermohle, C. J., Zegura, S. L., and Heathcote, G. M. (1983). Multiple observers, humidity, and choice of precision statistics: factors influencing craniometric data quality. *American Journal of Physical Anthropology*, **61**, 85–95.

Van Dongen, S., Molenberghs, G., and Matthysen, E. (1999). The statistical analysis of fluctuating asymmetry: REML estimation of a mixed regression model. *Journal of Evolutionary Biology*, **12**, 94–102.

Van Valen, L. (1962). A study of fluctuating asymmetry. *Evolution*, **16**, 125–42.

Washburn, S. L. (1951). The New Physical Anthropology. *Transactions of the New York Academy of Science*, **13**, 298–304.

Weiss, K. M. (1990). Duplication with variation: metameric logic in evolution from genes to morphology. *Yearbook of Physical Anthropology*, **33**, 1–24.

Wilder, H. H. (1920). *A Laboratory Manual of Anthropometry*. Philadelphia: P. Blakiston's Son and Company.

Winer, B. J., Brown, D. R., and Michels, K. M. (1991). *Statistical Principles in Experimental Design*, 3rd edn. New York: McGraw-Hill Book Company.

Wittwer-Backofen, U., Gampe, J., and Vaupel, J. W. (2004). Tooth cementum annulation for age estimation: results from a large known-age validation study. *American Journal of Physical Anthropology*, **123**, 119–29.

Woods, M. A., Robinson, Q. C., and Harris, E. F. (1990). Age-progressive changes in pulp widths and root lengths during adulthood: a study of American Blacks and Whites. *Gerodontology*, **9**, 41–50.

Workman, M. S., Leamy, L. J., Routman, E. J., and Cheverud, J. M. (2002). Analysis of quantitative trait locus effects on the size and shape of mandibular molars in mice. *Genetics*, **160**, 1573–86.

Yule, G. U. and Kendall, M. G. (1950). *An Introduction to the Theory of Statistics*, 14th edn. New York: Hafner.

Zar, J. H. (1999). *Biostatistical Analysis*, 4th edn. Upper Saddle River, NJ: Prentice Hall.

Endnotes

1. I have not seen a comment in the anthropological literature, but instrument companies offer machined blocks of known sizes (1 cm, 2 cm) so you can periodically confirm that your calipers read correctly.

2. A valuable source of statistical suggestions is the occasional series of Statistical Notes, primarily by J. M. Bland and D. G. Altman, in the *British Medical Journal* (articles exceed 50 pages and are easily found on the World Wide Web).
3. This has become a pejorative term in anthropological circles; it is used here because there is no satisfactory substitute.
4. DA normally refers to distinguishing between two groups, and multivariate DA (MDA) refers to distinguishing between more than two groups (and the number of canonical axes is one less than the number of groups).

Section II

Applications in assessing population health

4 *Using perikymata to estimate the duration of growth disruptions in fossil hominin teeth: issues of methodology and interpretation*

DEBBIE GUATELLI-STEINBERG

4.1 Introduction

Enamel hypoplasias are developmental defects of tooth enamel taking the form of pits, horizontal lines, grooves, or, occasionally, altogether missing enamel (FDI DDE Index, 1982, 1992). These defects result from disturbances to ameloblasts (enamel-producing cells) during the secretory phase of enamel formation (Goodman and Rose, 1990; Ten Cate, 1994). When systemic physiological stress, such as malnutrition or illness, disturbs enamel formation, all crowns forming during the period of stress are likely to develop enamel hypoplasias (Hillson, 1996). Once formed, these defects become permanent features of the crown, unless worn away by abrasion or attrition. For these reasons, and because teeth are the most abundant of skeletal remains (Hillson, 1996), enamel hypoplasias have become one of the most important sources of information about systemic physiological stress in fossil hominins (Bailey and Hublin, 2006; Bombin, 1990; Brennan, 1991; Brunet *et al.*, 2002; Guatelli-Steinberg 2003, 2004; Guatelli-Steinberg *et al.*, 2004; Hutchinson *et al.*, 1997; Moggi-Cecchi, 2000; Molnar and Molnar, 1985; Ogilvie *et al.*, 1989; Tobias, 1991; White, 1978).

Linear enamel hypoplasia (LEH) is the most common type of hypoplastic defect, taking the form of "furrows" on the enamel surface (Hillson and Bond, 1997). Of the different types of hypoplastic defects, LEH has the greatest potential to reveal information about the duration of enamel growth disturbances. This potential resides in several crucial facts about enamel formation and in the nature of LEH defects themselves.

Enamel grows in an incremental manner from the cusp of a tooth to its cervix (Aiello and Dean, 2002; Hillson, 1996). These incremental growth layers are

Technique and Application in Dental Anthropology ed. Joel D. Irish and Greg C. Nelson
Published by Cambridge University Press.

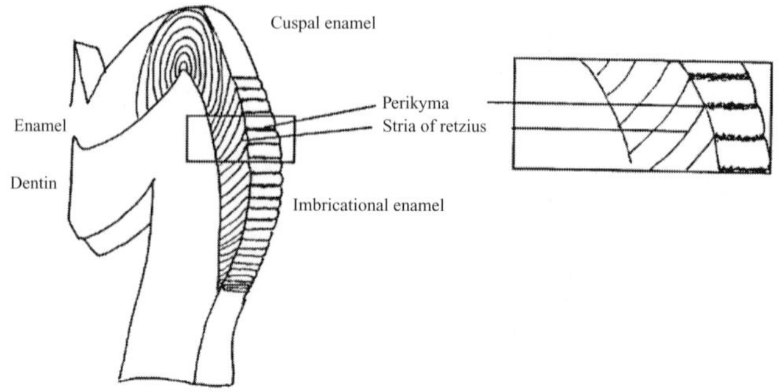

Figure 4.1 Relationship between striae of Retzius and perikymata in lateral (imbricational) enamel (Figure adapted from Ten Cate, 1994).

visible as dark lines, or striae of Retzius (more simply, striae), in transmitted light microscopy of thin sections (Aiello and Dean, 2002; Hillson, 1996). The exact period of growth represented by each stria can be determined by counting the daily growth increments, or cross striations, that lie between them (Aiello and Dean, 2002; Bromage, 1991; Fitzgerald, 1998; Hillson, 1996). The number of days represented by each stria, its periodicity, is constant within the teeth of an individual (Fitzgerald, 1998), but ranges in different individuals from 6–12 days (Smith *et al.*, in press), with an average of eight or nine days in modern humans, apes, and perhaps fossil hominins (Dean *et al.*, 2001a; Dean *et al.*, 2001b). In the cuspal region of the crown, enamel growth layers cover each other in a series of domes. However, on the sides of the tooth, in the lateral enamel, they outcrop onto the enamel surface as perikymata (Figure 4.1). In an LEH defect, growth disruptions cause ameloblasts to prematurely stop secreting enamel matrix, resulting in the exposure of wider than normal portions of Retzius planes at the enamel surface. Thus, perikymata are clearly associated with LEH defects, and can therefore be used to estimate the duration of enamel growth disruptions (Hillson and Bond, 1997).

In recent studies, I have attempted to use perikymata within LEH defects to estimate the duration of growth disruptions in fossil hominins (Guatelli-Steinberg, 2003, 2004; Guatelli-Steinberg *et al.*, 2004). In doing so, several issues associated with this method have become apparent. In addition, differences among hominin species in the estimated average duration of their growth disruptions have been found. In keeping with this volume's focus on technique and application, the present chapter discusses both the methodological and interpretative issues involved in using perikymata to estimate the duration of growth disruptions in fossil hominins.

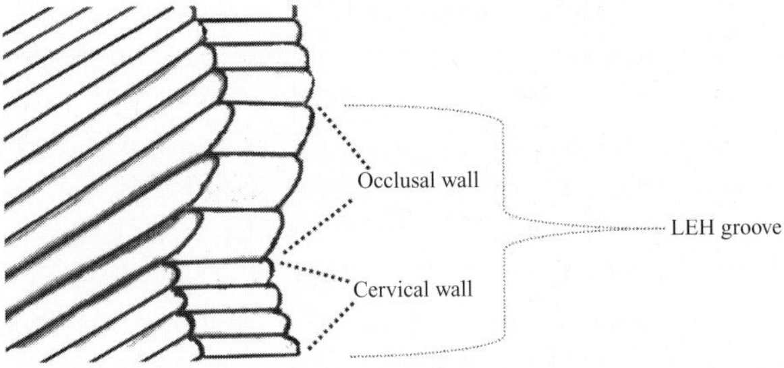

Figure 4.2 Occlusal and cervical walls of LEH (furrow-form) defects. Perikymata in the occlusal wall represent the actual period of growth disruption (adapted from Hillson and Bond, 1997).

4.2 Methodological issues

4.2.1 Counting perikymata within defects vs. measuring defect widths

Through microscopic investigation, Hillson and Bond (1997) determined that perikymata are more widely spaced than normal in the occlusal walls of hypoplastic furrows, and that these "occlusal wall" perikymata therefore reflect the period of disrupted growth. Perikymata in the cervical wall of a defect, instead, represent a return to normal growth (Hillson and Bond, 1997). Figure 4.2 is a diagram showing a linear defect's occlusal and cervical walls and the perikymata that comprise them. If perikymata can be seen within a defect on an actual tooth crown, then the duration of disrupted growth can be estimated. The defect depicted in Figure 4.2, with three perikymata in its occlusal wall, represents approximately 24–30 days of growth disruption (8–10 day perikymata periodicity).

Prior to Hillson and Bond's (1997) analysis, researchers employed the width of LEH defects as a measure of growth disruption duration (e.g. Blakey *et al.*, 1994; Ensor and Irish, 1995). However, underlying this practice is the assumption that enamel grows along the length of the crown at a constant rate, which it clearly does not (e.g. Reid and Dean, 2000, 2006). Enamel growth slows toward the cervix in humans, such that perikymata become increasingly more closely spaced as the cervix is approached. Hillson and Bond (1997) predicted that LEH widths would be influenced by this variation in perikymata spacing. Thus, a furrow consisting of 10 perikymata in the cervical part of the crown would be expected to be narrower than one with an identical number of perikymata in the occlusal region, where perikymata are more widely spaced.

Hillson and Bond's (1997) prediction that perikymata spacing can greatly influence defect widths is borne out in the analysis of Point Hope Inupiaq and Neandertal defects in Guatelli-Steinberg *et al.* (2004). For ready identification by non-Alaskan specialists, the Inupiaq were previously referred to by the generally recognizable term of Inuit (Guatelli-Steinberg *et al.*, 2004), but in this chapter the Northwest Alaska-specific term is used (Irish, personal communication, 2006). The Inupiaq remains, housed at the American Museum of Natural History, span five culture periods: Near Ipiutak (500–100 BC), Ipiutak (100 BC–500 AD), Birnirk (500–900 AD), Tigara (1300–1800 AD) and Recent (1700–present) (Schwartz *et al.*, 1995). The Neandertal sample consisted of: (1) 130 000-year-old dental remains from the Krapina rock shelter, housed at the Croatian Natural History Museum in Zagreb (Rink *et al.*, 1995), and (2) dental remains from Southern France, housed at various museums throughout Europe, spanning the time period of 65 to 41 MYA (Schwartz and Tattersall, 2002).

In Guatelli-Steinberg *et al.* (2004), perikymata counts were made within defects and compared with defect widths. Perikymata were counted between the occlusal and cervical borders of defects (Figure 4.3), and an average of three width measurements were taken along the length of defects (Figure 4.4). The average width of Neandertal defects ($n = 19$) was greater than that of Inupiaq defects ($n = 21$), although a t-test revealed that this difference was not statistically significant. On the other hand, a t-test on mean perikymata counts revealed that Neandertal defects ($n = 15$) had significantly *fewer* perikymata within them than Inupiaq defects ($n = 7$). Clearly, defect widths are not giving the same answer as perikymata counts about the relative duration of growth disruptions in Neandertal vs. Inupiaq.

The cause of the different results obtained from the perikymata count and defect width methods in the Neandertal vs. Inupiaq example becomes clear when one considers how perikymata are spaced in Neandertal and Inupiaq teeth. Many defects occur in the cervical regions of these teeth, where Inupiaq vs. Neandertal differences in perikymata spacing are at their greatest (Guatelli-Steinberg *et al.*, in press). Indeed, perikymata spacing (the number of perikymata per mm) was measured adjacent and incisal to these defects, and a t-test showed that Inupiaq perikymata were significantly more closely spaced than Neandertal perikymata (Guatelli-Steinberg *et al.*, 2004). The spacing difference can be seen in Figure 4.5. Even though Inupiaq defects have more perikymata within them, they do not appear wider than Neandertal defects because perikymata are more closely spaced on Inupiaq teeth than they are on Neandertal teeth.

This example supports Hillson and Bond's (1997) contention that width measurements are strongly influenced by perikymata spacing and therefore can lead to erroneous conclusions about the duration of stress episodes. Yet, while

A

B

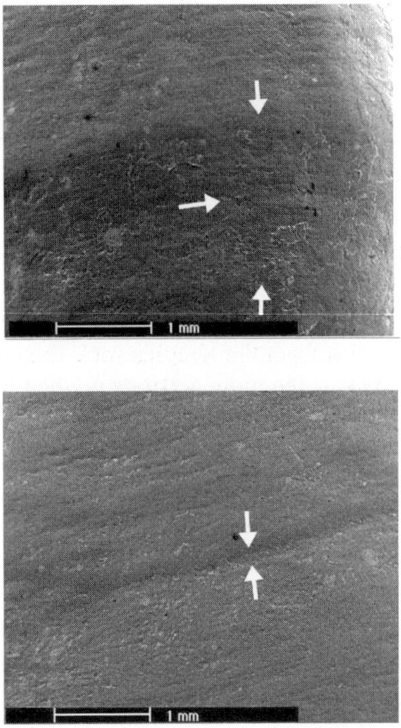

Figure 4.3 Two LEH defects in a Krapina Neandertal canine imaged under a scanning electron microscope. Image A shows a defect which has 25 perikymata, 12 in the occlusal wall. The right-facing arrow indicates the border between the occlusal and cervical defect walls. Image B shows a defect with 2 perikymata. The arrows indicate the borders of the defects.

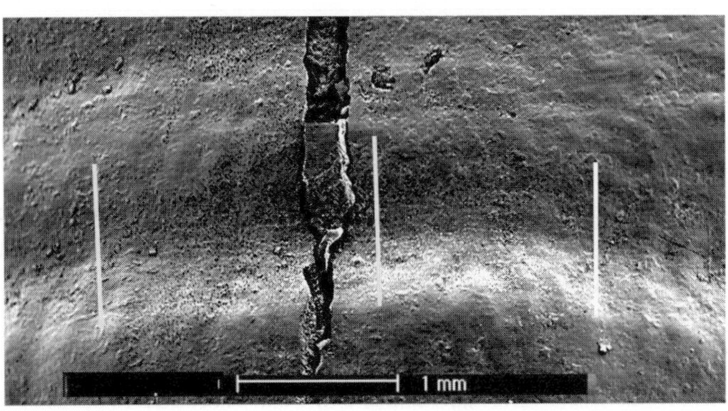

Figure 4.4 How defect widths were measured. White lines indicate the distances measured between defect borders as the defect curves around the crown.

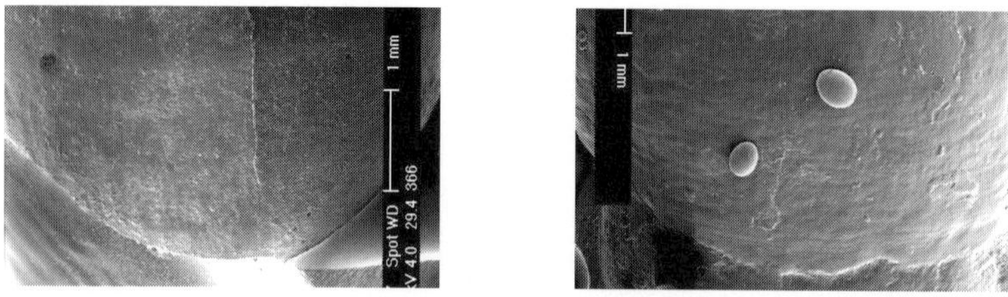

Figure 4.5 At the cervix of the tooth (the CEJ is at the bottom of each image), perikymata are more widely spaced in the Neandertal tooth on the right than they are in the Inupiaq tooth on the left.

counting perikymata within defects is the more accurate method, it is complicated by several factors. One of the major difficulties in employing perikymata to estimate the duration of growth disruptions in LEH defects is that perikymata are often not visible, or not continuously visible, within them, using either light or scanning electron microscopy (personal observation). Defect widths, on the other hand, are usually possible to measure. Of 44 Neandertal and Inupiaq defects identified in Guatelli-Steinberg *et al.* (2004), it was possible to measure widths for 40, but to count total perikymata for just 22. This difference suggests that if there was a way to make use of defect widths by taking into account differences in perikymata spacing, it would greatly increase the amount of data available to test hypotheses about stress episode duration. One way this might be done is to measure perikymata spacing adjacent to each defect, and to use this variable as a covariate to statistically control for perikymata spacing in the comparison of defect widths.

4.2.2 Additional methodological issues associated with counting perikymata within defects

The subjectivity involved in visual identification of defect borders may influence the number of perikymata counted within a defect; the same is true for measurements of defect width. Other researchers have dealt with this problem by using a measuring microscope to objectively define defect borders (Hillson 1992; Hillson and Jones, 1989; King *et al.*, 2002). Figure 4.6 depicts spacing between perikymata from a lower central incisor of a modern human juvenile (specimen courtesy of S. Hillson, data courtesy of R. Ferrell and S. Hillson). Measurements were smoothed using a five-day running average. Perikyma 1 occurs at the start of lateral enamel formation. Two counts, made by the same observer on separate days, are very similar except at the start of lateral enamel and at the cervix. Arrows denote major defects that were visible to the naked

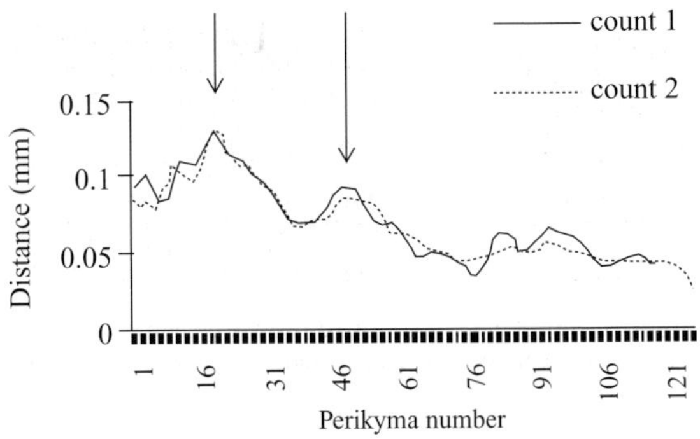

Figure 4.6 Plot of distances between perikymata numbered from first to last formed. Measurements were taken using a measuring microscope, courtesy of Rebecca Ferrell and Simon Hillson. The similarity of the two separate counts indicates that this method has high repeatability. Arrows denote the increase in perikymata spacing associated with two macroscopically identifiable defects.

eye, and are marked by an increase in perikymata spacing at their occlusal borders.

Up until this point, the discussion has focused on counting all perikymata within a defect. However, the preceding discussion emphasizes Hillson and Bond's (1997) observations that greater than normal perikymata spacing, representing disrupted growth, only occurs in the occlusal walls of defects. The occlusal wall of a defect can be identified by the wide perikymata spacing within the sloping occlusal wall, in contrast with the normally spaced perikymata in the sloping cervical wall (see Figures 4.2 and 4.3). The two walls meet at the bottom of a defect, such that the entire defect forms a "V." Isolating occlusal wall perikymata, however, is often difficult because the demarcation between the two walls of the defect, as well as changes in perikymata spacing, are often not clear, especially in defects comprised of very few perikymata. For example, in the two defects pictured in Figure 4.4, Defect A has 25 total perikymata, 12 of which are in the occlusal wall. Defect B has two perikymata within it and it is not clear, from this image, if there is an occlusal wall (which, in this case, would have to consist of a single perikyma). Thus, although there were 22 defects in which perikymata could be counted in Guatelli-Steinberg *et al.* (2004), there were only 13 which had clearly identifiable occlusal walls.

For comparing the *relative* duration of stress episodes in two different population samples, it is probably sufficient to use the total number of perikymata within defects. Furthermore, it seems reasonable to simply halve the number of total perikymata within defects to obtain an estimate of absolute stress episode duration. Table 4.1 gives occlusal and total perikymata counts within defects for which both could be counted (original data are in Guatelli-Steinberg *et al.*,

Table 4.1 *Perikymata counts in the occlusal walls and total perikymata counts within defects for 9 hypoplastic furrows. "K" stands for "Krapina." "P" stands for Point Hope Inupiaq*

Specimen number/tooth	Number of perikymata in occlusal wall	Total number of perikymata within defects
K "H" LRC	2	4
K 36 URC	5	10
K 76 URC	6	11
K 75 LRC	12	25
P 410 ULC	10	22
P 419 LRC	10	22
P 449 LLC	5	13
P 482 URC	4	10
P 511 ULC	3	7

2004). Note that occlusal wall perikymata counts are close to half of the total number.

Finally, variation in perikymata periodicity must be considered in estimating the duration of stress events. One way to take this variation into account is to consider a range of likely periodicities. Although periodicities vary widely among individuals, they appear to cluster around the values of 8, 9, and 10 in African apes and humans (Dean and Reid, 2001b). Stress episode duration can then be estimated by multiplying the number of perikymata within the occlusal walls of defects (or half the number of total perikymata) by these different likely mean values.

4.3 Results and interpretations of estimates of growth disruption duration in fossil hominins

4.3.1 Neandertal vs. Inupiaq

Enamel hypoplasias in Neandertals are of particular interest because several researchers have argued that Neandertals lived under conditions of nutritional stress (Jelinek, 1994) and were inefficient foragers (Soffer, 1994; Trinkaus, 1986, 1989; but see Sorensen and Leonard, 2001). Previous studies of developmental defects of enamel in Neandertals indicate that these hominins had relatively high frequencies of enamel hypoplasia (Brennan, 1991; Molnar and Molnar, 1985; Ogilvie *et al.*, 1989; Skinner, 1996), but Hutchinson *et al.* (1997) found that these high frequencies are matched by similar frequencies in

Table 4.2 *Estimated mean duration of growth disruptions in Neandertal and Point Hope Inupiaq teeth using three likely mean periodicities (8,9, and 10-day)*

Mean duration	8-day periodicity	9-day periodicity	10-day periodicity
Neandertal	29 days	33 days	37 days
Point Hope Inupiaq	58 days	66 days	73 days

various prehistoric foraging and horticultural populations. Neandertals were compared with Point Hope Inupiaq in Guatelli-Steinberg *et al.* (2004). Many of the Neandertal specimens included in that study derived from unstable (Hutchinson *et al.*, 1997) or cold environments (Schwartz and Tattersall, 2002), to which the marginal Arctic habitats of the Point Hope Inupiaq provide a modern analog. Stable isotope analyses also suggest that Neandertals may have been predominantly meat eaters (e.g. Bocherens *et al.*, 1999; Richards *et al.*, 2000), while the Inupiaq included a large portion of meat and fish in their diets (Larsen and Rainey, 1948). If Neandertals were less efficient foragers than the Point Hope Inupiaq, then they might be expected to have recorded in their enamel evidence of having withstood stress episodes of longer duration.

The evidence from counting perikymata within Neandertal defects, however, does not support this view. The mean total perikymata count within Inupiaq defects ($n = 7$) is 13.4 perikymata while it is 7.3 in Neandertal defects ($n = 15$), a statistically significant difference (t-test on logged values; see Guatelli-Steinberg *et al.*, 2004, for further detail). Actual disruption time averages can be estimated by halving the total perikymata count means and multiplying by periodicities of 8, 9, and 10 (Table 4.2). Note that even assuming a 10-day average periodicity for Neandertals, and an 8-day average periodicity for the Inupiaq, the average estimated disruption time for Neandertals is still less than that for the Inupiaq.

While these data do not provide support for the hypothesis that Neandertals were inefficient foragers, they must be interpreted with caution because of the small sample sizes involved. However, larger samples of Neandertals and Inupiaq were used in a comparison of LEH prevalence in the Guatelli-Steinberg *et al.* (2004) study, yet there was no statistically significant prevalence difference between the two groups. Still, it is possible that other differences between Neandertals and Inupiaq may account for these results. For example, the ameloblasts of Neandertals might have been less sensitive to disruption than those of the Inupiaq. In addition, a sample bias owing to the "osteological paradox" (Wood *et al.*, 1992) might be involved in that Neandertals and Inupiaq may have differed in their ability to survive stress episodes of long duration.

4.3.2 **Australopithecus *vs.* Paranthropus**

Differences between *Australopithecus* and *Paranthropus* in their cranio-facial and dental anatomy, as well as dental microwear, suggest that these two genera had different diets, with *Paranthropus* consuming harder, more brittle objects (Grine 1986; Grine and Kay, 1988). Recent isotopic (Sponheimer and Lee-Thorpe, 1999) and texture analysis (Scott, 2005) indicate, however, that there may have been significant dietary overlap between *Australopithecus africanus* and *Paranthropus robustus*. Sponheimer and Lee-Thorpe (1999) suggest that *A. africanus* and *P. robustus* may have eaten similar food items, but that the latter may have processed these foods more efficiently. Based on their texture analysis, Scott *et al.* (2005, p. 695) argue that *A. africanus* and *P. robustus* probably had "substantial overlap in the fracture properties of their preferred foods." These authors attribute the microwear differences previously found between these two species to microhabitats, seasonality, or fall-back food choices. Differences in critical fall-back food choices might explain why the isotopic signals of *A. africanus* and *P. robustus* are similar, while their cranio-facial and dental anatomy seem to be adapted to different types of foods.

If *P. robustus* was able to consume hard, brittle objects more efficiently than *A. africanus*, *P. robustus* might be expected to have been better buffered against seasonal scarcity of preferred resources. This in turn suggests a difference between the two in their experience of nutritional stress that might be reflected in their teeth as linear enamel hypoplasias.

Guatelli-Steinberg (2004) combined data from south and east African *Australopithecus* and from south and east African *Paranthropus* to enlarge sample sizes in an LEH comparison between these two genera. The *Australopithecus* sample was comprised of specimens of *A. africanus* from Sterkfontein and Makapansgat (housed at the Transvaal Museum or at the University of the Witwatersrand in South Africa), *A. anamensis* from Kanapoi and Allia Bay (Kenya National Museum), and *A. afarensis* from Laetoli (Kenya National Museum) and Hadar (National Museum of Ethiopia). The *Paranthropus* sample consisted of *P. robustus* and *P. crassidens* specimens from Swartkrans and Kromdrai (Transvaal Museum) and *P. boisei* specimens from Chesowanja, Peninj, Olduvai Gorge, Koobi Fora, and West Turkana (Kenya National Museum and the National Museum of Tanzania).

The two genera did not differ in LEH prevalence, but *Paranthropus* did have statistically significantly fewer defects per canine tooth than did *Australopithecus*. This latter result was expected because of the abbreviated lateral enamel formation times of *Paranthropus* relative to *Australopithecus* (Beynon and Dean, 1988; Bromage and Dean, 1985; Dean and Reid, 2001a; Dean *et al.*, 2001), which limit the number of stress episodes per tooth that *Paranthropus* teeth can

Table 4.3 *Estimated mean duration of growth disruptions in* Paranthropus *and* Australopithecus *teeth using three likely mean periodicities (8, 9, and 10-day)*

Mean duration	8-day periodicity	9-day periodicity	10-day periodicity
Paranthropus	17 days	20 days	22 days
Australopithecus	26 days	30 days	33 days

record. Variation in crown formation times across primate species is broadly related to the number of defects their canine teeth record (Guatelli-Steinberg, 2000).

Australopithecus ($n = 18$) and *Paranthropus* ($n = 10$) did, however, exhibit a statistically significant difference in the mean number of perikymata within their defects. The *Paranthropus* mean was 4.4 perikymata while that of *Australopithecus* was 6.6. As in the Neandertal vs. Inupiaq analysis, the mean number of perikymata within defects was halved and multiplied by periodicities of 8, 9, and 10 (Table 4.3).

The data in Table 4.3 suggest that the defects of *Australopithecus* recorded stress episodes of longer average duration than did those of *Paranthropus*, and this result appears to support the hypothesis that *Paranthropus* may have been better buffered than *Australopithecus* against nutritional stress. However, once again, there may be alternative explanations in possible taxonomic differences in the degree to which enamel growth is canalized or in the ability to survive stress episodes of long duration.

There is an additional complication in this comparison of stress episodes duration between *Australopithecus* and *Paranthropus*. The LEH defects of *Paranthropus* appear shallower than those of *Australopithecus*. This is very likely the result of differences between the two genera in the angles with which their Retzius planes meet the enamel surface. Retzius planes form more shallow angles with the enamel surface in *Paranthropus* than they do in *Australopithecus* (Beynon and Dean, 1988). Figure 4.7 depicts how this difference affects the depth of LEH defects: the shallower the angle between Retzius planes and the enamel surface, the shallower the hypoplastic furrow. Because *Paranthropus* defects are shallower, it is possible that a growth disruption has already begun before the occlusal wall of the defect begins to slope enough to be visually identifiable. Thus, the duration of shallow defects might be underestimated if their borders are identified visually, rather than by a measuring microscope. The *Paranthropus* vs. *Australopithecus* difference in the mean number of perikymata within defects therefore requires further investigation using a measuring microscope.

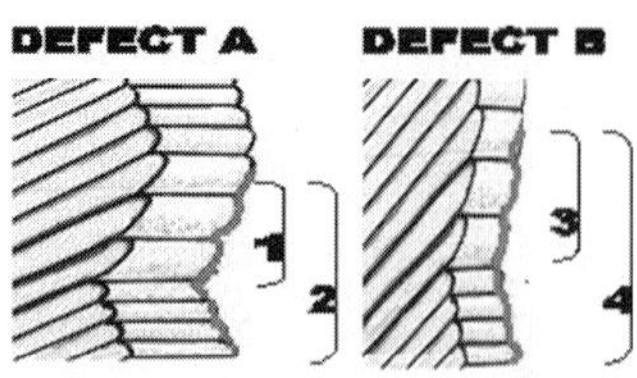

Figure 4.7 Effect of Retzius plane angles on the depth of hypoplastic defects. In defect A, the LEH groove is indicated by bracket 2; perikymata in the occlusal wall of the defect are indicated by bracket 1. In Defect B, occlusal wall perikymata are indicated by bracket 3 and the entire groove is indicated by bracket 4. Because the Retzius planes of Defect B are intersecting the enamel surface at shallower angles than they are in Defect A, the groove itself is also shallower.

4.4 Conclusions

To summarize, there are several methodological and interpretative issues associated with efforts to use perikymata within LEH defects to estimate the duration of the growth disruptions in fossil hominins. The greatest methodological limitation is that perikymata are often not visible, or are not continuously visible, between the borders of a hypoplastic furrow. This fact reduces sample sizes. In addition, the occlusal walls of the furrow are often difficult to isolate, although one way to deal with this difficulty (done here) is to estimate the number of perikymata in the occlusal wall by halving the total number of perikymata within a defect. In addition, a range of possible periodicities for perikymata must be considered.

The data presented here suggest that the mean duration of stress episodes was greater in Point Hope Inupiaq than in the Neandertals, and greater in *Australopithecus* than in *Paranthropus*. However, there are interpretive issues common to both sets of hominin comparisons discussed in this paper. There may be taxonomic differences in the responsiveness of ameloblasts to physiological stress and/or in the ability of different taxa to survive stress episodes of long duration. Finally, the difference in defect depth between *Australopithecus* and *Paranthropus* may bias perikymata counting within defects. These issues complicate the interpretation of perikymata counts within defects as direct indicators of the duration of stress episodes experienced by hominins.

Acknowledgments

My research on linear enamel hypoplasia in fossil hominins has been supported by Leakey Foundation grants as well as by internal grants from The Ohio State University. I thank Joel Irish and Greg Nelson for the invitation to participate in the symposium, and Rebecca Ferrell and Simon Hillson for their measuring microscope data. For research in Africa, I thank Donald Johanson and Bill Kimbel for granting me permission to study the Hadar fossils (both published and unpublished). Thanks are also due Mamitu Yilma of the National Museum of Ethiopia and the Ethiopian government for permitting me to conduct research at the NME. I am thankful to the governments of Kenya and Tanzania as well for allowing me to conduct research at the National Museums of Kenya and Tanzania, respectively. At these institutions, the following people were of great assistance: Christopher Kiarie, Paul Msemwa, and Eliwasa Maro. Heidi Fourie and Francis Thackery provided access to fossils at the Transvaal Museum in Pretoria, and their kindness is much appreciated. I am also grateful to Phillip Tobias, Beverley Kramer, and Kevin Kuykendall for providing access to the fossils at the University of the Witwatersrand in Johannesburg. Ian Tattersall, Jeff Schwartz, Henry McHenry, Ivy Pike, Jeffrey McKee and Terry Harrison advised me regarding the logistics of my research in East and South Africa. For research on Neandertals and Point Hope Inupiaq, I am grateful to the following people and institutions for access to their collections: Ian Tattersall and Ken Mowbray at the American Museum of Natural History; Jakov Radovčić of the Croatian Natural History Museum, Almutt Hoffman at the *Museum für Vor-Und Frühgeschichte Archäeologie Europas*; Veronique Merlin-Anglade and Guy Marchesseau at the *Musée du Perigord* in Périgueux, Henri De Lumley, Marie Antoinette De Lumley, Mr. Onorateni and Mr. Vourdain at the *Laboratoire d'Anthropologie of the Université de la Méditerranée*, and Phillipe Mennecier at the *Musée de l'Homme* in Paris. Thanks are also due Clark Spencer Larsen and Dale Hutchinson for loaning the Krapina replicas, Cathy Cooke and James Patrick Bell for making epoxy replicas, Cameron Begg and Hank Colijn of the Center for Electron Optics of The Ohio State University for their assistance, and the Ward family for their gracious hospitality. I thank the following people for advice regarding Neandertal collections: Shara Bailey, Jeff Schwartz, and Trent Holliday. I thank Bruce Floyd for his statistical advice and John Lukacs, Gary Schwartz, Simon Hillson, Donald Reid, Wendy Dirks, Christopher Dean, Rebecca Ferrell, and Jay Kelley for valuable discussions over the years. Finally, I thank Dan Steinberg for his steadfast support.

References

Aiello, L. and Dean, M. C. (2002). *An Introduction to Human Evolutionary Anatomy*. London: Academic Press.

Bailey, S. E. and Hublin, J.-J. (2006). Dental remains from the Grotte du Renne at Arcy-sur-Cure (Yonne). *Journal of Human Evolution*, **50**, 485–508.

Blakey, M. L., Leslie T. E., and Reidy, J. P. (1994). Frequency and chronological distribution of dental enamel hypoplasia in enslaved African Americans: a test of the weaning hypothesis. *American Journal of Physical Anthropology*, **95**, 371–84.

Beynon, D. and Dean, M. C. (1988). Distinct dental development patterns in early fossil hominids. *Nature*, **335**, 509–14.

Bombin, M. (1990). Transverse enamel hypoplasia on teeth of South African Plio-Pleistocene hominids. *Naturwissenschaften*, **77**, 128–9.

Bocherens, H., Billiou, D., Mariotti, A. *et al.* (1999). Paleoenvironmental and paleodietary implications of isotopic biogeochemistry of last interglacial Neanderthal and mammal bones in Scladina Cave (Belgium). *Journal of Archaeological Science*, **26**, 599–607.

Brennan, M. (1991). *Health and Disease in the Middle and Upper Paleolithic of Southwestern France: A Bioarchaeological Study*. Ph.D. Dissertation, New York University.

Bromage, T. G. (1991). Enamel incremental periodicity in the pig-tailed macaque: a polychrome fluorescent labeling study of dental hard tissues. *American Journal of Physical Anthropology*, **86**, 205–14.

Bromage, T. G. and Dean M. C. (1985). Re-evaluation of the age at death of immature fossil hominids. *Nature*, **317**, 525–7.

Brunet, M., Fronty, P., Sapanet, M., de Bonis L., and Viriot, L (2002). Enamel hypoplasia in a Pliocene Hominid from Chad. *Connective Tissue Research*, **43**, 94–7.

Dean, M. C. and Reid, D. J. (2001a). Perikymata spacing and distribution on hominid anterior teeth. *American Journal of Physical Anthropology*, **116**, 209–15.

Dean, M. C. and Reid, D. J. (2001b). Anterior tooth formation in *Australopithecus* and *Paranthropus*. In *Dental Morphology*, ed. A. Brook. Sheffield: University of Sheffield, pp. 135–43.

Dean, M. C., Leakey, M. G., Reid, D. J. *et al.* (2001). Growth processes in teeth distinguish modern humans from *Homo erectus* and earlier hominins. *Nature*, **414**, 628–31.

Ensor, B. E. and Irish, J. D. (1995). Hypoplastic area method for analyzing dental enamel hypoplasia. *American Journal of Physical Anthropology*, **98**, 507–18.

Fédération Dentaire Internationale (1982). An epidemiological index of developmental defects of dental enamel (DDE). *International Dental Journal*, **32**, 159–67.

Fédération Dentaire Internationale (1992). A review of the developmental defects of enamel index (DDE Index). *International Dental Journal*, **42**, 411–26.

Fitzgerald, C. M. (1998). Do enamel microstructures have regular time dependency? *Journal of Human Evolution*, **35**, 371–86.

Goodman, A. H. and Rose, J. C. (1990). Assessment of physiological perturbations from dental enamel hypoplasia and associated histological structures. *Yearbook of Physical Anthropology*, **33**, 59–110.

Grine, F. E. (1986). Dental evidence for dietary differences in *Australopithecus* and *Paranthropus*: a quantitative analysis of permanent molar microwear. *Journal of Human Evolution*, **15**, 783–822.

Grine, F. E. and Kay, R. F. (1988). Early hominid diets from quantitative image analysis of dental microwear. *Nature*, **333**, 765–8.

Guatelli-Steinberg, D. (2000). Linear enamel hypoplasia in gibbons (*Hylobates lar carpenteri*). *American Journal of Physical Anthropology*, **112**, 395–410.

Guatelli-Steinberg, D. (2003). Macroscopic and microscopic analyses of linear enamel hypoplasia in Plio-Pleistocene South African hominins with respect to aspects of enamel development and morphology. *American Journal of Physical Anthropology*, **120**, 309–22.

Guatelli-Steinberg, D. (2004). Analysis and significance of linear enamel hypoplasia in Plio-Pleistocene hominins. *American Journal of Physical Anthropology*, **123**, 199–215.

Guatelli-Steinberg, D., Larsen, C. S., and Hutchinson D. L. (2004). Prevalence and duration of linear enamel hypoplasia: a comparative study of Neanderthals and Inuit foragers. *Journal of Human Evolution*, **47**, 65–84.

Guatelli-Steinberg, D., Reid, D. J., Bishop, T. A., and Larsen, C. S. (in press). Imbricational enamel formation in Neandertals and recent modern humans. In *Dental Perspectives on Human Evolution: State of the Art Research in Dental Anthropology*, ed. S. Bailey and J.-J. Hublin. New York: Springer-Verlag.

Hillson, S. (1992). Impression and replica methods for studying hypoplasia and perikymata on human tooth crown surfaces from archaeological sites. *International Journal of Osteoarchaeology*, **2**, 65–78.

Hillson, S. (1996). *Dental Anthropology*. Cambridge: Cambridge University Press.

Hillson, S. and Bond, S. (1997). The relationship of enamel hypoplasia to the pattern of tooth crown growth: a discussion. *American Journal of Physical Anthropology*, **104**, 89–103.

Hillson, S. and Jones, B. K. (1989). Instruments for measuring surface profiles: an application in the study of ancient human tooth crown surfaces. *Journal of Archaeological Science*, **16**, 95–105.

Hutchinson, D. L., Larsen, C. S., and Choi, I. (1997). Stressed to the max? Physiological perturbation in the Krapina Neandertals. *Current Anthropology*, **38**, 904–14.

Jelinek, A. J. (1994). Hominids, energy, environment, and behavior in the Late Pleistocene. In *Origins of Anatomically Modern Humans*, ed. M. H. Nitecki and D. V. Nitecki. New York: Plenum Press, pp. 67–92.

King, T., Hillson, S. W., and Humphrey, L. T. (2002). A detailed study of enamel hypoplasia in a post-medieval adolescent of known age and sex. *Archives of Oral Biology*, **47**, 29–39.

Larsen, H. and Rainey, F. (1948). Ipiutak and the Arctic whale hunting culture. *Anthropological Papers of the American Museum of Natural History*, **42**, 1–276.

Moggi-Cecchi, J. (2000). Enamel hypoplasia in South African early hominids: A reappraisal. *American Journal of Physical Anthropology*, **30**, 230–1 (abstract).

Molnar, S. and Molnar, I. M. (1985). The prevalence of enamel hypoplasia among the Krapina Neandertals. *American Journal of Physical Anthropology*, **87**, 536–49.

Ogilvie, M. D., Curran, B. K., and Trinkaus, E. (1989). Prevalence and patterning of dental enamel hypoplasia among the Neandertals. *American Journal of Physical Anthropology*, **79**, 25–41.

Reid, D. J. and Dean, M. C. (2000). Brief communication: the timing of linear hypoplasias on human anterior teeth. *American Journal of Physical Anthropology*, **113**, 135–9.

Reid, D. J. and Dean, M. C. (2006). Population variation in human enamel formation. *Journal of Human Evolution*, **50**, 329–46.

Richards, M. P., Petit, P. B., Trinkaus, E. *et al.* (2000). Neanderthal diet at Vindija and Neanderthal predation: the evidence from stable isotopes. *Proceedings of the National Academy of Sciences*, **97**, 7663–6.

Rink, W. J., Schwartz, H. P., Smith, F. H., and Radovčić, J. (1995). ESR ages for Krapina hominids. *Nature*, **378**, 24.

Schwartz, J. H. and Tattersall, I. (2002). *The Human Fossil Record.* Vol. 1. New York: Wiley-Liss.

Schwartz, J. H., Brauer, J., and Gordon-Larsen, P. (1995). Brief communication: Tigaran (Point Hope, Alaska) tooth drilling. *American Journal of Physical Anthropology*, **97**, 77–82.

Scott, R. S., Ungar, P. S., Bergstrom, T. S. *et al.* (2005). Dental microwear texture analysis shows within-species dietary variability in fossil hominins. *Nature*, **436**, 693–5.

Skinner, M. (1996). Developmental stress in immature hominins from Late Pleistocene Eurasia: Evidence from enamel hypoplasia. *Journal of Archaeological Science*, **23**, 833–52.

Smith, T., Reid, D. J., Dean, M. C. *et al.* (in press). New perspectives on chimpanzee and human molar development. In *Dental Perspectives on Human Evolution: State of the Art Research in Dental Anthropology*, ed. S. Bailey and J.-J. Hublin. New York: Springer-Verlag.

Soffer, O. (1994). Ancestral lifeways in Eurasia: The Middle and Upper Paleolithic records. In *Origins of Anatomically Modern Humans*, ed. M. H. Nitecki and D. V. Nitecki. New York: Plenum Press, pp. 84–109.

Sorensen, M. V. and Leonard, W. R. (2001). Neandertal energetics and foraging efficiency. *Journal of Human Evolution*, **40**, 483–95.

Sponheimer, M. and Lee-Thorp J. A. (1999). Isotopic evidence for the diet of an early hominid, *Australopithecus africanus. Science*, **283**, 368–370.

Ten Cate, A. R. (1994). *Oral Histology: Development, Structure, and Function*, 4th edn. St. Louis: CV Mosby.

Tobias, P. V. (1991). *Olduvai Gorge Vol. 4: The Skulls, Endocasts, and Teeth of* Homo habilis. Cambridge: Cambridge University Press.

Trinkaus, E. (1986). The Neandertals and modern human origins. *Annual Review of Anthropology*, **15**, 193–218.

Trinkaus, E. (1989). The Upper Pleistocene transition. In *The Emergence of Modern Humans: Biocultural Adaptation in the Later Pleistocene*, ed. E. Trinkaus. New York: Cambridge University Press, pp. 42–6.

White, T. D. (1978). Early hominid enamel hypoplasia. *American Journal of Physical Anthropology*, **49**, 79–84.

Wood, J. W., Harpending, H. C., Weiss, K. M., and Milner, G. R. (1992). The osteological paradox: Problems of inferring prehistoric health from skeletal samples. *Current Anthropology*, **33**, 343–70.

5 *Micro spatial distributions of lead and zinc in human deciduous tooth enamel*

LOUISE T. HUMPHREY, TERESA E. JEFFRIES, AND
M. CHRISTOPHER DEAN

5.1 Introduction

Enamel is the hard crystalline external covering of teeth, and has a mineral component that closely resembles hydroxyapatite (Boyde, 1989; Brudevold and Soremark, 1967). The chemical constituents of hydroxyapatite are tolerant to substitution by a range of trace elements, and are readily incorporated into enamel formation at the time of environmental exposure. The composition of sub-surface enamel is fixed before tooth emergence, and is therefore able to provide a retrospective and relatively permanent record of the trace elements absorbed during the period of enamel formation. The information locked within this deep enamel can provide evidence of early nutrition, residential mobility, and exposure to toxic metals. The incorporation of some trace elements into enamel hydroxyapatite also has the potential to affect susceptibility to caries. The trace element composition of enamel has a broad relevance in disciplines ranging from dentistry and child health (Brown *et al.*, 2004; Dolphin *et al.*, 2005) to forensics (Gulson *et al.*, 1997a) and archaeology (Budd *et al.*, 2000). Two trace elements of particular interest are lead (Pb) and zinc (Zn).

Lead toxicity remains a major public health concern, particularly in relation to its neurological effects on infants and young children (Bellinger *et al.*, 1984; Goyer, 1996). Lead enters the body from contaminated food and drinking water, and inhaled air and dust, and accumulates gradually in calcified tissues. Non-food sources include lead emissions from gasoline, smelter emissions, lead-based paints and glazed food containers (Jarup, 2003). Mobilization of Pb from the mother's skeletal stores as a result of bone resorption during pregnancy and lactation is another potentially important source of Pb intake in the developing fetus and breastfed infant (Gulson *et al.*, 1997b; Gulson *et al.*, 1998; Manton *et al.*, 2003; Tellez-Rojo *et al.*, 2002). Tooth enamel has been considered to be

Technique and Application in Dental Anthropology ed. Joel D. Irish and Greg C. Nelson
Published by Cambridge University Press.

a reliable reservoir of biogenic Pb, reflecting environmental exposure during the period of enamel mineralization, and has been used widely to reconstruct exposure in modern and past populations (Budd *et al.*, 1998; Budd *et al.*, 2000; Gulson, 1996; Gulson and Wilson, 1994; Needleman *et al.*, 1972; Webb *et al.*, 2005).

Zinc is the most abundant essential trace metal in the body, and plays an important role in prenatal and postnatal growth, and cognitive and motor development (Bhatnagar and Taneja, 2001). Zinc deficiency leads to impaired immune function and lowered resistance to bacterial, viral, and fungal infections (Wellinghausen, 2001). The distribution of Zn in human teeth is of potential interest for the interpretation of dietary intake, particularly during the prenatal and early postnatal periods (Dolphin *et al.*, 2005). The status of zinc as a valid palaeodietary indicator has been questioned on theoretical grounds, in part because the relationship between zinc levels in mineralized tissues and dietary abundance is not straightforward. There is, however, some evidence to suggest that zinc levels in the bones of growing animals are lower under conditions of severe deficiency than during conditions of adequate zinc status (for a full discussion and review see Ezzo, 1994).

Previous work has demonstrated that the distribution of both Pb and Zn in human tooth enamel is non-homogeneous. In particular, concentrations of both Pb and Zn have been shown to increase in successive layers of enamel between the enamel-dentin junction and the enamel surface (Brudevold and Soremark, 1967; Brudevold and Steadman, 1956; Reitznerova *et al.*, 2000). Brudevold and Steadman (1956) reported high concentrations of Pb in the outermost layer of enamel, and rapidly decreasing levels in successive layers of sub-surface enamel. Concentrations in the surface layer of enamel were 6–10 times greater than in the deepest layers of enamel in permanent teeth. This trend was observed in erupted and un-erupted teeth, but the amount of surface Pb was lower in un-erupted teeth. For erupted teeth, surface Pb concentrations were higher in older age groups. Results indicated a substantial Pb acquisition prior to eruption, and further post-eruptive acquisition at the surface. A similar trend for concentrations to decrease with distance from the enamel surface was demonstrated for Zn in a large sample of permanent teeth from Augusta, Maine. The steepest reduction occurred between the outermost layers with concentrations close to the enamel surface occurring at levels up to ten times higher than those in the innermost enamel layers (Brudevold and Soremark, 1967). As with Pb, the tendency for concentrations to decrease with distance from the enamel surface is present in both erupted and un-erupted teeth, but overall Zn concentrations in the un-erupted teeth were lower than in erupted teeth, particularly in the outermost layer. The Maine study found no evidence of increasing concentration of Zn with age in the surface layers of enamel in erupted teeth, but it is possible that age related effects might be masked by differences in diet between age groups within the population studied (Brudevold and Soremark, 1967). More recently, Reitznerova and colleagues (2000) determined trace element concentrations in four enamel layers taken at 50, 100, 150 and 200 microns from the enamel surface. They reported changes in enamel composition to a depth of 100–150 microns from the enamel surface. Interestingly, concentrations of Pb and Zn in surface enamel were found to be higher in non-erupted teeth than in erupted teeth.

Studies of trace element concentrations within dental tissues have traditionally used a bulk sampling approach or have relied on the physical separation of different parts of a tooth prior to analysis (e.g. Brown *et al.*, 2004; Needleman *et al.*, 1972). Separation of successive layers of enamel from the enamel surface toward the enamel-dentine junction has been achieved by grinding (e.g. Brudevold and Steadman 1956) or acid dissolution (e.g. Reitznerova *et al.*, 2000). An alternative approach involved punching circular biopsies 500 microns in diameter from vertical tooth sections (Frank *et al.*, 1990).

Laser ablation inductively coupled plasma mass spectrometry (LA-ICP-MS) offers the opportunity to undertake *in situ* analysis of mineralized biological tissues and geological samples (Jeffries, 2004; Jeffries *et al.* 1998.) This preserves spatial and time dependent information within the sample (Lee *et al.*, 1999). The technique is relatively non-destructive so that a sample can be analyzed repeatedly and archived for future use. In recent years, numerous research groups have explored the potential of LA-ICP-MS for analysis of the spatial distribution of trace elements in dental tissues. For most studies of dental tissues the calcium signal has been simultaneously collected and used as an internal reference to normalize the elemental signal (Budd *et al.*, 1998; Humphrey *et al.*, in press; Kang *et al.*, 2004; Lee *et al.*, 1999).

To date, most previous LA-ICP-MS research on teeth has involved continuous ablation of an overlapping series of individual craters to produce a single transect across a longitudinal tooth section, with data collection in time-resolved analysis (TRA) mode (Budd *et al.*, 1998, Lee *et al.*, 1999). Budd and colleagues (1998) used LA-ICP-MS to derive continuous Pb profiles across sections of modern and archaeological human teeth. Results showed a consistent Pb peak close to the enamel surface and consistently low Pb within the core enamel. Lead enrichment was restricted to the outer 30 microns of enamel in both modern and archaeological teeth. Notably, a surface Pb peak was also present in an un-erupted permanent premolar. Lee and colleagues (1999) measured trends in metal concentration on either side of the neonatal line in longitudinal sections from human deciduous teeth. Data were collected as a single transect across longitudinal tooth sections in time-resolved analysis mode. The highest amounts of Pb and Zn were found within a few microns of the enamel surface. Zinc levels were found to be higher in postnatal enamel than in prenatal enamel and to increase gradually towards the enamel surface.

Kang and colleagues (2004) employed LA-ICP-MS to investigate micro spatial distributions of trace metals in a human deciduous upper central incisor. Normalized elemental intensity readings were obtained for seven rectangular areas, ablated from the polished surface of a half tooth section. Ablated regions included prenatal enamel, the neonatal line, postnatal enamel, the enamel–dentine junction, dentine, and the dentine–pulp junction. This study demonstrated heterogeneity in trace element composition within and between different parts of the tooth. In particular, elevated Zn and Pb levels were present in the dental pulp and at the neonatal line. Dolphin and colleagues (2005) compared normalized elemental intensities in prenatal and postnatal enamel in 38 exfoliated deciduous teeth donated by children from Solis Valley, Mexico. Two areas of enamel, one prenatal and one postnatal, were ablated in each tooth. The average normalized elemental intensities for both Pb and Zn were significantly higher in the (shallower) postnatal samples than in the (deeper) prenatal samples.

An alternative mode of analysis that can be undertaken using LA-ICP-MS involves *in situ* analysis of multiple discrete sampling points. This technique offers particular advantages for the analysis of dental tissues since the position of each sampling point can be accurately located and recorded relative to specific reference points within the sample (Humphrey *et al.*, in press). For teeth, relevant features include the enamel surface, the enamel–dentine junction, the neonatal line, and other prominent incremental growth structures in enamel and dentine. Visualization within the ablation chamber allows these and other features on the tooth to be identified and the position of sampling points can be determined relative to the features of interest. On-screen measuring tools allow distance measurements to be taken while the sample remains within the ablation chamber. 2D or 3D coordinates for the analysis points, tooth outline, and other relevant features can also be recorded at this stage. The technique allows systematic characterization of trace element distributions within a dental section, and interpretation of the results in relation to geometrical properties of the tooth and incremental growth structures.

In this study we employ a discrete multiple sampling strategy to investigate variation in Pb and Zn distributions in human deciduous tooth enamel. An understanding of underlying non-homogeneity of trace element distributions is an important prerequisite for studies that seek to reconstruct aspects of an individual's early life, including nutritional history, residential mobility, and exposure to pollutants. Specific aims were to: (1) compare patterns of surface enrichment in Pb and Zn, (2) compare the amount of surface enrichment in the occlusal and cervical parts of the tooth crown, and (3) investigate Pb and Zn distributions in sub-surface enamel.

5.2 Methods

Deciduous canines and second molars from six healthy European children were used for this study. All teeth were naturally shed and caries-free. Single teeth from four different individuals were analyzed, together with two teeth (a canine and molar) from each of two individuals. The sample included teeth from individuals who experienced a range of diets during the first few months of life, including exclusive breastfeeding, exclusive or predominant formula feeding from birth, or a period of exclusive breastfeeding followed by partial or complete replacement by formula feeding. The canine and second molar were selected because they occupy different positions within the oral cavity and both have a relatively prolonged residency within the oral environment, compared to other deciduous teeth. Accurate records for the age of gingival emergence and the age of exfoliation were not available for the teeth used in this study, so it was not possible to determine the duration of residency within the mouth for individual teeth.

On average the development and emergence of the second deciduous molars is slightly delayed relative to that of the deciduous canines. Deciduous canines initiate formation at 15–18 weeks after fertilization and complete formation of the enamel crown approximately nine months after birth, whereas second deciduous molars initiate enamel formation at 16–23.5 weeks after fertilization and complete enamel crown formation at approximately 10–11 months after birth (Hillson, 1996). Results from a longitudinal study of tooth emergence in healthy Finnish children suggest that clinical emergence of the deciduous canines takes place at approximately 1.5 years after birth, compared to 2.5 years for the deciduous second molar (Nyström, 1977). Data for the age of exfoliation of these teeth are not available, but the average age of emergence of the replacing permanent tooth gives an upper age limit. Within the same Finnish population (Nyström *et al.*, 2001), the permanent canines emerge at approximately 9.8 (female lower canines) to 11.4 years (male upper canines) and the permanent second premolars emerge at approximately 11.4 (female uppers and lowers) to 12.1 years (male uppers). The expected maximum residency time of deciduous canines and second molars in the mouth varies from approximately 8.2 years for female lower canines to 9.9 years for male upper canines.

Each tooth was sectioned longitudinally using a slow speed rotating Isomet (Buehler) diamond saw, and one cut face polished with three-micron aluminium oxide powder. The polished block face was fixed with epoxy resin adhesive to a glass microscope slide under pressure, and a mesiobuccal section, approximately 100 microns thick, was cut from the block together with the slide. The section was lapped planoparallel and polished in a Buehler slide holder. For each tooth the buccal enamel was analyzed. Discrete samples of enamel were ablated at regular intervals along trajectories running from the enamel–dentine junction to the enamel surface with an orientation approximately parallel to the direction of the enamel prisms. Rows of ablation points were spaced along the entire length of the tooth. Measurements were made between the center of each ablation point and the enamel surface, following a line roughly perpendicular to the enamel surface. The position of the neonatal line was recorded in each tooth section and ablation points were identified as prenatal (sample enamel that initiated formation prior to birth) or postnatal (sample enamel that initiated formation after birth). Prenatal sampling points are those situated between the neonatal line and the enamel–dentine junction, and postnatal sampling points are those situated between the neonatal line and the enamel surface.

LA-ICP-MS analyses were undertaken at the Natural History Museum using a New Wave Research UP213 aperture imaged frequency quintupled Nd:YAG laser ablation accessory operating at 213 nm coupled to a Thermo Elemental PlasmaQuad 3 quadrupole-based ICP-MS with enhanced sensitivity (s-option) interface. A mixed He:Ar sample carrier gas was used throughout. Discrete 30 μm diameter areas of the sectioned tooth were sampled during analysis. For each analysis data were collected for 120 seconds. During the first *c.* 60 seconds of collection, background data in the form of gas blank and electronic noise were acquired. The laser was then fired at the sample and data acquired for a further *c.* 60 seconds. Background data were subsequently subtracted from the ablation signal in the tooth. Data were collected in discrete runs of 20 analyses, beginning and ending with two analyses of the National Institute of Standards Technology (NIST) standard reference material SRM NIST612. Initial data processing and reduction, including selection and integration of background and ablated signal intervals, were performed off-line using LAMTRACE, a Lotus 123 macro-based spreadsheet created by Simon Jackson, Macquarie University, Australia. Further data processing including normalization of $^{208}Pb/^{43}Ca$ and $^{66}Zn/^{43}Ca$ ratios based on the measured ratio in NIST612 was performed using Microsoft Excel spreadsheet software. Analytical and instrumental operating conditions are presented in Table 5.1.

5.3 Results

A marked increase in elemental intensity occurs in the sampling points closest to the enamel surface on many of the trajectories, as shown in the examples in

Table 5.1 *Analytical and instrumental operating conditions*

ICP-MS		
Forward power		1350 W
Gas flows	Coolant	Ar: 13 l min^{-1}
	Auxiliary	Ar: 0.9 l min^{-1}
	Sample transport	He: 0.8 l min^{-1}
		Ar: 0.8 l min^{-1}
Laser		
Wavelength		213 nm
Pulse width (FWHM)		3 ns
Pulse energy		0.05 mJ per pulse
Energy density		3 J cm^{-2}
Energy distribution		Homogenized, flat beam, aperture imaged
Repetition rate		10 Hz
Spot size diameter		30 μm
Analysis protocol		
Scanning mode		Peak jumping, 1 point per peak
Acquisition mode		Time resolved analysis
Duration of analysis		120s (*c.* 60 s background, 60 s ablated signal)
Dwell times		10 ms all masses

Figure 5.1. For each example in the figure, the normalized elemental intensities for sampling points ablated along a single trajectory are joined by a line. On each trajectory data points are ordered from the enamel–dentine junction toward the enamel surface, with the value determined for the outermost sampling point shown on the right. The trajectories are ordered according to their position on the tooth, with those closest to the occlusal edge on the left, and those closest to the enamel cervix on the right. For Pb/Ca, a pronounced rise is typically observed in the outermost sampling points. The surface increase is often more pronounced toward the cervical end of the tooth and may be very low or absent in the most occlusally positioned trajectories, as shown in Figure 5.1c. The highest values for Zn/Ca also occur in the outermost sampling point on each trajectory, but normalized elemental intensities in the second closest sampling point to the enamel surface may also be noticeably higher than those in the deeper enamel. Surface Zn levels are typically enriched in all positions on the tooth crown, but peaks may be slightly lower in the most occlusal rows.

The relationship between the normalized elemental intensities and the distances between the sampling points and the enamel surface is shown in Figure 5.2 for two teeth. Normalized elemental intensities are relatively low in the deep enamel and rise sharply toward the enamel surface for both elements. The curvilinear trends shown in Figure 5.2 are typical of those observed

(a)

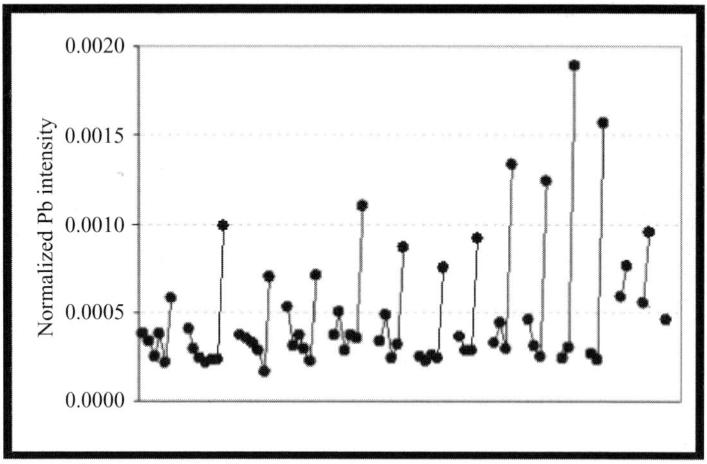

(b)

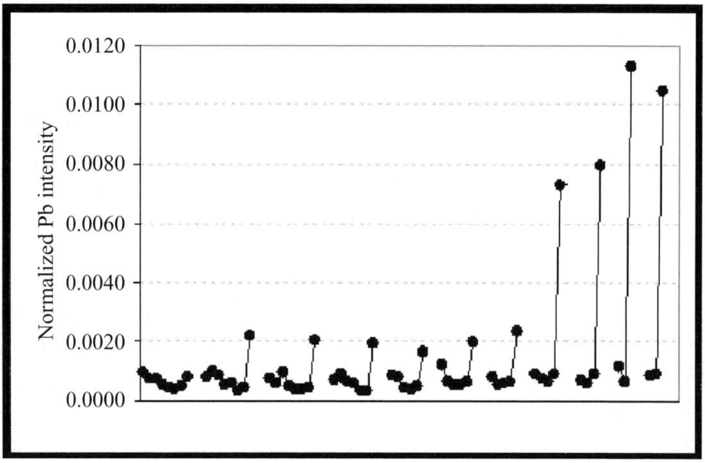

Figure 5.1 Normalized elemental intensities for discrete sampling points analyzed from thin sections of enamel from: (a) ^{208}Pb in molar from child 3; (b) ^{208}Pb in molar from child 5; (c) (^{66}Zn in molar from child 3; and (d) ^{66}Zn in molar from child 5. Each spot gives the result for a single sampling point. Lines connect the normalized elemental intensities for sampling points ablated along a single trajectory, running from the enamel–dentine junction towards the enamel surface. Data points are ordered from the enamel–dentin junction towards the enamel surface. Trajectories are ordered from those closest to the occlusal edge on the left to those closest to the enamel cervix on the right.

(c)

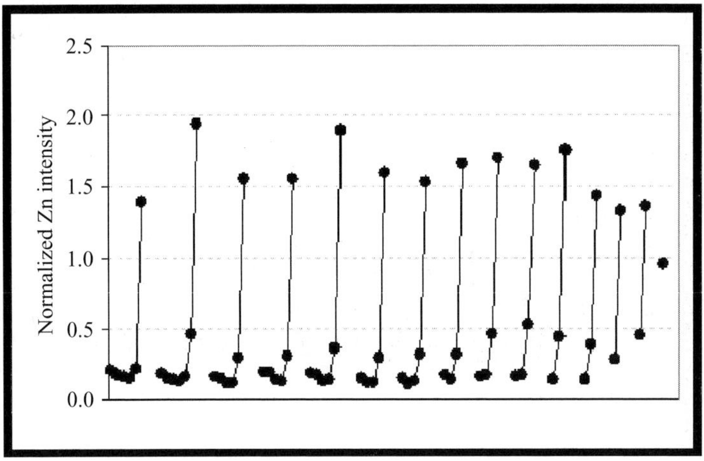

(d)

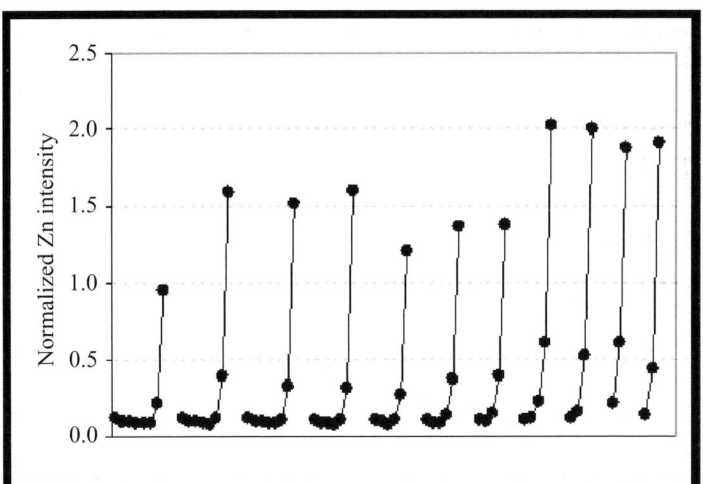

Figure 5.1 (*cont.*)

throughout the sample, but the depth of surface enrichment varies between teeth, and between elements within a tooth. The relationship between the normalized elemental intensities and the distance between the sampling point and the enamel surface within the sub-surface enamel in the same two teeth is illustrated in Figure 5.3, which shows only the lower range of values. As demonstrated by these examples, there is a trend in most teeth for normalized intensity ratios to fall to a minimum level within the sub-surface enamel and then increase slightly with increasing distance from the enamel surface.

(a)

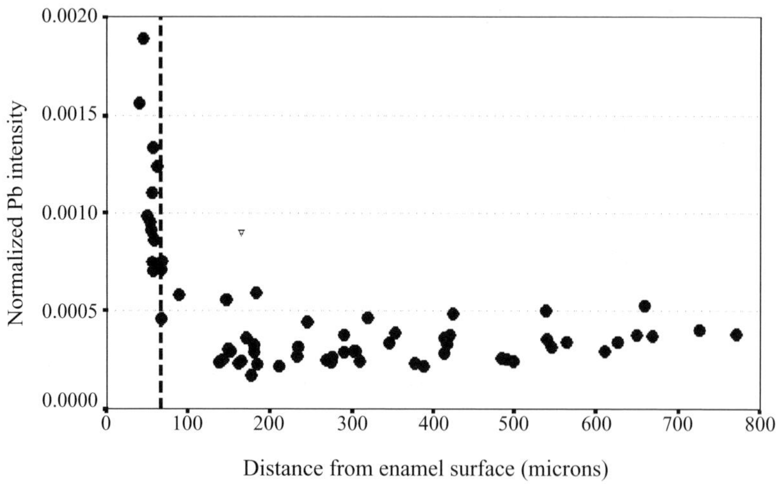

(b)

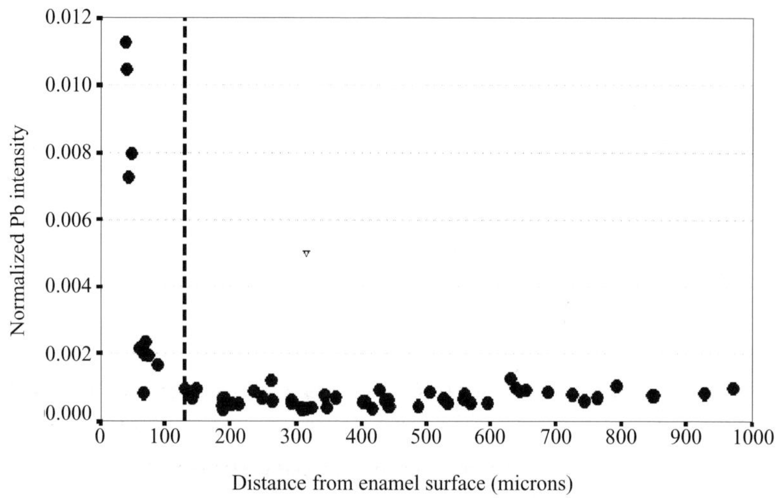

Figure 5.2 Normalized elemental intensities plotted against the minimum distance from the center of the sampling point to the enamel surface for: (a) ^{208}Pb in molar from child 3; (b) ^{208}Pb in molar from child 5; (c) ^{66}Zn in molar from child 3; and (d) ^{66}Zn in molar from child 5. Each spot gives the result for a single sampling point. The arrow points towards the distance from the enamel surface at which the lowest averaged elemental intensity occurs. The dotted line shows the depth to which the elemental intensity is enriched.

(c)

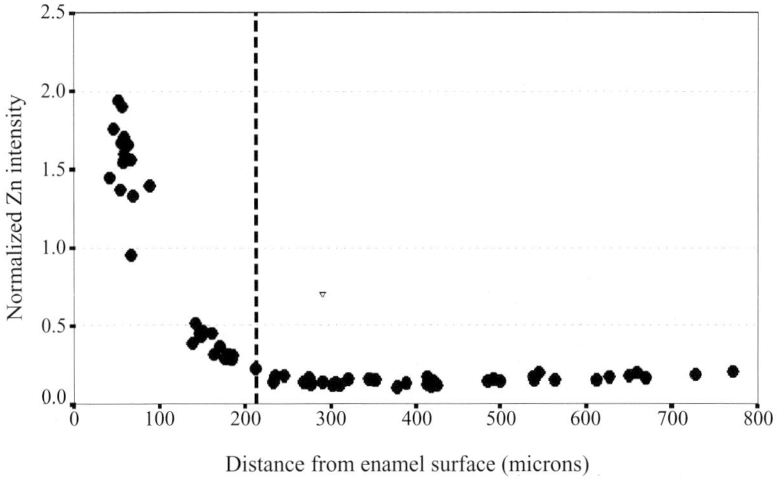

(d)

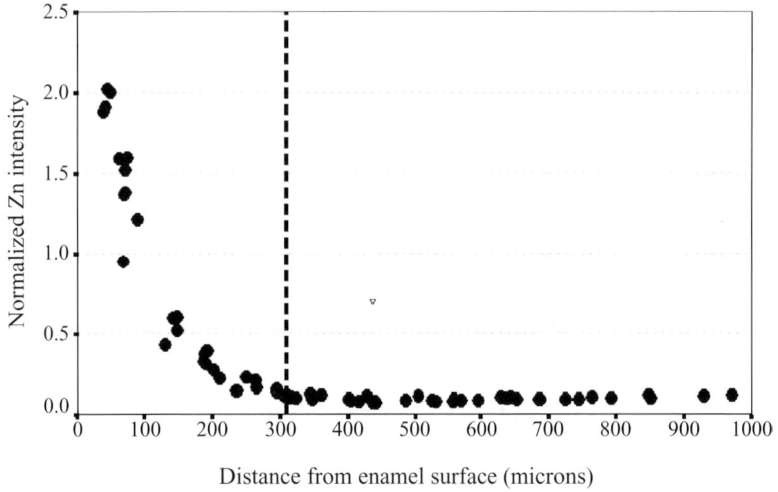

Figure 5.2 (*cont.*)

A straightforward data-smoothing calculation was used to determine the distance from the enamel surface at which the lowest normalized elemental intensity occurs. Data points were ordered according to their distance from the enamel surface, and a sliding average was calculated from the values for sets of five adjacent data points. At each distance from the enamel surface the average is based on the value at the distance indicated and the two values on either side within the ordered sequence. The lowest averaged normalized elemental

(a)

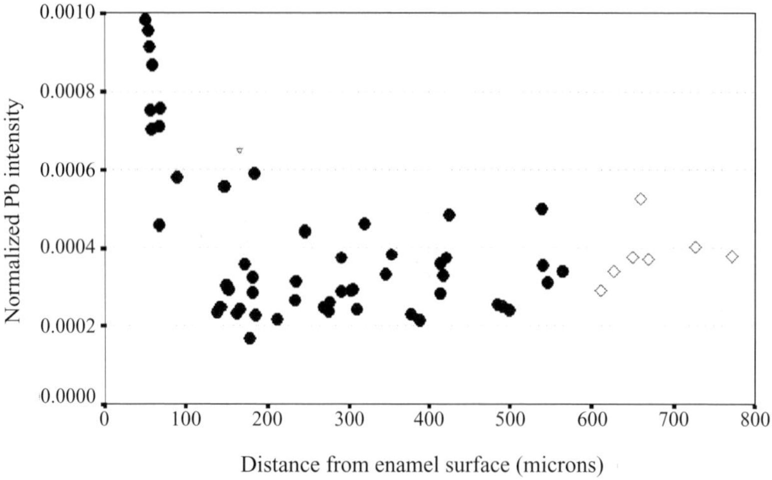

(b)

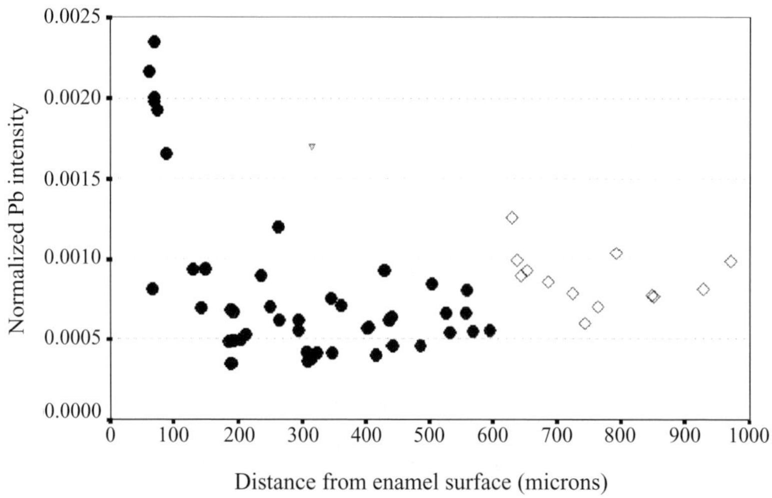

Figure 5.3 Normalized elemental intensities plotted against the minimum distance from the centre of the sampling point to the enamel surface for: (a) ^{208}Pb in molar from child 3; (b) ^{208}Pb in molar from child 5; (c) ^{66}Zn in molar from child 3; and (d) ^{66}Zn in molar from child 5. Each spot gives the result for a single sampling point. Sampling points located between the enamel–dentin junction and the neonatal line are shown as white diamonds. Sampling points located between the neonatal line and the enamel surface are shown as black circles. The arrow points towards the distance from the enamel surface at which the lowest averaged elemental intensity occurs.

(c)

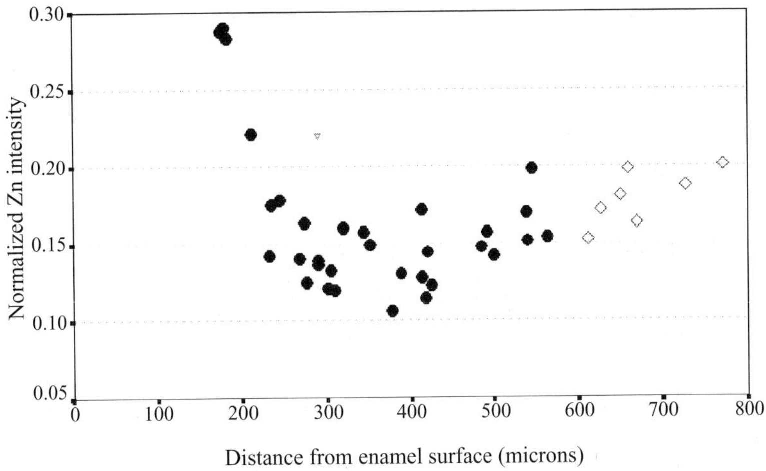

(d)

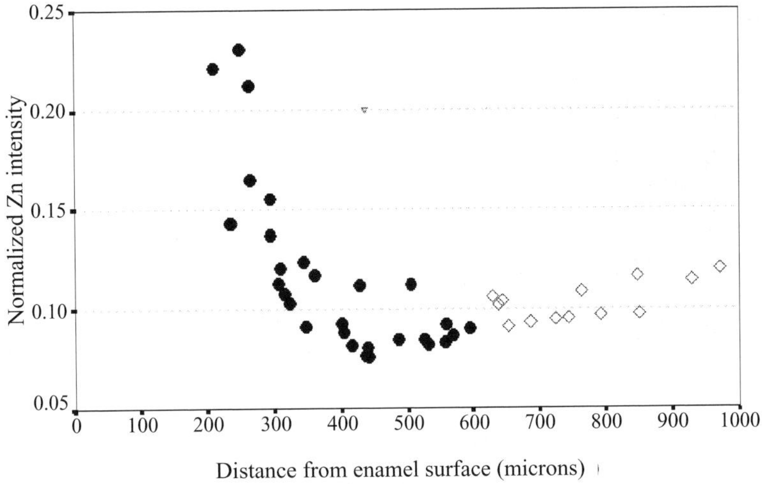

Figure 5.3 (*cont.*)

intensities for Pb and Zn, and the depths at which they occur, are presented in Tables 5.2 and 5.3. For each tooth the depth at which the lowest normalized elemental intensity occurs represents an objective estimate of distance from the enamel surface at which the underlying trend for normalized elemental intensities to decrease from the enamel surface is reversed. Arguably these depths also represent the maximum distance to which elemental enrichment from the enamel surface occurs. The distance from the enamel surface at which the

Table 5.2 *Distance of the lowest normalized elemental intensity from the enamel surface and depth of elevated normalized elemental intensity for Pb in eight human deciduous teeth*

	Tooth type	Lowest normalized elemental intensity[a]	Distance from enamel surface (μm)	Average normalized elemental intensity in deep enamel	Standard deviation	Depth of elevated normalized elemental intensity (μm)
Child 1	canine	0.000 75	437	0.000 93	0.000 14	123
Child 1	molar	0.000 67	461	0.000 99	0.000 47	84
Child 2	canine	0.000 40	180	0.000 58	0.000 20	68
Child 2	molar	0.000 48	270	0.000 62	0.000 14	152
Child 3	molar	0.000 27	165	0.000 33	0.000 09	68
Child 4	canine	0.000 70	201	0.001 02	0.000 55	72
Child 5	molar	0.000 45	315	0.000 71	0.000 21	131
Child 6	molar	0.000 22	602	0.000 29	0.000 13	284

[a] The lowest elemental intensity is based on an average of five adjacent values, calculated from a series of normalized elemental intensities ordered according to their distance from the enamel surface.

Table 5.3 *Distance of the lowest normalized elemental intensity from the enamel surface and depth of elevated normalized elemental intensity for Zn in eight human deciduous teeth*

	Tooth type	Lowest normalized elemental intensity[a]	Distance from enamel surface (μm)	Average normalized elemental intensity in deep enamel	Standard deviation	Depth of normalized elevated elemental intensity (μm)
Child 1	canine	0.128 95	332	0.140 82	0.015 24	236
Child 1	molar	0.105 98	317	0.123 58	0.019 09	270
Child 2	canine	0.099 31	447	0.107 07	0.010 84	289
Child 2	molar	0.101 03	396	0.114 39	0.015 13	297
Child 3	molar	0.128 70	290	0.152 57	0.025 97	212
Child 4	canine	0.093 22	318	0.107 67	0.009 74	222
Child 5	molar	0.084 82	437	0.095 21	0.012 92	309
Child 6	molar	0.095 91	463	0.112 46	0.016 48	304

[a] The lowest elemental intensity is based on an average of five adjacent values, calculated from a series of normalized elemental intensities ordered according to their distance from the enamel surface.

lowest averaged normalized elemental intensity occurs is marked by a downward arrow for individual teeth in Figures 5.2 and 5.3.

A second estimate of the depth of enrichment from the enamel surface was made based on the range of normalized elemental intensities within the core enamel. The average normalized elemental intensity within the core enamel was calculated as the average for all sampling points deeper than the point at which the lowest normalized elemental intensity occurs (Tables 5.2 and 5.3). Normalized elemental intensities that are more than two standard deviations above this core enamel average are considered to be elevated. The distance from the enamel surface within which all of the averaged normalized elemental intensities (based on five adjacent points in a depth ordered sequences as described above) fall more than two standard deviations above the core enamel average was identified for each element in each tooth (Tables 5.2 and 5.3). These distances represent more conservative estimates of the depth of surface enrichment and were used for comparisons between elements and tooth types. The depth to which surface enrichment occurs according to these calculations is marked by dotted line for individual teeth in Figure 5.2.

Elevated normalized elemental intensities occur to an average depth of $267.38 \pm 38.80\,\mu m$ for Zn and $122.75 \pm 72.70\,\mu m$ for Pb. Student's t-test was used to test the significance of this difference, using the assumption of unequal variance. The difference is highly significant ($P = 0.000$), confirming the impression gained from visual inspection for the plots for these two elements. For Pb, elevated normalized elemental intensities occur to an average depth of $87.67 \pm 30.65\,\mu m$ in the canines and $143.80 \pm 85.45\,\mu m$ in the molars. For Zn, elevated normalized elemental intensities occur to an average depth of $249.00 \pm 35.34\,\mu m$ in the canines and $278.4 \pm 40.05\,\mu m$ in the molars. For both Pb and Zn elevated normalized elemental intensities reach a deeper average depth in the molar than in the canines, but these differences are not statistically significant.

Within each tooth, the underlying trend for normalized elemental intensities to decrease with increasing distance from the enamel surface is reversed in the deepest enamel. The sampling points farthest from the enamel surface are typically the innermost sampling points on the trajectories closest to the occlusal edge of the tooth, since enamel thickness tends to be highest in the occlusal region and decreases cervically. The neonatal line is an accentuated line in enamel that reflects physiological disturbances associated with the birth process (Schour, 1936; Whittaker and Richard, 1978). It is present in all deciduous human teeth and separates enamel that initiates formation prior to birth from that which initiates formation after birth. The samples taken from enamel located between the neonatal line and the enamel–dentine junction are the innermost points on trajectories situated closest to the to the occlusal surface of the tooth.

Table 5.4 *Relationship between the position of prenatal enamel sampling points and the lowest element intensity relative to the enamel surface in eight human deciduous teeth*

	Tooth type	Number of points analyzed	Number of "prenatal" sampling points	Distance of "prenatal" sampling points from the enamel surface (μm)	Distance between outermost "prenatal" sampling point and lowest element intensity (μm)	
					Pb	Zn
Child 1	canine	64	5	488–571	51	156
Child 1	molar	64	5	667–895	206	350
Child 2	canine	64	7	475–645	295	28
Child 2	molar	64	7	704–904	434	308
Child 3	molar	64	7	612–771	447	322
Child 4	canine	64	5	477–586	276	159
Child 5	molar	63	13	631–928	316	194
Child 6	molar	95	16	517–871	−85	54

We examined normalized elemental intensities for sampling points on either side of the neonatal line to determine whether the changing trend within the deep enamel coincided with the transition from prenatal to postnatal onset of enamel formation.

The number and depth of "prenatal" sampling points varied for each tooth section according to the location of the neonatal line within the tooth (Table 5.4). The position of the neonatal line relative to the enamel–dentine junction varies between teeth according to the age of onset of enamel formation, the direction of the enamel prism tracks, and the amount of prism decussation and daily cross striation intervals (reflecting the rate of enamel secretion) during the secretory stage of prenatal enamel formation. The position of the neonatal line relative to the enamel surface reflects variation in each of these parameters during postnatal enamel matrix formation and the age at which individual ameloblasts complete enamel secretion. The position of the neonatal line relative to both the enamel–dentine junction and the enamel surface is influenced by the number of gestational weeks at which birth takes place (Skinner and Dupras, 1993). The amount of "prenatal" enamel available for sampling is also dependent to an extent on the amount of occlusal enamel lost through attrition.

The distance between the outermost "prenatal" sampling point and the depth at which the lowest normalized elemental intensity (μm) was calculated for Zn and Pb for each tooth. The results indicate that the lowest normalized elemental intensities for Pb and Zn did not correspond to the transition from prenatal to postnatal onset of enamel formation within a tooth (Table 5.4). For Zn, the lowest normalized elemental intensity occurred closer to the enamel surface than the outermost "prenatal" sampling point in all eight deciduous teeth. For Pb, the lowest normalized elemental intensity occurred closer to the enamel surface than the outermost "prenatal" sampling point in seven out of eight teeth. The lowest normalized elemental intensity for Pb in the deciduous molar for child 6 occurred deeper within the enamel than the outermost prenatal sampling point, but was less deep than the innermost postnatal sampling points.

5.4 Discussion

The most striking aspect of the distribution of Pb and Zn in this sample of human deciduous teeth is the enrichment in Ca-normalized elemental intensities at the enamel surface. Previous studies have demonstrated enrichment of Pb and Zn at the enamel surface in modern and archaeological teeth, but there has been no consensus concerning the depth to which enamel is enriched. Studies based on micro dissection recorded a decrease in Zn and Pb concentrations in successively deeper layers of enamel throughout the tooth crown in permanent teeth (Brudevold and Söremark, 1967). Other research has indicated that surface enrichment may be restricted to the outer 30 microns of enamel (Budd *et al.*, 1998). In this sample of exfoliated human deciduous teeth, a steep decline in normalized elemental intensities for Pb and Zn was recorded in enamel close to the enamel surface, followed by a more gradual decline away from the enamel surface. Markedly elevated elemental intensities were present in the outermost 267.38 ± 38.80 μm for Zn compared to only 122.75 ± 72.70 μm for Pb. There was a non-significant trend for elevated elemental intensities to extend farther from the enamel surface in deciduous second molars than in deciduous canines.

Three main theories have emerged to explain the relative enrichment in Pb and Zn of surface enamel from modern and archaeological teeth. Surface enhancement is at least partly attributable to the enamel formation process and/or exchanges between the enamel and surrounding tissues prior to gingival emergence. Evidence for this comes from several different studies that report that surface concentrations of Pb and Zn are already higher than sub-surface concentrations in un-erupted teeth (Brudevold and Soremark, 1967; Budd *et al.*, 1998; Reitznerova *et al.*, 2000). There is also evidence from some previous studies to suggest a further accumulation of heavy metals in the surface layers of enamel following emergence of the tooth into the mouth as a result of ion exchange within the oral environment. Surface concentrations of Pb and Zn were higher in erupted permanent teeth from lifelong residents of all age groups from a community in Maine (USA) than in un-erupted teeth from the same community (Brudevold and Soremark, 1967). Surface Pb concentrations (but not Zn) were also found to increase steadily between four successive age groups within this community suggesting a gradual accumulation of Pb with age. Another study of Pb concentrations in teeth from individuals from the Alsace (France) found significantly higher Pb concentrations in enamel sampled from just below the occlusal surface of permanent premolars or molars in older individuals than in younger individuals from both rural and urban communities (Frank *et al.*, 1990). Contrastingly, Reitznerova and colleagues (2000) reported lower trace element concentrations in the surface enamel of erupted teeth than those present in un-erupted teeth from a sample of East Slovakian individuals. They suggested that demineralization and remineralization of the enamel surface in erupted teeth could, under some circumstances, result in a net loss of micro-elements from the enamel surface. For archaeological teeth the third relevant parameter is diagenesis within the burial environment, which could in theory lead to an enhancement of surface trace-element concentrations (Waldron, 1981), or a reduction caused by losses into the burial environment (Budd *et al.*, 1998).

Other factors that may contribute to the observed trace element enrichment in surface tooth enamel are the position of the tooth within the oral cavity, the period between gingival emergence and tooth extraction or exfoliation (or death in the case of archaeological teeth), and the amount of enamel lost through attrition. In this study surface Pb levels were higher in the second deciduous molar than in the deciduous canine in both individuals for whom a direct comparison could be made, despite the fact that these teeth have a similar residency time in the oral cavity. However surface Zn levels were higher in the canine of one individual and in the molar of the second individual. Although not explicitly quantified in this study, a further preliminary observation is that surface enrichment of normalized elemental intensities tended to be lower in the occlusal regions of enamel than in the cervical region. This effect was more pronounced for Pb, for which elevated elemental intensities are fairly superficial, than for Zn, where elevated enamel intensities occur deeper within the enamel. This pattern may be the result of differences in the rate of attrition between the occlusal and cervical parts of the enamel. In other words, in regions of enamel that are exposed to the heaviest rates of wear, the loss of enriched surface enamel through attrition could occur more rapidly than the rate of subsequent absorption of these elements into the newly exposed enamel. Dental attrition could also be a factor in studies that have reported a lower concentration of Pb and Zn in erupted teeth than in non-erupted teeth (Reitznerova *et al.*, 2000).

A second consistent feature of the distribution of Pb and Zn in this sample of deciduous teeth is for normalized elemental intensities to reach a minimum value in the core region of enamel, and then increase slightly toward the enamel–dentine junction. This pattern has not been observed in previous studies of the distribution of Pb or Zn in human teeth, which may be, in part, due to differences in sampling approach. It is also possible that the trend observed here in deciduous teeth reflects circumstances that pertain during the formation of deciduous teeth, but not during the later formation period of the permanent teeth. Deciduous molars and canines initiate enamel formation during the second trimester of pregnancy, and continue to form during the period of marked dietary shifts that characterize the early postnatal period (Humphrey *et al.*, in press).

Prior to birth, fetal Zn and Pb are derived from the mother and therefore reflect maternal intake during pregnancy and mobilization from the mother's skeletal stores. The skeletal Pb contribution to maternal blood levels increases during pregnancy and is significantly greater during lactation (Gulson *et al.*, 1998). This is consistent with an expected increase in the amount of bone resorption and a change from trabecular bone resorption to cortical bone or whole skeleton resorption (Manton *et al.*, 2003). Increased mobilization of Pb from the mother's skeleton during the gestation period could lead to an increase in fetal Pb exposure with gestational age. The placenta can play an active (activation or inhibition) role in the transfer of trace metals between the mother and fetus as well as a gradient mode of action, and this may vary during the gestational period. The effect of the human placenta at the end of gestation can be determined from trace element concentrations in maternal and corresponding umbilical cord sera. In one such study, the concentration of Zn in umbilical cord sera was 148 % of that of the maternal sera, and the corresponding value for Pb was 50 % (Rossipal *et al.*, 2000). Analysis of postpartum scalp hair samples from mother and neonate pairs also demonstrated higher Zn and lower Pb concentrations in the neonate than in the mother (Razagui and Ghribi, 2005).

After birth, the only source of Zn intake for an exclusively breastfed infant is via the mother. Zinc concentrations in human milk exhibit a significant reduction during the course of lactation, with levels falling particularly steeply during the transition from colostrum to mature milk (Akanle *et al.*, 2001; Anderson, 1993; Dorea, 2000; Krachler *et al.*, 1998; Perrone *et al.*, 1993, 1994). Physiological levels of Zn in the infant might therefore be expected to decline during the period of exclusive breastfeeding, and then increase with the introduction of complementary foods. This pattern has been demonstrated in a mixed longitudinal study of Zn status in 186 full term and preterm infants. Leukocyte and plasma Zn levels in breastfed infants were high at birth, then declined gradually to a minimum level at four to six months of age, and increased to normal levels by nine months, following the introduction of complementary foods. Notably, formula-fed full term infants had significantly lower leukocyte Zn levels at three months of age than breastfed infants of the same age (Hemalatha *et al.*, 1997). For Pb the situation is more complex. Mobilization of Pb from the mother's skeleton increases during lactation, with maternal blood Pb levels reaching a maximum level several months after birth (Manton *et al.*, 2003). Despite this, studies of changes in breast milk composition have found a decrease in Pb concentrations during the lactation period (Krachler *et al.*, 1998; Perrone *et al.*, 1994). Following birth an infant is exposed to non-dietary sources of Pb, and they may increase with the development of hand-to-mouth coordination and independent mobility.

Taken together, the evidence from this study and previously published research suggests that several different mechanisms contribute to the deposition and loss of Zn and Pb in human tooth enamel throughout the life of the tooth.

(1) The comparatively low normalized elemental intensities present in the inner layers of enamel primarily reflect the incorporation of Pb and Zn into the apatite crystals during enamel formation. The amount and pattern of elemental distribution within this zone of enamel is likely to give the most accurate indication of environmental exposure during the period of tooth crown formation. This area of enamel is expected to yield the most reliable information concerning prenatal and postnatal nutrition, residential mobility, and exposure to toxic metals during the period of tooth crown formation. Interpretation of trace element distributions within this deep enamel will require a detailed understanding of the environmental, physiological and enamel formation processes that contribute to their patterning.

(2) The narrow sub-surface layer is the last part of the enamel to be fully mineralized, and may be susceptible to ionic exchange with surrounding body fluids for a longer period of time than the deeper enamel. It is also possible that some, as yet unexplained, aspect of the enamel maturation process results in the preferential accumulation of Pb and Zn in this late maturing zone of enamel.

(3) Following the completion of enamel maturation, but prior to gingival emergence, the surface enamel is in direct contact with tissue fluids, providing a possible means for incorporation of Pb and Zn into the surface layer of enamel through ionic exchange. Penetration of these ions into the enamel is likely to be limited, but may be greater for Zn than for Pb.

(4) Following gingival emergence, trace metals continue to accumulate in the surface and near-surface enamel as a result of exchanges within the oral environment brought about by de- and remineralization of surface enamel caused by pH fluctuations. Surface enrichment may vary between teeth and between different surfaces of the same tooth as a result of differential susceptibility to attrition. Other factors that may contribute to variation between teeth from one individual are

differences in age of emergence (and exfoliation), and hence the time spent within the oral cavity and different localities within the mouth. It has not yet been possible to quantify the separate contribution of pre- and post-eruptive deposition to surface enrichment, but such a study could, in theory, be conducted using teeth donated by individuals who migrated between global regions with different prevailing Pb isotope compositions at the age of gingival emergence of a particular tooth.

(5) Diagenetic changes within the burial environment could result in a net loss or a gain of Pb and Zn from the enamel surface.

5.5 Summary

Analysis of human tooth enamel using laser ablation inductively coupled plasma mass spectrometry (LA-ICP-MS) provides a basis for systematic evaluation of variation in normalized elemental intensities in relation to tooth crown geometry. An understanding of non-homogeneity in trace element distributions is an important prerequisite for studies that seek to reconstruct aspects of an individual's early life, including nutritional history, residential mobility and exposure to heavy metals. In this chapter, a discrete multiple sampling strategy was used to investigate variation in Pb and Zn distributions in enamel from exfoliated deciduous teeth. Normalized elemental intensities for Pb and Zn are relatively low in the deep enamel and rise steeply towards the enamel surface. Markedly elevated elemental intensities occur deeper within the enamel for zinc than for lead (267.38 ± 38.80 μm for Zn compared to 122.75 ± 72.70 μm for Pb). Parameters that may contribute to this surface enrichment include enamel formation processes, amount of time within the oral cavity, and differences in rates of attrition between teeth and enamel surfaces. A second consistent feature of the distribution of lead and zinc in this sample of deciduous teeth is for normalized elemental intensities to reach a minimum value in the core region of enamel and then increase slightly towards the enamel–dentine junction. This transition does not relate to the position of the neonatal line, so cannot be directly related to differences between prenatal and postnatal exposure.

Acknowledgments

We would like to thank Joel Irish and Greg Nelson for the invitation to contribute to this volume. We thank Paul Cooper, Jonathon Cornish, Christopher Mayes, Stephanie Mayes, Raquel Garcia-Sanchez, Helen Liversidge, Christophe Soligo, Tom Stringer and Tony Wighton for helpful discussions, technical support and advice. We thank Joel Irish, Greg Nelson and another reviewer for helpful comments on an earlier version of this chapter.

References

Akanle, O. A., Balogun, F. A., Owa, J. A. and Spyrou, N. M. (2001). Variations in trace element concentrations in breast milk with stages of lactation. *Journal of Radioanalytical and Nuclear Chemistry*, **249**, 71–5.

Anderson, R. R. (1993). Longitudinal changes of trace-elements in human-milk during the 1st 5 months of lactation. *Nutrition Research*, **12**, 499–510.

Bellinger, D. C., Needleman, H. L., Leviton, A. *et al.* (1984). Early sensory-motor development and prenatal exposure to lead. *Neurobehavioral Toxicology and Teratology*, **6**, 387–402.

Bhatnagar, S. and Taneja, S. (2001). Zinc and cognitive development. *British Journal of Nutrition*, **85**, S139-45.

Boyde, A. (1989). Enamel. In *Handbook of Microscopic Anatomy, Vol. 6: Teeth*. Berlin: Springer, pp. 309–473.

Brown, C. J., Chenery, S. R. N., Smith, B. *et al.* (2004). Environmental influences on the trace element content of teeth – implications for disease and nutritional status. *Archives of Oral Biology*, **49**, 705–17.

Brudevold, F. and Söremark, R. (1967). Chemistry of the mineral phase of enamel. In *Structural and chemical organisation of teeth, Vol. 2*, ed. A. E. W. Miles. London: Academic Press, pp. 247–77.

Brudevold, F. and Steadman, L. T. (1956). The distribution of lead in human enamel. *Journal of Dental Research*, **35**, 430–37.

Budd, P., Montgomery, J., Cox, A. *et al.* (1998). The distribution of lead within ancient and modern human teeth: implications for long-term and historical exposure monitoring. *Science of the Total Environment*, **220**, 121–36.

Budd, P., Montgomery, J., Evans, J., and Barreiro, B. (2000). Human tooth enamel as a record of the comparative lead exposure of prehistoric and modern people. *Science of the Total Environment*, **263**, 1–10.

Dolphin, A. E., Goodman, A. H., and Amarasiriwardena, D. D. (2005). Variation in elemental intensities among teeth and between pre- and postnatal regions of enamel. *American Journal of Physical Anthropology*, **128**, 878–88.

Dorea, J. G. (2000). Zinc in human milk. *Nutrition Research*, **20**, 1645–87.

Ezzo, J. A. (1994). Zinc as a paleodietary indicator – an issue of theoretical validity in bone-chemistry analysis. *American Antiquity*, **59**, 606–21.

Frank, R. M., Sargentinimaier, M. L., Turlot, J. C., and Leroy, M. J. F. (1990). Comparison of lead levels in human permanent teeth from Strasbourg, Mexico City, and rural zones of Alsace. *Journal of Dental Research*, **69**, 90–3.

Goyer, R. A. (1996). Results of lead research: prenatal exposure and neurological consequences. *Environmental Health Perspectives*, **104**, 1050–4.

Gulson, B. L. (1996). Tooth analyses of sources and intensity of lead exposure in children. *Environmental Health Perspectives*, **104**, 306–12.

Gulson, B. L., Jameson, C. W., and Gillings, B. R. (1997a). Stable lead isotopes in teeth as indicators of past domicile – A potential new tool in forensic science? *Journal of Forensic Sciences*, **42**, 787–91.

Gulson, B. L., Jameson, C. W., Mahaffey, K. R. *et al.* (1997b). Pregnancy increases mobilization of lead from maternal skeleton. *Journal of Laboratory and Clinical Medicine*, **130**, 51–62.

Gulson, B. L., Mahaffey, K. R., Jameson, C. W. *et al.* (1998). Mobilization of lead from the skeleton during the postnatal period is larger than during pregnancy. *Journal of Laboratory and Clinical Medicine*, **131**, 324–9.

Gulson, B. L. and Wilson, D. (1994). History of lead-exposure in children revealed from isotopic analyses of teeth. *Archives of Environmental Health*, **49**, 279–83.

Hemalatha, P., Bhaskaram, P., Kumar, P. A., Khan, M. M., and Islam, M. A. (1997). Zinc status of breastfed and formula-fed infants of different gestational ages. *Journal of Tropical Pediatrics*, **43**, 52–4.

Hillson, S. (1996). *Dental Anthropology*. Cambridge: Cambridge University Press.

Humphrey, L. T., Dean, M. C., and Jeffries, T. E. (in press). An evaluation of changes in strontium/calcium ratios across the neonatal line in human deciduous teeth. In *Dental Perspectives on Human Evolution: State of the Art Research in Dental Anthropology*, ed. S. Bailey and J.-J. Hublin. New York: Springer.

Jarup, L. (2003). Hazards of heavy metal contamination. *British Medical Bulletin*, **68**, 167–82.

Jeffries, T. E. (2004). Laser ablation inductively coupled plasma mass spectrometry. In: *Wilson and Wilson's Comprehensive Analytical Chemistry, Vol. XLII: Non-Destructive Microanalysis of Cultural Heritage Materials*, ed. K. Janssens and R. Van Grieken. Amsterdam: Elsevier, pp. 313–58.

Jeffries, T. E., Jackson, S. E., and Longerich, H. P. (1998). Application of a frequency quintupled Nd: YAG source ($\lambda = 213$ nm) for laser ablation inductively coupled plasma mass spectrometric analysis of minerals. *Journal of Analytical and Atomic Spectrometry* **13**, 935–40.

Kang, D., Amarasiriwardena, D., and Goodman, A. H. (2004). Application of laser ablation-inductively coupled plasma-mass spectrometry (LA-ICP-MS) to investigate trace metal spatial distributions in human tooth enamel and dentine growth layers and pulp. *Analytical and Bioanalytical Chemistry*, **378**, 1608–15.

Krachler, M., Li, F. S., Rossipal, E., and Irgolic, K. J. (1998). Changes in the concentrations of trace elements in human milk during lactation. *Journal of Trace Elements in Medicine and Biology*, **12**, 159–76.

Lee, K. M., Appleton, J., Cooke, M., Keenan, F., and Sawicka-Kapusta, K. (1999). Use of laser ablation inductively coupled plasma mass spectrometry to provide element versus time profiles in teeth. *Analytica Chimica Acta*, **395**, 179–85.

Manton, W. I., Angle, C. R., Stanek, K. L. *et al.* (2003). Release of lead from bone in pregnancy and lactation. *Environmental Research*, **92**, 139–51.

Needleman, H. L. Tuncay, O. C., and Shapiro, I. M. (1972). Lead levels in deciduous teeth of urban and suburban American children. *Nature*, **235**, 111–12.

Nyström, M. (1977). Clinical eruption of deciduous teeth in a series of Finnish children. *Proceedings of the Finnish Dental Society*, **73**, 155–61.

Nyström, M., Kleemola-Kujala, E., Evälahti, M., Peck, L., and Kataja, M. (2001). Emergence of permanent teeth and dental age in a series of Finns. *Acta Odontologica Scandinavica*, **59**, 49–56.

Perrone, L., Dipalma, L., Ditoro, R., Gialanella, G., and Moro, R. (1993). Trace-element content of human-milk during lactation. *Journal of Trace Elements and Electrolytes in Health and Disease*, **7**, 245–7.

Perrone, L., Dipalma, L., Ditoro, R., Gialanella, G., and Moro, R. (1994). Interaction of trace-elements in a longitudinal-study of human-milk from full-term and preterm mothers. *Biological Trace Element Research*, **41**, 321–30.

Razagui, I. B. A. and Ghribi, I. (2005). Maternal and neonatal scalp hair concentrations of zinc, copper, cadmium, and lead – relationship to some lifestyle factors. *Biological Trace Element Research*, **106**, 1–27.

Reitznerova, E., Amarasiriwardena, D., Kopcakova, M., and Barnes, R. M. (2000). Determination of some trace elements in human tooth enamel. *Fresenius Journal of Analytical Chemistry*, **367**, 748–54.

Rossipal, E., Krachler, M., Li, F., and Micetic-Turk, D. (2000). Investigation of the transport of trace elements across barriers in humans: studies of placental and mammary transfer. *Acta Paediatrica*, **89**, 1190–5.

Schour, I. (1936). Neonatal line in enamel and dentin of human deciduous teeth and first permanent molar. *Journal of the American Dental Association*, **23**, 1946–55.

Skinner, M. and Dupras, T. (1993). Variation in birth timing and location of the neonatal line in human enamel. *Journal of Forensic Sciences*, **38**, 1383–90.

Tellez-Rojo, M. M., Hernandez-Avila, M., Gonzalez-Cossio, T. *et al.* (2002). Impact of breastfeeding on the mobilization of lead from bone. *American Journal of Epidemiology*, **155**, 420–8.

Waldron, H. A. (1981). Postmortem absorption of lead by the skeleton. *American Journal of Physical Anthropology*, **55**, 395–8.

Webb, E., Amarasiriwardena, D., Tauch, S. *et al.* (2005). Inductively coupled plasma-mass (ICP-MS) and atomic emission spectrometry (ICP-AES): versatile analytical techniques to identify the archived elemental information in human teeth. *Microchemical Journal*, **81**, 201–8.

Wellinghausen, N. (2001). Immunobiology of gestational zinc deficiency. *British Journal of Nutrition*, **85**, S81–6.

Whittaker, D. K. and Richard, D. (1978). Scanning electron microscopy of the neonatal line in human enamel. *Archives of Oral Biology*, **23**, 45–50.

6 *The current state of dental decay*

SIMON HILLSON

6.1 Introduction

Dental caries is one of the most commonly recognized diseases in archaeological collections of human remains. Several decades of intensive clinical research have elucidated the mechanisms that underlie it, and its common pattern of occurrence in living people. After two centuries of high caries rates, it seems that the disease is now on the decline. It is less often appreciated that the high rates of the twentieth century were, in any case, an anomaly in archaeological terms. Not only were caries rates much lower throughout the great bulk of human existence, but the nature of the disease was different as well. The present chapter presents an overview of this pervasive and important dental disease – from cause and effect, to variation through time and among populations – and provides context for the remaining papers in this section.

6.2 The nature of dental caries

Dental caries is a progressive demineralization of dental enamel, cement, and dentin. It is the cumulative effect of changes in the pH environment of dental plaque deposits on the surface of the teeth. The pH varies during the day. It is lowered by the production of organic acids (especially lactic acid) through the fermentation of carbohydrates by the plaque bacteria, and raised again toward neutral pH by the clearance of fermentable carbohydrates from the mouth and through the buffering effect of saliva. The mineral component of dental tissues is in a chemical equilibrium with ions in solution in the plaque fluid that changes with the pH. As the pH lowers (i.e. the plaque fluid becomes more acidic) the mineral component starts to dissolve. As pH returns to neutral, the dental tissue remineralizes because the saliva, and thus also the plaque fluid, is saturated with calcium and phosphate ions. Caries is a result of an overall imbalance of low and neutral pH episodes during the day. If low pH phases predominate, there is a net loss of tooth mineral – that is, a lesion of dental caries develops.

Technique and Application in Dental Anthropology ed. Joel D. Irish and Greg C. Nelson
Published by Cambridge University Press.

The balance can change, however, and the lesion may be halted, or even remineralize, if the environment of the overlying dental plaque is altered.

Six factors influence dental caries: (1) the nature of dental tissues and tooth surfaces, (2) the bacterial community present in the plaque, (3) the interstitial matrix between the bacteria (mostly produced by the bacteria themselves), (4) the plaque fluid that occupies the spaces in the plaque and bathes the bacteria and the tooth surface, (5) the saliva that bathes the surface of the plaque, and (6) the nature of the diet that arrives in the mouth and adheres, at least briefly, to the surface of teeth and plaque.

6.2.1 *Dental tissues and tooth surfaces*

Many characteristics of the teeth have an effect on caries. Fluoride ions are incorporated into the mineral component of dental tissues, either from the water supply or by the use of fluoride toothpaste and mouthwash. Fluoride has a strongly protective effect against caries (Thylstrup and Fejerskov, 1994; Williams and Elliott, 1989), partly because the pH point at which there is a net loss of tooth mineral is lower, and perhaps because it inhibits the plaque bacteria. Since it was first added to water and toothpaste in the 1950s, fluoride has been a major factor in caries epidemiology. It also occurs naturally in drinking water, so one requirement for any archaeological caries study is, therefore, also to consider fluoride levels in the regional groundwater.

Another important factor is the structure of the dental tissues. When erupted into the mouth, the newly formed dental enamel is not completely mineralized (Hillson, 1996). Teeth are therefore at their most vulnerable to caries when they first erupt. In addition, dentitions that are affected by the developmental defects of enamel hypoplasia are associated with higher caries rates (Mellanby, 1934). These defects are common, so this possibility also needs to be checked. Within the enamel, microscope sections show that the lesion spreads along lines of existing growth layerings (Jones and Boyde, 1987). Particular points on the crown surface, such as the contact points with neighboring teeth or the occlusal fissures, provide protection for plaque deposits and show a much higher rate of lesions than other sites on the crown (Batchelor and Sheiham, 2004; Sheiham, 1997; Thylstrup and Fejerskov, 1994).

Tooth wear has an effect that is seen particularly in archaeological jaws (Hillson, 2000; Hillson, 2001). To some extent rapid wear might remove tissue affected by carious lesions, but it seems to have functioned more by creating new sites at which lesions could develop. In the past it was also a major factor in continuous eruption of teeth, which exposed the root surfaces above the gingivae. Even after all the teeth have erupted into the mouth, eruption continues slowly throughout adult life (Whittaker *et al.*, 1985, 1990, 1982). In living people, the rate is very slow and, as the teeth also wear down slowly, the face often increases in height through life by a few millimeters. In the past, both the wear rate and eruption rate was much faster, in what appears to have been a mechanism to keep the teeth in occlusion as wear progressed.

Carious lesions also develop in different ways in the different dental tissues. The whole character of a crown lesion that starts in the enamel changes once it penetrates into the dentine underneath (Schüpbach *et al.*, 1992; Thylstrup and Fejerskov, 1994). There is also some evidence to suggest that the cement (and dentine rapidly follows because the cement layer is thin) coating the root surface is less resistant to caries than the enamel of the crown (Hoppenbrouwers *et al.*, 1987; Lingström *et al.*, 2000). The pH below which there is a net loss of mineral seems to be considerably higher. This may be an important point in the interpretation of the archaeological record (below).

6.2.2 *The bacterial community of the dental plaque*

Plaque is a complex association of many different species of bacteria. They work together in attaching themselves, in building the deposit, and in providing different parts of the battery of enzymes that break down the variety of biomolecules that come their way from the saliva, other mouth fluids, and from the human diet. They are, however, in competition with one another. The plaque community has a complex ecology (Marsh and Martin, 1992), and different species rise to dominance depending on the environment in which the community finds itself (pH, oxygen, etc.). For example, the most common species in plaque from a relatively exposed crown surface are different from those in plaque from contact areas between neighboring teeth, and both are different from the plaque found on exposed root surfaces. In plaque overlying carious lesions on the tooth crown, there is a particular dominance of *Streptococcus mutans*, *Lactobacillus* spp. and a group known as low-pH non-*mutans* streptococci (Lingström *et al.*, 2000; van Houte, 1994). All three of these groups are tolerant of low pH and, therefore, have a selective advantage over other bacterial forms in these conditions. They are also particularly efficient at fermenting dietary carbohydrates. It therefore seems that a plaque deposit becomes potentially cariogenic when there is sufficient carbohydrate provided regularly in the diet to confer a selective advantage on the low pH bacteria. Once they have risen to dominance, the plaque is capable of producing organic acids more rapidly. Patients with a history of many carious lesions have plaque deposits that are often characterized by the low-pH-loving bacteria, and they are much less common in patients with few lesions. Plaque deposits overlying root surface lesions also tend not to have so many low-pH bacteria, and this is another reason why the higher susceptibility of dental tissues at this point (above) may be important.

6.2.3 The dental plaque matrix

The matrix holds the plaque deposit together and adheres to the tooth surface. It is made partly from components derived from saliva, but is often made by the bacteria themselves. A variety of polymers are made from sugars, particularly sucrose (below), and, as might be expected, *Streptococcus mutans* is one of the main manufacturers. The sugars come from dietary carbohydrates. Plaque grows more rapidly in a diet containing sucrose because *mutans* streptococci can make a more voluminous matrix (van Houte, 1994). It may also be that the greater spacing of bacteria, produced with copious matrix, allows more channels from the plaque surface to the tooth, along which sugars from the diet can diffuse.

6.2.4 The plaque fluid

Plaque deposits are highly organized and have a definite surface membrane. Within this, and occupying the spaces in the matrix, is the plaque fluid. It contains dissolved gases, sugars, and amino acids, the organic acids produced by the fermentation of sugars, and a variety of other components. It shows strong gradients, from the plaque surface to the base of the deposit on the tooth, and from place to place within the deposit. It is the pH balance of the plaque fluid that is responsible for dental caries; however, this balance varies in a very localized way so that a carious lesion can be initiated at one point on the crown surface, while the neighboring enamel is not affected. The pH also varies from minute to minute, particularly as a result of variation in the fermentable carbohydrate available to the plaque bacteria. When sugary food is eaten, the sugar rapidly diffuses into the plaque and is made available to the bacteria, which ferment it to produce organic acids. The pH can lower markedly within minutes (Thylstrup and Fejerskov, 1994; van Houte, 1994). Gradually, the sugar clears from the mouth, and is used up by the bacteria, so the pH returns toward neutral. Consuming a sugary drink or meal containing fermentable carbohydrates, therefore, results in an episode of low plaque fluid pH lasting up to an hour or more.

6.2.5 *The saliva*

Saliva bathes all surfaces of the teeth, gingivae, and plaque (Lenander-Lumikari and Loimaranta, 2000). It is buffered to an approximately neutral pH and, thus, provides the basis on which plaque fluid pH returns to neutral after a sugar-eating episode. It also contains a number of antibacterial factors and mechanisms, so the size and location of plaque deposits must involve a balance with the saliva. Food, including carbohydrates, is cleared from the mouth at least partly by the action of saliva. It is notable, for example, that the lingual surfaces of the lower incisors and canines are one of the least common locations for carious lesions, and it is these surfaces that are closest to the openings of the submaxillary and sublingual salivary gland ducts that are situated under the tongue (Lingström, *et al.*, 2000). Patients with xerostomia – lower than normal salivary flow – often experience high caries rates.

6.2.6 *The human diet*

Most proteins and fats in the food that we eat seem to have little effect on the plaque. They are long chain molecules that are unable to diffuse across the plaque surface membrane and into the fluid. Bacteria certainly produce a battery of enzymes that can metabolize proteins, but these are mostly adapted to the proteins found in the saliva. Milk products (particularly cheese) have a protective effect against caries (Bowen and Pearson, 1993). They contain the protein casein, which does seem to be metabolized by plaque bacteria. In addition, they may affect the adhesion of food to the teeth and plaque, and provide a source of calcium and phosphorus ions for remineralization. Carbohydrates (Garrow *et al.*, 2000) consist of sugars, short-chain carbohydrates (SCC), starches, and non-starch polysaccharides (NSP). SCC and NSP are unlikely to be fermentable by plaque bacteria (Lingström *et al.*, 2000). Sugars are small molecules that can diffuse directly into the plaque fluid and are rapidly fermented by the bacteria. All common dietary sugars seem to be potentially cariogenic, but the most strongly related to caries is sucrose. This is also the most common dietary sugar. There is a wealth of epidemiological studies linking sucrose consumption to caries (Navia, 1994; Rugg-Gunn, 1993; Sheiham, 1983; Thylstrup and Fejerskov, 1994). During the Second World War, for example, those countries such as Britain and Japan that had sugar rationing (but starchy food supplies were maintained) experienced a marked reduction in caries among children. Caries only became common in children again after the war, when rationing ended. Similarly, groups of people who had lived without a supply of sugar in their diet, but then started to gain access to supplies of sweetened foods, such as the East Greenland or Canadian Inuit, or Tristan da Cunha islanders, showed a marked increase in caries.

Starches are long molecules, polymers of sugar units. They are too big to diffuse directly into the plaque fluid but, if broken down by enzymes, release sugars that do so (Lingström *et al.*, 2000). An enzyme called amylase is present in saliva and is produced by some bacteria; it rapidly breaks down starches into sugars, particularly maltose, that can be fermented by plaque bacteria. One limiting factor in the production of sugars from starch in the diet is that the latter is held within plant cells inside microscopic water-insoluble granules. In raw starchy foods, these granules are intact and the starch is not available for breakdown. Cooking and grinding rupture the granules and release the starches (called gelatinization), but this varies greatly with the temperature reached and the amount of water in the mixture (Garrow *et al.*, 2000).

There is experimental evidence that eating starch can produce episodes of low plaque pH, but these vary greatly between foods. Generally speaking, starchy foods lower the pH less rapidly and to a lesser extent than sugars, but it remains low for longer. The length of this low pH episode is longer for bread than rice, potatoes or pasta (Mörmann and Mühlemann, 1981; Mundorff *et al.*, 1990; Mundorff-Shrestha *et al.*, 1994). This has to do with the degree of gelatinization and consistency of the food. With industrial cooking processes, the more processed the food, the lower and longer the pH depression. Starches can therefore potentially produce carious lesions, but there has been relatively little epidemiological work focusing on this aspect. In any case, many foods contain mixtures of starch and sugar, so it is hard to separate their effects.

Generally speaking, starch is not regarded as cariogenic, although diets in which starches are mixed with sugars seem to be even more cariogenic than sugar on its own. In a study of Papua New Guinea, people whose entire source of carbohydrate was sago (which has effectively no sugar) had variable caries rates: high in some villages, low in others (Schamschula *et al.*, 1978). This was presumably related to different ways in which food was prepared and eaten. A final feature of diet that is thought to have a large effect on caries rates is the frequency with which food is eaten during the day. If fermentable carbohydrates are introduced into the mouth only at mealtimes, two or three times a day, then they are less cariogenic than when also introduced at snacks in between meals. Even diets supplemented with sugar may produce little caries if this is given only at mealtimes. It thus appears that regular and frequent consumption of carbohydrates, rather than the amount, is the most important factor in making a sustained shift in the balance between tooth mineral and plaque fluid toward net mineral loss.

6.3 Caries sites

Carious lesions do not occur randomly over the tooth surface. Particular sites on the surface are much more susceptible than others. First among these are the fissure systems of the occlusal surfaces in molar and premolar crowns. These features are narrow – narrower than a brush bristle – so no amount of care in cleaning can remove the plaque. Their depth also brings them close to the enamel–dentine junction, so a lesion that starts inside can develop rapidly into a large cavity. Another prime site is just under the contact point between neighboring teeth. Regular flossing can keep this clear, but how many children can be persuaded to do that? In adults, two processes progressively expose the root surfaces. One is the development of periodontal disease, and the other is continuous eruption of the teeth in a mechanism that adjusts for wear. The adult pattern of periodontal disease is a common cause of recession of the gums and underlying bone in modern people, but there is less evidence that it was a major factor in ancient populations. In most living populations, wear is a relatively minor factor and continuous eruption occurs at a slow rate. In the past, however, wear was much more rapid and the continuous eruption seems to have progressed at a similarly high rate. Whatever the mechanism, the root surfaces exposed above the gum line are susceptible to dental caries.

The lesions of dental caries, for the most part, develop slowly (Pine and ten Bosch, 1996; Thylstrup and Fejerskov, 1994). They start as a focus of demineralization that is invisible from the surface. In the enamel, the first surface sign is a tiny white or brown spot. This grows gradually, its surface becomes rough, and it eventually breaks down to form a cavity. A great deal of demineralization has gone on under the surface, often including the dentine, before this stage is reached. Root surface lesions are usually first seen as an area of brown stain. The surface becomes softened and eventually breaks down to form a broad depression.

In both crown and root, the lesion may develop very slowly over many years. This is particularly true of the root surface. The lesion may also remain stable, or even remineralize. Even a large lesion involving much of the tooth may only be progressing slowly. Where the pulp has been exposed it becomes inflamed and, as often happens, may die. This allows bacteria, or the products of the inflammatory process, to emerge from the apical foramen at the root tip. In this situation, the periodontal tissues that support the tooth may become inflamed. This process is known as periapical inflammation which, if acute, is very painful. The simplest remedy is to extract the tooth, and this operation has considerable antiquity. Many archaeological jaws, however, have evidence of chronic periapical inflammation where the tooth has not been extracted, and it is clear that the situation persisted for some time before death (Hillson, 2000, 2001). Chronic inflammation of this type would not necessarily have been painful, although there might well have been acute phases, so the need for extraction might not be so pressing. The full development of a carious lesion, therefore, usually takes many years. Even in the absence of fillings and other dental treatment, it does not necessarily lead to the type of toothache that would cause the sufferer to have the tooth extracted. Just occasionally, modern children show a condition called "rampant" caries, which is rapidly progressive; yet this is usually associated with very frequent consumption of sugar-rich snacks and drinks.

6.4 Twentieth century caries

During the second half of the twentieth century, a great deal of research was carried out on dental caries. It concentrated on the permanent teeth of children because these were seen to be most important in maintaining a lifetime of functional teeth. Throughout most of the twentieth and nineteenth centuries, caries was very common in children who went on to lose many teeth early in their adult lives, so it was seen as a serious problem. It became apparent that carious lesions were not randomly distributed, but showed a clear pattern (Batchelor and Sheiham, 2004; Sheiham, 1997). Some children were particularly caries-prone and had many lesions, while others were much less affected. The caries rate of a group of children was, therefore, often greatly affected by a relatively small number of children in the total group. Similarly, some teeth were much more frequently affected than others. Indeed, some particular points on the tooth crowns were especially at risk. From this came the idea of a hierarchy of caries lesion sites (Table 6.1).

The site most at risk is the occlusal fissure system of the permanent first molars and, in the lower first molars, the pit or depression that is sometimes present on the buccal side of the crown. Next come the fissure systems and buccal pits of the second molars and second premolars, together with the lingual pits of the upper first molars. After that, it is the occlusal fissures of the first premolars, lingual pits of upper second molars and upper second incisors, and crown contact points of first molars. Last of all are the contact points of the second molars, premolars, and incisors. Canines are only rarely involved. Susceptibility is therefore arranged like a pyramid, with the first molar fissures at its apex. In low caries-rate groups of people, very few children have lesions, and these are found particularly at the most susceptible sites. In progressively higher caries-rate groups, more individual children have caries lesions in their mouths, and they are found in less susceptible sites farther down the susceptibility pyramid.

Table 6.1 *The pyramid of caries susceptibility in children's permanent tooth crowns*[a]

Susceptibility	2nd molars	1st molars	2nd premolars	1st premolars	Canines	2nd incisors	1st incisors
Most		Fissures and lower pits					
	Fissures and lower pits	Upper pits	Fissures				
	Upper pits	Contacts and other surfaces		Fissures		Upper pits	
	Other surfaces		Contacts and other surfaces	Upper contacts and other surfaces		Other surfaces	Upper any surface, lower contacts
Least				Lower contacts and other surfaces	Any surface		Lower other surfaces

[a] Data from Batchelor and Sheiham (2004). Only potential caries sites on the permanent tooth crowns of children are included. Some potential caries sites have different susceptibilities in upper and lower teeth and are indicated in the table. "Fissures" means fissures of the occlusal surface. "Pits" means the extensions of the fissure system to the buccal side of lower molars and lingual side of upper molars that results in a marked depression in some teeth (but this potential caries site is not present in all teeth in all individuals). There is sometimes a similar pit on the lingual surface of upper second incisors and in rare cases upper first incisors. "Contacts" refers to the points at which neighboring teeth in the same jaw meet. The potential site is just below the contact point. "Other surfaces" are anything else – usually buccal/labial or lingual surfaces along the line of the gingivae. The most susceptible sites are found in any study group that has caries. The least susceptible sites are found commonly only in groups with high caries rates.

Only the highest-rate groups have many lesions in sites at the base. This pattern may partly be due to the eruption sequence – earlier erupting teeth such as first molars spending more of their crucial poorly mineralized years in childhood, when people tend to eat more sugary snacks. It must also, however, be related to the position of teeth in the mouth relative to salivary gland ducts, to the traps for plaque made by fissures and pits in the crown, and to the cleaning effects of the lips, cheeks, and tongue.

Deciduous teeth have been less studied, but they follow a similar pattern (Evans and Lo, 1992), with the majority of carious lesions occurring in the fissures of deciduous molars and the pit of the second deciduous molar (its form is similar to the permanent first molar). Children with a history of caries in their deciduous dentition tend also to develop lesions in their following permanent teeth (Skeie *et al.*, 2006), although this trend does not always follow.

Childhood caries of this type dominated city populations of the twentieth century. Rural populations tended to have lower rates than urban, and less well-off socioeconomic groups higher rates than the more prosperous (Källestål and Wall, 2002; Locker, 2000; Peres *et al.*, 2005; Sheiham, 1997; Thomson *et al.*, 2004). During the last years of the twentieth century, caries rates showed a sustained decline (Carvalho *et al.*, 2004) that has continued into the twenty-first century. This may partly be due to fluoridation of water supplies and the increased use of fluoride toothpaste, but it cannot all be explained in this way. Similarly, there is little evidence that fermentable carbohydrates in the diet have decreased. The caries rate decline is paralleled by a general improvement in health, so it seems to be part of a broader social change that is not yet properly understood.

There have been fewer studies that follow caries into adult life, at least partly because dental treatment makes such a difference to the progress of the disease. Some, however, have been carried out in groups of people who have had little access to dentists – studies of the "natural history of caries" – for example in rural Kenya (Manji *et al.*, 1989, 1991). One of the most noticeable features of caries is its strong patterning with age. In Figure 6.1, it can be seen that the children and young adults, in general, had the pattern of caries described above, in which the molars are much more affected than the other teeth. Lesions were mostly confined to the enamel, although a few penetrated to the dentine and pulp, and thus represented a more advanced stage of the disease. In older age groups, the general proportion of molars affected by caries did not increase, but those in the premolars, canines, and incisors did, so that more of the dentition was involved, even though the molars remained the most important site. Enamel-only lesions continued to be present, either as slowly developing existing lesions or as new lesions. At the same time, more deeply penetrating dentine- and pulp-exposing lesions became more common. From the late 20s and early 30s, root

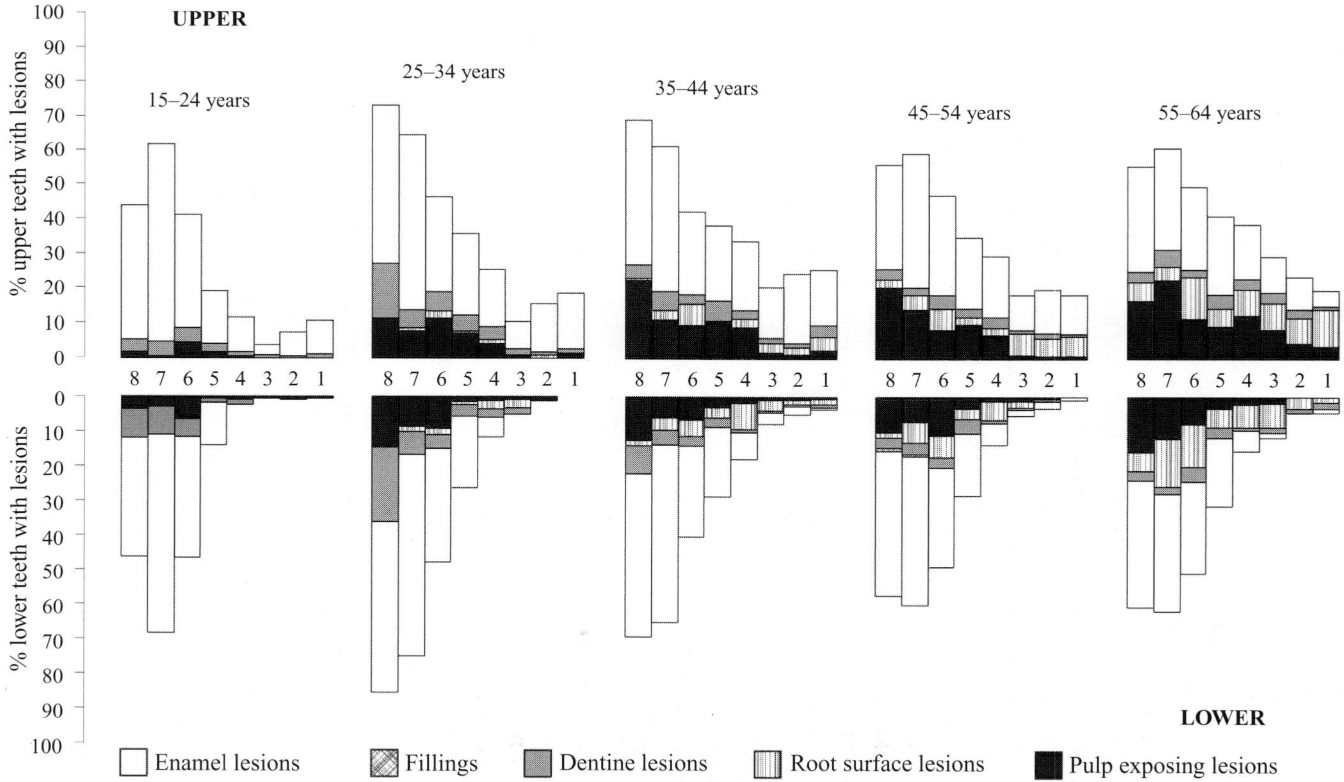

Figure 6.1 Dental caries in different permanent tooth classes (numbered from 8 for third molar to 1 for first incisor) for 10-year age groups of recent rural Kenyan people. Upper dentition is above the line and lower below. The different patterns of shading represent different types of caries as indicated by the key. Re-drawn using figures scaled from Figure 4.7, page 86 in Manji *et al.* (1991).

surface caries made its appearance as these surfaces became exposed, and the proportion of teeth affected by root caries increased steadily in older groups. It should be remembered that these figures are for the teeth surviving in the mouth. Other teeth almost certainly would be extracted if pulp-exposing lesions led to periapical inflammation (that can produce the most violent toothache) – so the proportion of pulp-exposing lesions is almost certainly an underestimate. Teeth must also have been lost, particularly in older age groups, through periodontal disease. It is for this reason that tooth loss is not included in the graph. Of the remaining teeth, a considerable proportion was affected by caries in all age groups; for example 50–70 % of molars were affected.

The twentieth century pattern was, therefore, one in which the crowns of deciduous and permanent teeth, particularly the molars, were commonly affected in children from the youngest age. The proportion of surviving molars affected did not increase greatly in adulthood but, with increasing age, more premolars, canines, and incisors became involved. The enamel of the crown was the focus of carious lesions in children, particularly the occlusal fissures of the molars, but in progressively older age groups a larger proportion of lesions penetrated the dentine and pulp, and root surface caries became more and more important. The dietary context within which this pattern of disease developed was one of high carbohydrate consumption – with much sugar, starch, and a high frequency of snacks between meals, so that there were many "caries incidents" throughout the day. A similar pattern of dental caries can be seen in, for example, Londoners of the nineteenth century (personal observation in specimens from the Museum of London) or a small town in northern England (see Figure 6.2).

6.5 Pre-nineteenth/twentieth century agriculturalists

With the long-term chronology of archaeology, it is possible to see that the twentieth century pattern of caries is an anomaly – a product of the ready availability of refined sugars, surplus of carbohydrate that allows frequent snacks, and diet and behavior that produces very little wear during an entire lifetime. Throughout the whole of human history before this, the experience of caries was very different. That is not to say that carbohydrates were not available. Since the origins of agriculture, cereals, rice, and maize, for example, have been dietary staples. They are, however, rich in starches and relatively poor in sugars (even though they are still present, depending on the way in which cereal-based foods are prepared; Table 6.2).

In addition, tooth wear in the past proceeded at a much greater rate. There is no clear answer as to why this should be or, to put it another way, why our

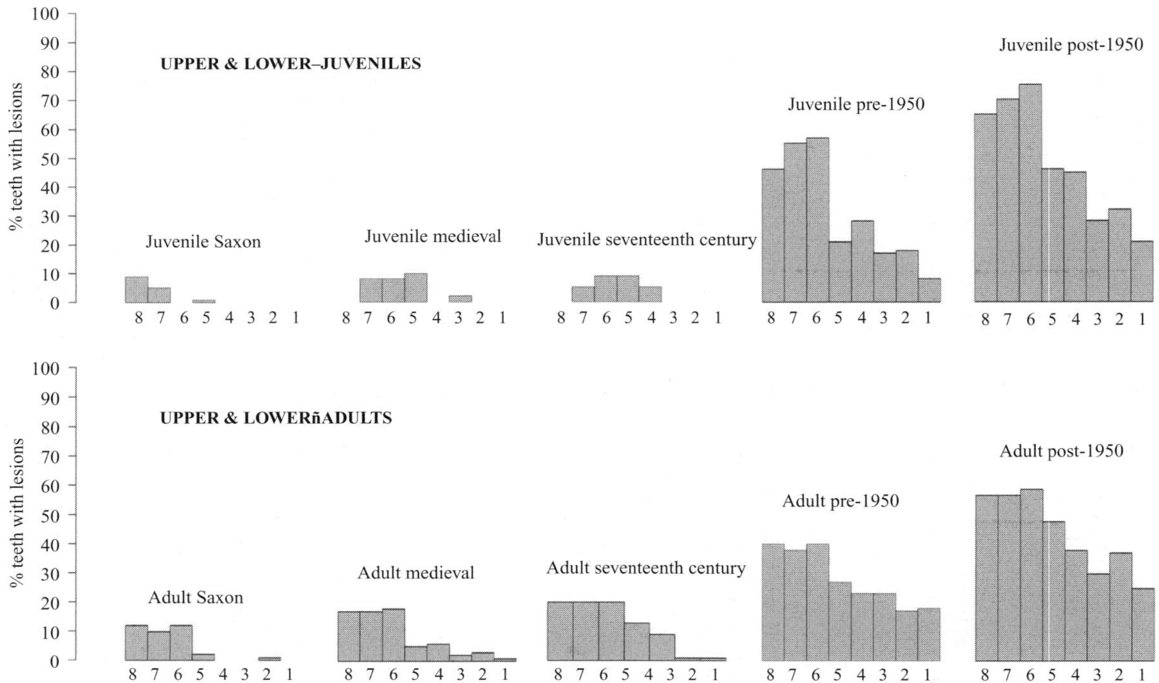

Figure 6.2 Dental caries in different permanent tooth classes (numbered from 8 for third molar to 1 for first incisor) for juveniles (before third molar eruption completed) and adults (after) in archaeological collections from England. Scaled from graphs of Corbett and Moore (1976). Upper and lower teeth are combined because they were not separated in the original publication. It was also not possible to derive separate percentages for different caries type in different tooth classes so the bars show only the percentage of teeth in each category with carious lesions. All dentitions are from archaeological assemblages excavated in England. Anglo Saxons were a combined group from the Midlands, southern, and eastern England. Details were not given for the sites in the later medieval group. The seventeenth-century group came from a plague pit (AD 1665) in London. The nineteenth-century dentitions came from a cemetery at Ashton-under-Lyne in Lancashire. They were divided into pre-1850 and post-1850 groups.

Table 6.2 *Starch and sugar composition of some foods*[a]

	Starch (mean g per 100 g fresh weight)	Total sugars (mean g per 100 g fresh weight)
Maize tortilla[b]	29.7	0.8
Wheat tortilla[b]	30.9	2.3
Brown leavened bread	41.3	3.0
Spaghetti (white)	21.7	0.5
Rice (white)	30.9	0.0
Potato (old)	14.5	1.0
Sweet corn kernels	16.6	9.6
Peas (raw)[c]	7.0	2.3
Chocolate chip cookies[c]	30.6	31.5
Potato chips	52.6	0.7
Jam doughnut[c]	30.0	18.8

[a] Various maize and wheat breads are included. They include more sugar than other ways of eating cereal such as pasta, or other staples such as rice and potato. Sweet corn is included to contrast with maize prepared in other ways and peas, because they were important in the European medieval diet. At the bottom of the table are examples of modern snack foods, which often contain large quantities of sugar.
[b] from Sánchez-Castillo *et al.* (2000)
[c] from Food Standards Agency and Institute of Food Research (2002)

own tooth wear is so slow. Grinding stones do indeed add grit to cereals and, if this is not removed after the milling, would add abrasives to the mouth. Ancient Egyptian bread, for example, was full of grit (Leek, 1972). Similarly, if there is much dietary fiber, this is likely to increase the chewing time required. Dental work must play a role too, as restorations and crowns, in effect, continuously replace the surfaces that would have been worn in earlier times. In addition, people probably used their teeth more in everyday jobs, to grip items, crack nuts, and so on. Whatever the reason, by the time third molars were erupted and fully in wear, early medieval British people (Brothwell, 1989; Miles, 1958, 1962) had a state of wear in the rest of their dentition greater than that reached in a whole modern lifetime. By middle age, there was often little remaining of many of their tooth crowns. Coupled with this was a much faster rate of continuous eruption to adjust for the tooth height lost by wear. The root surfaces must have been rapidly exposed by this mechanism, whether or not periodontal disease was an important factor.

The largest detailed study of dental caries carried out on such high wear-rate agriculturalists was that of Moore and Corbett (1971, 1973, 1975; Corbett and Moore, 1976), based on medieval collections in England. The important innovations that they made (so far as archaeological studies were concerned) were to give separate counts of lesions for different teeth in the mouth, for different age groups, and to distinguish between root surface and crown caries. In Figure 6.2, prepared using Moore and Corbett's figures, it is possible to compare medieval, seventeenth-century, and nineteenth-century people. The biggest change is among children. The nineteenth-century children in their study, as in the twentieth-century pattern described above, had just as high of a caries rates as the adults – the main difference being that in adults the caries rates were more evenly spread through the different teeth of dentition. In the medieval and seventeenth-century children, caries rates were very low and concentrated in the molars. In adults, caries rates were about twice as high as those for children and involved more different tooth types, but they were still only a fraction of the nineteenth-century rates. One of the noticeable things about a medieval collection of jaws is how often carious lesions are associated with heavily worn teeth in adults. The main site in these teeth is along the cemento-enamel junction. Moore and Corbett noted that although the cavity was too large to see the initial site of the lesion in many cases, in those cases where this was possible it tended to be the root surface rather than the crown. Carious lesions seem to follow interfaces such as the cemento-enamel junction and enamel–dentine junction. It is, thus, quite common to see lesions in the worn surface of an occlusal wear facet. This would be an uncommon lesion site in twentieth-century clinical practice.

Historical sources make it clear that the main diet of medieval England was bread, with various salad and vegetable foods that would have contributed little to the carbohydrate component (Carlin, 1998; Dyer, 1998). Sugary foods were beyond the reach of most. There are variations around the world, but many other archaeological agriculturalist groups must have been characterized by this high wear rate, high starch, low sugar environment. It can be seen, for example, in the agriculturalists of eastern North America before contact with Europe. Figure 6.3 shows a similar caries distribution throughout the dentition for collections from the US Georgia Bight coastline studied by Larsen *et al.* (1991). They included hunter-gatherer groups before the adoption of agriculture. The later agriculturalists show a very similar distribution of caries to the medieval English, with few lesions in juvenile dentitions and also low rates in adults. They are thought to have practiced maize agriculture, although still supplemented by a range of gathered, hunted, and fished foods. With the arrival of Spanish missionaries (early contact group) there was little change in the pattern of caries, but the late contact group, representing much better established missions, shows much higher rates. The authors of the study suggested that this was due to a greater reliance on maize. The Georgia Bight study shows higher rates than the English medieval assemblages. This may to some extent be due

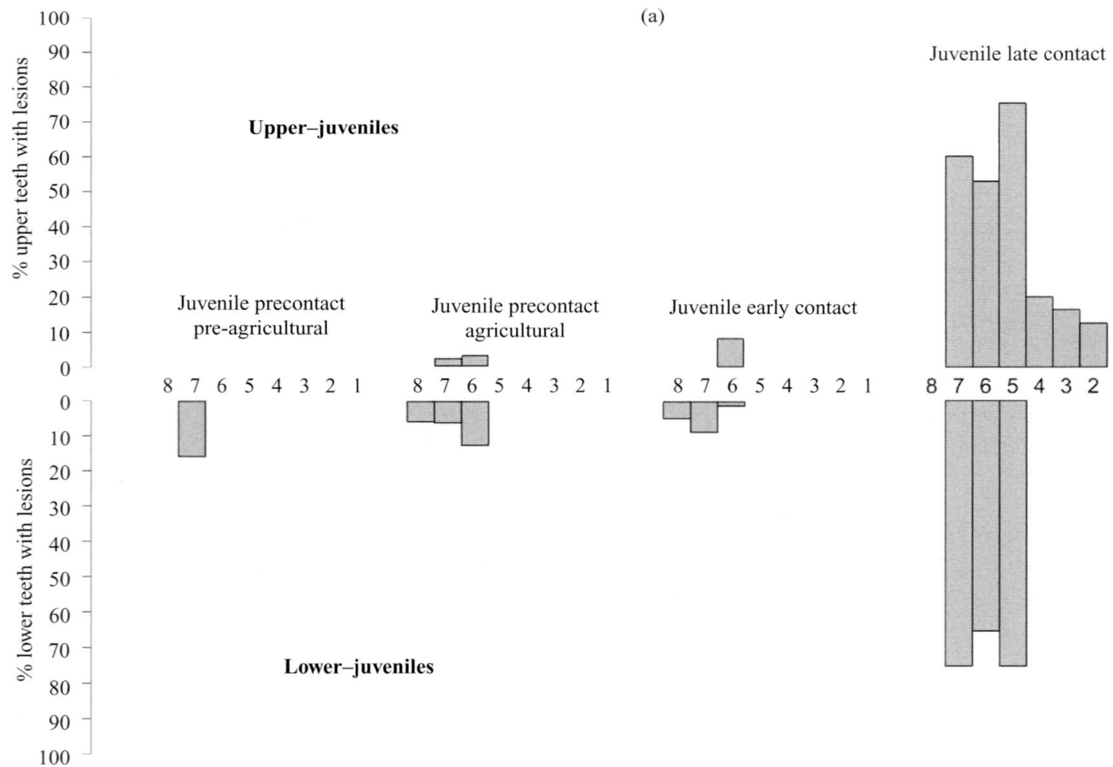

Figure 6.3 Dental caries in different permanent tooth classes (numbered from 8 for third molar to 1 for first incisor) for juveniles (before third molar eruption completed) and adults (after) in archaeological collections from the Georgia Bight, USA. Assemblages from several different sites were combined. Precontact pre-agricultural (1000 BC–AD 1150) comprised 13 different assemblages representing people who fished, hunted, and gathered food from the sea, estuaries, and neighboring land. Precontact agricultural (AD 1150–1550) comprised 11 assemblages representing people who are thought to have used cultivated food. Early contact (AD 1607–1680) is the period of the first Spanish mission outposts and was represented by one site, Santa Catalina de Guale on St Catherines Island. Late contact (AD 1680–1702) is the period in which the missions became more established and was represented by another single site, Santa Cataline de Guale de Santa Maria on Amelia Island.

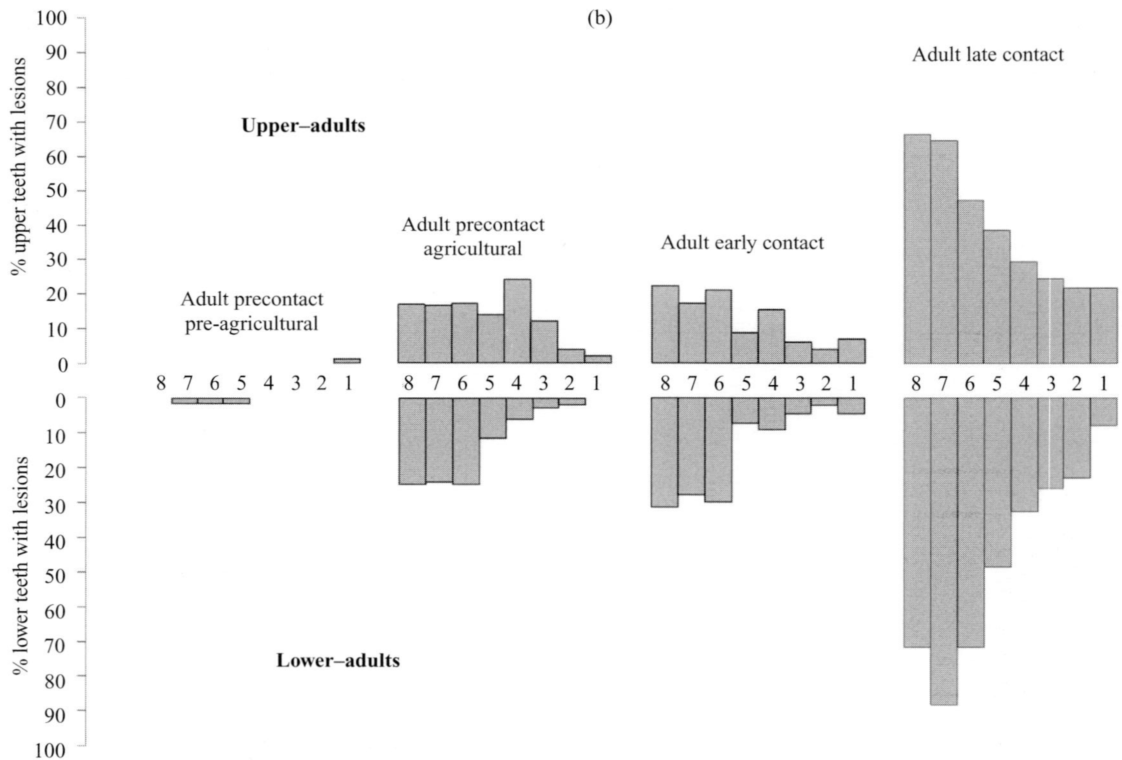

Figure 6.3 (*cont.*)

to different methodology, and in any archaeological study there are variations that may be due to the nature of the collections on which caries rates are based.

6.6 Hunter-gatherer caries

The other observation that can be made from Figure 6.3 is that caries rates were much lower in the pre-agriculturalist hunter-gatherers than in the agriculturalists (even though the latter probably included many hunted and gathered resources in their diet). Before the adoption of agriculture, in which sources of carbohydrate were cultivated, dental caries was a rare condition. Middle and late Pleistocene cases worldwide can be counted on the fingers of two hands. Neandertal examples (Trinkaus *et al.*, 2000) include the Aubesier 5 deciduous upper first molar (Vaucluse, France), the fissures of a third molar in the Banyoles 1 mandible, and the lingual pit of the Kebara 1 upper second incisor (Tillier *et al.*, 1995). Early modern human examples include Qafzeh 3 and Skhul 2 (Soggnaes, 1956), and Upper Palaeolithic examples include Cro-Magnon 4, Les Rois 50–4, Les Rois R51–5 (Trinkaus *et al.*, 2000), the Pavlov 1 third molar, and possibly the Dolní Vestonice 13 first molars (Trinkaus *et al.*, 2001; Trinkaus *et al.*, 2005). The Middle Pleistocene Kabwe (Broken Hill) skull is a completely exceptional case, with gross carious lesions affecting many teeth (Bartsiokas and Day, 1993; Koritzer and St Hoyme, 1979; Puech *et al.*, 1980). Caries is consistently present in Mesolithic and Neolithic dentitions, but only a few percent of potential lesion sites actually have carious lesions (Fitzgerald and Hillson, 2004; Smith, 1972; Smith *et al.*, 1984).

Dentists visited recent hunter-gatherer groups before they adopted a diet based on cultivated carbohydrate-rich plant foods, and wrote detailed accounts. These include the East Greenland (Davies and Pedersen, 1955; Pedersen, 1938, 1947, 1949, 1966) and Canadian Inuit (Costa, 1980a, 1980b, 1982; Mayhall, 1970, 1977, 1978; Tomenchuk and Mayhall, 1979), aborigine people of Central Australia (Barrett, 1953, 1956; Campbell, 1925, 1928, 1937, 1938a, 1938b, 1938c, 1939; Campbell and Barrett, 1953; Campbell and Gray, 1936; Campbell and Lewis, 1926; Campbell and Moore, 1930; Cran, 1959, 1960; Moody, 1960), and the San Bushmen of southern Africa (van Reenen, 1964, 1966, 1982). The experience of dental caries differed widely among groups, depending on the available gathered food resources; however, they all shared one common feature – an extremely rapid rate of tooth wear, even greater than that of the medieval agriculturalists.

The Inuit showed particularly extensive wear so that, by early middle age, the crowns of many teeth had almost completely been lost to wear. Recent hunter-gatherers also showed a strong wear gradient, with greatest wear in the incisors and least in the third molars. Indeed, in dentitions where the incisors were worn down to the roots, the occlusal fissures could still survive in the third molar crowns. This pattern seems to have related to the heavy use made of teeth not only for feeding, but also for holding and making things. Among Inuit who gained most of their nutrition from marine resources and, therefore, had almost no source of carbohydrates, caries was practically non-existent. Rarely, it could be found in the fissures of the little-worn third molars. Teeth were lost when they became worn out. Continuous eruption pushed them up into the mouth as they were worn, and eventually there was only a small fragment of root left that became loose and could be pulled out. Caries and periodontal disease were almost never causes of tooth loss.

The aborigine people of Central Australia studied in the 1920s to 1950s by dentists from the University of Adelaide had a very different experience of caries. While rare in children, it became common in the worn teeth of older adults. Not much detail on the character of the lesions was published, but they appear to have been associated particularly with fractured surfaces rather than root surface lesions. The pulp chambers were frequently exposed, giving rise to chronic periapical inflammatory conditions, although this does not seem to have been associated with tooth loss. The source of carbohydrates in Central Australia seems to have been buried tubers that could be gathered.

San Bushmen studied by Van Reenen (references above) had a similar dental condition and, once again, they gathered buried tubers rich in starch. It is therefore reasonable to suggest that ancient hunter-gatherers might show a similar variation in caries rates. Palaeolithic and Mesolithic assemblages, however, are closest to the Inuit pattern of very low caries rates in all age groups. This implies that they were obtaining very little in the way of gathered starch or sugar-rich foods. It fits well with the stable isotopes evidence that Neandertals and Upper Palaeolithic people in Europe obtained most of their protein from meat and fish. Their isotope signatures look more like those of top carnivores than of omnivores (Richards and Hedges, 2000; Richards *et al.*, 2000, 2001). Once again, this emphasizes how recent a phenomenon the agriculturalist diet is, with its associated pattern of caries.

6.7 Conclusions

In terms of human evolutionary history, dental caries was, for the most part, a rare condition. The oldest known stone artifacts are perhaps 2.5 million years old, and the earliest cereal agriculture in western Asia appeared around 10 000 years ago. It is only after this point in the record that carious lesions appear at all consistently, and this represents 0.4 % of known tool-making history. Before this, it seems that sources of gathered plant foods rich in carbohydrates, or other sources such as honey, were rare or at least not regularly found. Even after the adoption of agriculture with stores of carbohydrate-rich foods providing regular supplies of starch, caries rates for the most part were low and involved adults more than children. The pattern of caries since the nineteenth century, in which many children are affected and there is a lifelong experience of the condition, is even more anomalous (some 0.008 % of tool-making history) and must represent the ready availability of foods containing refined sugar.

References

Barrett, M. J. (1953). Dental observations on Australian aborigines: Yuendumu, Central Australia, 1951–52. *Australian Journal of Dentistry*, **57**, 127–38.

Barrett, M. J. (1956). Dental observations on Australian aborigines: water supplies and endemic dental fluorosis. *Australian Dental Journal*, **1**, 87–92.

Bartsiokas, A., and Day, M. C. (1993). Lead poisoning and dental caries in the Broken Hill hominid. *Journal of Human Evolution*, **24**, 243–9.

Batchelor, P. A. and Sheiham, A. (2004). Grouping of tooth surfaces by susceptibility to caries: a study in 5–16-year-old children. *BMC Oral Health*, 4(2).

Bowen, W. H., and Pearson, S. K. (1993). Effect of milk on cariogenesis. *Caries Research*, **27**, 461–6.

Brothwell, D. R. (1989). The relationship of tooth wear to aging. In *Age Markers in the Human Skeleton*, ed. M. Y. Iscan. Springfield: Charles C. Thomas, pp. 303–16.

Campbell, T. D. (1925). *Dentition and Palate of the Australian Aboriginal*. Publications under the Keith Sheridan Foundation. Adelaide: University of Adelaide.

Campbell, T. D. (1928). Adelaide University field anthropology: Central Australia, No. 5, dental notes. *Transactions of the Royal Society of Southern Australia*, **52**, 28.

Campbell, T. D. (1937). Dental observations on the teeth of Australian aborigines, Hermannsberg, Central Australia. *Australian Journal of Dentistry*, **41**, 1–6.

Campbell, T. D. (1938a). Observations on the teeth of Australian aborigines, Cockatoo Creek, Central Australia. *Australian Journal of Dentistry*, **42**, 41.

Campbell, T. D. (1938b). Observations on the teeth of Australian aborigines, Mount Liebig, Central Australia. *Australian Journal of Dentistry*, **42**, 85.

Campbell, T. D. (1938c). Observations on the teeth of Australian aborigines, River Diamantina, South Australia. *Australian Journal of Dentistry*, **42**, 121.

Campbell, T. D. (1939). Food, food values and food habits of the Australian aborigines: a changing environment and food pattern. *Australian Journal of Dentistry*, **43**, 1–15.

Campbell, T. D. and Barrett, M. J. (1953). Dental observations on Australian aborigines: a changing environment and food pattern. *Australian Dental Journal*, **57**, 1–6.

Campbell, T. D. and Gray, J. H. (1936). Observations on the teeth of Australian aborigines. *Australian Journal of Dentistry*, **40**, 290–5.

Campbell, T. D. and Lewis, A. J. (1926). The aborigines of South Australia: dental observations recorded at Ooldea. *Australian Journal of Dentistry*, **30**, 371.

Campbell, T. D. and Moore, A. P. R. (1930). Adelaide University Field Anthropology, Koonibba, South Australia, dental notes. *Australian Journal of Dentistry*, **34**, 123–7.

Carlin, M. (1998). Fast food and urban living standards in medieval Europe. In *Food and Eating in Medieval Europe*, ed. M. Carlin and J. T. Rosenthal. London: Hambledon Press, pp. 27–51.

Carvalho, J. C., D'Hoore, W., and Van Nieuwenhuysen, J. P. (2004). Caries decline in the primary dentition of Belgian children over 15 years. *Community Dentistry and Oral Epidemiology*, **32**, 277–82.

Corbett, M. E., and Moore, W. J. (1976). Distribution of dental caries in ancient British populations: IV The nineteenth century. *Caries Research*, **10**, 401–14.

Costa, R. L. (1980a). Age, sex, and antemortem loss of teeth in prehistoric Eskimo skeletal samples from Point Hope and Kodiak Island, Alaska. *American Journal of Physical Anthropology*, **53**, 579–87.

Costa, R. L. (1980b). Incidence of caries and abscesses in archeological Eskimo skeletal samples from Point Hope and Kodiak Island, Alaska. *American Journal of Physical Anthropology*, **52**, 501–14.

Costa, R. L. (1982). Periodontal disease in the prehistoric Ipiutak and Tigara skeletal remains from Point Hope, Alaska. *American Journal of Physical Anthropology*, **59**, 97–110.

Cran, J. A. (1959). The relationship of diet to dental caries. *Australian Dental Journal*, **4**, 182–90.

Cran, J. A. (1960). The histological structure of the teeth of Central Australian aborigines and the relationship to dental caries incidence. *Australian Dental Journal*, **5**, 100–4.

Davies, T. G. H. and Pedersen, P. O. (1955). The degree of attrition of the deciduous teeth and the first permanent molars of primitive and urbanised Greenland natives. *British Dental Journal*, **99**, 35–43.

Dyer, C. (1998). Did the peasants really starve in Medieval Europe. In *Food and Eating in Medieval Europe*, ed. M. Carlin and J. T. Rosenthal. London: Hambledon Press, pp. 53–72.

Evans, R. W. and Lo, E. C. M. (1992). Effects of school dental care service in Hong Kong – primary teeth. *Community Dentistry and Oral Epidemiology*, **20**, 193–5.

Fitzgerald, C. M. and Hillson, S. W. (2004). Testing hypotheses for dental reduction in Late Pleistocene and Early Holocene hominids. *American Journal of Physical Anthropology*, **Suppl. 38**, 95.

Food Standards Agency and Institute of Food Research. (2002). *McCance and Widdowson's The Composition of Foods*, 6th edn. Cambridge: Royal Society of Chemistry.

Garrow, J. S., James, W. P. T., and Ralph, N. G. A. (2000). *Human Nutrition and Dietetics*. Edinburgh: Churchill Livingstone.

Hillson, S. (1996). *Dental Anthropology*. Cambridge, Cambridge University Press.

Hillson, S. W. (2000). Dental pathology. In *Biological Anthropology of the Human Skeleton*, ed. M. A. Katzenberg and S. R. Saunders. New York: John Wiley & Sons, Inc., pp. 249–86.

Hillson, S. W. (2001). Recording dental caries in archaeological human remains. *International Journal of Osteoarchaeology*, **11**, 249–89.

Hoppenbrouwers, P. M. M., Driessens, F. C. M., and Borggreven, J. M. P. M. (1987). The mineral solubility of human tooth roots. *Archives of Oral Biology*, **32**, 319–22.

Jones, S. J. and Boyde, A. (1987). Scanning microscopic observations on dental caries. *Scanning Microscopy*, **1**, (1991–2002).

Källestål, C., and Wall, S. (2002). Socio-economic effect on caries. Incidence data among Swedish 12–14-year-olds. *Community Dentistry and Oral Epidemiology*, **30**, 108–14.

Koritzer, R. T., and St Hoyme, L. E. (1979). Extensive caries in early man circa 110 000 years before present. *Journal of the American Dental Association*, **99**, 642–3.

Larsen, C. S., Shavit, R., and Griffin, M. C. (1991). Dental caries evidence for dietary change: an archaeological context. In *Advances in Dental Anthropology*, ed. M. A. Kelley, and C. S. Larsen. New York: Wiley-Liss, pp. 179–202.

Leek, F. F. (1972). Teeth and bread in ancient Egypt. *Journal of Egyptian Archaeology*, **58**, 126–32.

Lenander-Lumikari, M., and Loimaranta, V. (2000). Saliva and dental caries. *Advances in Dental Research*, **14**, 40–7.

Lingström, P., van Houte, J., and Kasuya, T. (2000). Food starches and dental caries. *Critical Reviews in Oral Biology and Medicine*, **11**, 366–80.

Locker, D. (2000). Deprivation and oral health: a review. *Community Dentistry and Oral Epidemiology*, **28**, 161–9.

Manji, F., Fejerskov, O., and Baelum, V. (1989). Pattern of dental caries in an adult rural population. *Caries Research*, **23**, 55–62.

Manji, F., Fejerskov, O., Baelum, V., Luan, W. M., and Chen, X. (1991). The epidemiological features of dental caries in African and Chinese populations: implications for risk assessment. In *Volume 1. Dental Caries. Markers of High and Low Risk Groups and Individuals Risk Markers for Oral Diseases*, ed. N. W. Johnson. Cambridge: Cambridge University Press, pp. 62–9.

Marsh, P., and Martin, M. (1992). *Oral Microbiology*, 3rd edn. London: Chapman and Hall.

Mayhall, J. T. (1970). The effect of culture change upon the Eskimo dentition. *Arctic Anthropology*, **7**, 117.

Mayhall, J. T. (1977). Cultural and environmental influences on the Eskimo dentition. In *Orofacial Growth and Development*, ed. A. A. Dahlberg and T. M. Graber. The Hague: Mouton, pp. 215–27.

Mayhall, J. T. (1978). Canadian Inuit caries experience 1969–73. *Journal of Dental Research*, **54**, 1245.

Mellanby, M. (1934). *Diet and Teeth: An Experimental Study. Part III. The Effect of Diet on the Dental Structure and Disease in Man.* Medical Research Council, Special Report Series, No 191. London: His Majesty's Stationery Office.

Miles, A. E. W. (1958). The assessment of age from the dentition. *Proceedings of the Royal Society of Medicine*, **51**, 1057–60.

Miles, A. E. W. (1962). Assessment of the ages of a population of Anglo-Saxons from their dentitions. *Proceedings of the Royal Society of Medicine*, **55**, 881–6.

Moody, J. E. H. (1960). The dental and periodontal conditions of aborigines at settlements in Arnhem Land and adjacent areas. In *Records of the*

American-Australian Scientific Expedition to Arnhem Land: Anthropology and Nutrition, ed. C. R. Mountford. Melbourne: Melbourne University Press, pp. 60–71.

Moore, W. J. and Corbett, M. E. (1971). Distribution of dental caries in ancient British populations: I Anglo-Saxon period. *Caries Research*, **5**, 151–68.

Moore, W. J. and Corbett, M. E. (1973). Distribution of dental caries in ancient British populations: II Iron Age, Romano-British and Medieval periods. *Caries Research*, **7**, 139–53.

Moore, W. J., and Corbett, M. E. (1975). Distribution of dental caries in ancient British populations: III The 17th Century. *Caries Research*, **9**, 163–175.

Mörmann J. E. and Mühlemann H. R. (1981). Oral starch degradation and its influence on acid production in human dental plaque. *Caries Research*, **15**, 166–75.

Mundorff, S. A., Featherstone, J. D. B., Bibby, B. G. *et al.* (1990). Cariogenic potential of foods. I. Caries in the rat model. *Caries Research*, **24**, 344–55.

Mundorff-Shrestha, S. A., Featherstone, J. D. B., Eisenberg, A. D. *et al.* (1994) Cariogenic potential of foods. II. Relationship of food composition, plaque microbial counts, and salivary parameters to caries in the rat model. *Caries Research*, **28**, 106–15.

Navia, J. M. (1994). Carbohydrates and dental health. *American Journal of Clinical Nutrition*, **59**, 719S–27S.

Pedersen, P. O. (1938). Investigations into the dental conditions of about 3000 ancient and modern Greenlanders. *Dental Record*, **58**, 191–8.

Pedersen, P. O. (1947). Dental investigations of Greenland Eskimos. *Proceedings of the Royal Society of Medicine*, **40**, 726–32.

Pedersen, P. O. (1949). The East Greenland Eskimo dentition. *Meddelelser om Grønland*, **142**, 1–244.

Pedersen, P. O. (1966). Nutritional aspects of dental caries. *Odontologisk Revy*, **17**, 91–100.

Peres, M. A., Latorre, M. R. D. O., Sheiham, A. *et al.* (2005). Social and biological early life influences on severity of dental caries in children aged 6 years. *Community Dentistry and Oral Epidemiology*, **33**, 53–63.

Pine, C. M. and ten Bosch, J. J. (1996). Dynamics of and diagnostic methods for detecting small carious lesions. *Caries Research*, **30**, 381–8.

Puech, P. F., Albertini, H., and Mills, N. T. W. (1980). Dental destruction in the Broken-Hill man. *Journal of Human Evolution*, **9**, 33–9.

Richards, M. P. and Hedges, R. E. M. (2000). FOCUS: Gough's Cave and Sun Hole Cave human stable isotope values indicate a high animal protein diet in the British Upper Palaeolithic. *Journal of Archaeological Science*, **27**, 1–3.

Richards, M. P., Pettitt, P. B., Stiner, M. C., and Trinkaus, E. (2001). Stable isotope evidence for increasing dietary breadth in the European mid Upper Paleolithic. *Proceedings of the National Academy of Sciences USA*, **98**, 6528–32.

Richards, M. P., Pettitt, P. B., Trinkaus, E. *et al.* (2000). Neanderthal diet at Vindija and Neanderthal predation: the evidence from stable isotopes. *Proceedings of the National Academy of Sciences USA*, **97**, 7663–6.

Rugg-Gunn, A. J. (1993). *Nutrition and Dental Caries*. Oxford Medical Publications. Oxford: Oxford University Press.

Sánchez-Castillo, C. P., Dewey, P. J. S., Lara, J. J. *et al.* (2000). The starch and sugar content of some Mexican cereals, cereal products, pulses, snack foods, fruits and vegetables. *Journal of Food Composition and Analysis*, **13**, 157–170.

Schamschula, R. G., Barmes, D. E., Keyes, P. H., and Gulbinat, W. (1978). *WHO Study of Dental Caries Etiology in Papua New Guinea*. Publication 40. Geneva: World Health Organization.

Schüpbach, P., Lutz, F., and Guggenheim, B. (1992). Human root caries: histopathology of arrested lesions. *Caries Research*, **26**, 153–64.

Sheiham, A. (1983). Sugars in dental decay. *Lancet*, **1**, 282–4.

Sheiham, A. (1997). Impact of dental treatment on the incidence of dental caries in children and adults. *Community Dentistry and Oral Epidemiology*, **25**, 104–12.

Skeie, M. S., Raadal, M., Strand, G. V., and Espelid, I. (2006). The relationship between caries in the primary dentition at 5 years of age and permanent dentition at 10 years of age – a longitudinal study. *International Journal of Paediatric Dentistry*, **16**, 152–60.

Smith, P. (1972). Diet and attrition in the Natufians. *American Journal of Physical Anthropology*, **37**, 233–8.

Smith, P., Bar-Yosef, O., and Sillen, A. (1984). Archaeological and skeletal evidence for dietary change during the late Pleistocene/early Holocene in the Levant. In *Palaeopathology at the Origins of Agriculture*, ed. M. N. Cohen and G. J. Armelagos. New York: Academic Press, pp. 101–36.

Soggnaes, R. F. (1956). Histological evidence of developmental lesions in teeth originating from Paleolithic, prehistoric, and ancient man. *American Journal of Pathology*, **32**, 547–77.

Thomson, W. M., Poulton, R., Milne, B. J. *et al.* (2004). Socioeconomic inequalities in oral health in childhood and adulthood in a birth cohort. *Community Dentistry and Oral Epidemiology*, **32**, 345–53.

Thylstrup, A., and Fejerskov, O. (1994). *Textbook of Clinical Cariology*. Copenhagen: Munksgaard.

Tillier, A. M., Arensburg, B., Rak, Y., and Vandermeersch, B. (1995). Middle Palaeolithic dental caries: new evidence from Kebara Mount Carmel, Israel. *Journal of Human Evolution*, **29**, 189–92.

Tomenchuk, J. and Mayhall, J. T. (1979). A correlation of tooth wear and age among modern Igloolik Eskimos. *American Journal of Physical Anthropology*, **51**, 67–78.

Trinkaus, E., Formicola, V., Svoboda, J., Hillson, S. W., and Holliday, T. W. (2001). Dolní Vestonice 15: Pathology and persistence in the Pavlovian. *Journal of Archaeological Science*, **28**, 1291–1308.

Trinkaus, E., Hillson, S. W., Franciscus, R. G., and Holliday, T. W. (2005). Skeletal and dental paleopathology. In *Early Modern Human Evolution in Central Europe*, Human Evolution Series, ed. E. Trinkaus and J. Svoboda. Oxford: Oxford University Press, pp. 419–58.

Trinkaus, E., Smith, R. J., and Lebel, S. (2000). Dental caries in the Aubesier 5 Neandertal primary molar. *Journal of Archaeological Science*, **27**, 1017–21.

van Houte, J. (1994). Role of micro-organisms in caries etiology. *Journal of Dental Research*, **73**, 305–26.

van Reenen, J. F. (1964). Dentition, jaws and palate of the Kalahari Bushman. *Journal of the Dental Association of South Africa*, **19**, 1–44, 67.
van Reenen, J. F. (1966). Dental features of a low-caries primitive population. *Journal of Dental Research*, **45**, 703–13.
Van Reenen, J. F. (1982). The effects of attrition on tooth dimensions of San Bushmen. In *Teeth: Form, Function, and Evolution*, ed. B. Kurtén. New York: Columbia University Press, pp. 182–203.
Whittaker, D. K., Daniel, A. T., Williams, J. T., Rose, P., and Resteghini, R. (1985). Quantitative assessment of tooth wear, alveolar-crest height and continuing eruption in a Romano-British population. *Archives of Oral Biology*, **30**, 493–501.
Whittaker, D. K., Griffiths, S., Robson, A., Roger Davies, P., and Thomas, G. (1990). Continuing tooth eruption and alveolar-crest height in an eighteenth-century population from Spitalfields, East London. *Archives of Oral Biology*, **35**, 81–5.
Whittaker, D. K., Parker, J. H., and Jenkins, C. (1982). Tooth attrition and continuing eruption in a Romano-British population. *Archives of Oral Biology*, **27**, 405–9.
Williams, R. A. D. and Elliott, J. C. (1989). *Basic and Applied Dental Biochemistry*. 2nd edn. Dental Series. Edinburgh: Churchill Livingstone.

7 *Dental caries prevalence by sex in prehistory: magnitude and meaning*

JOHN R. LUKACS AND LINDA M. THOMPSON

7.1 Introduction

The focus of this chapter is to determine if there is a significant relationship between sex and oral disease in human prehistory.[1] The idea that dental caries prevalence may be etiologically complex and multifactorial in nature is not new (Mandel, 1979). Nevertheless, significant advances in understanding the mechanisms of cariogenesis continue (Featherstone, 1987, 2000), and the epidemiological study of dental caries continues to broaden, embracing geographically and culturally more diverse populations. Less widely appreciated is the frequently reported finding that females display worse dental health than males, especially in epidemiological studies of living populations (Haugejorden, 1996). While some anthropologists are well aware of the tendency for women to exhibit worse dental health than men (Larsen, 1998; Walker and Hewlett, 1990), a systematic global survey of sex differences in dental pathology in prehistory has not been conducted. The present meta-analysis tested for a gender bias in oral health by gathering, critically evaluating, and statistically summarizing data on sex differences in dental caries for a global sample of early historic and prehistoric skeletal series.

A recent evaluation of the etiological role of saliva, sex hormones, and women's reproductive life histories highlighted sex differences in dental prevalence for the Guanches of Tenerife, in the Canary Islands (Lukacs and Largaespada, 2006). This meta-analysis of sex differences in caries prevalence derives directly from the first author's research in South Asia and the Canary Islands, which found that females' caries rates were consistently greater than that of males (Lukacs, 1996). The goal here is to determine if dental caries rates in past populations are consistently sex dimorphic, with females routinely tending to exceed males in caries prevalence. Will the results of an extensive global survey of prehistoric samples support or contradict the assertion that "[c]aries is more common in women than men and shows a stronger age-related development" (Hillson, 2000, p. 263)? Do studies of dental health conducted on skeletal

Technique and Application in Dental Anthropology ed. Joel D. Irish and Greg C. Nelson
Published by Cambridge University Press.

samples from different continents, cultures, and time periods reveal a systematic patterning by sex? If results of the present study are consistent with the expectation of a female bias, then consideration will be given to recent developments in understanding the multifactorial nature of caries etiology. Emphasis will focus on etiological factors that have an evolutionary basis and involve reproductive function, relative fertility, and hormonal fluctuations – factors that may synergistically predispose women to poorer oral health and higher caries rates than men.

Epidemiological surveys of dental caries in living populations consistently report higher mean age-specific scores for decayed, missing, and filled teeth (DMFT) for women than for men (Sauerwein, 1974). This differential expression by sex has been recognized by dental anthropologists. "In almost all clinical studies of caries, females show higher rates than males, and there frequently seems to be a bias against the burial and survival of female remains in archaeology" (Hillson, 2000, p. 261). The extent of this gender bias in dental caries in modern populations may be unknown or unappreciated among many biological anthropologists. For example, a meta-analysis of sex differences in dental caries experience using the D(M)FT[2] index revealed that between 1946 and 1959, in the "pre-fluoride era," nine separate clinical research teams reporting on six age groups (12 through 17 years) consistently found that females had higher D(M)FT scores (10.1, $n = 4496$) than males (8.7, $n = 4281$). After standardizing percentages to control for differences in age distribution, the relative gender difference in D(M)FT was 16.8 % (Haugejorden, 1996). The same study reported mean D(M)FT scores for a "post-fluoride" (1983–93) era sample, with similar results. In the post-fluoride sample, nine different clinical research teams reported on a Euro-American sample of 12–17 year olds and found that females (5.7, $n = 19\,674$) consistently out-scored men (4.9, $n = 20\,229$) in mean D(M)FT; the relative gender difference was 13.7 % after standardizing for heterogeneity in age and sample size – only slightly less than in the earlier study. Is the female bias in caries experience – so clearly documented by clinical researchers like Haugejorden – unambiguously evident in documents describing dental health among prehistoric peoples of the world? Knowledge of whether dental caries prevalence by sex is geographically uniform or displays significant variability in space and time may inform us of the relative contribution that different factors make to the observed prevalence patterns. We contend that now is an opportune time to conduct a meta-analysis on dental caries prevalence by sex in prehistory because new and more detailed reports on the paleopathology of poorly known regions are now available (Cohen, 2007; Oxenham and Tayles, 2006). Furthermore, the clinical samples included in Haugejorden's (1996) large survey were predominantly adolescent Americans and Europeans and from industrialized nations. We recognize the need for a similar survey of dental caries rates by sex among non-industrial, non-Western populations representing a wide range of different natural and cultural settings. Such a study of sex differences in dental caries prevalence among a global sample of living population from rural and urban settings is now in progress.

7.2 Materials and methods

This study relies upon the original research of investigators whose goals include documenting the oral health of early historic and prehistoric people from the prevalence of pathological lesions of the teeth and jaws. The objectives of such studies are wide ranging, and may include an understanding of the relationship between oral health and a variety of inter-related variables including: ecology, subsistence, and diet. Differences in the frequency of dental diseases in past populations are often studied with the objective of understanding how similar or different the living conditions and general health were among sub-groups of a population, such as citizens and slaves (Sakashita *et al.*, 1997), urban and rural communities (Henneberg, 1998), citizens vs. warrior Samurai (Oyamada *et al.*, 2004), and high versus low status groups (Cucina and Tiesler, 2003). This meta-analysis is based on data from the published literature on dental health in prehistory, and from personal research on dental health in prehistoric South Asia. Any such broad-based comparative analysis risks criticism on several critical issues. A study of the type we conducted must be concerned with aspects of sample size and composition, as well as methodological issues related to data collection and analysis. In scrutinizing each study, special attention was given to: (1) sample size and composition, (2) data collection, and (3) data analysis.

With regard to the first component, the size and representativeness of the entire sample, relative equality of sub-samples by sex, and demographic aspects of male and female sub-samples – especially age structure – were evaluated. For the second, evidence of the researcher's precision in the recognition and diagnosis of caries lesions is often not explicitly stated (no assessment of intra-observer variance). A wide range of methods is used to report dental caries rates, and the basis for calculating caries prevalence is not always described in detail, nor are the methods used routinely identified. Lastly, with regard to the third component, inter-group comparative assessment using data gathered by different researchers rarely addresses the potentially significant issue of inter-observer variance (Jackes and Lubell, 1996). In Southeast Asia, for example, a high level of inter-observer consistency is evident in data for the same series by different observers (Domett, 2001; Tayles, 1999; Tayles *et al.*, 2000), while reports on dental caries among Mesolithic Iberian samples reveal significant differences between investigators (Frayer, 1987; Jackes and Lubell, 1996). Statistical methods are not routinely employed in evaluating the significance of sex differences in caries prevalence. The diversity of statistical techniques may

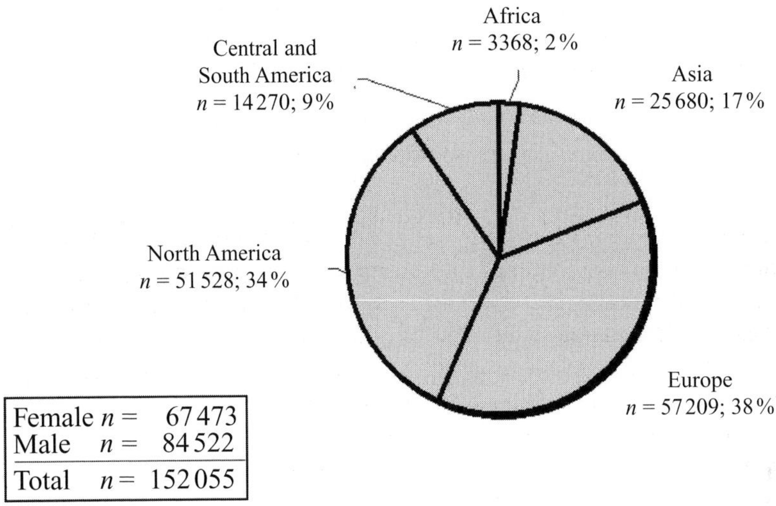

Figure 7.1 Dental sample by continent.

involve the application of inappropriate methods or render direct comparison of results problematic.

The size and composition of samples in studies comprising this meta-analysis are depicted in Figures 7.1 and 7.2. The number of teeth observed by investigators in each continent is presented proportionately with pie chart (Figure 7.1). The relative representation of female and male samples is given in Figure 7.2, which shows that male dental samples consistently outnumber those of females in many studies included here. Whether the preponderance of males represents a bias against the burial and survival of female remains in archaeological sites, or a methodological bias toward sexing remains as male, is unknown.

Approximately one-third of the studies consulted for this survey do not report dental caries prevalence by sex. Justification for omitting sex as a variable in the analysis is frequently not provided (Cornero and Puche, 2000; Maczel *et al.*, 1997; Thornton 1995; Vodanovic *et al.*, 2005), yet in many cases poor preservation, postmortem damage, or incompleteness of specimens precludes accurate sex estimation (Kerr *et al.*, 1988, 1990; Reeves, 2000; Watt, *et al.*, 1997). Several analyses report no significant sex difference in the frequency or type of dental caries, yet neither sex-specific caries rates nor results of the statistical analysis are presented (Molnar and Molnar, 1985; Schollmeyer and Turner, 2004; Smith, 2000).

When caries prevalence is reported by sex, statistical analysis is often omitted from analysis, and small differences in caries rates are reported as firm

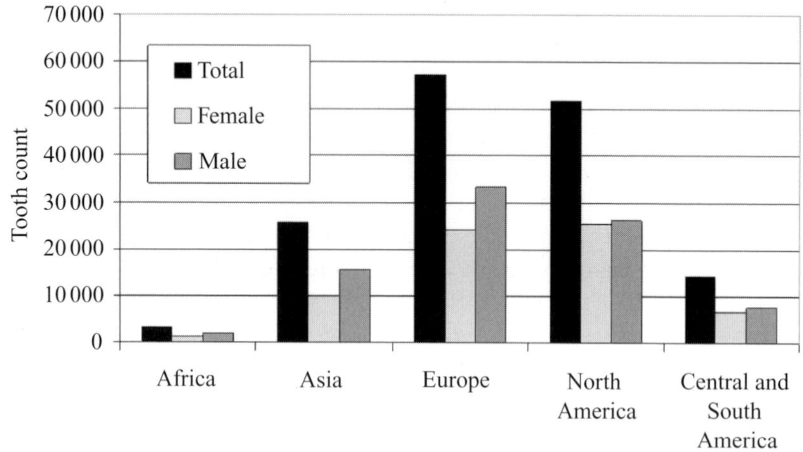

Figure 7.2 Dental sample by sex.

or unequivocal evidence of meaningful inter-sex variation in oral pathology (Hutchinson, 2004; Yu-Zhu 1982). Frequently, assertions of a sex difference in caries rate are found to be unsubstantiated when a chi-square (χ^2) test of independence is administered. A skeptical investigator wishing to statistically test data reported by others may be stymied in completing an analysis because caries data often are incompletely presented.

We followed five main steps in conducting this meta-analysis:

(1) The anthropological, archaeological, and clinical literature was searched for reports on dental health in early historic and prehistoric skeletal samples that might contain data on dental caries. The prime criterion was that reports presented dental caries data by sex.
(2) Analytical methods and techniques used in observing and recording dental caries data were reviewed for agreement with standardized and widely accepted methods (i.e. Hillson, 2000; Hillson, 2001; Lukacs, 1989).
(3) Data on dental caries prevalence were included in the analysis only if the methods of reporting were clearly and explicitly stated, and sample size was clearly specified.
(4) Data on caries rates by sex were entered into an Excel database in three ways:
    (a) The tooth count method. The most common method for reporting caries prevalence is also the most basic; the numbers of carious teeth, total teeth, and percentage with caries are entered by sex. This method often included variations that enhanced precision for reporting of caries frequency including, for example, by

tooth class (I, C, P, M), tooth group (anterior, posterior), or jaw (maxilla, mandible). Additional precision was achieved by reporting of carious lesions by tooth surface (occlusal, mesial, distal, bucco-lingual; interproximal, etc.), size (pin-point, one-quarter, half, three-quarters, or entire crown destroyed) and location (fissure, coronal, cervical, root). Data were systematically reduced to composite summary rates for female and male samples.

(b) The corrected tooth count method. Various reporting methods attempt to accommodate and correct for antemortem tooth loss or differential representation (taphonomic) or susceptibility to caries of different tooth groups (Costa, 1980; Duyar and Erdal, 2003; Erdal and Duyar 1999; Lukacs, 1995). The application of such methods requires unjustifiable assumptions; however, other techniques require few assumptions, are sensitive to differences in subsistence, and are population specific. Caries correction factors may require more detailed observation, diagnosis of non-carious dental lesions, and data collection than some investigators typically employ. Yet increased attention to detail is essential, since the etiological pathway to antemortem tooth loss can only be inferred from a study sample when the complex and interrelated processes of dental disease are understood (Lukacs, 1995). We believe that correction factors yield more precise estimates of true caries rates, especially in groups suffering from high rates of AMTL. No attempt was made to assess the appropriateness of caries correction factors, except to determine whether investigators systematically applied such methods to both sexes. When studies reported caries rates using both methods (i.e. observed tooth count and corrected caries rate), we examined the sex-specific results of each for level of agreement.

(c) The individual prevalence method. In addition to one or both of the above methods, many studies report results of caries by individual (specimen). In this method, caries prevalence is calculated from the number of individuals afflicted with one or more caries divided by the number of individuals in the study group. This method is most appropriate and yields the most accurate results when applied to large and well preserved skeletal series comprised of complete specimens. As specimens become more fragmentary and poorly preserved, the method becomes less useful and may be misleading. In fragmentary remains, the label "individual" may apply to specimens with as many as 32 teeth, or as few as one or two teeth. In such cases, the individual method then becomes unreliable and potentially biased, and the tooth count is preferred because of its greater accuracy and potential for statistical analysis (Douglas, 2006).

(5) The analysis of data for sex differences in caries prevalence was then conducted using the following approach. If the original report did not test for significant sex differences in caries rates, we applied the standard χ^2 test of independence (or Fisher's Exact Test if $n < 5$ for any cell) using SAS – PC 9.1. The apparent sex difference in caries rate was compared with the outcome of the test of independence. Next, samples were sorted by country and by continent, and descriptive statistics were computed for mean caries prevalence by sex. Summary statistics were compiled by sex for each caries reporting method separately (using the data analysis package in Excel). Descriptive statistics were then computed for the global sample, for composite New and Old World samples, and for each continental sample. A paired-samples, one-tailed t-test was used to test for significant differences in mean caries prevalence by sex. The analysis was conducted for each reporting method, and separately for samples grouped by country, by hemisphere (Old and New World samples), and for the pooled global sample.

7.3 Results

The results are presented in three parts. First, the analysis of tooth count caries data are presented. Second, the findings of the individual count analysis are described. Finally, we present an in-depth analysis of caries prevalence from Asia to illustrate general patterns and the effect of using the caries correction factor.

7.3.1 Tooth count caries prevalence by sex

Mean dental caries prevalence is presented by sex for continental samples in Table 7.1 and Figure 7.3; the sites, data, and sources from which data were culled are listed in Appendix 7.1. The number of reports that could be included in the analysis is comparable for Asia ($n = 43$), Europe ($n = 38$), and North America ($n = 44$), and represents a broad geographical and temporal array of archaeological sites. By contrast, Africa ($n = 9$) and Central and South America ($n = 12$) are not as well represented. Figure 7.3 reveals that for all continental samples, the mean caries prevalence for females is greater than for males. In Africa and Europe, the inter-sex difference is small and not significant, while in Asia, North America, and Central and South America, the sex difference in caries is significantly higher among females (t-test results in Table 7.1). For continental samples, mean caries prevalence among females averages 3.6 % greater than in males, and ranges from a low of 0.8 % (Europe) to a high of 5.4 %

Table 7.1 *Mean dental caries prevalence by sex and continent (tooth count, observed)*

			Female		Male		Statistical test	
	Raw sex diff.	n	0 %	Var.	0 %	Var.	one-tail, P_t	Result
Old World								
Africa	F > M	9	13.3	0.015	8.5	0.004	0.0828	F = M
Asia	F > M	43	10.9	0.009	8.1	0.007	0.0011	F > M
Europe	F > M	38	9.5	0.003	8.7	0.003	0.0678	F = M
OW summary	F > M	90	10.4	0.007	8.6	0.005	0.0005	F > M
New World								
North America	F > M	44	15.5	0.016	11.5	0.008	0.0001	F > M
Central and South America	F > M	14	15.1	0.009	9.7	0.002	0.0053	F > M
NW summary	F > M	58	15.5	0.014	11.1	0.007	<0.0000	F > M
Global sample	F > M	142	12.5	0.011	9.7	0.006	<0.0000	F > M

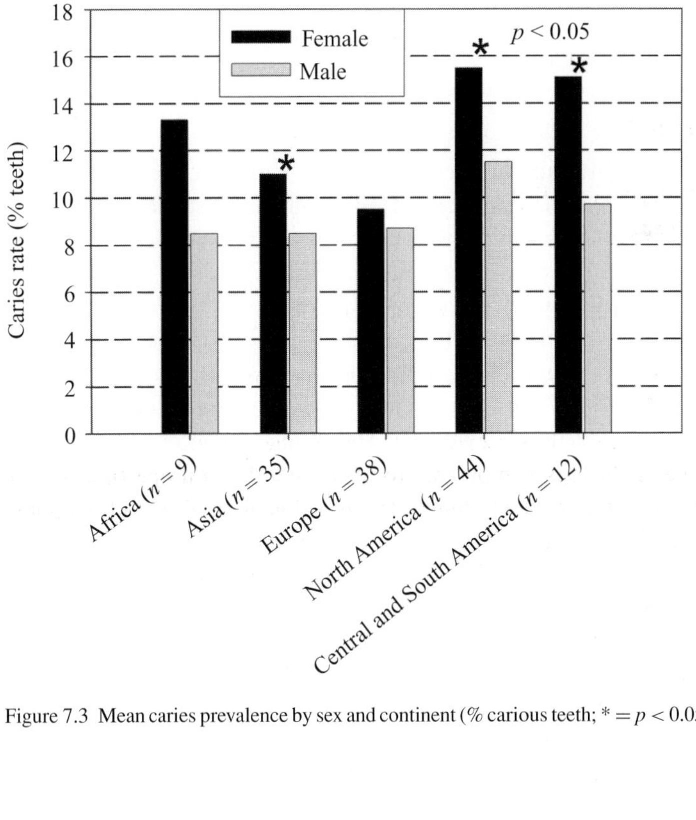

Figure 7.3 Mean caries prevalence by sex and continent (% carious teeth; * = $p < 0.05$).

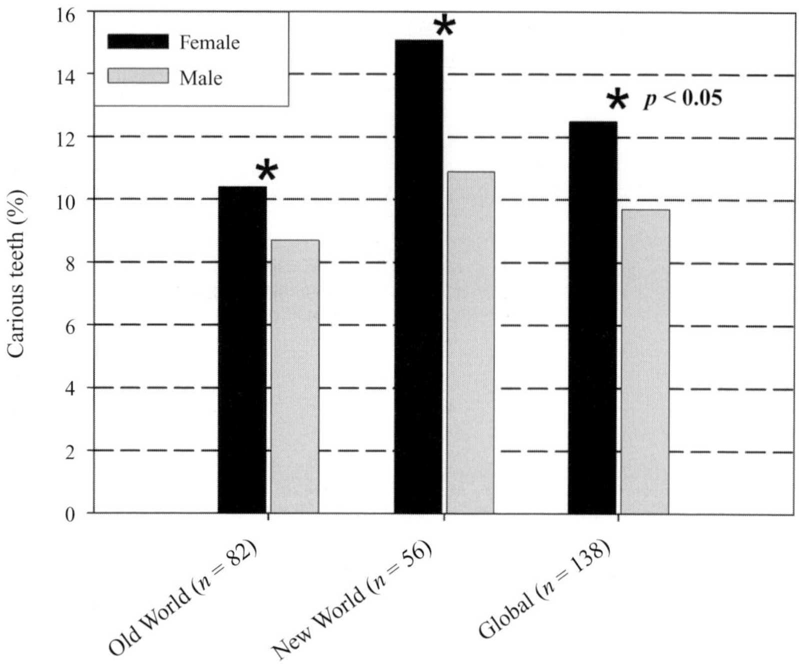

Figure 7.4 Mean caries prevalence: global summary (% carious teeth; * = $p < 0.05$).

(Central and South America). The sex difference in caries for the African sample is large (F – M = 4.8 %), but does not attain statistical significance due to the small sample size and high variance for the female caries rate. The European sample exhibits the smallest difference in mean caries prevalence by sex.

Continental samples were pooled and analyzed by hemisphere and as a global composite sample in Table 7.1 and Figure 7.4. This comparison reveals that females have significantly higher mean caries prevalence than males in pooled Old and New World samples, and in the composite global sample. All differences are statistically significant, and females display caries rates that are 1.8 % (Old World) to 4.4 % (New World) higher than males (see Table 7.1 for data and test results). These data provide strong support for the existence of a sex difference in dental caries prevalence in early historic and prehistoric human populations. While caries rates based on tooth count observation have numerous limitations that make direct comparison between studies problematic, we find the presence of a consistently patterned sex difference in different continents and time periods convincing. Furthermore, like other investigators we regard estimates of caries prevalence based on the tooth count method amenable to statistical analysis due to enhanced sample sizes and, consequently, a more reliable

Table 7.2 *Mean dental caries prevalence by sex and continent (individuals)*

	Raw sex diff.	n	Female 0%	Female Var.	Male 0%	Male Var.	Statistical test one-tail, P_t	Statistical test Result
Old World								
Africa	F < M	7	37.0	0.030	37.7	0.072	0.4376	F = M
Asia	F > M	18	53.3	0.030	49.2	0.022	0.1495	F = M
Europe	F > M	19	52.6	0.069	45.9	0.040	0.0229	F > M
OW summary	F > M	44	50.4	0.049	45.8	0.036	0.0198	F > M
New World								
North America	F > M	15	39.5	0.075	38.6	0.078	0.4575	F = M
Mesoamerica	F < M	10	59.3	0.070	63.7	0.027	0.2292	F = M
NW summary	F > M	25	47.4	0.080	43.4	0.071	0.3364	F = M
Global sample	F > M	69	50.8	0.065	47.9	0.051	0.0400	F > M

indicator of population dental health. In our analysis the results of tooth count caries prevalence provide the most convincing evidence of a female sex bias in dental caries prevalence in past populations.

7.3.2 *Individual count caries prevalence by sex*

The analysis of dental caries prevalence by sex based on individual (specimen) count data is presented in Table 7.2 and Figure 7.5. Some investigators report caries prevalence by tooth-count and by individual-count methods; others may prefer one method over the other. Consequently, some sites or samples are included in both tooth count and individual count analyses, yet many studies report results in only one format. The tooth-count method is most common; far fewer studies report dental caries prevalence by percentage of individuals affected and data reported in this manner are inconsistent or incomplete. Percentages may be given without an indication of the number of individuals affected or the total number of specimens observed. Nevertheless, a similar pattern is evident in the number of samples included in our survey: Asia ($n = 18$), Europe ($n = 19$) and North America ($n = 15$) received more study than either Africa ($n = 7$) or Mesoamerica ($n = 10$) (see also Appendix 7.2). Figure 7.5 shows that in Asia and Europe, caries is more prevalent among females than males; however, this result is significant only for Europe (see Table 7.2 for data and test results). Mean caries prevalence by sex is nearly equal for Africa and North America, while among Mesoamerican samples males exhibit higher mean caries prevalence than females. The continental samples are aggregated

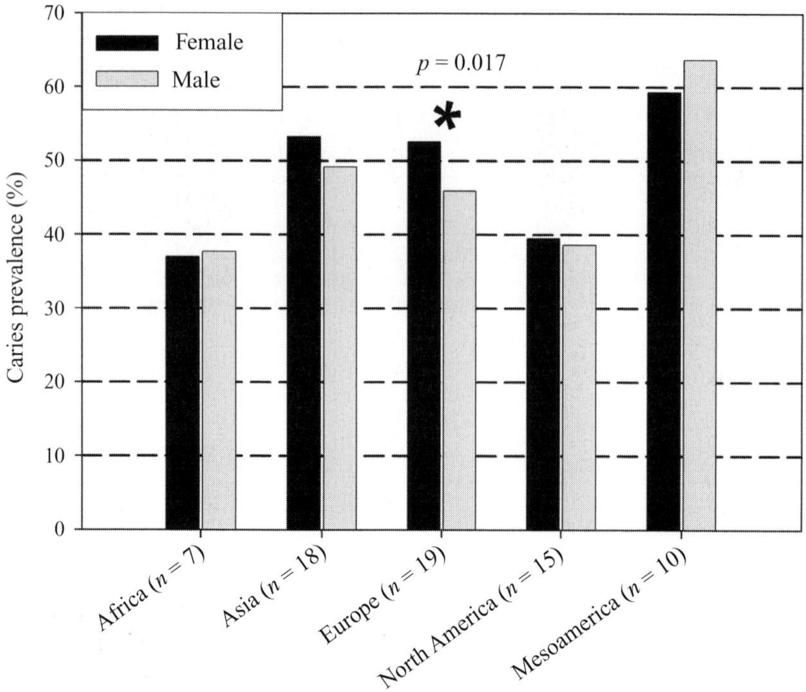

Figure 7.5 Mean caries prevalence by sex and continent (% individuals; * = $p < 0.05$).

into Old and New World samples, and into a global sample in Figure 7.6. In these comparisons, mean caries rates for Old World and global samples are significantly greater among women than men by 4.6 % and 2.9 %, respectively. The New World sample shows females with greater caries prevalence than males, but the result is not significant (see Table 7.2 for data and test results). In sum, the assessment of sex differences in caries prevalence using the individual method yielded less consistent results than the tooth-count method.

7.3.3 *Sex and caries in Asia: correction factors and statistical significance*

Data for dental caries prevalence by sex in Asia is presented in Table 7.3. This table includes site or sample name, method of calculation used in the study (obs. – observed or corr. – corrected), the perceived sex bias in caries prevalence, female and male caries rates in tooth-count and corrected tooth-count formats (where available), the p value derived from a χ^2 test (or Fisher's Exact Test when appropriate) of significance for sex differences in caries rate, whether a

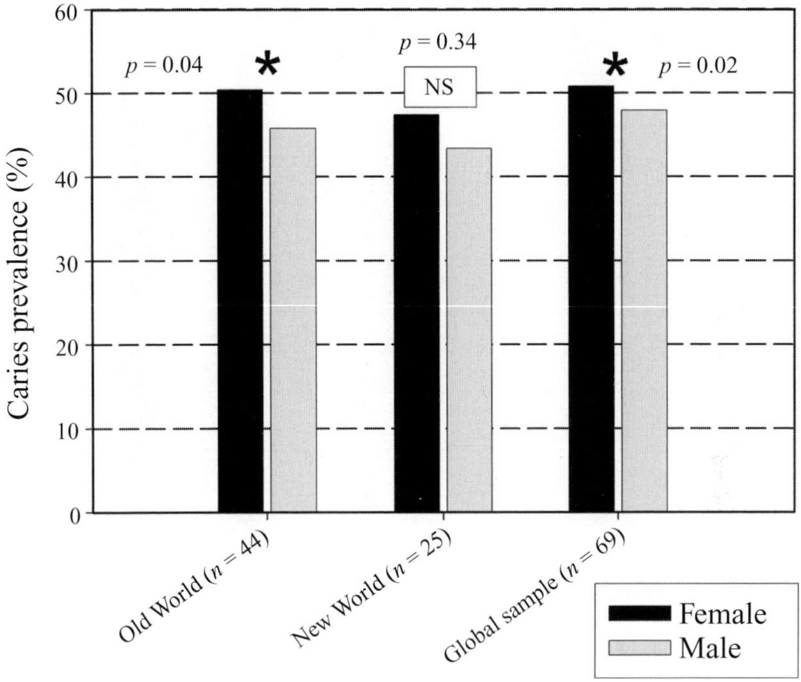

Figure 7.6 Mean caries prevalence by sex: global summary (% individuals; * = $p < 0.05$).

significant difference in caries rate exists, and the source from which the data were derived. Table 7.3 reveals several common themes: (1) the perception that females have higher caries rates than males is frequently taken at face value as real, yet the difference is often invalidated by *post hoc* application of a χ^2 test of independence, (2) the use of caries correction factors typically magnifies the inter-sex difference in caries rate, and (3) female caries rates are significantly greater than male rates for most cultures, subsistence systems, and time periods.

Inter-sex differences in caries prevalence of more than 10 % are commonly not statistically significant. For example, while 10 of 14 (71.4 %) East Asia and Pacific samples suggest females have greater caries prevalence than males, when the appropriate test of independence is conducted (χ^2 or Fisher's Exact Test) no significant difference was found in caries prevalence for the majority of samples. Statistical analysis reveals only two cases ($n = 14$; 14.3 %) in East Asia and the Pacific for which females display significantly greater caries rates than males. This outcome derives from the combined effect of the small and disparate size of male and female samples. Consequently, data evaluation

Table 7.3 *Caries prevalence by sex in Asia*

Site or group name	Method	Abs. diff. by sex	Female a	Female *n*	Female %	$p_{\chi 2}$	Male a	Male *n*	Male %	Stats diff. by sex	Source
China ($n=7$)											
Yin-Shang (citizens)	obs.	F > M	19	419	4.5	0.469	25	684	3.7	M = F	Sakashita *et al.*, 1997
Beiliu (Yangshao)	obs.	M > F	1	46	2.2	0.617	3	46	6.5	M = F	
Jiangzhai (Yangshao)	obs.	F > M	6	163	3.7	0.325	5	255	2.0	M = F	Pechenkina *et al.*, 2002
Shijia (Yangshao)	obs.	F > M	2	45	4.4	1.000	5	134	3.7	M = F	
Kangjia (Longshan)	obs.	M >F	15	54	27.7	0.840	27	92	29.3	M = F	
Xicun (West Zhao)	obs.	F > M	2	155	1.3	1.000	2	217	0.9	M = F	
Yangshao	obs.	F > M	9	173	5.2	0.1421	23	775	3.0	F = M	Yu-Zhu, 1982
Japan ($n=3$)											
Jomon	obs.	F > M	42	322	13.0	**0.000**	59	892	6.6	**F > M**	Turner, 1979
Mashiki (Okinawa)	obs.	F > M	49	221	22.2	**0.000**	20	191	10.5	**F > M**	Oyamada *et al.*, 1996
Kyushu	obs.	F > M	81	317	25.6	0.110	106	510	20.8	M = F	
Pacific Islands ($n=4$)											
Apurguan (Guam)	obs.	M > F	11	512	2.1	0.4368	22	772	2.8	M = F	Douglas *et al.*, 1997
Easter Island (20–29)	obs.	M > F	53	234	22.6	0.0733	63	209	30.1	M = F	
(30–39)	obs.	F > M	15	54	27.8	0.8501	45	170	26.5	M = F	Owsley *et al.*, 1985
(40+)	obs.	F > M	24	53	45.3	0.1507	57	166	34.3	M = F	
East Asia & Pacific Islands – % F > M		71.4 %								14.3 %	
Thailand ($n=11$)											
Ban Chiang (all)	obs.	M > F	29	489	5.9	0.109	45	527	8.5	M = F	Pietrusewsky and Douglas, 2002
Ban Chiang – early	obs.	M > F	9	198	4.5	0.154	24	310	7.7	M = F	
Ban Chiang – late	obs.	M > F	22	316	7.0	0.469	21	244	8.6	M = F	Douglas, 1996
(Khok Phanom Di)[a]	obs.	F > M	85	557	15.3	**<0.0001**	40	540	7.4	**F > M**	
	cor	F > M	142	676	21.0	**<0.0001**	44	569	7.7	**F > M**	

Table 7.3 (*cont.*)

Site or group name	Method	Abs. diff. by sex	Female a	Female *n*	Female %	$p_{\chi 2}$	Male a	Male *n*	Male %	Stats diff. by sex	Source
(Ban Lum Khao)	obs.	F > M	30	445	6.7	**0.0004**	7	400	1.8	**F > M**	
	cor	F > M	42	472	8.9	**<0.0001**	8	417	1.9	**F > M**	
Noen U-Loke	obs.	M > F	9	281	3.2	0.506	14	331	4.2	M = F	
	cor.	M > F	9	305	2.9	0.252	16	341	4.7	M = F	Tayles *et al.*, 2000
Non Nok Tha (all)	cor.	F > M	28.3	682	4.1	0.192	18.7	676	2.8	M = F	
NNT early	obs.	M > F	5	382	1.3	0.542	6	284	2.1	M = F	
NNT late	obs.	F > M	14	244	5.7	0.082	8	292	2.7	M = F	Douglas, 1996, 2006
Ban Lum Khao	obs.	F > M	32	477	6.7	**<0.01**	8	408	2.0	**F > M**	
	cor.	F > M	43	508	8.5	**<0.0001**	9	436	2.1	**F > M**	
Ban Na Di	obs.	F > M	12	147	8.2	**<0.03**	12	368	3.3	**F > M**	
	cor.	F > M	19	178	10.7	**0.0004**	12	375	3.2	**F > M**	
Khok Phanom Di	obs.	F > M	96	656	15.6	**<0.01**	43	625	6.9	**F > M**	
	cor.	F > M	169	799	21.2	**<0.0001**	49	666	7.4	**F > M**	
Nong Nor	obs.	F > M	44	472	9.3	**<0.01**	22	545	4.0	**F > M**	Domett, 2001
	cor.	F > M	48	512	9.4	**0.0005**	23	563	4.1	**F > M**	
Vietnam (*n* = 3)											
Da But		F > M	7	333	2.1	0.528*	7	445	1.6	M = F	Oxenham *et al.*, 2006
Ma & Ca River		F > M	14	294	4.8	**0.013**	7	435	1.6	**F > M**	
Red River		M > F	0	51	0.0	0.091*	3	168	1.8	M = F	
Southeast Asia % F > M		57.1 %								35.7 %	
South Asia (*n* = 5)											
Damdama	obs.	F > M	6	359	1.8	**0.020***	1	523	0.2	**F > M**	
	cor.	F > M	17	398	4.3	**0.000***	1	530	0.2	**F > M**	

(*cont*).

Table 7.3 (*cont.*)

Site or group name	Method	Abs. diff. by sex	Female a	Female n	Female %	$p_{\chi 2}$	Male a	Male n	Male %	Stats diff. by sex	Source
Mahadaha	obs.	F > M	1	62	1.6	0.558*	2	199	1.0	M = F	
	cor.	F > M	5	85	5.9	**0.027***	2	199	1.0	**F > M**	Lukacs, 1996 (Table 2)
Mehrgarh (MR 2)	obs.	F > M	21	433	4.8	**0.005**	6	433	1.4	**F > M**	
	cor.	F > M	28	456	6.1	**0.001**	8	437	1.8	**F > M**	
Harappa	obs.	F > M	29	288	10.1	0.129	18	281	6.4	F = M	
	cor.	F > M	60	339	17.7	**0.012**	31	294	10.5	**F > M**	
Sarai Khola	obs.	F > M	15	297	5.1	0.564	21	503	4.2	F = M	Lukacs *et al.*, 1989
Southwest Asia ($n = 7$)											
Bahrain											
Bronze Age	obs.	F > M	16	77	20.8	**0.043**	19	171	11.1	**F > M**	
Iron Age	obs.	M = F	1	13	7.7	1.000*	3	21	14.3	M = F	Littleton and Frohlich, 1989
Islamic Period	obs.	M = F	27	132	20.5	0.2279	43	275	15.6	M = F	
Teppe Hissar											
WG 1	cor.	F > M	75	561	13.4	**0.0255**	112	1146	9.8	**F > M**	Hemphill, 2006 this volume
WG 2	cor.	M > F	40	288	13.9	0.8612	64	446	14.3	M = F	
WG 3	cor.	F > M	135	473	28.5	**<0.0001**	102	835	12.2	**F > M**	
WG 4	cor.	F > M	72	420	17.1	**<0.0001**	44	543	8.1	**F > M**	
South & Southwest Asia% F > M		75 %								66.7 %	
All – Asia% F > M		67.5 %								37.5 %	

[a] Neither Khok Phanom Di nor Ban Lum Khao (Tayles *et al.*, 2000) are counted in tabulations since these series were more recently analyzed with larger sample sizes by Domett (2001).

must carefully assess the meaning of statistical significance vs. the probability of meaningful biological significance. Table 7.3 shows that for each region of Asia, the apparently greater female bias in caries prevalence is diminished when appropriate statistical testing is conducted.

Caries correction factors have been more commonly used in the analysis of Asian caries rates, especially in South and Southeast Asia, than in other regions of the world. The result of employing such correction factors is evident in Table 7.3 in several ways: (1) the magnitude of inter-sex difference increases, often dramatically, (2) the strength of the association between sex and caries increases, as indicated by a decrease in the associated *p* value, and (3) though observed tooth-count data indicate that sex differences are not significant, use of the correction factor may result in a difference in caries prevalence that is significant (e.g. at Harappa and Mahadaha). Since a significant component of antemortem tooth loss in women is due to caries, and correction factors address this, corrected caries prevalence estimates are regarded as more accurately estimating true inter-sex differences in caries prevalence than observed (uncorrected) tooth-count figures. The relationship between observed (tooth count) and corrected (tooth count) caries rates for Southeast Asia is presented in Figure 7.7 to illustrate the significance of employing correction factors in caries research (data from Domett, 2001; Douglas, 2006; and Tayles *et al.*, 2000).

Recent research on the oral pathology of prehistoric Asian populations from Central Asia and Southeast Asia lends general support to the hypothesis that women's oral health tends to be poorer than men's. An analysis of dental health by socio-economic status and sex at Tepe Hissar, Iran (4200–2000 BC) was based on a total sample of 235 skeletons – 88 female and 147 males (Hemphill, 2006, this volume). When caries prevalence is calculated by sex for all individuals in the composite sample at Tepe Hissar, females display a significantly higher caries rate (65 %) than males (42 %). Within this sample, Hemphill identified four wealth groups on the basis of quality and quantity of grave goods: (1) poor, (2) affluent poor, (3) near rich, and (4) rich. Using the observed tooth-count caries rates, females were found to have significantly higher caries prevalence in three of the four wealth groups (see Table 7.3 for data). Only among the affluent poor was the sex difference in caries rate not significant.

A recent analysis of change in oral health status upon the adoption and intensification of agriculture in Southeast Asia addressed the issue of sex differences in caries rates (Oxenham *et al.*, 2006). This synthetic regional analysis includes results from Thai skeletal series studied by others, including Ban Chiang (Douglas, 1996; Pietrusewsky and Douglas, 2002), Ban Lum Khao, Ban Na Di, and Khok Phanom Di (Domett, 2001; Tayles *et al.*, 2000), Noen U-Loke (Tayles *et al.*, 2000), Non Nok Tha (Douglas, 1996, 2006), Nong Nor (Domett, 2001; Tayles *et al.*, 1998), as well as new data for three samples from Vietnam:

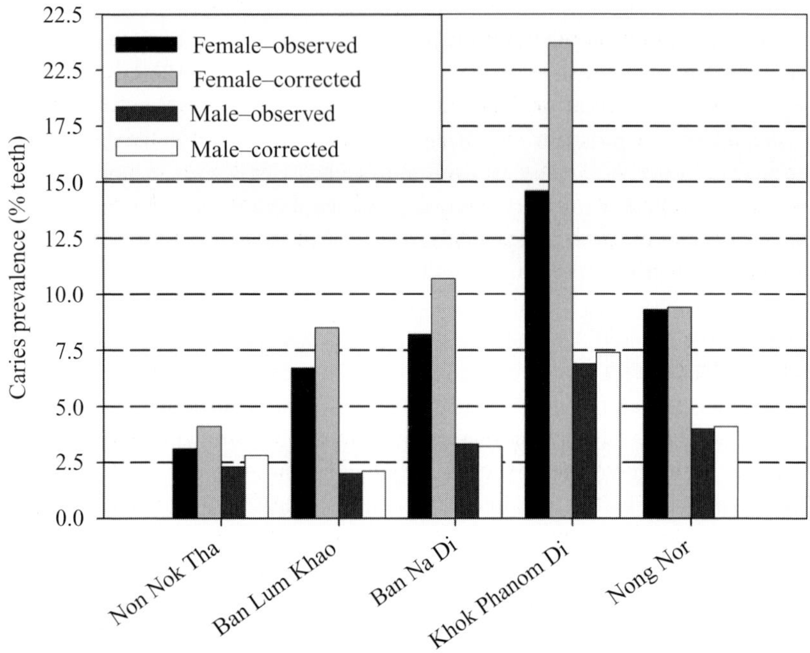

(Data sources: Domett, 2001; Douglas, 2006; Tayles *et al.*, 2000)

Figure 7.7 Caries prevalence by sex in Southeast Asia: The effect of applying the caries correction factor (Lukacs, 1996;% carious teeth).

Da But, Ma and Ca Rivers, and Red River (Oxenham *et al.*, 2006). Three important results derive from this synthetic analysis: (1) longevity may not be a key factor in the etiology of caries in Southeast Asia, (2) no obvious correlation exists between putative subsistence pattern and caries rates, and most critical for this investigation, (3) in two-thirds of samples studied (8/12), females displayed a higher rate of dental caries than males. The female bias in caries prevalence was statistically significant in four of the eight samples. The authors characterize this as being not unexpected, and list the standard variables – earlier dental eruption among females, pregnancy, sex differences in diet or eating frequency – as potential causal agents (Oxenham *et al.*, 2006).

By contrast, a recent re-assessment of dental pathology at Non Nok Tha that employed the "dental pathology profile" (Lukacs, 1989), found no significant difference in caries prevalence by sex for either the composite sample or for early or late groups analyzed separately (Douglas, 2006; see data in Table 7.3). While men had overall poorer dental health than women at Non Nok Tha, females experienced a greater decline in dental health through time. Douglas

(2006) finds this result consistent with a sexual division of labor, where females are involved in more agricultural and food processing activities, and have greater and more frequent access to softer, processed foods than men.

Subjecting the Asian evidence for sex differences in caries rates to close scrutiny permits a greater awareness of the complex and cross-cutting nature of variables involved here and in other continental samples. However, it also allows us to better appreciate the general pattern of sex difference in dental caries as documented in the global meta-analysis – women's oral health is consistently poorer than men's.

7.4 Discussion

Few anthropological studies of oral health in prehistoric or early historic skeletal series directly address the issue of sex differences. One comprehensive and comparative analysis of sex dimorphism in dental pathology of ancient populations included observations on dental caries in European (Greek and British), African (Nubian), and native North American (Gran Quivira) samples (Burns, 1982). This analysis employed observations on tooth surfaces rather than whole teeth, and used multivariate statistical methods. Burns found the sex dimorphic nature of caries experience extremely complex and variable within and between groups (e.g. by age, jaw, tooth position, and surface affected). Nevertheless, the first of several significant findings from this study was that female sub-groups tend to be more carious than male sub-groups (Burns, 1982). We re-analyzed sex differences in percentage of carious tooth surfaces for eight of Burns' data sets (Late Roman and Byzantine Greece; Iron Age, Romano-British, and medieval England; and Middle and Late Puebloan, Gran Quivira) and found that females exhibited significantly more carious tooth surfaces than males in four samples (Iron Age and Romano-British, England; Middle Puebloan, Gran Quivira; Sudanese Nubia), female and male caries prevalence was not significantly different in three samples (Byzantine Greece, medieval England, and Late Pueblo, Gran Quivira), and male caries prevalence exceeded female caries rate in one sample (Late Roman, Greece).

Many studies were not included in the statistical component of this meta-analysis due to small or unstated sample size (e.g. Gualandi, 1992; Hutchinson, 2002; Saul, 1975, 1982; White, 1997) or because they reported caries rate by sex in a less common manner – average number of caries per individual (per mouth; e.g. Angel, 1971a; Costa, 1980; Hallein, 1996; Rathbun, 1987; Smith, 2000). In his pioneering study of the people of Middle Bronze Age Lerna (Greece), Angel reported a greater average number of carious lesions per mouth among females (2.5) than among males (1.8; Angel, 1971b). Furthermore, when other indicators of dental health and demography are considered, he states that, "Lerna women have worse teeth than men, if one makes allowance for their younger age at death, because of the pregnancy drain on health . . ." (Angel 1971b, p. 89). With this observation we shift the focus of attention to caries etiology, and especially to potential factors that may contribute to sex differences in cariogenesis.

Approximately 40 % of the studies reporting sex differences in dental caries prevalence do not offer an explanation for the difference, assert that the cause of the difference is unknown, or contend that this outcome is a random effect. The most commonly identified mechanisms responsible for sex differences in dental caries include: (1) girls' teeth erupt earlier than boys' and therefore are exposed earlier and for a longer period of time to a cariogenic oral environment, (2) culture-based dietary differences between females (more carbohydrates) and males (more protein), and (3) sex dimorphic activity or behavior that differentially increases risk for one sex (females) over the other. In the latter case, women's role in preparing and cooking food, as well as their proximity to food storage and preparation areas of the home, are common explanations for the higher prevalence of caries in women.

While pregnancy is sometimes offered as an explanation for the greater frequency of caries in females, others contend that sex differences in the timing of eruption or pregnancy cannot explain the variation seen in caries between the sexes (Larsen, 1997). We agree that sex differences in the timing of dental emergence are small and have been shown not to play a significant role in cariogenesis (Mansbridge, 1959). Elsewhere we provide extensive documentation for the way in which female life-history events, including puberty, menstruation, and especially pregnancy have an effect on the caries experience of women (Lukacs and Largaespada, 2006). The multifaceted nature of proximate mechanisms that predispose women to higher caries rates than men include fluctuation in estrogen levels during menses and pregnancy, changes in biochemical composition of saliva during pregnancy, and lower rate of saliva flow. Confounding factors include those with a theoretical basis in evolutionary theory, including food cravings and aversions, and suppression of the immune-response system during pregnancy (Figure 7.8). The relative importance of these factors and the mechanisms by which they contribute to poorer dental health among women are now under investigation in collaboration with researchers at Oregon State University (Cheyney, 2007) and the University of Alberta (Vallianatos, 2007).

In his review of sex differences in diet and dental health among prehistoric and modern hunters and gatherers, Walker (1988) considered differences in the timing of dental eruption and factors associated with pregnancy (e.g. gingivitis, periodontal disease, mineral balance). He concluded that behavioral variables, such as sex differences in diet and activity pattern, were paramount in explaining variation in caries prevalence by sex. If physiological factors such as eruption timing and pregnancy played a significant role in cariogenesis, he argued, we

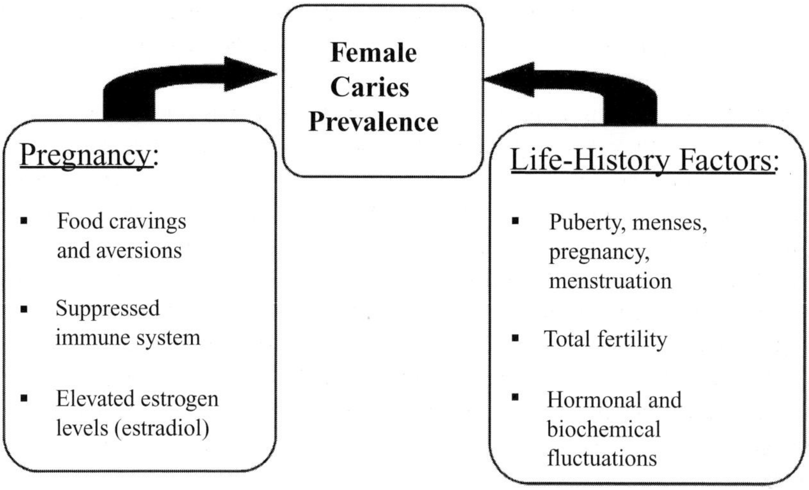

Figure 7.8 Mechanisms by which pregnancy and reproductive life history impact female caries prevalence.

would expect to find a more consistent patterning of sex differences in dental health that cross-cut sociocultural differences (Walker, 1988). Most often, when pregnancy or hormonal fluctuations are mentioned as factors contributing to higher caries rates in women the assertion is brief, without elaboration and potential causal mechanisms remain unstated. For example, in the analysis of caries in the Spitalfields collection, Whittaker and Molleson (1996, p. 60) state, that "[s]ignificant differences in caries . . . were noted between males and females, the females in each case having a slightly higher prevalence. The reasons for this are not are not clear but may be related to dietary or hormonal differences." Some suggest that physiological stress due to pregnancy or lactation are responsible, yet the details regarding how dental health is impacted may be vaguely, incompletely, or speculatively proposed, with no mention of a specific mechanism provided. Occasionally, specific mechanisms are proposed as "proximate" causal agents, including specific hormones: cortisol, estrogen generally, or estradiol in particular. More recent research gives specific attention to hormones and pregnancy in the etiology of caries in women. For example, following the lead of Wing and Brown (1979) and Little (1973), Burgess (1999) suggested that elevated cortisol levels in females, at adolescence and during pregnancy, stimulate connective tissue to produce proteolytic enzymes that have an effect on enamel quality and resistance to demineralization. In the analysis of dental pathology among Sudanese Nubians, Beck (1988) found that women's caries prevalence was greater than men's, and that pregnancy influenced caries rate through folate deficiency, an elevated cortisol level, and lowered salivary pH. Collectively, these factors were regarded as partly responsible for coining the phrase "a tooth is lost for every child." Sex differences in caries rates among the ancient inhabitants of Gran Canaria are partly accounted for by the idea that cariogenic micro-organisms in saliva may increase during pregnancy along with a decrease in saliva pH and its buffer effect (Delgado-Darias *et al.*, 2005; Laine, 2002). We anticipate that new insights into saliva–plaque interaction, and the nature of oral bacterial biofilms, will reveal important inter-group differences (by sex, socio-economic status, and ethnic identity) that will contribute to a better understanding of inter-group differences in caries experience (Kolenbrander and Palmer, 2004; Marsh, 2004, Tabak, 2006).

7.5 Conclusions

This meta-analysis suggests that a sex differential in caries experience exists in prehistory, and exhibits a strong and often significant tendency to impact females more than males. An important causal factor contributing to this sex bias in caries prevalence is women's reproductive role in society. Women's life-history events, including puberty, menses, and pregnancy, involve recurring events and complex changes in hormone levels, physiological state, and immunological competence that directly impact their predisposition to dental caries. Traditional anthropological explanations for sex differences in dental caries include fundamental differences in diet, food preparation, frequency of consumption, division of labor, and other aspects of a behavioral and cultural nature. Though these factors are paramount, the mechanisms and pathways through which women's reproductive and evolutionary biology influence caries susceptibility require a higher level of attention from anthropologists.

Acknowledgments

An abridged version of this chapter was presented at the sixteenth European Paleopathology Conference in Santorini, Greece on August 30, 2006. A Bray Fellowship (2005–7) from the University of Oregon, College of Arts and Sciences to JRL defrayed research expenses and conference travel. Thanks to Missy Cheyney (Oregon State University) and Helen Vallianatos (University of Alberta) for offering critical comments on an earlier draft of this manuscript, and to Brian Hemphill (California State University, Bakersfield) for sharing pre-publication data on Tepe Hissar. We thank Joel Irish and Greg Nelson for the invitation to contribute an original research article to this anthology of recent research in dental anthropology.

Appendix 7.1 Samples, data and sources for tooth-count caries rates by sex

Sample/site name	Country	Antiquity	Female			Male			Data source
			n – car.	*n* – obs.	% car.	*n* – car.	*n* – obs.	% car.	
AFRICA (*n* = 9)									
Nubian A-Group	Egypt	3100–2500 BC	5	150	3.3	9	373	2.4	Beckett and Lovell, 1994
Nubian C-Group	Egypt	2000–1500 BC	19	204	9.3	8	128	6.3	
Faraoskop	South Africa	2300–1900 BP	7	26	26.9	4	84	4.8	
Oakhurst	South Africa	10 000–4 000 BP	2	21	9.5	19	122	15.6	Sealy, 1992
Griqua	South Africa	18th–19th century	8	210	3.8	22	295	7.5	
Kakamas	South Africa	18th–19th century	5	384	1.3	8	433	1.8	
Riet River	South Africa	18th–19th century	25	454	5.5	21	484	4.3	Morris, 1992
R Cemetery	Sudan	AD 550–1450			34.1			17.2	
S Cemetery	Sudan	AD 550–750			25.7			16.3	Beck, 1988
ASIA (*n* = 44)									
Apurguan	Guam	AD 1000–1521	11	512	2.1	22	772	2.9	Douglas, Pietrusewsky *et al.*, 1997
Australian Sample	Australia	not given	67	1440	4.7	129	2752	4.7	
Iron Age	Bahrain	750–500 BC	1	13	7.7	3	21	14.3	
Islamic Period	Bahrain	AD 1250–1520	27	132	20.5	43	275	15.6	Littleton and Frohlich, 1989
Mid-Bronze Age	Bahrain	2500–1700 BC	16	77	20.8	19	171	11.1	
Anyang Citizens	China	1400–1100 BC	19	419	4.5	25	684	3.7	Sakashita, Inoue *et al.*, 1997
Beiliu	China	7000–6000 BP	1	46	2.2	3	46	6.5	
Jiangzhai	China	7000–6000 BP	6	163	3.7	5	255	2.0	
Kangjia	China	5000–4000 BP	15	54	27.8	27	92	29.3	
Shijia	China	6000–5000 BP	2	45	4.4	5	134	3.7	
Xicun	China	3800–2200 BP	2	155	1.3	2	217	0.9	Pechenkina, Benfer *et al.*, 2002
Yangshao Culture	China	5000–6000 BP	9	173	5.2	23	775	3.0	
Hane dune site (Marquesas)	French Polynesia	AD 275–1635	4	14	28.6	5	29	17.2	Pietrusewsky, 1976

(*cont.*)

Appendix 7.1 *(cont.)*

			Female			Male			
Sample/site name	Country	Antiquity	*n* – car.	*n* – obs.	% car.	*n* – car.	*n* – obs.	% car.	Data source
Mehrgarh	India	Chalcolithic era	21	433	4.9	6	433	1.4	
Damdama	India	Mesolithic era	6	359	1.7	1	523	0.2	Lukacs, 1996
Mahadaha	India	Mesolithic era	1	62	1.6	2	199	1.0	
Tepe Hissar – WG 1	Iran	4500–1750 BC	34	306	11.1	42	649	6.5	
Tepe Hissar – WG 2	Iran	4500–1750 BC	21	222	9.5	22	268	8.2	
Tepe Hissar – WG 3	Iran	4500–1750 BC	53	275	19.3	43	493	8.7	Hemphill, 2006, 2007
Tepe Hissar – WG 4	Iran	4500–1750 BC	33	252	13.1	26	366	7.1	
Jomon	Japan	ca 1000 BC	42	322	13.0	59	892	6.6	Turner 1979
Kyushu	Japan		81	317	25.6	106	510	20.8	Oyamada, Manabe *et al.*, 1996
Mashiki	Japan		49	221	22.2	20	191	10.5	
Easter Is 30–39	Pacific Is		15	54	27.8	45	170	26.5	
Easter Is 39+	Pacific Is		24	53	45.3	57	166	34.3	Owsley, Miles *et al.* 1985
Easter Island 20–29	Pacific Is		53	234	22.7	63	209	30.1	
Harappa	Pakistan	Bronze Age	29	288	10.1	18	281	6.4	Lukacs 1992
Sarai Khola	Pakistan	1000 BC	15	297	5.1	21	503	4.2	Schultz *et al.*, 1996; Lukacs *et al.*, 1989
Nebira	Papua New Guinea	AD 1000–1600	3	24	12.5	2	32	6.3	Douglas, Pietrusewsky, *et al.* 1997
Ban Chiang	Thailand	composite	29	489	5.9	45	482	8.5	Pietrusewsky and Douglas, 2002
Ban Chiang	Thailand	early	9	198	4.5	24	310	7.7	
Ban Chiang	Thailand	late	22	316	7.0	21	244	8.6	Douglas 1996
Ban Lum Khao	Thailand	1000–500 BC	30	445	6.7	7	400	1.8	
Khok Phanom Di	Thailand	2000–1500 BC	85	557	15.3	40	540	7.4	Tayles, Domett *et al.*, 2000
Noen U-Loke	Thailand	300 BC–AD 300	9	281	3.2	14	331	4.2	
Ban Lum Khao	Thailand	1000–500 BC	32	477	6.7	8	408	2.0	
Ban Na Di	Thailand	600–400 BC	12	147	8.2	12	368	3.3	

			Female			Male			
Sample/site name	Country	Antiquity	n – car.	n – obs.	% car.	n – car.	n – obs.	% car.	Data source
Khok Phanom Di	Thailand	2000–1500 BC	96	656	14.6	43	625	6.9	
Nong Nor	Thailand	1100–700 BC	44	472	9.3	22	545	4.0	Domett, 2001
Non Nok Tha	Thailand	early	5	382	1.3	6	284	2.1	
Non Nok Tha	Thailand	late	14	244	5.7	8	292	2.7	Douglas, 2006
Red River	Vietman		0	51	0.0	3	168	1.8	
Da But	Vietnam		7	333	2.1	7	445	1.6	Oxenham, Nguyen *et al.*, 2006
Ma & Ca River	Vietnam		14	294	4.8	7	435	1.6	
CENTRAL & SOUTH AMERICA ($n = 12$)									
La Tolita	Ecuador	200 BC–AD 400	4	189	2.1	2	121	1.7	Ubelaker, 1997
Copan-Maya (20–34 yrs)	Honduras	AD 700–900	22	80	27.5	41	376	10.9	
Copan-Maya (35 + yrs)	Honduras	AD 700–900	84	229	36.7	60	313	19.2	
Copan-Maya (all ages)	Honduras	AD 700–900	110	416	26.4	102	713	14.3	Whittington 1989, 1999
Classic Maya (pooled)	Mexico	AD 250–900	27	377	7.2	32	605	5.3	Cucina and Tiesler 2003
Classic Maya (high)	Mexico	AD 250–900	8	91	8.8	3	214	1.4	
Classic Maya (low)	Mexico	AD 250–900	12	175	6.9	18	285	6.3	
Postclassic (Oaxaca)	Mexico	AD 950–1519	475	9693	4.9	603	9030	6.7	Hodges 1989
Chribaya Alta	Peru	AD 900–1350	240	1197	20.1	79	741	10.7	Burgess, 1999
El Yaral	Peru	AD 960–1265	49	450	10.9	34	428	7.9	
Pachacamac	Peru	Pre-Columbian	188	1168	16.1	235	1559	15.1	Stewart, 1931
San Geronimo	Peru	AD 900–1350	141	717	19.7	42	439	9.6	Burgess, 1999
EUROPE ($n = 38$)									
Clopton	Britain	12th–14th century	33	304	10.9	62	486	12.8	Tattersall, 1968
Prehistoric Series	Croatia	5300–400 BC	23	280	8.2	15	222	6.8	
Antique Series	Croatia	4th century AD	65	704	9.2	90	934	9.6	
Early Medieval Series	Croatia	6th–8th century AD	129	1176	11.0	97	1050	9.2	

(*cont.*)

Appendix 7.1 *(cont.)*

			Female			Male			
Sample/site name	Country	Antiquity	*n* – car.	*n* – obs.	% car.	*n* – car.	*n* – obs.	% car.	Data source
Historic Series	Croatia	14th–17th century AD	66	727	9.1	110	932	11.8	
Late Medieval Series	Croatia	11th–13th century AD	63	711	8.9	92	771	11.9	Slaus, 2002
Non-lime Antique Series	Croatia	4th century AD	79	674	11.7	67	800	8.4	
Zmajevac	Croatia	4th century AD	54	507	10.7	56	526	10.6	Slaus *et al.*, 2004
Bronze AgeUnitice Culture	Czech Republic	1500 BC	82	379	21.6	179	654	27.4	Cechova, 1998
Libice Culture	Czech Republic	9th–10th century AD	69	601	11.5	48	609	7.9	
Oskobrh–Gothic Era	Czech Republic	14th–15th century AD	47	558	8.4	56	601	9.3	
Oskobrh -Renaissance Era	Czech Republic	16th–17th century AD	60	249	24.1	38	199	19.1	
Prague	Czech Republic	10th–12th century AD	38	538	7.1	76	581	13.1	
Nova Raca	Croatia	14th–17th century AD	32	361	8.9	50	404	12.4	Slaus, 1997
Aebelholt Abbey–Defective	Denmark	AD 1180–1561	128	1831	7.0	133	2671	5.0	
Aebelholt Abbey–Perfect	Denmark	AD 1180–1561	98	1720	5.7	235	3644	6.4	Brinch and Moller-Christensen, 1949
Tirup Cemetery	Denmark	AD 1100–14th century	26	463	5.6	29	702	4.1	Boldsen, 1997
Cirencester	England	3rd century AD/ Romano-British	47	869	5.4	120	2382	5.0	Wells, 1982
English Skeletal Sample	England	18th century	157	908	17.3	176	1344	13.1	Krogman, 1938
Kapolna	Hungary	11th century AD	50	368	13.6	32	312	10.3	Frayer, 1984
Var	Hungary	9–11th century AD	11	341	3.2	54	851	6.3	
Mesocsat	Hungary	385 BC–AD 100	27	563	4.8	14	456	3.1	Ery, 1971
Tengelic	Hungary	10th century AD			7.3			6.1	Ubelaker and Pap, 1998

Appendix 7.1 *(cont.)*

			Female			Male			
Sample/site name	Country	Antiquity	*n* – car.	*n* – obs.	% car.	*n* – car.	*n* – obs.	% car.	Data source
Isola Sacra (NIS)	Italy	1st–3rd century AD	11	251	4.4	24	621	3.9	
La Selvicciola (SLV)	Italy	7th century AD	50	316	15.8	65	596	10.9	
Lucus Feroniae (LFR)	Italy	1st–3rd century AD	27	457	5.9	30	485	6.2	Manzi, Salvadei *et al.*, 1999
Metaponto–rural	Italy	6th–3rd century BC	81	1324	6.1	40	753	5.3	
Metaponto–urban	Italy	6th–3rd century BC	225	1033	21.8	117	908	12.9	Henneberg, 1998
Molise	Italy	1st–4th century AD	69	495	13.9	94	511	18.4	Bonfiglioli *et al.*, 2003
Vallerano (Roman Suburbium)	Italy	2nd–3rd century AD	14	494	2.8	13	562	2.3	Cucina, Vargiu *et al.*, 2006
Western Liguria	Italy	4th century BC	20	178	11.2	17	225	7.6	Formicola, 1986
Cabeco da Arruda	Portugal	7170–6880 BP	20	284	7.0	5	129	3.9	
Moita do Sebastiao	Portugal	7170–6880 BP	18	218	8.3	22	297	7.4	Frayer, 1987
Gran Canaria (Canary Islands)	Spain	2500 BP to contact	354	1786	19.8	567	3843	14.8	Delgado-Darias, Velasco-Vázquez *et al.*, 2005
Lund	Sweden	Middle Ages			7.2			5.3	Olsson and Sagne, 1976
Early Upper Paleolithic	Various	before 27 000 BP	0	135	0.0	0	199	0.0	
Late Upper Paleolithic	Various	27 000 BP–Mesolithic	4	215	1.9	5	461	1.1	
Mesolithic	Various	Mesolithic era	73	1988	3.7	44	2482	1.8	Frayer, 1989
NORTH AMERICA (*n* = 44)									
Belleville	Canada	AD 1821–1874	718	1997	36.0	715	2651	27.0	Saunders, 1997
Archaic Tennessee Valley	US	6000–500 BC	47	1609	2.9	46	1805	2.5	Smith, 1982
Black Mesa (Posterior Mandible)	US	AD 800–1150			45.0			32.7	
Black Mesa (Posterior Maxilla)	US	AD 800–1150			41.9			36.8	Martin, Goodman *et al.*, 1991

(cont.)

Appendix 7.1 *(cont.)*

			Female			Male			
Sample/site name	Country	Antiquity	*n* – car.	*n* – obs.	% car.	*n* – car.	*n* – obs.	% car.	Data source
Canada Verde (California)	US	3000–4000 BP	121	784	15.4	108	934	11.6	
Skull Gulch A (California)	US	1820–900 BP	21	150	14.0	6	101	5.9	
Skull Gulch B (California)	US	AD 1100–1500	33	530	6.2	26	404	6.4	Walker and Erlandson, 1986
Classic Hopewellian (Klunk Mound)	US	500 BC–AD 500	28	183	15.3	13	297	4.4	Herrala, 1961
Colonial–Civil War (Blacks)	US	AD 1675–1879	12	293	4.1	18	783	2.3	
Colonial–Civil War (Whites)	US	AD 1675–1879	6	143	4.2	29	1208	2.4	Angel, 1976
Florida–Gulf Coast	US	AD 1525–1550	31	524	5.9	13	434	3.0	Hutchinson and Norr, 2006
Florida Gulf coast (Palmer site)	US	AD 500–800	1	59	1.7	2	54	3.7	Hutchinson, 2004
Gran Quivira (Early)	US	AD 1315–1400	33	90	36.7	11	76	14.5	Swanson, 1976
Gran Quivira (Late)	US	AD 1550–1672	62	464	13.4	43	320	13.4	
Gran Quivira (Middle)	US	AD 1400–1550	58	263	22.1	27	255	10.6	
Grasshopper Pueblo	US	AD 1275–1400	414	2214	18.7	288	1433	20.1	Fenton, 1998
Highland Beach (Florida)	US	AD 600–1200	17	947	1.8	4	642	0.6	Isler, Schoen *et al.*, 1985
Indian Knoll (S. Archaic)	US	3350 BC			6.2			0.4	Herrala, 1961
Ipiutak (Alaska)	US	AD 1409–1829	36	390	9.2	97	532	18.2	
Jones Point (Alaska)	US	pre-white contact	27	790	3.4	28	776	3.6	

Appendix 7.1 *(cont.)*

			Female			Male			
Sample/site name	Country	Antiquity	*n* – car.	*n* – obs.	% car.	*n* – car.	*n* – obs.	% car.	Data source
Tigara (Alaska)	US	AD 1540 -1740	106	2349	4.5	88	2026	4.3	Costa, 1980
Kellogg site (Mississippi)	US	AD 1000–1540	17	42	40.5	12	44	27.3	Sims, Danforth *et al.*, 1992
Lenape Indians	US	late 17th–early 18th C.			16.0			12.0	Hrdlicka, 1916
Middle Mississippi (Angel Village)	US	AD 1200–1400	60	471	12.7	53	513	10.3	Herrala, 1961
Middle Mississippi (Spoon River)	US	AD 1200–1400	14	297	4.7	68	868	7.8	
Monroe County Poorhouse (New York)	US	AD 1826–1863	155	1618	9.6	168	1611	10.4	Sutter, 1995
Moundville Cheifdom (Alabama)	US	AD 1050–1550	386	2082	18.5	283	1293	21.9	Powell, 1988
New Orleans Slaves (15–29 yrs)	US	AD 1720–1810	14	63	22.2	8	52	15.4	
New Orleans Slaves (30+ yrs)	US	AD 1720–1810	3	17	17.6	31	119	26.1	Owsley *et al.*, 1987
Old Copper (N. Archaic)	US	5600 BC	1	97	1.0	1	232	0.4	Herrala, 1961
Old Walpi (Arizona)	US	AD 1300–1700	61	882	6.9	46	825	5.6	Ryan, 1977
Post-agricultural (Georgia coast)	US	AD 1150–1550	263	1688	15.6	145	1295	11.2	Larsen, 1983; Larsen, Shavit *et al.*, 1991
Pre-agricultural (Georgia coast)	US	pre 1150	12	1016	1.2	4	617	0.6	
Pueblo II (Arizona)	US	AD 1000–1150	8	93	8.6	8	132	6.1	
Pueblo III (early & middle) (Arizona)	US	AD 1150–1250	16	114	14.0	16	143	11.2	
Pueblo III (late) (Arizona)	US	AD 1250–1350	57	293	19.5	47	281	16.7	

(cont.)

Appendix 7.1 *(cont.)*

			Female			Male			
Sample/site name	Country	Antiquity	*n* – car.	*n* – obs.	% car.	*n* – car.	*n* – obs.	% car.	Data Source
Puerco Pueblo III (Arizona)	US	AD 1150–1250	4	53	7.5	14	143	9.8	Ryan, 1977
RI-1000 (Rhode Island)	US	AD 1650–1670	135	337	40.1	58	248	23.4	Kelley *et al.*, 1987
Southeast-inner Coast (Hopwell, NC)	US	AD 1400	23	90	25.6	7	56	12.5	Higginbotham, 1999
Southeast-inner Coast (Jordan's Lndg)	US	AD 1280–1425	1	65	1.5	2	49	4.1	
Southeast-outer Coast (Baum, NC)	US	AD 1300–1400	23	139	16.5	20	264	7.6	
Toqua (Tennessee)	US	AD 1250–1600	142	1071	13.3	121	1083	11.2	Smith, 1986
Upper Mississippi (Oakwood Mound)	US	AD 1600–1650	39	221	17.6	15	182	8.2	
Upper Mississippi (Sauk)	US	AD 1790–1810			2.9			2.5	Herrala, 1961
Voegtly Cemetery (Pennsylvania)	US	AD 1833–1861	352	881	40.0	335	1451	23.1	Ubelaker, Jones *et al.*, 2003

Appendix 7.2 Samples, data and sources for individual-count caries rates by sex

		Female			Male			
Sample/site name	Country	n – car.	n – obs.	% car.	n – car.	n – obs.	% car.	Data source
AFRICA ($n = 7$)								
Nubian A-Group	Egypt	3	10	30.0	3	23	13.0	
Nubian C-Group	Egypt	7	18	38.9	5	15	33.3	Beckett and Lovell, 1994
various sites	Egypt	49	314	15.6	43	374	11.5	Hillson, 1979
Oakhurst	South Africa	2	3	66.7	7	8	87.5	Sealy, 1992
Griqua	South Africa	4	9	44.4	7	14	50.0	
Kakamas	South Africa	4	20.5	19.5	4	19	21.1	Morris, 1992
Riet River	South Africa	9	20.5	43.9	10	21	47.6	
ASIA ($n = 18$)								
Australian Skeletal Sample	Australia			35.0			31.5	Krogman 1938
Iron Age	Bahrain	4	16	25.0	5	13	38.5	
Islamic Period	Bahrain	8	9	88.9	16	20	80.0	Littleton and Frohlich, 1989
Mid-Bronze Age	Bahrain	12	18	66.7	27	66	40.9	
Damdama	India	4	15	26.7	1	20	5.0	
Mahadaha	India	1	4	25.0	3	10	30.0	Lukacs 1996
Harappa	India	10	16	62.5	6	17	35.5	Lukacs 1992
Tepe Hissar – WG 1	Iran	12	28	42.9	23	58	39.7	Hemphill, 2006
Tepe Hissar – WG 2	Iran	4	15	26.7	10	21	47.6	
Tepe Hissar – WG 3	Iran	16	22	72.7	15	35	42.9	
Tepe Hissar – WG 4	Iran	12	18	66.7	12	27	44.4	
Commoners	Japan	20	31	64.5	18	36	50.0	
Samurai	Japan	15	31	48.4	26	40	65.0	Oyamada *et al.*, 2004
Sarai Khola (Iron Age)	Pakistan	7	15	43.9	12	21	57.1	Lukacs *et al.*, 1989; Schultz *et al.*, 1996

(*cont.*)

Appendix 7.2 *(cont.)*

		Female			Male			
Sample/site name	Country	*n* – car.	*n* – obs.	% car.	*n* – car.	*n* – obs.	% car.	Data source
Ban Chaing	Thailand	13	31	41.9	17	29	58.6	Pietrusewsky and Douglas, 2002
Ban Lum Khao	Thailand	14	24	58.3	5	19	26.3	
Khok Phanom Di	Thailand	24	36	66.7	15	31	48.4	Tayles *et al.*, 2000
Noen U-Loke	Thailand	6	19	31.6	7	23	30.4	
EUROPE ($n = 19$)								
Aebelholt Abbey – Defective	Denmark	47	90	52.2	63	135	46.7	
Aebelholt Abbey – Perfect	Denmark	29	58	50.0	72	124	58.1	Brinch and Moller-Christensen, 1949
Iron Age	Denmark		111			147		
M/L Neolithic	Denmark		117			198		
Middle Ages	Denmark		35			66		Bennike, 1985
Tirup Cemetery	Denmark	13	51	25.5	21	73	28.8	Boldsen, 1997
Viking Period	Denmark		41			43		Bennike, 1985
Romano-British (Baldock)	England	32	50	64.0	26	42	61.9	Thornton, 1991
English Skeletal Sample	England			88.2			65.0	Krogman, 1938
Kapolna	Hungary	24	32	75.0	11	25	44.0	Frayer, 1984
Var	Hungary	6	21	28.6	19	45	42.2	Frayer, 1984
Isola Sacra (NIS)	Italy	7	21	33.3	16	43	37.2	
La Selvicciola (SLV)	Italy	12	17	70.6	22	31	71.0	
Lucus Feroniae (LFR)	Italy	14	25	56.0	12	25	48.0	Manzi *et al.*, 1999
Metaponto – rural	Italy	43	64	67.2	18	34	52.9	
Metaponto – urban	Italy	72	90	80.0	48	75	64.0	Henneberg, 1998
Western Liguria	Italy	8	8	100.0	6	10	60.0	Formicola, 1986
Muge	Portugal	14	29	48.3	11	28	39.3	Frayer, 1987
Gran Canaria (Canary Islands)	Spain	105	156	67.3	190	290	65.5	Delgado-Darias *et al.*, 2005

Appendix 7.2 *(cont.)*

		Female			Male			
Sample/site name	Country	n – car.	n – obs.	% car.	n – car.	n – obs.	% car.	Data source
Lund	Sweden			54.5			52.1	Olsson and Sagne, 1976
Early Upper Paleolithic	Various	0	10	0.0	0	12	0.0	
Late Upper Paleolithic	Various	2	16	12.5	4	28	14.3	
Mesolithic	Various	26	98	26.5	19	123	15.4	Frayer, 1989
MESOAMERICA ($n = 10$)								
Barton Ramie	Belize	7	20	35.0	12	18	66.7	Willey, 1965
Cuello	Belize	8	8	100.0	31	36	86.1	
Lubaantan	Belize	4	6	67.0	3	5	60.0	Saul, 1975
Tipu	Belize	43	47	92.0	42	59	71.2	Danforth, 1997
Altar de Sacrificious	Guatemala	9	10	90.0	20	23	87.0	Saul, 1972
Classic Period (Oaxaca Valley)	Mexico	24	58	41.4	27	59	45.8	
Formative Period (Oaxaca Valley)	Mexico	27	77	35.1	35	82	42.7	
Postclassic Period (Oaxaca Valley)	Mexico	16	58	27.6	35	88	39.8	Hodges, 1989
Oaxaca (intensive agriculture)	Mexico	35	70	50.0	66	103	64.1	
Oaxaca(non-intensive agrcult)	Mexico	22	40	55.0	29	43	67.4	Hodges, 1987
NORTH AMERICA ($n = 15$)								
Archaic Tennessee Valley	US	20	59	33.9	25	62	40.3	Smith, 1982
Arikara (Northern Plains)	US	43	78	55.1	61	92	66.3	
Chumash (California)	US	95	218	43.6	66	166	39.8	Hollimon, 1992, 2000
Dunning Cemetery/Poorhouse (Illinois)	US	11	25	44.0	14	25	56.0	Grauer *et al.*, 1998
Etowah – mounds	US	2.4	9	26.7	4.2	11	38.2	
Etowah – village	US	5.1	11	46.1	4.32	12	36.0	Blakely, 1995

(cont.)

Appendix 7.2 *(cont.)*

		Female			Male			
Sample/site name	Country	*n* – car.	*n* – obs.	% car.	*n* – car.	*n* – obs.	% car.	Data source
Florida / post-contact (Tatham md)	US	13	36	36.1	7	25	28.0	Hutchinson and Norr, 2006
Indeterminates (Alabama)	US	26	720	3.6	17	856	2.0	Rabkin, 1942
Koger Island (Alabama)	US	24	261	9.2	15	332	4.5	Rabkin, 1942
Postagricultural (Georgia coast)	US	75	108	69.4	47	80	58.8	
Preagricultural (Georgia coast)	US	8	75	10.7	3	49	6.1	Larsen, 1980, 1983
RI-1000 (Rhode Island)	US	17	18	94.4	10	11	90.9	Kelley *et al.*, 1987
Shell Mound (Alabama)	US	8	343	2.3	6	393	1.5	Rabkin, 1942
Texas Indians	US	67	181	37.0	69	212	32.5	Goldstein, 1948
Toqua (Tennessee)	US	29	36	80.6	29	37	78.4	Smith, 1986

References

Angel, J. L. (1944). Greek teeth: Ancient and modern. *Human Biology*, **16**, 283–297.

Angel, J. L. (1971a). Early Neolithic skeletons from Catal Huyuk: Demography and pathology. *Anatolian Studies*, **21**, 77–98.

Angel, J. L. (1971b). *The People of Lerna: Analysis of a Prehistoric Aegean Population*. Princeton, N J, American School of Classical Studies at Athens.

Angel, J. L. (1976). Colonial to Modern Skeletal Change. *American Journal of Physical Anthropology*, **45**, 723–35.

Armelagos, G. J. (1998). Introduction: sex, gender and health status in prehistoric and contemporary populations. In *Sex and Gender in Palaeopathological Perspective*, ed. A. L. Grauer and P. Stuart-Macadam. Cambridge: Cambridge University Press, pp. 1–10.

Beck, R. (1988). *The dental pathology of medieval-Christian Sudanese-Nubians from the Batn-El-Hajar*. Ph.D. Dissertation, University of Colorado.

Beckett, S. and Lovell, N. C. (1994). Dental disease evidence for agricultural intensification in the Nubian C-Group. *International Journal of Osteoarchaeology*, **4**, 223–40.

Bennike, P. (1985). *Paleopathology of Danish Skeletons: A Comparative Study of Demography, Disease, and Injury*. Denmark: Akademisk Forlag.

Blakely, R. L. (1995). Social organization at Etowah: a reconsideration of paleodemographic and paleonutritional evidence. *Southeastern Archaeology*, **14**, 46–59.

Boldsen, J. L. (1997). *Estimating Patterns of Disease and Mortality in a Medieval Danish Village. Integrating Archaeological Demography: Multidisciplinary Approaches to Prehistoric Population*. Occasional Paper No. 24. Carbondale, Illinois: Board of Trustees, Southern Illinois University. Center for Archaeological Investigations, pp. 229–41.

Bonfiglioli, B., Brasili, P., and Belcastro, M. G. (2003). Dental alveolar lesions and nutritional habits of a Roman Imperial Age population (first–fourth century AD), Quadrella (Molise, Italy). *Homo*, **54**, 36–56.

Brinch, O. and Moller-Christensen, V. (1949). On comparative investigations into the occurence of dental caries in archaeological skulls. *Odontologisk Tidskrift*, **57**, 357–73.

Burgess, S. D. (1999). *Chiribayan skeletal pathology on the south coast of Peru: patterns of production and consumption*. Ph.D. Dissertation, University of Chicago.

Burns, P. E. (1982). *A study of sexual dimorphism in the dental pathology of ancient peoples*. Ph.D. Dissertation, Arizona State University.

Cechova, L. (1998). *Dental Caries in the Period From the Bronze Age Up to the Modern Times in Bohemia*. Praha, Czech Republic: Univerzity Karlovy.

Cheyney, M. (2007). Effects of pregnancy on women's dental health: evolutionary and etiological perspectives. *American Journal of Physical Anthropology* (2007) Annual Meeting Suppl. 44, 87.

Cohen, M. N. (2007). *Ancient Health*. Gainesville: University Press of Florida.

Cornero, S. and Puche, R. C. (2000). Diet and nutrition of prehistoric populations at the alluvial banks of the Parana River. *Medicina*, **60**, 109–14.

Costa, R. L. Jr. (1980). Incidence of caries and abscesses in archaeological Eskimo skeletal samples from Point Hope and Kodiak Island, Alaska. *American Journal of Physical Anthropology*, **52**, 501–14.

Cucina, A. and Tiesler, V. (2003). Dental caries and antemortem tooth loss in the Northern Peten area, Mexico: a biocultural perspective on status differences among the classic Maya. *American Journal of Physical Anthropology*, **122**, 1–10.

Cucina, A., Vargiu, R., Mancinelli, D. *et al.* (2006). The Necropolis of Vallerano (Rome, second–third Century AD): an anthropological perspective on the Ancient Romans in the Suburbium. *International Journal of Osteoarchaeology*, **16**, 104–17.

Danforth, M. E. (1997). Gender and health among the Colonial Maya of Tipu, Belize. *Ancient Mesoamerica*, **8**, 13–22.

Delgado-Darias, T., Velasco-Vázquez, J., Arnay-de-la-Rosa, M., Martín-Rodrìguez, E., and González-Reimers, E. (2005). Dental caries among the prehispanic population from Gran Canaria. *American Journal of Physical Anthropology*, **128**, 560–8.

Domett, K. M. (2001). *Health in Late Prehistoric Thailand*. BAR 946. Oxford, England: Archaeopress. British Archaeological Reports International Series.

Douglas, M. T. (1996). *Paleopathology in human skeletal remains from the pre-metal, Bonze, and Iron Ages, northeast Thailand*. Ph.D. Dissertation, University of Hawaii.

Douglas, M. T. (2006). Subsistence change and dental health in the people of Non Nok Tha, northeast Thailand. In *Bioarchaeology of Southeast Asia*, ed. M. Oxenham and N. Tayles. Cambridge: Cambridge University Press, pp. 191–219.

Douglas, M. T., Pietrusewsky, M., and Ikehara-Quebral, R. M. (1997). Skeletal biology of Apurguan: A precontact Chamarro site on Guam. *American Journal of Physical Anthropology*, **104**, 291–313.

Duyar, I. and Erdal, Y. S. (2003). A new approach for calibrating dental caries frequency of skeletal remains. *Homo*, **54**, 57–70.

Erdal, Y. S. and Duyar, I. (1999). A new correction procedure for calibrating dental caries frequency. *American Journal of Physical Anthropology*, **108**, 237–40.

Ery, K. (1971). The anthropological examination of a tenth century population at Tengelic, Hungary. *Anthropologia Hungarica*, **10**, 49–89.

Featherstone, J. D. B. (1987). The mechanism of dental decay. *Nutrition Today*, **22**, 10–16.

Featherstone, J. D. B. (2000). The science and practice of caries prevention. *Journal of the American Dental Association*, **131**, 887–99.

Fenton, T. W. (1998). *Dental conditions at Grasshopper Pueblo: evidence for dietary change and increased stress*. Ph.D. Dissertation, University of Arizona.

Formicola, V. (1986). The dentition of the Neolithic sample from western Liguria (Italy). *Ossa*, **13**, 97–107.

Frayer D. W. (1984). Tooth size, oral pathology, and class distinctions: evidence from the Hungarian Middle Ages. *Anthropologiai Közlemények*, **28**, 47–54.

Frayer, D. W. (1987). Caries and oral pathologies at the Mesolithic sites of Muge (Cabeco da Arruda and Moita do Sebastiao). *Trabalhos de Antropologia e Etnologia*, **27**, 9–25.

Frayer, D. W. (1989). Oral pathologies in the European Upper Paleolithic and Mesolithic. In *People and Culture in Change: Proceedings of the Second Symposium on Upper Paleolithic, Mesolithic and Neolithic Populations of Europe and the Mediterranean Basin*, ed. I. Hershkovitz. London: BAR International Series No. 508, pp. 255–81.

Goldstein, M. S. (1948). Dentition of Indian Crania from Texas. *American Journal of Physical Anthropology*, **6**, 63–84.

Grauer, A. L., McNamara, E. M., and Houdek, D. V. (1998). A history of their own: patterns of death in a nineteenth century poorhouse. In *Sex and Gender in Paleopathological Perspective*, ed. A. L. Grauer and P. Stuart-Macadam. Cambridge: Cambridge University Press, pp. 149–63.

Gualandi, P. B. (1992). Food habits and dental disease in an Iron-Age population. *Anthropologischer Anzeiger*, **50**, 67–82.

Hallein, Y. K. (1996). *Pathological dental conditions in two Sudanese Nubian cemeteries with an emphasis on periodontal infections.* Ph.D. Dissertation, University of Colorado.

Haugejorden, O. (1996). Using the DMF gender difference to assess the "major" role of fluoride toothpastes in the caries decline in industrialized countries: a meta-analysis. *Community Dentistry and Oral Epidemiology*, **24**, 369–75.

Hemphill, B. E. (2006). Wealth, status and gender at Bronze Age Tepe Hissar: an investigation of intra-cemetery variation in dental pathology prevalence in prehistoric Iran. *American Journal of Physical Anthropology*, **129**, 102–3.

Hemphill, B. E. (2007). Dental pathology prevalence and pervasiveness at Tepe Hissar: statistical utility for investigating inter-relationships between wealth, gender, and status. In *Technique and Application in Dental Anthropology*, ed. J. D. Irish and G. C. Nelson, Cambridge: Cambridge University Press, 178–215.

Henneberg, R. J. (1998). *Dental Health and Affiliations of Inhabitants of the Ancient Greek Colony of Metaponto, Italy (sixth to third century BC).* Ph.D. Thesis, University of Witwatersrand, Johannesburg, South Africa.

Herrala, E. A. (1961). *The incidence of dental caries and alveoloclasta in a number of prehistoric American Indian groups of the Middle West.* Ph.D. Dissertation, Indiana University.

Higginbotham, L. C. (1999). *Gender-specific dental health patterns in late Prehistoric populations from the southeastern coast.* Greenville, M. A. Thesis, East Carolina University.

Hillson, S. W. (1979). Diet and dental disease. *World Archaeology*, **11**, 147–62.

Hillson, S. W. (2000). Dental pathology. In *Biological Anthropology of the Human Skeleton*, ed. M. A. Katzenberg and S. R. Saunders. New York: Wiley-Liss, Inc., pp. 249–86.

Hillson, S. W. (2001). Recording dental caries in archaeological human remains. *International Journal of Osteoarchaeology*, **11**, 249–89.

Hodges, D. C. (1987). Health and agricultural intensification in the prehistoric Valley of Oaxaca, Mexico. *American Journal of Physical Anthropology*, **73**, 323–32.

Hodges, D. C. (1989). *Agricultural Intensification and Prehistoric Health in the Valley of Oaxaca, Mexico*. Ann Arbor, MI: University of Michigan, No. 22.

Hollimon, S. E. (1992). Health consequences of sexual division of labor among Native Americans: the Chumash of California and the Arikara of the Northern Plains. In *Exploring gender through archaeology*, ed. C. Claasen. Madison, Wisconsin: Prehistory Press, pp. 81–8.

Hollimon, S. E. (2000). Sex, health and gender roles among the Arikara of the northern plains. In *Reading the Body: Representations and Remains in the Archaeological Record*, ed. A. E. Rautman. Philadelphia: University of Pennsylvania Press, pp. 25–37.

Hrdlicka, A. (1916). Physical anthropology of the Lenape or Delawares and of the Eastern Indians in general. *Bureau of American Ethnology Bulletin*, 48.

Hutchinson, D. L. (2002). *Foraging, Farming and Coastal Biocultural Adaptation in Late Prehistoric North Carolina*. Gainesville: University Press of Florida.

Hutchinson, D. L. (2004). *Bioarchaeology of the Florida Gulf Coast*. Gainesville: University Press of Florida.

Hutchinson, D. L. and Norr, L. (2006). Nutrition and health in late prehistoric central Gulf Coast Florida. *American Journal of Physical Anthropology*, **129**, 375–86.

Isler, R., Schoen, J., and Iscan, M. Y. (1985). Dental pathology of a prehistoric population in Florida. *Florida Scientist*, **48**, 139–46.

Jackes, M. and Lubell, D. (1996). Dental pathology and diet: second thoughts. In *Nature et Culture, Actes du Colloque international de Liège, December 1993. Etudes et Recherches Archéologiques de l'Université de Liège*, **68**, 457–80.

Kelley, M., Barrett, T., and Saunders, S. D. (1987). Diet, disease, and transition in northeast native Americans. *Man in the Northeast*, **33**, 113–25.

Kerr, N. W., Bruce, M. F., and Cross, J. F. (1988). Caries experience in the permanent dentition of late Mediaeval Scots. *Archives of Oral Biology*, **33**, 143–8.

Kerr, N. W., Cross, J. F., and Bruce, M. F. (1990). Caries experience in Mediaeval Scots. *American Journal of Physical Anthropology*, **83**, 69–76.

Kolenbrander, P. E. and Plamer, R. J. Jr. (2004). Human oral bacterial biofilms. In *Microbial Biofilms*, ed. M. Ghannoum & G. A. O'Toole, pp. 85–117. Washington, D. C.: ASM Press.

Krogman, W. M. (1938). The role of urbanization in the dentitions of various population groups. *Zeitschrift fur Rassenkunde*, **7**, 41–72.

Laine, M. A. (2002). Effect of pregnancy on periodontal and dental health. *Acta Odontologica Scandinavica*. **60**, 257–64.

Larsen, C. S. (1980). *Prehistoric human biological adaptation: a case study from the Georgia coast.* Ph.D. Dissertation, University of Michigan.

Larsen, C. S. (1983). Behavioural implications of temporal change in cariogenesis. *Journal of Archaeological Science*, **10**, 1–8.

Larsen, C. S. (1997). *Bioarchaeology: Interpreting Behavior from the Human Skeleton*. Edinburgh: Cambridge University Press.

Larsen, C. S. (1998). Gender, health and activity in foragers and farmers in the American southeast: implications for social organization in the Georgia Bight. In *Sex and Gender in Paleopathological Perspective*, ed, A. L. Grauer and P. Stuart-Macadam. Cambridge: Cambridge University Press, pp. 165–87.

Larsen, C. S., Shavit, R., and Griffin, M. C. (1991). Dental caries evidence for dietary change: an archaeological context. In *Advances in Dental Anthropology*, ed. M. A. Kelley and C. S. Larsen. New York: Wiley-Liss, Inc., pp. 179–202.

Little, K. (1973). *Bone Behavior*. London: Academic Press.

Littleton, J. and Frohlich, B. (1989). Analysis of dental pathology and diet on historic Bahrain. *Paleorient*, **15**, 59–75.

Lukacs, J. R. (1989). Dental paleopathology: methods for reconstructing dietary patterns. In *Reconstruction of Life from the Skeleton*, ed. M. Y. Iscan and K. A. R. Kennedy. New York: Alan R. Liss, Inc., pp. 261–86.

Lukacs, J. R. (1992). Dental paleopathology and agricultural intensification in South Asia: new evidence from Bronze Age Harappa. *American Journal of Physical Anthropology*, **87**, 133–50.

Lukacs, J. R. (1995). The "caries correction factor": a new method of calibrating dental caries rates to compensate for antemortem loss of teeth. *International Journal of Osteoarchaeology*, **5**, 151–6.

Lukacs, J. R. (1996). Sex differences in dental caries rates with the origin of agriculture in South Asia. *Current Anthropology*, **37**, 147–53.

Lukacs, J. R. and Largaespada, L. (2006). Explaining sex differences in dental caries rates: Saliva, hormones and "life history" etiologies. *American Journal of Human Biology*, **18**, 540–55.

Lukacs, J. R., Schultz, M., and Hemphill, B. E. (1989). Dental pathology and dietary patterns in Iron Age Pakistan. In *South Asian Archaeology 1985*, ed. K. Frifelt and P. Sorensen. London: Curzon Press, pp. 475–98.

Maczel, M., Kocsis, G. S., Marcsik, A., and Molnár, E. (1997). Dental disease in the Hungarian conquest period. *Bulletin et mémoires de la Société d'Anthropologie de Paris*, **9**, 457–70.

Mandel, I. D. (1979). Dental caries. *American Scientist*, **67**, 680–8.

Mansbridge, J. N. (1959). Sex differences in the prevalence of dental caries. *British Dental Journal*, **106**, 303–8.

Manzi, G., Salvadei, L., Vienna, A., and Passarello, P. (1999). Discontinuity of life conditions at the transition from the Roman Imperial Age to the early Middle Ages: example from central Italy evaluated by pathological dento-alveolar lesions. *American Journal of Human Biology*, **11**, 327–41.

Marsh, P. D. (2004). Dental plaque as a microbial biofilm. *Caries Research*, **38**, 204–11.

Martin, D. L., Goodman, A. H., Armelagos, G. L., and Magennis, A. L. (1991). Diet and dental health. In *Black Mesa Anasazi Health: Reconstructing Life from Patterns of Death and Disease*, ed. D. L. Martin, A. H. Goodman, G. L. Armelagos, and A. L. Magennis. Carbondale, IL: Southern Illinois University, pp. 165–206 and 327–41.

Molnar, S. and Molnar, I. (1985). Observations of dental disease among prehistoric populations of Hungary. *American Journal of Physical Anthropology*, **67**, 51–64.

Morris, A. G. (1992). *The Skeletons of Contact: a Study of Protohistoric Burials from the Lower Orange River Valley, South Africa*. Johannesburg: Witwatersrand University Press.

Olsson, G. S. S. and Sagne, S. (1976). Studies of caries prevalence in a medieval population. *Dento Maxillo Facial Radiology*, **5**, 12–18.

Owsley, D. W., Miles, A.-M., and Gill, G. W. (1985). Carious lesions in permanent dentitions of protohistoric Easter Islanders. *Journal of the Polynesian Society*, **94**, 415–22.

Owsley, D. W., Orser, C. E. Jr., Mann, R. W., Moore-Jansen, P. H., and Montgomery, R. I. (1987). Demography and pathology of an urban slave population from New Orleans. *American Journal of Physical Anthropology*, **74**, 185–97.

Oxenham, M., Nguyen, L. C., and Nugyen, K. T. (2006). The oral health consequences of the adoption and intensification of agriculture in Southeast Asia. In *Bioarchaeology of Southeast Asia*, ed. M. Oxenham and N. Tayles. Cambridge: Cambridge University Press, pp. 263–89.

Oxenham, M. and Tayles, N., eds. (2006). *Bioarchaeology of Southeast Asia*. Cambridge: Cambridge University Press.

Oyamada, J., Manabe, Y., Kitagawa, Y., and Rokutanda, A. (1996). Dental morbid condition of hunter-gatherers on Okinawa Island during the middle period of the prehistoric shell midden culture and of agriculturalists in northern Kyushu during the Yayoi period. *Anthropological Science*, **104**, 261–80.

Oyamada, J., Kitagawa, Y., Manabe, Y., and Rokutanda, A. (2004). Dental pathology in the Samurai and commoners of early modern Japan. *Anthropological Science*, **112**, 235–46.

Pechenkina, E., Benfer, R. A. Jr., and Zhijun, W. (2002). Diet and health changes at the end of the Chinese Neolithic: the Yangshao/Longshan transition in Shaanxi Province. *American Journal of Physical Anthropology*, **117**, 15–36.

Pietrusewsky, M. (1976). *Prehistoric Human Skeletal Remains from Papua New Guinea and the Marquesas*. Vol. 7. Asian and Pacific Archaeology Series. University of Hawaii at Manoa: Social Sciences and Linguistics Institute.

Pietrusewsky, M. and Douglas, M. T. (2002). *Ban Chiang, A Prehistoric Village Site in Northeast Thailand I: The Human Skeletal Remains*. Museum of Archaeology and Anthropology, Monograph Number 111. Philadelphia: University of Pennsylvania.

Powell, M. L. (1988). *Status and Health in Prehistory*. Washington, D C: Smithsonian Institution,

Rabkin, S. (1942). Dental conditions among prehistoric Indians of northern Alabama. *Journal of Dental Research*, **21**, 211–22.

Rathbun, T. A. (1987). Health and disease at a South Carolina plantation: 1840–1870. *American Journal of Physical Anthropology*, **74**, 239–53.

Reeves, M. (2000). Dental health at early historic Fusihatchee Town: biocultural implications of contact in Alabama. In *Bioarchaeological Studies of Life in the Age of Agriculture: A View from the Southeast*, ed. P. Lambert. Tuscaloosa: University of Alabama Press, pp. 78–95.

Ryan, D. J. (1977). *The paleopathology and paleoepidemiology of the Kayenta Anasazi Indians in northeastern Arizona*. Ph.D. Dissertation, Arizona State University.

Sakashita, R., Inoue, M., Inoue, N., Pan, Q., and Zhu, H. (1997). Dental disease in the Chinese Yin-Shang Period with respect to relationships between citizens and slaves. *American Journal of Physical Anthropology*, **103**, 401–8.

Sauerwein, E. (1974). *Kariologie*. Stuttgart: G. Thieme.

Saul, F. P. (1972). The human skeletal remains of Altar de Sacrificios. In *The Altar de Sacrificios excavations; general summary and conclusions*, ed. G. R. Willey. Cambridge, MA: Peabody Museum, pp. 1–123.

Saul, F. P. (1975). Human remains from Lubaantun. In *Lubaantun*, ed. N. Hammond. Cambridge, MA: Harvard University, pp. 389–410.

Saul, F. P. (1982). Human Remains from Tancah, Mexico. In *On the Edge of the Sea: Mural Paintings at Tancah-Tulum, Quintana Roo, Mexico*, ed. A. G. Miller. Washington, DC: Dumbarton Oaks Research Library and Collection, pp. 115–28.

Saunders, S. R. (1997). Dental caries in nineteenth century upper Canada. *American Journal of Physical Anthropology*, **104**, 71–87.

Schollmeyer, K. G. and Turner, C. G., II (2004). Dental caries, prehistoric diet, and the pithouse-to-pueblo transition in southwestern Colorado. *American Antiquity*, **69**, 569–82.

Schultz, M., Lukacs, J. R., Schwartz, P., and Hemphill, B. E. (1996). Results of paleopathological investigations in Iron Age skeletons from Sarai Khola (Pakistan). *Homo*, **47**, 85–110 (in German).

Sealy, J. C. (1992). Diet and dental caries among later Stone Age inhabitants of the Cape Province, South Africa. *American Journal of Physical Anthropology*, **88**, 123–34.

Sims, D. C., Danforth, M. E., Giliberti, J. A., Montana, A. M., and McMakin, T. (1992). Analysis of diet in the Mississippian populations at Kellogg Village, Mississippi, using dental indicators. *Mississippi Archaeology*, **27**, 44–59.

Slaus, M. (1997). Dental Disease in the Late Medieval Population from Nova Raca, Croatia. *Collegium Antropologicum*, **21**, 561–72.

Slaus, M. (2002). *The Bioarchaeology of Continental Croatia: An analysis of human skeletal remains from the prehistoric to post-medieval periods*. Oxford, England: Archaeopress B.A.R.

Slaus, M., Peina-Slaus, N., and Brki, H. (2004). Life stress on the Roman Limes in continental Croatia. *Homo*, **54**, 240–63.

Smith, M. O. (1982). *Patterns of association between oral health status and subsistence: a study of Aboriginal skeletal populations from the Tennessee Valley area.* Ph.D. Dissertation, University of Tennessee.

Smith, M. O. (1986). Caries frequency and distribution in the Dallas skeletal remains from Toqua. *Tennessee Anthropologist*, **11**, 145–55.

Smith, S. K. (2000). Skeletal and dental evidence for social status in late Bronze Age Athens. In *Paleodiet in the Aegean*, ed. S. J. Vaughan and W. D. E. Coulson. Weiner Laboratory Monograph 1, Oxford: Oxbow Books, pp. 105–13.

Stewart, T. D. (1931). Dental caries in Peruvian skulls. *American Journal of Physical Anthropology*, **15**, 315–25.

Sutter, R. C. (1995). Dental pathologies among inmates of the Monroe County poorhouse. In *Bodies of Evidence: Reconstructing History through Skeletal Analysis*, ed. A. L. Grauer. New York: Wiley-Liss, Inc., pp. 185–96.

Swanson, C. E. (1976). *Dental pathologies in Gran Quivira.* Ph.D. Dissertation, Arizona State University.

Tabak, L. A. (2006). In defense of the oral cavity: the protective role of the salivary secretions. *Pediatric Dentistry*, **28**, 110–17.

Tattersall, I. (1968). Dental Paleopathology of Medieval Britain. *Journal of the History of Medicine and Allied Sciences*, **23**, 380.

Tayles, N. (1999). *Report of the Research Committee. LXI. The Excavation of Khok Phanom Di, a Prehistoric Site in Central Thailand, Vol. V: The People*. London: Society of Antiquaries.

Tayles, N., Domett, K. M., and Hunt, V. (1998). The people of Nong Nor. In *University of Otago Studies in Prehistoric Anthropology, 18: The Excavation of Nong Nor, a Prehistoric Site in Central Thailand*, ed. C. Higam and R. Thosarat. Dunedin: University of Otago Press, pp. 321–68.

Tayles, N., Domett, K. M., and Nelsen, K. (2000). Agriculture and dental caries? The case of rice in prehistoric Southeast Asia. *World Archaeology*, **32**, 68.

Thornton, F. (1991). Dental disease in a Romano-British skeletal population from Baldock, Hertfordshire. *International Journal of Osteoarchaeology*, **1**, 273–77.

Thornton, F. (1995). Change in oral pathology through time of Nile Valley populations predynastic to Roman. In *The Archaeology of Death in the Ancient Near East*, ed. S. Campbell and A. Green. Oxford: Oxbow Books, pp. 41–4.

Turner, C. G., II. (1979). Dental anthropological indications of agriculture among the Jomon people of central Japan. *American Journal of Physical Anthropology*, **51**, 619–36.

Ubelaker, D. H. (1997). *Skeletal Biology of Human Remains from La Tolita, Esmeraldas Province, Ecuador*. Smithsonian Contributions to Anthropology, No 41. Washington, DC: Smithsonian Institution Press.

Ubelaker, D. H. and Pap, I. (1998). Skeletal evidence for health and disease in the Iron Age of northeastern Hungary. *International Journal of Osteoarchaeology*, **8**, 231–51.

Ubelaker, D. H., Jones, E. B., and Landers, D. B. (2003). *Human Remains from Voegtly Cemetery, Pittsburgh, Pennsylvania*. Smithsonian Contributions to Anthropology, No. 46. Washington, DC: Smithsonian Institution Press.

Vallianatos, H. (2007). Food cravings and aversions in pregnancy: a Darwinian perspective on gender differences in dental health. *American Journal of Physical Anthropology*, Suppl. 44, 235–6.

Vodanovic, M., Brkic, H., Slaus, M., and Demo, Z. (2005). The frequency and distribution of caries on the mediaeval population of Bijelo Brdo in Croatia. *Archives of Oral Biology*, **50**, 669–80.

Walker, P. L. (1988). Sex differences in the diet and dental health of prehistoric and modern hunter-gatherers. *Proceedings of the VI European Meeting of the Paleopathology Association*, Madrid: Universidad Compultense de Madrid, pp. 249–60.

Walker, P. L. and Cook, D. C. (1998). Brief communication: gender and sex: vive la difference. *American Journal of Physical Anthropology*, **106**, 255–9.

Walker, P. L. and Erlandson, J. (1986). Dental evidence for prehistoric dietary change on the northern Channel Islands, California. *American Antiquity*, **51**, 375–83.

Walker, P. L. and Hewlett, B. (1990). Dental health, diet and social status among central African foragers and farmers. *American Anthropologist*, **92**, 383–98.

Watt, M. E., Lunt, D. A., and Gilmour, W. H. (1997). Caries prevalence in the permanent dentition of a Mediaeval population from the southwest of Scotland. *Archives of Oral Biology*, **42**, 601–20.

Wells, C. (1982). The Human Burials. In *Romano-British Cemeteries at Cirencester*, ed. A. McWhirr, L.Viner and C. Wells. Cirencester, England: Cirencester Excavation Committee, pp. 146–52.

White, C. D. (1997). Ancient diet at Lamanai and Pacbitun: Implications for the ecological model of collapse. In *Bones of the Ancient Maya: Studies of Ancient Skeletons*, ed. S. L. Whittington and D. M. Reed. Washington, DC: Smithsonian Institution Press, pp. 171–80.

Whittaker, D. K. and Molleson, T. (1996). Caries prevalence in the dentition of a late eighteenth century population. *Archives of Oral Biology*, **41**, 55–61.

Whittington, S. L. (1989). *Characteristics of demography and disease in low status Maya from classic period Copan, Honduras.* Ph.D. Dissertation, Pennsylvania State University.

Whittington, S. L. (1999). Caries and antemortem tooth loss at Copán: implications for commoner diet. In *Reconstructing Ancient Maya Diet*, ed. C. D. White. Salt Lake City: University of Utah Press, pp. 151–67.

Willey, G. R. (1965). The human skeletal remains. In *Prehistoric Maya Settlements in the Belize Valley*, ed. G. R. Willey, W. R. Bullard Jr., J. B. Glass, and J. C. Gifford. Cambridge, MA: Peabody Museum, pp. 530–58.

Wing, E. S. and Brown, A. B. (1979). *Paleonutrition: Method and Theory in Prehistoric Foodways*. Orlando: Academic Press.

Yu-Zhu, Z. (1982). Dental disease of Neolithic age skulls excavated in Shaanxi Province. *Chinese Medical Journal*, **95**, 391–6.

Endnotes

1. We define sex as a person's biological identity and regard gender as one aspect of a person's social identity (Armelagos, 1998; Walker and Cook, 1998). Estimation of an individual's sex from the human skeleton constitutes the basis for this study, not social indicators of gender.
2. Since the age groups included in the study were 12–17 year olds, the missing (M) component of the DMFT index was irrelevant, hence D(M)FT.

8 *Dental pathology prevalence and pervasiveness at Tepe Hissar: statistical utility for investigating inter-relationships between wealth, gender and status*

BRIAN E. HEMPHILL

8.1 Introduction

This contribution demonstrates how dental pathology analysis can be used to document differences in dental health that likely stem from social stratification. The case study is based on a sample of human remains from Tepe Hissar, Iran. Reflecting the overall theme of this volume, the primary emphasis of this study is to explore how dental disease prevalence based on individual counts, coupled with a new method for assessment of pervasiveness controlled for subsequent proliferation after initial insult among individuals, yields greater insight into intra-populational differences in dietary behavior.

Advances in applying analytical chemistry to archaeologically derived skeletal material has led to an upswing in studies that employ carbon and nitrogen stable isotope analysis of bone collagen to determine whether differences in dietary behavior may be found within ancient populations. These studies often couple sex identification with the artifacts associated with individuals to determine if dietary differences correspond to assumed differences in wealth status (Ambrose *et al*., 2003; Dürrwächter *et al*, 2006; Jay and Richard, 2006; Le Huray and Schutkowsky, 2005; Murray and Schoeninger, 1988; Ubelaker *et al*, 1995).

While such studies provide a powerful tool for assessing the impact of social divisions in past populations, it is sometimes impossible to perform destructive analyses. In such cases, alternative procedures to determine whether elites suffered less from disease (Hatch and Geidel, 1983; Robb *et al*., 2001; Storey, 1998), or enjoyed longer lives have been employed (Cook, 1981; Šlaus, 2000; Storey, 1998; Sullivan, 2004).

Technique and Application in Dental Anthropology ed. Joel D. Irish and Greg C. Nelson
Published by Cambridge University Press.

A popular alternative strategy is to evaluate the impact of social divisions through assessment of dental pathology. Walker and Hewlett (1990) examined dental health, diet, and social stratification among modern Central African Pygmies and Bantu. They found significant differences in the frequency of carious teeth between men and women, Pygmy leaders and non-leaders, and Pygmies and neighboring Bantus. They interpreted these differences as the product of socially mediated variation in access to animal protein relative to carbohydrate-rich plant foods.

Two recent studies have extended this research design to evaluate prehistoric samples. Sakashita and coworkers (1997) compared tooth count frequencies of caries, antemortem tooth loss, and alveolar resorption among 82 citizens recovered from Yin-Shang period tombs at Anyang to 183 slaves recovered from "sacrificial pits." While no significant differences were found between younger individuals, older individuals among the citizens suffered from significantly higher pervasion of antemortem tooth loss and periodontal disease. Cucina and Tiesler (2003) used tooth-count frequencies of caries and antemortem tooth loss among classic period Maya of the northern Peten to document sex discrimination in dietary preferences; among elite members the males consumed a more diversified diet, while there was an absence of sex-based differences among low-status individuals (see also Storey, 1999; Whittington, 1999).

Dental pathology affliction is commonly analyzed by individual and/or by tooth. There are advantages and limitations to each method. Individual counts of disease prevalence are justifiable on the grounds that individuals are the unit upon which natural selection and social selection – manifested via gender roles and social status – ultimately act. Lukacs (1992, p. 137) laments that, "when a prehistoric sample is subdivided by age and sex the number of individuals often becomes quite small, precluding reliable statistical analysis." This is true, but the difficulties extend beyond significance testing because individual counts, as a dichotomous measure, give rise to several difficulties. First, as a dichotomous variable, the relationship between individual count-based disease prevalence and wealth cannot be assessed by means of ordinary least squares (OLS) regression. The reason is that dichotomous variables violate an array of assumptions underlying OLS associated with distributions and levels of measurement (Agresti and Finlay 1997). Second, in an attempt to preserve the individual as the unit of selection, the researcher is forced to ignore potentially important information that may be obtained from the extent, or "pervasiveness" of specific dental diseases suffered by individuals. It is likely that the pervasiveness of dental disease experienced by individuals provides related, but unique information about dietary behavior which, when coupled with individual count-based dental disease prevalence, provides greater insight into the impact of differential social selection on the health and lifeways of members of past societies.

Some have advocated tooth counts as a superior method for capturing information about disease affliction, and for increasing sample sizes to improve statistical performance (Cucina and Tiesler, 2003; Hemphill *et al.*, 1991; Lukacs, 1989, 1992; Sakashita *et al.*, 1997; Walker and Hewlett, 1990). Unfortunately, direct tooth-count comparisons suffer several difficulties that arise from the fact that subsequent proliferation of dental disease throughout the dentition from initial insult does not represent separate independent events (Ibsen and Phelan, 2005). Quite the contrary, increased liability to proliferation represents an instance of positive autocorrelation (Bowerman and O'Connell, 1987). Consequently, one cannot employ statistical measures that assume event independence. Further, this non-independence artificially inflates the degrees of freedom used in statistical tests, thereby increasing the likelihood of committing Type I errors (Heiman, 2000). Hence, despite much potential, tooth-count comparisons are either eschewed, or performed in a manner that renders interpretation unreliable.

This study sets forth a new methodology that solves these inherent difficulties related to non-independence of tooth-count based assessments; yet it still preserves the individual as the relevant unit of analysis, while demonstrating that comparisons between relatively small samples yield meaningful results.

8.2 Materials and methods

8.2.1 Materials

The transition from the Chalcolithic to Middle Bronze Age in Iran witnessed the rise of complex cities, inter-site differentiation within regions, development of social stratification, and formation of an extensive trade network (Dyson and Tosi, 1989; Hole, 1987b; Johnson, 1987). It spanned the Indo-Iranian borderlands, linking together an array of local populations in Iran, south central Asia, and the Indus Valley (Jarrige, 1994; Kohl, 1978).

Tepe Hissar, 150 miles east-northeast of Tehran (Figure 8.1), represents the largest known site in the Damghan region of northeastern Iran. Situated along an important trade route (Dyson and Remsen, 1989; Hole, 1987a; Howard, 1989; Piggott, 1989), Tepe Hissar was occupied for nearly three millennia, encompassing at least three major (Schmidt, 1933, 1937; but see Howard, 1989) periods of occupation from the early Chalcolithic (*c.* 4590 BC) to the Middle Bronze Age (*c.* 1705 BC) (Dyson and Lawn, 1989; Howard, 1989; Tosi *et al.*, 1992; Voigt and Dyson, 1992).

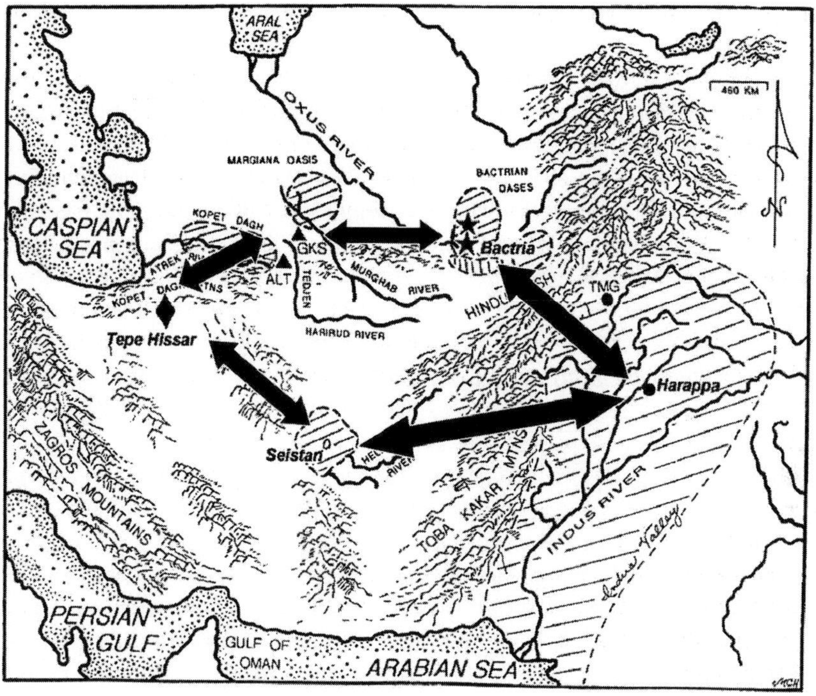

Figure 8.1 Geographic location of Tepe Hissar. Arrows represent bidirectional trade network spanning northeastern Iran, south Central Asia, Afghanistan, Indus Valley and southern Iran as described by Jarrige (1994).

Excavations by Erich Schmidt in 1931–2 led to the recovery of 1637 burials (Nowell, 1989; Schmidt, 1933, 1937) and a large number of burial goods. These burials were not recovered from a formal cemetery, but from beneath house floors throughout the settlement (Dyson and Remsen, 1989; Schmidt, 1933, 1937). The remains of nearly 300 individuals are curated at the University of Pennsylvania. Some 235 have been identified by sex, have dental and/or gnathic remains, and are accompanied by burial records that document associated burial goods, or the lack thereof.

8.2.2 *Methods: determination of wealth status*

Burial accoutrements were divided into nine categories. A wealth score was determined for each burial by weighting the relative value of each item found in association with the burial and summing them. The value for each category of object was calculated by scaling its relative rarity to the frequency of the most common accoutrement category.

The relationship between dental disease and wealth was analyzed with wealth considered as both a continuous (wealth score) and ordinal variable (wealth group). When considered as a continuous variable, disease occurrence relative to wealth score was assessed by means of ANOVA. When considered as an ordinal variable, disease prevalence relative to wealth group is assessed by means of logistic regression, ANOVA, independent samples t-tests, paired samples t-tests, and Kruskal–Wallis *H*-tests.

8.2.3 Methods: analysis of dental pathology

Dental and gnathic remains were assessed for seven pathological conditions according to Lukacs (1989). These include abscessing (Absc), antemortem tooth loss (AMTL), caries, hypercementosis (Hyper), hypoplasia (Hypo), pulp exposures (PulpX) and alveolar resorption (Resorp). Teeth affected by pulp exposures were further examined to determine whether pulp exposure was caused by excessive wear (PulpXW) or by caries (PulpXC). The relative contribution of wear and caries to pulp exposure was used in conjunction with the rate of AMTL to calculate the caries correction factor (CariesC) to provide a more accurate estimate of caries prevalence (Lukacs, 1992).

The following methodology was developed to avoid the problems of dichotomous variables used in individual-count assessments of disease prevalence; it also addresses the problem of non-independence caused by subsequent proliferation of dental disease after initial insult with tooth count assessments of disease pervasiveness, while preserving the semi-overlapping utility of both approaches.

Assessment of sex differences, differences by wealth status, and the interaction of sex and wealth status on dental disease prevalence by individual count are accomplished with logistic regression. Logistic regression avoids the assumptions of distributions and levels of measurement that plague OLS regression. Further, logistic regression permits the prediction of discrete outcomes, such as sex or wealth group, from a set of variables that may be continuous, discrete, dichotomous, or mixes thereof (Tabachnick and Fidell, 2001). Since disease prevalence by individual count represents independent events, and since Lilliefors tests uniformly reveal significant departures from normality for all variables (Hemphill, unpublished manuscript), assessment of statistical significance of differences between sexes, wealth status, and the interaction of sex and wealth status was based on Mann–Whitney U-tests. Tests for significance of individual count differences in disease prevalence across all wealth groups were accomplished with Kruskal–Wallis *H*-tests.

The methodology for assessment of tooth-count differences in disease pervasiveness was more complicated. The first step involved testing each disease to determine whether subsequent proliferation after initial insult was a significantly dependent event. This was accomplished by coding individuals so that the number of teeth affected is a continuous variable. Ordinary least squares regression was used to test the relationship between affected individuals and the number of teeth affected. Residuals obtained from testing the null hypothesis that subsequent proliferation is unrelated to initial insult were tested for significant positive autocorrelation with Durban–Watson's d according to the method of Bowerman and O'Connell (1987).

Once dependency of subsequent proliferation is established, the goal is to preserve information about the severity of affliction by individual (pervasiveness) without inflating the degrees of freedom underlying statistical significance tests. The initial problem is that the number of teeth affected for the number of teeth possible to assess is a percentage value for each sample and each sub-sample. Hence, there is no variance. A second problem is that such percentages become increasingly volatile as the number of observations per individual decrease and as sample sizes differ between samples compared. The following procedure, known as random reiterative assignment (RRA), is a randomized-block experimental design (Keppel, 1991; Shadish *et al.*, 2002) developed by the author to avoid the issues of non-variance and sample-size heterogeneity.

RRA involves drawing a series of equal number random samples of individuals by sex and by wealth group to match $n-1$ individuals for the disease with the fewest observations by wealth group and by sex (in the current study, AMTL among females of wealth group 2, where $n = 15$ observations). A total of 15 random samples of identical size were drawn for both males and females from the four wealth groups defined below. Each individual within these random samples was assigned a number and randomly shuffled in sequence. Each shuffle was reiterated 15 times. The distribution of the proportion of affected teeth in 25 randomly drawn and reshuffled samples was tested for normality with Lilliefors (1967) test. If significant departure from normality was detected, the data were ranked and each reiteration provides the basis of sequential assignment by individual for a series of Wilcoxon signed-rank T-tests. A total of 25 Wilcoxon signed rank T-tests were conducted between randomly selected and unique pairwise contrasts between reshuffled randomly drawn samples.

Because all 25 Wilcoxon signed-rank T-tests were performed on identical size random samples from the same two population sets, the overall significance of differences between contrasted samples was obtained from the average of the 25 T-tests. Since random numbers were generated in accordance with the triple modulo method of Wichmann and Hill (1982), this procedure offers the additional benefit of generating meta-samples by sex and by wealth group that have normally distributed variances and where heterogeneity of variances can be tested with Bartlett's chi-square. If the meta-samples yield contrasts with non-heterogeneous variances, then contrasts across all wealth groups are valid.

In essence, RRA provides a means to test the null hypothesis that two blocks of randomly drawn and randomly shuffled samples are derived from the same original population. RRA nullifies the non-independence of subsequent disease proliferation after initial insult because members of both groups experience the same liability for proliferation. Hence, in accordance with *ceteris peribus*, individuals of both groups are identical in sample size, in likelihood of being selected, and liability for subsequent disease proliferation; they differ only in regard to the treatment (i.e. sex, wealth status) under investigation (Shadish *et al.*, 2002). By following these steps, RRA preserves the individual basis of dental pathology data, yet permits assessment of differences in severity (pervasiveness) of affliction, without artificially inflating the degrees of freedom between contrasts, which render significance testing invalid.

8.3 Results

8.3.1 Gender and wealth

Schmidt (1937) reported the 782 individuals excavated during the 1932 field season by period (no such tally was made for the 1931 field season in his 1933 report). Age status was determined using Oetteking's age categories (see Schmidt, 1937); sex was identified for 484 individuals. A comparison of the 235 individuals used in the current study to the 484 sex-identified individuals recovered by Schmidt shows the current sample to be non-representative (Hemphill, unpublished manuscript). The samples are almost exclusively adult-aged individuals. Therefore, it is unlikely that differential age at death represents a significant factor contributing to differences in prevalence or pervasiveness between samples.

When considered by sex, there is a slight over-representation of females in the current sample, but this difference is not significant ($\chi^2 = 1.767; p = 0.184$). The current sample diverges in regard to occupational period ($\chi^2 = -2.974$; $p = 0.031$). This divergence is due to a vast under-representation of Period 1 and 2 individuals, especially males. The current sample, while representative by sex, should be viewed as biased toward the latest occupation at Tepe Hissar. Hence, interpretations based on the study sample reflect differences in dental health when occupation of this site attained its greatest internal complexity and greatest participation in inter-regional trade. As such, the study sample should provide an extra sensitive indicator of the effects of social stratification.

Wealth scores among females range from 0 to 286, with an average of 12.4, while wealth scores among males range from 0 to 206, with an average of

Table 8.1 *Analysis of variance between dental disease and wealth score*[a]

		All		Females		Males	
Pathology	Count[b]	*F*	*p*	*F*	*p*	*F*	*p*
Abscessing	I	3.530	0.062	1.501	0.224	1.689	0.196
	T	5.082	0.025	1.075	0.303	4.640	0.033
Antemortem Loss	I	1.352	0.246	0.523	0.472	0.852	0.358
	T	2.530	0.113	0.662	0.418	2.524	0.114
Caries	I	0.084	0.772	1.258	0.265	0.271	0.604
	T	0.658	0.418	0.680	0.412	0.244	0.622
Hypercementosis	I	2.939	0.088	0.752	0.388	2.373	0.126
	T	2.284	0.132	0.432	0.513	2.458	0.119
Hypoplasia	I	0.115	0.735	0.436	0.511	0.124	0.725
	T	1.033	0.310	0.054	0.816	2.234	0.137
Pulp Exposures	I	0.467	0.495	0.587	0.446	0.016	0.899
	T	2.168	0.142	0.885	0.350	1.386	0.241
Alveolar Resorption	I	0.631	0.428	0.771	0.383	0.020	0.888
	T	0.985	0.322	0.441	0.508	0.445	0.506

[a] Wealth score considered as a continuous variable.
[b] Counts are by individual (I) and by tooth (T).

8.6. An independent-samples t-test reveals no significant difference in wealth scores between males and females ($t = 0.898, p = 0.371$). The composition of wealth, however, is not the same. Burial furniture accompanying males includes significantly greater numbers of copper, lapis lazuli, and silver objects, while female graves feature a significantly greater number of ceramics (Hemphill, unpublished manuscript).

8.3.2 *Wealth score and dental disease*

ANOVA identifies few significant relationships between wealth score and pathology affliction regardless of whether consideration is by individual, tooth, across the entire sample, or sex (Table 8.1). Scatterplots reveal this is due to an inverse quadratic distribution in which individuals with low and high wealth scores tend to manifest dental pathologies less than individuals accompanied by intermediate scores. To deal with such a distribution, this continuous variable – wealth score – was divided into four ordinal categories (wealth groups) to provide numerical balance among burials accompanied by grave goods (Table 8.2). A paired-samples t-test reveals no significant difference in the proportion of males and females found in each wealth group ($t = -2.598$, $p = 0.081$). These wealth groups will be referred to either by number, or as the "poor" (group 1), "affluent poor" (group 2), "near rich" (group 3), and "rich"

Table 8.2 *Number of individuals by wealth group and by sex*

		Females		Males		Total	
Group	Wealth Range[a]	*n*	%	*N*	%	*n*	%
1	0	29	33.0	60	40.8	89	37.9
2	1	16	18.2	22	15.0	38	16.2
3	1.1–9.9	23	26.1	37	25.2	60	25.5
4	>10	20	22.7	28	19.0	48	20.4
TOTAL		88	100.0	147	100.0	235	100.0

[a] Wealth Range represents the range in wealth scores, as calculated according to the methodology described in the text, encompassed by the wealth group.

(group 4). Individual count and tooth counts of pathological afflictions overall and by wealth group are provided in Tables 8.3 and 8.4 for males and females, respectively.

An examination of whether initial affliction of dental disease results in a significant trend (autocorrelation) for subsequent proliferation of the disease throughout the remaining dental elements possessed by an individual is presented in Table 8.5. The tests permit rejection of the null hypothesis for all diseases with alpha at 0.10 and all diseases, except pulp exposures, with alpha at 0.05. These results confirm that disease pervasiveness, as revealed through tooth-count measures, are not independent events.

8.3.3 Gender and dental disease

Examination of disease prevalence by sex, regardless of wealth (Figure 8.2), reveals that males exceed females for three afflictions (i.e. Absc, Hyper, Resorp), females exceed males for two (Caries, Hypo), and there is near parity for the remaining two afflictions (AMTL, PulpX). With alpha set at 0.10, Mann–Whitney U-tests (Table 8.6) indicate that sex difference in disease prevalence is statistically significant for antemortem tooth loss, caries, and hypoplasia. In all three cases, females are more often affected than males. Assessment of disease pervasiveness confirms that females significantly exceed males in the number of teeth affected by hypoplastic defects, caries, the corrected caries rate (CariesC) and in the number of caries-induced pulp exposures (PulpXC). Males, however, suffer from significantly more abscesses. Only for the number of pulp exposures is there near parity between the sexes (Figure 8.3). When considered in tandem, dental prevalence and pervasiveness reveal that, although fewer wealth-group pooled females than males suffered AMTL, when these females were affected,

Table 8.3 *Dental pathology affliction among males*

		Group 1			Group 2			Group 3			Group 4			Overall		
Pathology[a]	Count	*p*	*n*	%	*P*	*n*	%	*P*	*n*	%	*p*	*n*	%	*p*	*n*	%
Absc	I	33	59	55.9	15	22	68.2	20	35	57.1	9	25	36.0	77	141	54.6
	T	113	1124	10.1	54	447	12.1	80	759	10.5	18	481	3.7	265	2811	9.4
AMTL	I	31	59	52.5	12	22	54.6	19	37	51.4	9	27	33.3	71	145	49.0
	T	146	1146	12.7	64	446	14.4	109	835	13.1	42	543	7.7	361	2970	12.2
Caries	I	23	58	39.7	10	21	47.6	15	35	42.9	12	27	44.4	60	141	42.6
	T	42	649	6.5	22	268	8.2	43	493	8.7	26	366	7.1	133	1776	7.5
CariesC	T	112	1146	9.8	64	446	14.3	102	835	12.3	44	543	8.1	322	2970	10.8
Hyper	I	21	58	36.2	12	21	57.1	24	35	68.6	8	27	29.6	65	141	46.1
	T	70	704	9.9	46	290	15.9	74	548	13.5	33	389	8.5	223	1931	11.6
Hypo	I	37	55	67.3	15	20	75.0	22	33	66.7	21	27	77.8	95	135	70.4
	T	167	557	30.0	55	243	22.6	94	441	21.3	66	332	19.9	382	1573	24.3
PulpX	I	30	58	51.7	9	21	42.9	21	35	60.0	14	27	51.9	74	141	52.5
	T	54	668	8.1	20	270	7.4	46	495	9.3	26	364	7.1	146	1797	8.1
PulpXC	T	26	54	48.2	13	20	65.0	25	46	54.4	11	26	42.3	75	146	51.4
PulpXW	T	28	54	51.8	7	20	35.0	21	46	45.6	15	26	57.3	71	146	48.6
Resorp	I	19	59	32.2	7	22	31.8	12	35	34.3	6	25	24.0	44	141	31.2
	T	69	1132	6.1	27	439	6.2	51	777	6.6	16	480	3.3	163	2828	5.8

[a] absc = Abscessing, AMTL = Antemortem tooth loss, Caries = Caries, CariesC = Caries corrected, Hyper = Hypercementosis, Hypo = Hypoplasia, PulpX = Pulp exposures, PulpXC = Caries-induced pulp exposures, PulpXW = Wear-induced pulp exposures, Resorp = Alveolar resorption.

Table 8.4 *Dental pathology affliction among females*

		Group 1			Group 2			Group 3			Group 4			Overall		
Pathology[a]	Count	*p*	*n*	%	*P*	*n*	%	*P*	*n*	%	*p*	*n*	%	*p*	*n*	%
Absc	I	11	28	39.3	6	16	37.5	13	23	56.5	7	19	36.8	37	86	43.0
	T	33	546	6.0	15	296	5.07	46	486	9.5	23	406	5.7	117	1754	6.8
AMTL	I	12	28	42.9	4	15	26.7	16	22	72.7	9	19	47.4	41	84	48.8
	T	65	561	11.6	25	288	8.7	107	473	22.6	56	420	13.3	253	1742	14.5
Caries	I	15	28	53.6	13	16	81.3	14	21	66.7	12	18	66.7	54	83	65.1
	T	34	306	11.1	21	222	9.5	53	275	19.3	33	252	13.1	141	1055	13.4
CariesC	T	75	561	13.3	40	288	13.8	135	473	28.4	72	420	17.2	322	1742	18.5
Hyper	I	10	28	35.7	5	16	31.3	11	21	52.4	6	18	33.3	32	83	38.6
	T	25	339	7.4	19	249	7.6	36	312	11.5	13	254	5.1	93	1154	8.1
Hypo	I	19	27	70.4	15	16	93.8	17	20	85.0	15	19	79.0	66	82	80.5
	T	75	290	25.9	74	217	34.1	81	265	30.6	56	256	21.9	286	1028	27.8
PulpX	I	13	28	46.4	6	16	37.5	14	21	66.7	10	18	55.6	43	83	51.8
	T	24	310	7.7	8	224	3.6	42	282	14.9	20	259	7.7	94	1075	8.74
PulpXC	T	15	24	62.5	6	8	75.0	32	42	76.2	14	20	70.0	67	94	71.3
PulpXW	T	9	24	37.5	2	8	25.0	10	42	23.8	6	20	30.0	27	94	28.7
Resorp	I	6	28	21.4	6	16	37.5	7	23	30.4	5	19	26.3	24	86	27.9
	T	14	550	2.6	14	305	4.6	15	483	3.1	10	411	2.4	53	1749	3.0

[a] Pathology abbreviations same as Table 8.3 above.

Table 8.5 *Tests for significant autocorrelation of residuals obtained from ordinary least squares regression of null hypothesis of non-dependence of subsequent proliferation of dental disease after initial insult (tooth count, sexes pooled)*

Pathology	n^a	d^b	p^c
Absc	114	1.974	0.013
AMTL	112	1.922	0.020
Caries	114	2.667	0.003
Hyper	97	1.970	0.015
Hypo	161	1.971	0.015
PulpX	117	2.182	0.091
Resorp	68	1.983	0.009

[a] Number of individuals is limited to those affected by the disease.
[b] Durbin–Watson's *d* is their test statistic for autocorrelation.
[c] *p* values associated with Durbin–Watson's *d* do not follow linearly from one pathology to another due to differences in the number of observations and in the number of non-singular (i.e. single unaccompanied insults by individual) categories of subsequent affliction.

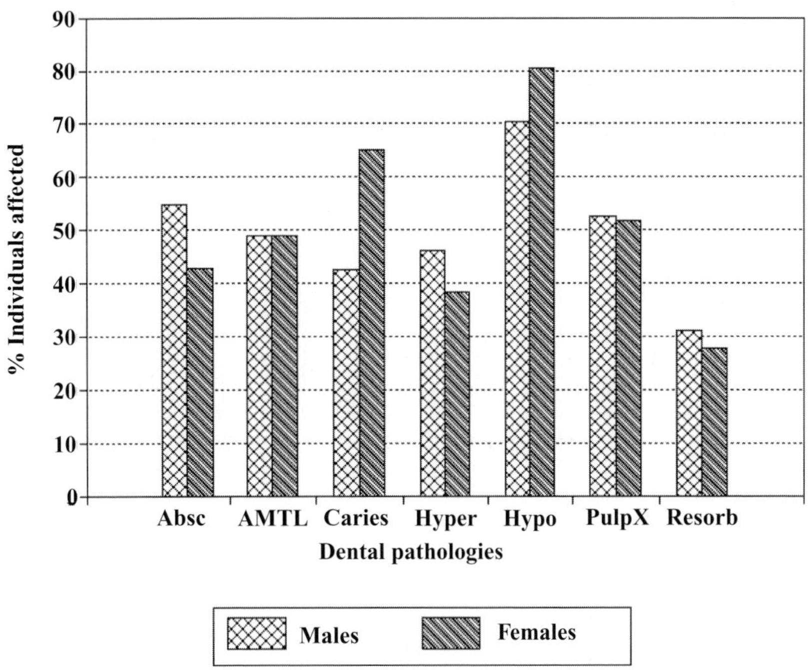

Figure 8.2 Dental pathology prevalence by sex, regardless of wealth status (individual count).

Table 8.6 *Mann–Whitney U-tests of dental pathology affliction by sex (wealth groups pooled)*

	Individual count			Tooth count	
Pathology	U^a	p	Pathology	U	p
Absc	−5360.5	0.091	Absc	−5241.5	0.067
AMTL	−6175.0	0.058	AMTL	6346.0	0.882
Caries	7168.5	0.001	Caries	7453.0	0.000
			CariesC	8285.0	0.000
Hyper	−5410.0	0.272	Hyper	−5504.5	0.671
Hypo	6095.0	0.099	Hypo	6379.0	0.058
PulpX	−5812.0	0.922	PulpX	5868.5	0.969
			PulpXC	8228.0	0.002
Resorp	−5863.0	0.599	Resorp	−5666.5	0.308

[a]Positive values reflect higher values among females; negative values reflect higher values among males.

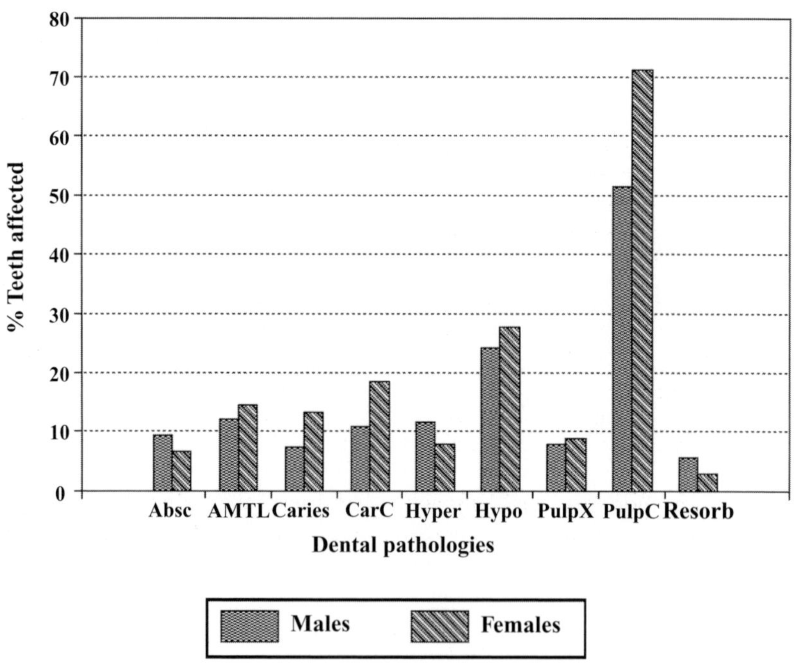

Figure 8.3 Dental pathology pervasiveness by sex, regardless of wealth status (tooth count).

Table 8.7 *Kruskal–Wallis* H-*tests of dental disease affliction across all wealth groups with sexes pooled*[a]

			Wealth group			
Prevalence			1	2	3	4
Individual Count						
Pathology	H	*p*	Rank score			
Absc	4.681	0.197	2	3	4	1
AMTL	6.252	0.100	3	2	4	1
Caries	3.797	0.284	1	4	2	3
Hyper	12.876	0.005	2	3	4	1
Hypo	3.737	0.291	1	4	2	3
PulpX	4.066	0.254	2	1	4	3
Resorp	1.604	0.658	2	4	3	1
Summary score	9.147	0.027	1.857	3.000	3.286	1.857
			Wealth group			
Pervasiveness			1	2	3	4
Tooth Count						
Pathology	H	*p*	Rank			
Absc	6.676	0.083	2	3	4	1
AMTL	7.144	0.067	3	2	4	1
Caries	3.288	0.349	1	2	4	3
CariesC	6.273	0.099	1	2	3	4
Hyper	10.615	0.014	2	3	4	1
Hypo	5.943	0.144	4	3	2	1
PulpX	3.289	0.281	3	1	4	2
PulpXC	3.853	0.278	1	3	4	2
Resorp	2.567	0.463	2	4	3	1
Summary score	14.951	0.002	2.111	2.571	3.571	1.778

[a] Here and in all subsequent tables, tooth counts are not direct tooth counts, but represent the proportion of teeth affected from meta-samples of individuals drawn through random reiterative assignment as described in the text.

AMTL was more pervasive. Inspection of CariesC and PulpXC rates suggests the driving force behind this increased pervasion of AMTL among females is carious activity.

8.3.4 Wealth group and dental disease

Sex-pooled comparisons of disease prevalence and pervasiveness across all wealth groups with Kruskal–Wallis *H*-tests yield similar, but not identical results (Table 8.7). Both reveal significant differences across wealth groups for AMTL

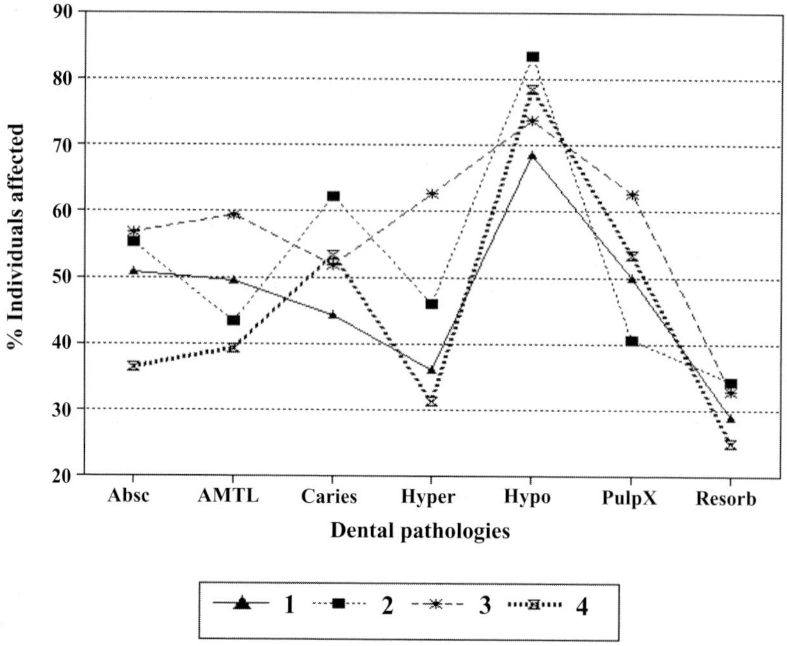

Figure 8.4 Dental pathology prevalence by wealth group with sexes pooled (individual count).

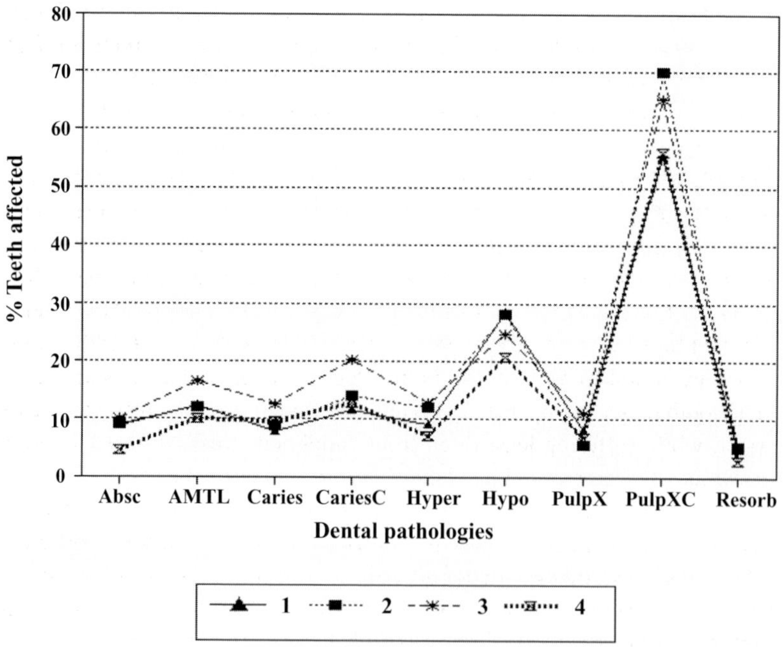

Figure 8.5 Dental pathology pervasiveness by wealth group with sexes pooled (tooth count).

and hypercementosis, but differences in the pervasiveness of abscessing and the corrected caries rate are also significant. Rank-order comparisons across wealth groups also yield differences in comparisons of disease prevalence and pervasiveness. While Kruskal–Wallis *H*-tests indicate that the relationship between wealth group and overall dental health by rank order is significant, regardless of whether prevalence ($H = 9.147$, $p = 0.027$) or pervasiveness ($H = 14.951$, $p = 0.002$) serves as the basis of comparison, and with both identifying the richest and the poorest at Tepe Hissar as having enjoyed the best overall dental health while those of intermediate wealth suffered most, the patterning is not the same.

Assessment of disease prevalence yields a fundamental dichotomy in dental health, in which the poorest and wealthiest experienced equally good overall dental health, while that experienced by the affluent poor and near rich was both far inferior and nearly equivalent to one another. By contrast, disease pervasiveness indicates that overall dental health among the wealthy exceeded that of the poor. This outcome is even more intriguing given that the two additional pathologies not considered by the individual count method (Caries C, PulpXC) yield higher scores among the wealthy (4, 2) than among the poor (1, 1). Turning to those of intermediate wealth, the roughly equivalent but inferior dental health among the affluent poor and the near rich is not confirmed. Rather, disease pervasiveness reveals that the near rich had markedly worse dental health than their affluent poor counterparts. The most influential factor behind this difference is the extensive pervasiveness of caries among the near rich.

Further insights into dietary differences between the poorest and the wealthiest at Tepe Hissar are revealed when prevalence and pervasiveness are considered in tandem. With sexes pooled, lowest prevalence of caries and hypoplasia suggest that the poor likely consumed a low-sugar diet and suffered the least childhood stress (Figure 8.4). With lowest prevalence for abscessing, antemortem tooth loss, hypercementosis and alveolar resorption, the richest individuals at Tepe Hissar experienced good overall dental health, but suffered from rather high levels of caries and hypoplasia. Yet, when examined by tooth, the poor are found to possess dentitions where hypoplastic defects and antemortem tooth losses are pervasive (Figure 8.5). Taken together, results indicate the poor, while suffering least often from childhood stress, suffered severely when afflicted.[1] For the wealthy, the reverse appears to be the case.

When consideration is limited to males, Kruskal–Wallis *H*-tests identify significant differences in dental disease affliction among members of different wealth groups, regardless of prevalence or pervasiveness (Table 8.8). Significant differences in disease prevalence are limited to one disease, hypercementosis ($p = 0.008$). Although a Kruskal–Wallis *H*-test fails to find a significant relationship between overall dental health and wealth group ($H = 4.078$, $p = 0.253$)

Table 8.8 *Kruskal–Wallis* H-*tests of dental disease affliction across all wealth groups (males only)*

			Wealth group			
Prevalence *Individual Count*			1	2	3	4
Pathology	H	*p*	Rank score			
Absc	4.402	0.221	2	4	3	1
AMTL	4.076	0.253	3	4	2	1
Caries	0.614	0.893	1	4	2	3
Hyper	11.779	0.008	2	3	4	1
Hypo	1.695	0.638	2	3	1	4
PulpX	1.345	0.718	2	1	4	3
Resorp	1.088	0.780	3	2	4	1
Summary	*H*	*p*	2.143	3.000	2.857	2.000
Score	4.078	0.253				
			Wealth group			
Pervasiveness *Tooth Count*			1	2	3	4
Pathology	H	*p*	Rank			
Absc	7.557	0.056	2	4	3	1
AMTL	6.364	0.095	2	4	3	1
Caries	0.396	0.941	1	3	4	2
CariesC	4.042	0.257	2	4	3	1
Hyper	10.365	0.016	2	4	3	1
Hypo	3.309	0.346	4	3	2	1
PulpX	1.521	0.677	3	2	4	1
PulpXC	1.708	0.635	2	4	3	1
Resorp	2.711	0.438	2	3	4	1
Summary	*H*	*p*				
score	23.938	0.000	2.222	3.444	3.222	1.111

in disease prevalence, it is apparent that dental health is, again, best among the poorest and richest. Relatively few poor males have caries or hypercementosis, a moderate number experienced alveolar resorption, while many poor males suffered antemortem tooth losses (Figure 8.6). This pattern is likely indicative of a broad-spectrum, low-sugar diet of coarse food. Rich males, on the other hand, suffered rarely from abscessing, antemortem tooth loss, hypercementosis, or alveolar resorption. Nevertheless, rich males were most often affected by childhood stress, and by a relatively high prevalence of caries and pulp exposures. In a reversal of results obtained with sexes pooled, rank-order scores of prevalence

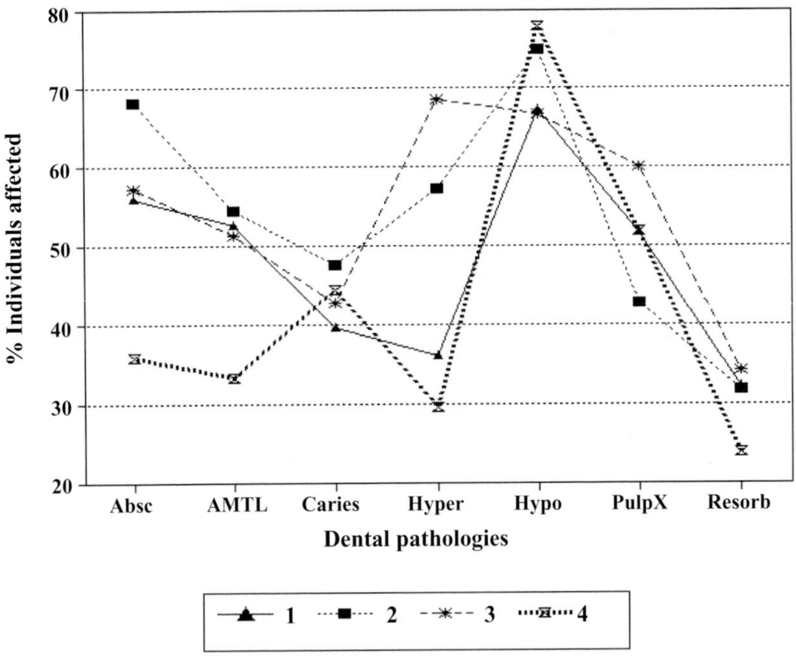

Figure 8.6 Dental pathology prevalence among males by wealth group (individual count).

indicate that the worst overall dental health occured among males of the affluent poor, rather than the near rich.

Kruskal–Wallis *H*-tests of dental disease pervasiveness among males yield significant differences across all wealth groups for abscessing, antemortem tooth loss, and hypercementosis. For all three pathologies, this difference is largely due to the disparity in pervasiveness between rich males (low) and males among the affluent poor (high). A Kruskal–Wallis *H*-test of summary scores reveals a strong association between overall dental health and wealth group ($H = 23.938$, $p = 0.000$) assessed by pervasiveness. It is clear that, with the lowest pervasiveness for eight diseases, rich males enjoyed the best dental health of all males. Poor males experienced the next best overall dental health with one exception, hypoplasia. In fact, a clear pattern of hypoplasia affliction is present wherein each increase in social status is associated with a decrease in pervasiveness. Thus, as noted for the sex-pooled comparisons, it appears that although poor males (Figure 8.7) suffered growth disruptions least often, they also suffered most severely when affected. Rich males, on the other hand, were often affected by bouts of growth disruption, but with mild

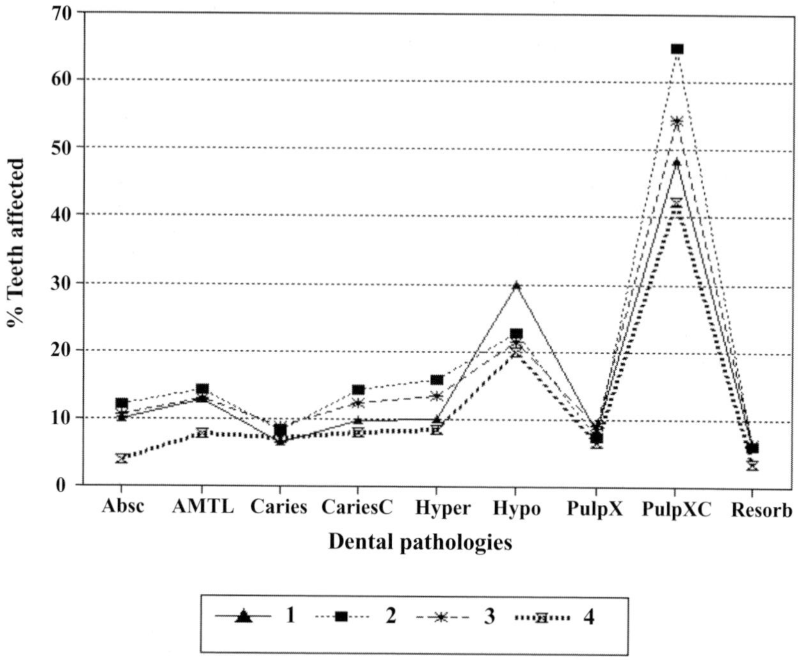

Figure 8.7 Dental pathology pervasiveness among males by wealth group (tooth count).

severity. Males among the affluent poor and the near rich appear to have borne the brunt of inferior dental health at Tepe Hissar, garnering between them the two highest ranked scores in prevalence for all diseases, except hypoplasia and pulp exposures.

When the impact of differential wealth is examined among females, a Kruskal–Wallis *H*-test of wealth group differences in summary scores reveals that, regardless of whether disease prevalence ($H = 8.264$, $p = 0.041$) or pervasiveness ($H = 15.469$, $p = 0.001$) serves as the basis of comparison, the best dental health again appears to have been experienced by the poorest and the richest individuals (Table 8.9). When assessed by prevalence (Figure 8.8), poor females – in a reversal to males – enjoyed even better dental health than wealthy females; however, like their male counterparts, relatively few females among the poor suffered from caries or hypoplasia. Apart from the poorest females, hypoplasia prevalence yields a consistent trend in which decreased prevalence co-occurs with each improvement in wealth status. Yet, despite this trend, it is clear that elevated social position notwithstanding, females among the near rich,

Table 8.9 *Kruskal–Wallis* H-*tests of dental disease affliction across all wealth groups (females only)*

			Wealth group			
Prevalence			1	2	3	4
Individual Count						
Pathology	H	*p*	Rank score			
Absc	2.809	0.422	3	2	4	1
AMTL	9.044	0.029	2	1	4	3
Caries	3.522	0.318	1	4	2.5	2.5
Hyper	3.092	0.378	3	1	4	2
Hypo	3.677	0.299	1	4	3	2
PulpX	3.273	0.351	2	1	4	3
Resorp	1.549	0.671	1	4	3	2
Summary	*H*	*p*				
score	8.264	0.041	1.857	2.429	3.500	2.214
			Wealth group			
Pervasiveness			1	2	3	4
Tooth Count						
Pathology	H	*p*	Rank			
Absc	3.164	0.367	3	1	4	2
AMTL	7.769	0.051	2	1	4	3
Caries	3.080	0.379	2	1	4	3
CariesC	7.480	0.058	1	2	4	3
Hyper	2.173	0.537	2	3	4	1
Hypo	6.258	0.100	2	4	3	1
PulpX	3.230	0.357	3	1	4	2
PulpXC	1.453	0.693	1	3	4	2
Resorp	1.909	0.591	2	4	3	1
Summary	*H*	*p*				
score	15.469	0.001	2.000	2.222	3.778	2.000

with the highest rank scores in prevalence for four of seven diseases, suffered markedly worse dental health relative to all other females at Tepe Hissar.

A somewhat different picture emerges when disease prevalence serves as the basis of comparison (Figure 8.9). Now, both the poorest and the wealthiest females appear to have enjoyed equivalent overall dental health, followed closely by the affluent poor. Indeed, affluent poor females appear to have experienced nearly equivalent dental health to their richest and poorest counterparts. Yet, two glaring exceptions to this pattern, elevated pervasion of hypoplasia and

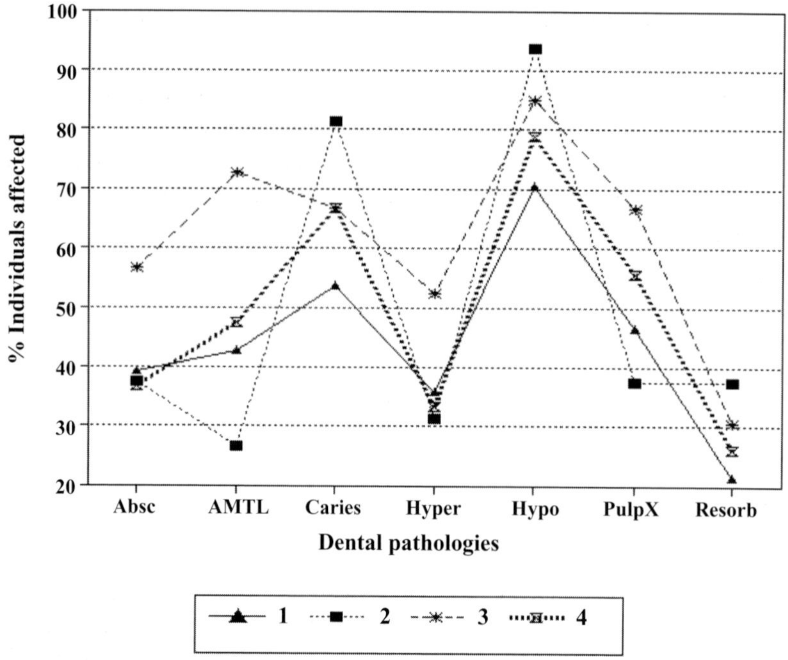

Figure 8.8 Dental pathology prevalence among females by wealth group (individual count).

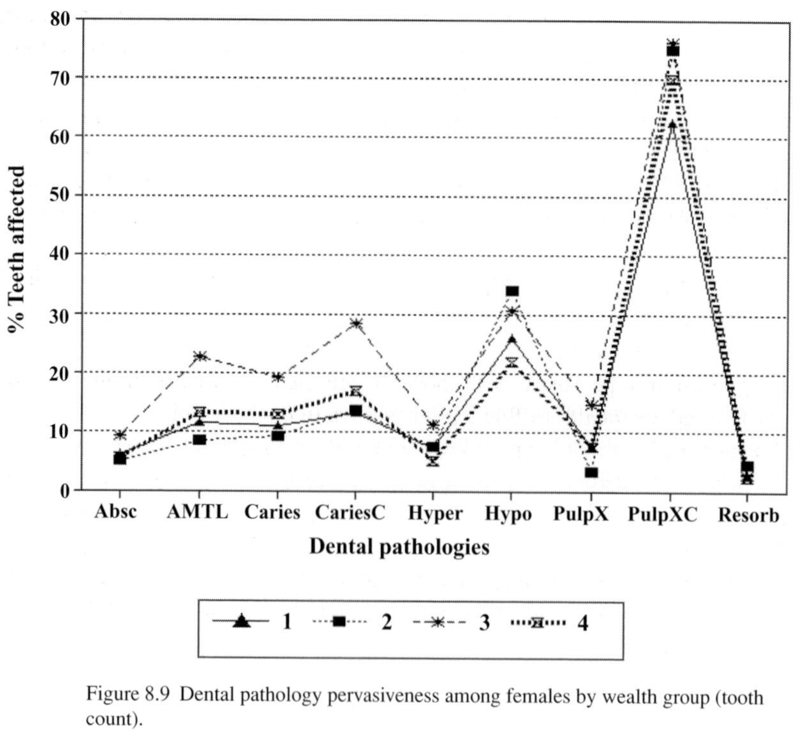

Figure 8.9 Dental pathology pervasiveness among females by wealth group (tooth count).

alveolar resorption, hint at levels of childhood stress and poor dietary quality not found among the wealthiest and poorest females. Marked by the highest rank scores for all but two diseases (hypoplasia, alveolar resorption), disease pervasiveness confirms that females among the near rich suffered markedly worse dental health than any other females.

8.3.5 Sex differences in dental disease across wealth groups

Examination of sex differences in dental pathology prevalence and pervasiveness between wealth groups yields similar, but by no means identical, results. With alpha levels at 0.10, logistic regression (Table 8.10) reveals that more significant differences in dental disease prevalence occur between the poor and those of intermediate wealth (groups 2 and 3), than with the richest at Tepe Hissar. Logistic regression finds that, relative to the poorest, a significantly greater number of affluent poor suffered from caries and hypoplasia. Similarly, a significantly greater number of near rich suffered from hypercementosis and pulp exposures relative to the poor. In striking contrast, logistic regression fails to identify a single disease that affected a significantly greater or lesser number among the poor relative to their counterparts among the wealthy.

Wilcoxon signed-rank tests of dental disease pervasiveness between wealth groups with sexes pooled reveal that the greatest differences occur with the richest, rather than poorest (Table 8.11). A total of eight contrasts were found significant with alpha set at 0.10, and all but two involve contrasts in which the richest experienced less pervasive dental disease. Of the six remaining significant contrasts, all but one (hypoplasia between members of wealth groups 1 and 4) reflect significantly less pervasive disease among the wealthy compared to those of intermediate wealth. Half of the 42 possible pairwise comparisons indicate a reduction in dental disease prevalence with an increase in wealth status, while half indicate the opposite. Intriguingly, the bulk of those that indicate a reduction involve contrasts with the wealthiest ($19/21 = 90.5\,\%$), while those that reflect the opposite (i.e. increased pervasiveness) involve contrasts between the poorest at Tepe Hissar with those of intermediate wealth, or among those of intermediate wealth (affluent poor relative to the near rich).

Few significant differences are identified when dental disease prevalence is considered across wealth groups by sex (Table 8.12). The only significant difference occurs for hypercementosis between individuals of wealth groups 1 and 3. Among both males and females, a significantly greater number of near-rich individuals of wealth group 3 suffered from hypercementosis (males: group $1 = 36.2\,\%$, group $3 = 68.6\,\%$; females: group $1 = 35.7\,\%$, group $3 = 52.4\,\%$).

Table 8.10 *Logistic regression analysis of dental disease prevalence across wealth groups with sexes pooled (individual count)*

	Group 2[a]				Group 3				Group 4			
Path.	*C*[b]	*SE*[c]	Wald[d]	*p*	*C*	*SE*	Wald	*p*	*C*	*SE*	Wald	*p*
Absc	0.188	0.390	0.233	0.630	0.255	0.341	0.558	0.455	−0.583	0.380	2.354	0.125
AMTL	−0.249	0.395	0.397	0.529	0.400	0.341	1.379	0.240	−0.419	0.370	1.278	0.258
Caries	0.730	0.403	3.289	0.070	0.305	0.344	0.784	0.376	0.367	0.369	0.988	0.320
Hyper	0.411	0.399	1.060	0.303	1.084	0.356	9.282	0.002	−0.221	0.393	0.318	0.573
Hypo	0.842	0.506	2.766	0.096	0.257	0.392	0.431	0.511	0.514	0.429	1.433	0.231
PulpX	−0.383	0.398	2.428	0.119	0.511	0.350	3.155	0.076	0.134	0.369	0.027	0.869
Resorp	0.254	0.416	0.394	0.530	0.189	0.367	0.292	0.589	−0.190	0.421	0.639	0.424

[a] The omitted category for all models is wealth group 1. Hence, values reflect the contrast between the omitted category (wealth group 1) and the named category.
[b] C represents the coefficient used to provide parameter estimates. In the first instance, individuals of wealth group 2 are 18 % more likely to experience abscessing than individuals of wealth group 1.
[c] SE represents the standard error.
[d] Wald is the Wald test, which is functionally equivalent to a *z*-score (Tabachnick and Fidell 2001).

Table 8.11 *Wilcoxon signed-rank tests of dental disease pervasiveness between wealth groups with sexes pooled and random reiterative assignment (tooth count)*

	G1 vs. G2[a]		G1 vs. G3		G1 vs. G4		G2 vs. G3		G2 vs. G4		G3 vs. G4	
Path.	T^b	p	T	p	T	P	T	p	T	p	T	p
Absc	−1.557	0.157	−2.341	0.028	0.734	0.519	−0.930	0.409	1.923	0.060	2.521	0.021
AMTL	0.764	0.479	−1.664	0.129	0.454	0.673	−0.903	0.417	0.974	0.385	1.423	0.194
Caries	−1.089	0.290	−0.426	0.680	−0.942	0.385	−0.720	0.784	−0.344	0.752	0.550	0.567
Hyper	−1.352	0.242	−1.150	0.315	0.438	0.665	−0.536	0.518	1.065	0.343	0.722	0.138
Hypo	−1.457	0.179	0.446	0.671	2.453	0.023	0.795	0.447	3.629	0.000	2.500	0.023
PulpX	0.543	0.609	−1.596	0.221	0.559	0.598	−1.092	0.319	−0.396	0.703	1.337	0.211
Resorp	−1.964	0.097	−1.068	0.357	0.639	0.559	0.730	0.482	2.134	0.044	1.029	0.321

[a]G stands for wealth group. Hence, in the first instance, G1 vs. G2 indicates a contrast between members of wealth group 1 against members of wealth group 2.
[b]Positive T values indicate that frequencies are higher in the first group contrasted, while negative values indicate that frequencies are higher in the second group contrasted.

Table 8.12 *Sex-controlled logistic regression analysis of dental disease prevalence across wealth groups (individual count)*

	Group 2[a]				Group 3				Group 4			
Path.	C^b	*SE*	Wald	*p*	*C*	*SE*	Wald	*p*	*C*	*SE*	Wald	*p*
Absc	0.237	0.394	0.363	0.547	0.293	0.344	0.725	0.394	−0.538	0.383	1.980	0.159
AMTL	−0.250	0.396	0.400	0.527	0.400	0.341	1.371	0.242	−0.420	0.371	1.280	0.258
Caries	0.666	0.412	2.616	0.106	0.273	0.352	0.602	0.438	0.316	0.378	0.697	0.404
Hyper	0.451	0.402	1.258	0.262	1.109	0.358	9.594	0.002	−0.197	0.394	0.250	0.617
Hypo	0.794	0.509	2.429	0.119	0.236	0.394	0.360	0.549	0.478	0.432	1.225	0.268
PulpX	−0.381	0.399	0.911	0.340	0.512	0.351	2.130	0.144	0.135	0.369	0.133	0.715
Resorp	0.271	0.417	0.421	0.516	0.202	0.368	0.301	0.583	−0.173	0.423	0.167	0.683

[a]The omitted category for all models is wealth group 1. Hence, values reflect the contrast between the omitted category (wealth group 1) and the named category.
[b]Positive values indicate higher prevalence in named wealth group; negative values indicate higher values in wealth group 1. All abbreviations are identical to those used in Table 8.9 above.

Results from sex-segregated Wilcoxon signed-rank tests of disease prevalence are more illuminating. With alpha at 0.10, these tests yield eight significant differences among males (Table 8.13), and every one involves a contrast with the wealthiest at Tepe Hissar. Three significant differences occur between rich males and both affluent-poor and near-rich males, respectively. Two significant differences separate rich from poor males, while no significant differences occur between affluent-poor and near-rich males. Intriguingly, significant differences in hypoplasia severity, as quantified by pervasiveness, occur only between the wealthiest males and those of intermediate wealth. A majority of pairwise comparisons (27/42 = 64.3 %) indicate disease pervasiveness decreases as wealth status increases. Improvement in dental health is especially evident among the wealthiest males where all but one contrast (20/21 = 95.2 %) is marked by a decrease in pervasiveness. Those that run counter to this pattern involve contrasts between the poor males and males of intermediate wealth. It appears that, while advancement in social status paid clear benefits with regard to less pervasive dental disease among the wealthy, males of intermediate wealth – especially those of the affluent poor – suffered more pervasive dental disease than their poor counterparts.

Sex-segregated Wilcoxon signed-rank tests of dental disease prevalence among females (Table 8.14) yield 11 significant differences with alpha at 0.10. In an absolute mirror image to results obtained among males, the majority of significant differences (8/11) involve the poorest females at Tepe Hissar. The greatest number (4) occurs between poor and near rich females, followed by two significant differences between the poor and affluent poor, and between the poorest and wealthiest females, respectively. A single significant difference separates affluent-poor females from near rich and from the richest females, as well as near rich from the richest females. Unlike males, where significant differences in hypoplasia pervasiveness only occur between the wealthiest and those of intermediate wealth, such differences constitute nearly half of all significant differences among females, and separate females in all but one of the six possible contrasts by wealth group. Only the contrast between affluent-rich and near-rich females fails to yield a significant difference in hypoplasia pervasiveness. Fewer pairwise contrasts among females (22/42 = 52.4 %) reflect less pervasive dental disease accompanying increases in wealth status than among males (64.3 %). Similarly, the wealthiest females do not exhibit the near universal improvement in disease prevalence (16/21 = 76.2 %) enjoyed by the wealthiest males (95.2 %). Like males, the majority of contrasts that run counter to the pattern of less pervasive disease with increases in wealth status involve those between the poor females and females of intermediate wealth. But, unlike males, it is females of the near rich, rather than females among the affluent poor, who suffered the greatest increase in disease pervasiveness.

Table 8.13 *Wilcoxon signed-rank tests of dental disease pervasiveness among males between wealth groups with random reiterative assignment (tooth count)*

	G1 vs. G2[a]		G1 vs. G3		G1 vs. G4		G2 vs. G3		G2 vs. G4		G3 vs. G4	
Path.	T^b	p	T	p	T	P	T	p	T	p	T	p
Absc	−1.201	0.305	−0.868	0.416	2.156	0.074	0.523	0.617	3.170	0.002	2.678	0.013
AMTL	−0.615	0.569	−0.409	0.695	2.188	0.062	0.543	0.613	2.627	0.022	2.111	0.076
Caries	−0.658	0.549	−0.292	0.778	−0.751	0.517	−0.447	0.385	0.542	0.612	0.552	0.614
Hyper	−1.731	0.150	−1.432	0.266	1.052	0.391	0.553	0.458	2.179	0.094	2.227	0.042
Hypo	0.538	0.613	1.589	0.148	1.730	0.115	1.501	0.170	1.761	0.102	0.574	0.595
PulpX	0.736	0.521	−0.863	0.476	0.852	0.445	−0.587	0.599	0.418	0.688	0.770	0.480
Resorp	−1.061	0.384	−1.031	0.389	1.224	0.284	−0.331	0.750	1.579	0.122	1.676	0.122

[a] Abbreviations identical to those described for Table 8.10 above.

Table 8.14 *Wilcoxon signed-rank tests of dental disease pervasiveness among females between wealth groups with random reiterative assignment (tooth count)*

	G1 vs. G2[a]		G1 vs. G3		G1 vs. G4		G2 vs. G3		G2 vs. G4		G3 vs. G4	
Path.	T^b	p	T	p	T	P	T	p	T	p	T	p
Absc	0.971	0.342	−3.077	0.002	1.322	0.196	1.472	0.158	0.889	0.392	0.297	0.773
AMTL	0.578	0.580	−2.475	0.019	−1.714	0.097	−1.656	0.125	1.054	0.330	0.286	0.778
Caries	0.835	0.414	−0.757	0.463	−0.994	0.341	−0.433	0.407	0.373	0.717	0.389	0.704
Hyper	−0.294	0.772	−0.359	0.729	−0.884	0.391	−0.597	0.794	−0.738	0.477	0.262	0.798
Hypo	−2.472	0.016	−2.294	0.025	1.834	0.072	−0.623	0.540	3.368	0.001	3.283	0.001
PulpX	0.190	0.851	−2.287	0.028	0.284	0.783	−1.173	0.234	−0.275	0.789	1.137	0.267
Resorp	−1.716	0.095	−0.573	0.574	0.775	0.477	1.758	0.092	1.327	0.223	0.743	0.495

[a] Abbreviations identical to those described for Table 8.13 above.

Table 8.15 *Logistic regression analysis of sex differences in dental disease prevalence within wealth groups (individual count)*

Pathology	C^a	*SE*	Wald	*p*
Absc	−0.466	0.233	2.765	0.096
AMTL	0.015	0.278	0.003	0.958
Caries	0.895	0.288	9.634	0.002
Hyper	−0.351	0.292	1.444	0.230
Hypo	0.509	0.339	2.249	0.134
PulpX	−0.017	0.281	0.004	0.983
Resorp	−0.165	0.304	0.294	0.588

[a]Negative values indicate that females tend to be marked by lower disease prevalence relative to males within wealth groups, while positive values indicate that females tend to be marked by higher disease prevalence.

8.3.6 Sex differences in dental disease across wealth groups

Examination of sex differences in dental pathology prevalence and prevalence within wealth groups yields few significant differences. Logistic regression (Table 8.15) reveals that males tend to suffer more from abscessing, regardless of wealth group, while the opposite is true for caries. A nearly significant difference ($p = 0.134$) was obtained for hypoplasia prevalence. Females, with the exception of the poorest, suffer more hypoplasia than their male counterparts in each of the three remaining wealth groups.

Wilcoxon signed-rank tests of sex differences in disease pervasiveness within wealth groups (Table 8.16) identify no significant differences between the poorest, affluent poor, and richest males and females. It is only among the near rich that sex differences in disease pervasiveness attain statistical significance. Among the near rich, females suffered significantly more caries and hypoplastic defects than their male counterparts. Despite the dearth of significant differences, examination of the directionality of disease pervasiveness (as reflected by positive or negative T-values) yields an intriguing pattern. Among the poor and affluent poor, males experience more pervasive affliction than females for six and five diseases, respectively. However, among the near rich and rich, females suffer more pervasive affliction for four and five diseases, respectively.

8.4 Discussion

The results of this research provide confirmation that, once the non-independence of subsequent disease proliferation throughout the dentition is

Table 8.16 *Wilcoxon signed-rank tests of dental disease pervasiveness between males and females within wealth groups with random reiterative assignment (tooth count)*

	Group 1		Group 2		Group 3		Group 4	
Pathology	T^a	p	T	p	T	p	T	p
Absc	−0.911	0.410	−1.573	0.144	−0.719	0.496	0.954	0.351
AMTL	−0.590	0.612	−0.855	0.472	1.119	0.324	1.436	0.177
Caries	1.047	0.349	1.203	0.260	2.010	0.059	1.618	0.122
Hyper	−0.404	0.738	−0.719	0.452	−0.736	0.491	−0.761	0.471
Hypo	−0.527	0.622	1.405	0.180	1.957	0.068	0.470	0.650
PulpX	−0.483	0.653	−0.536	0.611	0.510	0.633	0.330	0.756
Resorp	−0.926	0.384	−0.603	0.581	−0.990	0.359	−0.297	0.766

[a] Positive values indicate higher frequencies for females; negative values indicate higher values among males.

taken into account through random reiterative assignment (RRA), analysis of dental disease pervasiveness in tandem with prevalence yields greater insight into the impact of social stratification on overall dental health than a consideration of disease prevalence alone. Results of prevalence and pervasiveness may be compared between males and females across all wealth groups, across all wealth groups with sexes pooled and by sex, by wealth group with sexes pooled and by sex, and between males and females within wealth groups.

Examination of sex differences in dental disease without consideration of wealth status reveals that fewer females suffered from antemortem tooth loss than males. Yet, when prevalence and pervasiveness are considered together, it is clear that while fewer females did suffer antemortem tooth losses, when they were affected it was more pervasive. Assessment of the corrected caries rate and caries-induced pulp exposures suggest the likely cause behind increased pervasiveness of antemortem tooth losses among females was caries.

Additional insight into the impact of dental disease across all wealth groups with sexes pooled is also obtained when disease prevalence is considered in conjunction with disease pervasiveness. This is because these two approaches yield similar, but by no means identical, results. Both identify the richest and the poorest as having the best overall dental health, while those in between suffered most. Examination of disease prevalence suggests that the poorest and wealthiest experienced equally good overall dental heath, while the affluent poor and near rich had nearly equivalent and far worse dental health. Yet, pervasiveness permits refinement of this observation; overall dental health among the wealthiest was actually somewhat better than that experienced by the poor, despite the fact that the wealthy suffered from a higher corrected caries rate and more caries-induced pulp exposures. This is because the wealthy, when afflicted by dental disease, suffered less pervasively than their poor counterparts. Similarly, a consideration of disease pervasiveness offers further refinement of dental health status among those of intermediate wealth. The roughly equivalent, but inferior overall dental health is not confirmed. Rather, the near rich are identified as experiencing markedly worse dental health than the affluent poor, largely because of more extensive carious activity.

As noted in the results, a consideration of prevalence and pervasiveness together reveals that while the poor experienced the lowest prevalence of hypoplasia by individual, they suffered the most pervasive affliction when affected. The opposite occurs among the wealthiest at Tepe Hissar. Hence, it appears the poor were generally able to secure adequate and fairly well-balanced foods for their children. However, on occasion, the poor either lost access to these resources or their children fell seriously ill, and when they did, they were severely stressed. The wealthy, on the other hand, appear to have been able to secure adequate, although perhaps less well-balanced food for their children. Consequently, stress experienced by children among the wealthy, although recurrent, was mild.

Assessment of overall dental health across wealth groups yields additional insight into the nature of dental disease among males and females when pathology prevalence results are considered with those of pervasiveness. Among males, it is clear that the slightly better overall dental health identified by disease prevalence among wealthy males was further enhanced by exceedingly low pervasiveness. That is, wealthy males reaped a double benefit; fewer males among the wealthy suffered from dental disease and, with the sole exception of hypoplasia, when affected, pervasiveness was mild. Further, consideration of pathology prevalence and pervasiveness reveals that the slightly inferior dental health experienced by affluent poor males relative to their near-rich counterparts involved more individuals suffering from disease, as well as more pervasive disease when affected. Assessments of dental disease among females yields results that initially appear contradictory. Disease prevalence identifies the poor as possessing better overall dental health than the wealthy. By contrast, disease pervasiveness indicates that the poor and the wealthy enjoyed equivalent overall dental health. Such findings reveal that overall dental health among poor and rich females was achieved in different ways. Fewer poor individuals suffered from hypoplasia, pulp exposure, and resorption than their wealthy counterparts. Yet, despite fewer individuals being affected by these diseases, the poor consistently suffered more extensively when affected.

Examinations of dental disease affliction between wealth groups with sexes pooled also attest to the importance of considering both disease prevalence and pervasiveness. If consideration is limited to prevalence, contrasts among individuals across wealth groups only reveal that those of intermediate wealth suffered more often from dental disease than the wealthy or poor. However, when disease pervasiveness is also included, it is apparent that the driving force behind this pattern is the remarkably less extensive disease experienced by the wealthiest at Tepe Hissar. Further, coupling disease prevalence with pervasiveness makes clear that increases in social status from poor to intermediate wealth status led to increases in the extent, as well as number of individuals affected. Further still, disease prevalence indicates that the downward trend in dental health continued as individuals of intermediate wealth moved from the affluent poor to the near rich. Taken as a whole, and in conjunction with one another, these results indicate that that the costs of social aspiration – both in disease prevalence and pervasion – weighed heaviest on the near rich of wealth group 3.

The utility of coupling prevalence and pervasiveness is clearly demonstrated from an assessment of the impact of wealth status by sex on overall dental health. While disease prevalence merely shows that a significantly greater number of near-rich males and females suffered from hypercementosis than their poor counterparts, examination of disease pervasiveness reveals how changes in wealth status affected males and females at Tepe Hissar in profoundly different ways. For males, increases in wealth status clearly paid greatest benefits for the wealthy; these benefits focus on those diseases that reflect longstanding good dental health, such as low prevalence and pervasiveness of abscessing, antemortem tooth losses, caries and hypercementosis. Among males, it was those of intermediate wealth who suffered from elevated prevalence of dental disease; and among them, males of the affluent poor rather than the near rich suffered most from inferior overall dental health. In contrast, apart from the wealthiest, increases in wealth status among females most often led to deterioration in dental health. Females of intermediate wealth suffered significantly higher dental disease pervasiveness relative to wealthy, and especially, poor females. In a striking departure from the pattern seen among males, it appears that rampantly pervasive disease was especially atrocious among those closest to the brass ring, females of the near rich.

Combining assessments of disease prevalence and pervasiveness also yields greater insight when interpreting patterns of sex differences within wealth groups. Assessment of prevalence merely reveals that more females suffered from caries and hypoplasia than males, regardless of wealth status. For the former, this difference is statistically significant. Examination of sex differences within wealth groups in disease pervasiveness yields a consistent pattern in which it is clear that, apart from the poor, each increase in wealth group resulted in clear benefits for males. For females, except the wealthiest at Tepe Hissar, each increase in wealth status led to poorer and poorer dental health, as dental disease became more and more pervasive when they moved from the poor, to affluent poor, to near rich.

8.5 Conclusions

This research demonstrates the utility of coupling examinations of dental pathology prevalence with dental pathology pervasiveness. By accounting for the non-independence of subsequent disease proliferation throughout the dentition after initial insult, the latter approach yields meaningful and statistically valid results. Together, these methods reveal that increases in wealth did not lead to a simple monotonic improvement in dental health at Tepe Hissar. Rather, the efforts of the poor to improve their social status, as reflected by the richness of their burial accoutrements, came at the price of compromised dental health. Importantly, the pattern of who bore the brunt of these costs differed between males and females. Poor males suffered from worse dental health than poor females, and of all males, the affluent poor suffered the worst dental health. Yet, each increase in wealth status conferred clear and significant improvements in dental health. This was not the case for females. Except for the wealthiest, each increase in wealth status led to commensurate declines in dental health as females moved from the poor to the affluent poor to the near rich. As such, it appears that the brunt of social aspiration in increasing wealth, as expressed by sacrifices in dental health and hence poor nutrition and hygiene, was borne by women.

This study has broad research implications for the health, social stratification and dietary patterns of ancient lifeways. Significant information can be recovered using small, effective sample sizes by using the innovative statistical analyses described in this chapter. It is hoped that further research employing these methods will help elucidate the biological impacts of social stratification, and give more comprehensive insight into the social, economic, and gendered lifeways experienced by peoples of the past.

Acknowledgments

Financial support for this research was provided by a faculty research grant from the University Research Council at Vanderbilt University. The author thanks Phil Walker for stimulating this research in an engaging conversation during the airplane ride to California from the meetings in Milwaukee, when we discussed the frustrating problems caused by the non-independency of dental disease proliferation. Thanks go to Robin Shirer Högnäs for assistance with the logistic regression analysis and to Jaymie Brauer for insightful suggestions on an earlier draft of this paper. I appreciate Joel Irish and Greg Nelson inviting me to participate in this edited volume. Special thanks also go to Janet Monge at the University of Pennsylvania for making the Tepe Hissar collection available for study and for tracking down the original burial records that proved vital in making this investigation possible.

References

Agresti, A. and Finlay, B. (1997). *Statistical Methods for the Social Sciences*. Upper Saddle River, NJ: Prentice Hall.

Ambrose, S. H., Buikstra, J., and Kreuger, H. W. (2003). Status and gender differences in diet at Mound 72, Cahokia, revealed by isotopic analysis of bone. *Journal of Anthropological Archaeology*, **22**, 217–26.

Blakey, M. L. and Armelagos, G. J. (1985). Deciduous enamel defects in prehistoric Americans from Dickson Mounds: prenatal and postnatal stress. *American Journal of Physical Anthropology*, **66**, 371–80.

Bowerman, B. L. and O'Connell, R. T. (1987). *Time Series Forecasting: Unified Concepts and Computer Implementation*, 2nd edn. Boston: Duxbury Press.

Cook, D. C. (1981). Mortality, age structure and status in the interpretation of stress indicators in prehistoric skeletons: a dental example from the Lower Illinois Valley. In *The Archaeology of Death*, ed. R. Chapman, I. Kinnes and K. Randsborg. Cambridge: Cambridge University Press, pp. 134–44.

Cucina, A. and Tiesler, V. (2003). Dental caries and antemortem tooth loss in the northern Peten area, Mexico: a biocultural perspective on social status differences among the Classic Maya. *American Journal of Physical Anthropology*, **122**, 1–10.

Dürrwächter, C., Craig, O. E., Collins, M. J., Burger, J., and Alt, K. W. (2006). Beyond the grave: variability in Neolithic diets in Southern Germany? *Journal of Archaeological Science*, **33**, 39–48.

Dyson, R. H. Jr. and Lawn, B. (1989). Key stratigraphic and radiocarbon elements for the 1976 Hesār sequence. In *Tappeh Hesār: Reports of the Restudy Project, 1976*, ed. R. H. Dyson, Jr. and S. M. Howard. Florence: Casa Editrice Le Lettere, p. 143.

Dyson, R. H. Jr. and Remsen, W. C. S. (1989). Observations on architecture and stratigraphy at Tappeh Hesār. In *Tappeh Hesār: Reports of the Restudy Project, 1976*, ed. R. H. Dyson, Jr. and S. M. Howard. Florence: Casa Editrice Le Lettere, pp. 69–109.

Dyson, R. H. Jr. and Tosi, M. (1989). Introduction. In *Tappeh Hesār: Reports of the Restudy Project, 1976*, ed. R. H. Dyson, Jr. and S. M. Howard. Florence: Casa Editrice Le Lettere, pp. 1–6.

Ensor, B. E. and Irish, J. D. (1995). The hypoplastic area method for analyzing dental enamel hypoplasia. *American Journal of Physical Anthropology*, **98**, 507–17.

Guatelli-Steinberg, D. and Lukacs, J. R. (1999). Interpreting sex differences in enamel hypoplasia in human and non-human primates: developmental, environmental, and cultural considerations. *Yearbook of Physical Anthropology*, **42**, 73–126.

Hatch, J. W. and Geidel, R. A. (1983). Tracing status and diet in prehistoric Tennessee. *Archaeology*, **36**, 56–9.

Heiman, G. W. (2000). *Basic Statistics for the Behavioral Sciences*. Boston: Haughton Mifflin.

Hemphill, B. E., Lukacs, J. R., and Kennedy, K. A. R. (1991). Biological adaptations and affinities of Bronze Age Harappans. In: *Harappa Excavations 1986–1990: A Multidisciplinary Approach to Third Millennium Urbanism*, ed. R. Meadow. Madison: Prehistory Press, pp. 137–82.

Hillson, S. (1998). Crown diameters, tooth crown development, and environmental factors in growth. In *Human Dental Development, Morphology, and Pathology: A Tribute to Albert A. Dahlberg*, ed. J. R. Lukacs. Eugene: University of Oregon Antropological Papers No. 54, pp. 17–28.

Hillson, S. and Bond, S. (1997). The relationship of enamel hypoplasia to the pattern of tooth crown growth: a discussion. *American Journal of Physical Anthropology*, **104**, 89–103.

Hole, F. (1987a). Archaeology of the village period. In *The Archaeology of Western Iran*, ed. F. Hole. Washington, DC: Smithsonian Institution Press, pp. 29–78.

Hole, F. (1987b). Settlement and society in the village period. In *The Archaeology of Western Iran*, ed. F. Hole. Washington, DC: Smithsonian Institution Press, pp. 79–105.

Howard, S. M. (1989). The stratigraphic sequence of the main mound at Tappeh Hesār, 1976. In *Tappeh Hesār: Reports of the Restudy Project, 1976*, eds. R. H. Dyson, Jr. and S. M. Howard. Florence: Casa Editrice Le Lettere, pp. 55–68.

Hutchinson, D. L. and Larsen, C. S. (1988). Determination of stress episode duration from linear hypoplasias: a case study from St. Catherine's Island, Georgia. *Human Biology*, **60**, 93–110.

Hutchinson, D. L. and Larsen, C. S. (1990). Stress and lifeway change: the evidence from enamel hypoplasias. In *The Archaeology of Mission Santa Catalina de Guale: 2. Biocultural Interpretations of a Population in Transition*, ed. C. S. Larsen. New York: American Museum of Natural History, Anthropological Papers No. 68, pp. 50–65.

Ibsen, O. A. C. and Phelan, J. A. (2005). *Oral Pathology for the Dental Hygienist*, 4th edn. Philadelphia: W. B. Saunders.

Jarrige, J.-F. (1994). The final phase of the Indus occupation at Nausharo and its connections with the following cultural complex of Mehrgarh VIII. In *South Asian Archaeology 1993*, ed. A. Parpola and P. Koskikallio. Helsinki: Annales Academie Scientiarum Fennicae B 271, pp. 295–313.

Jay, M. and Richards, M. P. (2006). Diet in the Iron Age cemetery population at Wetwang Slack, East Yorkshire, UK: carbon and nitrogen stable isotope evidence. *Journal of Archaeological Science*, **33**, 653–62.

Johnson, G. A. (1987). Nine thousand years of social change in western Iran. In *The Archaeology of Western Iran*, ed. F. Hole. Washington, DC: Smithsonian Institution Press, pp. 283–91.

Keppel, G. (1991). *Design and Analysis: A Researcher's Handbook*, 3rd edn. Englewood Cliffs, NJ: Prentice-Hall.

Kohl, P. L. (1978). The balance of trade in southwestern Asia in the mid-3rd millennium B.C. *Current Anthropology*, **19**, 463–92.

Larsen, C. S. and Hutchinson, D. L. (1999). Osteopathology of Carson Desert foragers: reconstructing prehistoric lifeways in the western Great Basin. In *Prehistoric Lifeways in the Great Basin Wetlands: Bioarchaeological Reconstruction and Interpretation*, ed. B. E. Hemphill and C. S. Larsen. Salt Lake City: University of Utah Press, pp. 184–202.

Le Huray, J. D. and Schutkowsky, H. (2005). Diet and social status during the La Tène period in Bohemia: Carbon and nitrogen stable isotope analysis of bone collagen from Kutná Hora-Karlov and Radovesice. *Journal of Anthropological Archaeology*, **24**, 135–47.

Lilliefors, H. W. (1967). On the Kolmogorov-Smirnov test for normality with mean and variance unknown. *Journal of the American Statistical Association*, **64**, 399–402.

Lukacs, J. R. (1989). Dental paleopathology: methods for reconstructing dietary patterns. In *Reconstruction of Life from the Skeleton*, ed. K. A. R. Kennedy and M. I. Iscan. New York: Alan R. Liss, pp. 261–86.

Lukacs, J. R. (1992). Dental pathology and agricultural intensification in South Asia: new evidence from Bronze Age Harappa. *American Journal of Physical Anthropology*, **87**, 133–50.

Murray, M. L. and Schoeninger, M. J. (1988). Diet, status, and complex social structure in Iron Age Central Europe: Some contributions from bone chemistry. In *Tribe and Polity in Late Prehistoric Europe: Demography, Production and Exchange in the Evolution of Complex Social Systems*, ed. D. B. Gibson and M. N. Geselowitz. New York: Plenum Press, pp. 155–76.

Nowell, G. W. (1989). An evaluation of the Tappeh Hesār 1931–1932 skeletal sample. In *Tappeh Hesār: Reports of the Restudy Project, 1976*, ed. R. H. Dyson, Jr. and S. M. Howard. Florence: Casa Editrice Le Lettere, pp. 131–32.

Piggott, V. C. (1989). Archaeo-metallurgical investigations at Bronze Age Tappeh Hesār, 1976. In *Tappeh Hesār: Reports of the Restudy Project, 1976*, ed. R. H. Dyson, Jr. and S. M. Howard. Florence: Casa Editrice Le Lettere, pp. 25–33.

Radlanski, R. J. Seidl, W., and Steding, G. (1995). Prism arrangement in human dental enamel. In *Aspects of Dental Biology: Palaeontology, Anthropology and Evolution*, ed. J. Moggi-Cecchi. Florence: International Institute for the Study of Man, pp. 33–49.

Robb, J., Bigazzi, R., Lazzarini, L., Scarsini, C., and Sonego, F. (2001). Social "status" and biological "status": a comparison of grave goods and skeletal indicators from Pontecagnano. *American Journal of Physical Anthropology*, **115**, 213–22.

Sakashita, R., Inoue, M., Inoue, N., Pan, Q., and Zhu, H. (1997). Dental disease in the Chinese Yin-Shang period with respect to relationships between citizens and slaves. *American Journal of Physical Anthropology*, **103**, 401–8.

Schmidt, E. F. (1933). Tepe Hissar excavations 1931. *The Museum Journal*, **XXIII**, 323–483.

Schmidt, E. F. (1937). *Excavations at Tepe Hissar, Damghan*. Philadelphia: University of Pennsylvania Press.

Shadish, W. R., Cook, T. D., and Campbell, D. T. (2002). *Experimental and Quasi-Experimental Designs for Generalized Causal Inference*. Boston: Houghton Mifflin.

Šlaus, M. (2000). Biocultural analysis of sex differences in mortality profiles and stress levels in the Late Medieval population from Nova Rača, Croatia. *American Journal of Physical Anthropology*, **111**, 193–209.

Storey, R. (1998). The mothers and daughters of a patrilineal civilization: the health of females among the Late Classic Maya of Copan, Honduras. In *Sex and Gender in Paleopathological Perspective*, ed. A. L. Grauer and P. Stuart-Macadam. Cambridge: Cambridge University Press, pp. 133–48.

Storey, R. (1999). Late Classic nutrition and skeletal indicators at Copán, Honduras. In *Reconstructing Ancient Maya Diet*, ed. C. D. White. Salt Lake City: University of Utah Press, pp. 83–100.

Suckling, G., Elliot, D. C., and Thurley, D. C. (1986). The macroscopic appearance and associated histological changes in the enamel organ of hypoplastic lesions of sheep incisor teeth resulting from induced parasitism. *Archives of Oral Biology*, **31**, 427–39.

Sullivan, A. (2004). Reconstructing relationships among mortality, status, and gender at the medieval Gilbertine priory of St. Andrew, Fishergate, York. *American Journal of Physical Anthropology*, **124**, 330–45.

Tabachnick, B. G. and Fidell, L. S. (2001). *Using Multivariate Statistics*, 4th edn. Needham Heights, MA: Allyn and Bacon.

Tosi, M., Sahmirzadi, S. M., and Joyenda, M. A. (1992). The Bronze Age in Iran and Afghanistan. In *History of Civilizations of Central Asia. Volume I The Dawn of Civilization: Earliest Times to 700 B. C.*, ed. A. H. Dani and V. M. Masson. Paris: UNESCO, pp. 191–223.

Ubelaker, D. H., Katzenberg, M. A., and Doyon, L. G. (1995). Status and diet in precontact highland Ecuador. *American Journal of Physical Anthropology*, **97**, 403–11.

Voigt, M. M. and Dyson, R. H., Jr. (1992). Iran. In *Chronologies in Old World Archaeology, Volume I*, 3rd edn., ed. R. W. Ehrlich. Chicago: University of Chicago Press, pp. 125–53.

Walker, P. L. and Hewlett, B. S. (1990) Dental health, diet, and social status among central African foragers and farmers. *American Anthropologist*, **92**, 383–98.

Whittington, S. L. (1999). Caries and antemortem tooth loss at Copán. Implications for commoner diet. In *Reconstructing Ancient Maya Diet*, ed. C. D. White. Salt Lake City: University of Utah Press, pp. 151–67.

Wichmann, B. A. and Hill, I. D. (1982). Algorithm AS 183: an efficient and portable pseudo-random number generator. *Applied Statistics*, **31**, 188–90.

Endnote

1. Severity and duration of stress, as indicated by hypoplastic defects, have been assessed in a variety of ways. Blakey and Armelagos (1985), Hutchinson and Larsen (1988,

1990), Ensor and Irish (1995), Larsen and Hutchinson (1999), and Suckling *et al.* (1986) all use the width of linear defects as a measure of the duration and/or severity of stress. However, as pointed out by Guatelli-Steinberg and Lukacs (1999), inferring the duration or intensity of stress from defect width suffers from a number of problems including, but not limited to, positioning of the defect on the enamel surface (Hillson 1998; Hillson and Bond 1997) and the geometry of enamel formation (Radlanski *et al.* 1995). Given these limitations, it was decided to assess "severity" of stress by the proportion of teeth affected. In doing so, assessment of the severity of stress during childhood (via hypoplasia) was scored in a similar manner to determining the severity of carious infection; that is, by the proportion of teeth affected per individual, rather than by the size and/or location of carious lesions (see Lukacs 1989).

Section III
Applied life and population history

9 *Charting the chronology of developing dentitions*

GARY T. SCHWARTZ AND M. CHRISTOPHER DEAN

9.1 Introduction

A primary goal of paleoanthropology, and indeed all sub-fields of paleontology, is to breathe life, metaphorically speaking, into fossilized remains of extinct species. Parsing out details of the phylogeny of a particular group of extinct organisms, inferring diet from comparative functional analyses of dentognathic remains, reconstructing locomotor repertoires, and sorting out brain/body size scaling relationships, etc., are but a few of the more prominent examples of how researchers make "fossils speak to us" from across vast stretches of time. Ever since the pioneering work of Schultz (1935, 1960), however, primatologists and paleoanthropologists have endeavored to reconstruct aspects of extinct species' schedule of growth, development, maturation, etc. – referred to as life history. Life history, simply put, is the schedule of key events in an organism's life cycle (e.g. gestation length, maternal–infant mass ratio, pre- and postnatal growth rates, age/weight at weaning, age at first reproduction, reproductive span, number of offspring per litter, inter-birth interval, etc.) that enable some individuals of a species to avoid predators or other mortality risks more effectively, or that in some way contribute to overall fitness (Godfrey *et al.*, 2002; Ross, 1998). Thus, life history is the "direct outcome of the interaction between developmental variables (e.g. growth rate, age at skeletal maturation) and demographic variables (survival, reproduction, population growth, life-cycle stage census counts, etc.)" (Godfrey *et al.*, 2002, p. 117).

When viewed in this light, it might seem impossible to infer such reproductive, physiological, and even behavioral parameters from fossilized remains. Fortunately, for most species of primates many important life-history events are highly correlated with one particular skeletal phenomenon: the eruption age of the permanent first molar (Smith, 1989a). As a result, studies of the timing of dental developmental events, including the age at M1 emergence, have figured prominently in a number of paleoanthropological investigations aiming to reconstruct the life history of fossil primates and hominins (e.g. Beynon *et al.*,

Technique and Application in Dental Anthropology ed. Joel D. Irish and Greg C. Nelson
Published by Cambridge University Press.

1998; Dean *et al.*, 2001; Dirks *et al.*, 2002; Godfrey *et al.*, 2001, 2004; Kelley and Smith, 2003; Mann, 1974; Schwartz *et al.*, 2005; Smith, 1986, 1989a, 1989b, 1992, 2000; Smith *et al.*, 1994; Zihlman *et al.*, 2004).

At the core of many of these studies lies a reconstruction of the pattern and pace of a developing dentition – most often illustrated as a bar chart of crown and root development. Often such bar charts are based on observations of dental emergence patterns, radiographic assessments of tooth crown and root development (e.g. Anemone *et al.*, 1996; Kuykendall, 1996; Kuykendall *et al.*, 1992; Liversidge *et al.*, 1999; Smith, 1991), or computed tomography (e.g. Conroy and Kuykendall, 1995; Conroy and Vannier, 1991a, 1991b). More recently, new techniques have emerged for mapping the growth of individual teeth, and entire dentitions, that can be applied to fossils and which complement and even clarify life-history inferences derived from studies of dental eruption, body weight, skeletal dimensions, etc. (e.g. Beynon *et al.*, 1998; Dean *et al.*, 2001; Dirks *et al.*, 2002; Schwartz *et al.*, 2002). Our goal in this chapter is to describe the means by which a bar chart illustrating the initiation, duration, and completion of an entire dentition, referred to as a dental chronology, is produced. To do so, we provide two examples: one from a recent analysis of the developing dentition of the giant sub-fossil lemur, *Megaladapis edwardsi* (Schwartz *et al.*, 2005), the other from the developing dentition of a juvenile gorilla (Schwartz *et al.*, 2006).

9.2 Tooth growth

The cells that secrete dental hard tissues leave a record of their activity in the form of incremental lines in both enamel and dentine. Over the last two decades, analyses of these incremental lines have facilitated fascinating insights into the evolutionary history of primate growth and development (e.g. Beynon and Dean, 1988; Beynon *et al.*, 1991a, 1991b, 1998; Dean, 1987, 1998; Dean *et al.*, 1993, 2001; Dean and Reid, 2001; Dirks, 1998; Dirks *et al.*, 2002; Kelley and Smith, 2003; Ramirez Rozzi and Bermudez de Castro 2004; Reid *et al.*, 1998; Schwartz *et al.*, 2002, 2005; Smith *et al.*, 2003a).

The incremental lines preserved as dental tissues appear in two forms: short- and long-period. Short-period lines, or cross striations, are daily representing the body's circadian rhythm. Long-period lines (also termed striae of Retzius) are of unknown etiology, and have a range between 2–12 days apart within primates (Smith *et al.*, 2003b). One fascinating detail about these growth lines is that the long-period incremental markings in enamel manifest themselves on the tooth crown surface as perikymata. Metabolic and physiological disturbances during the growth period are recorded in developing teeth as accentuated striae

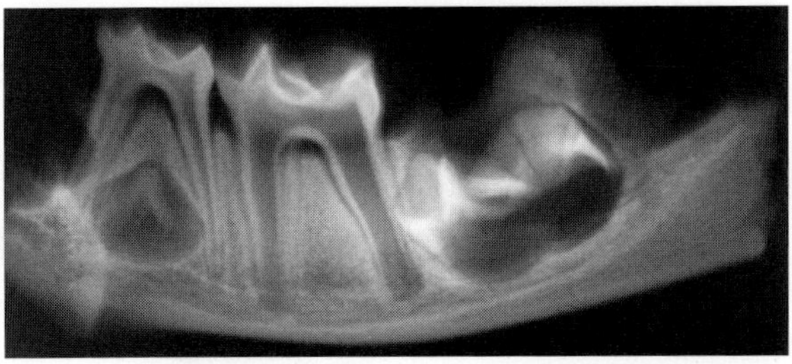

Figure 9.1a Radiograph of the left hemi-mandible of a juvenile specimen of *Megaladapis edwardsi* (UA 4620) illustrating the erupted dp_4 and M_1, the P_4 developing within the crypt deep to the dp_4, and also the M_2 (nearly crown complete) in the crypt posterior to M_1.

of Retzius (or sometimes as Wilson bands[1]) occasionally surfacing as upsets in the regular spacing and appearance of external perikymata; these are referred to as hypoplastic lesions. Such lesions (i.e. enamel defects) have been viewed as reliable markers of overall "health," and lie at the core of population studies on nutrition and disease patterns in humans and non-human primates (see Guatelli-Steinberg, 2001 for a review). These accentuated striae are the key to reliably constructing a chronology of dental development from histological sections of teeth.

9.3 Material and methods

The chronology of molar crown development in *Megaladapis edwardsi* was examined using a left hemi-mandible of a juvenile specimen (UA 4620) from Beloha Anavoha, a sub-fossil site in southwestern Madagascar. An X-ray of this specimen reveals the dp_4, a developing P_4 within its crypt beneath the dp_4, an erupted M_1, and a partially formed (i.e. crown incomplete) M_2 still seated within an exposed crypt (Figure 9.1a).

A series of teeth (maxillary and mandibular permanent I1-M2) were also extracted from a hemi-mandible and hemi-maxilla of a captive juvenile western lowland gorilla (*Gorilla gorilla gorilla*); the corresponding X-ray is presented in Figure 9.1b.

For each specimen, the intact teeth were removed from the alveolus, cleaned, and molded prior to sectioning. Each molar was also embedded in a polyester resin or coated with cyanoacrylate to reduce the risk of splintering during sectioning. A series of 180–200 μm thick ground sections were made using a Buehler® diamond-wafering blade saw (*Megaladapis*) or a Logitech PM30 annular blade saw (*Gorilla*). For *Megaladapis*, sections were made through the

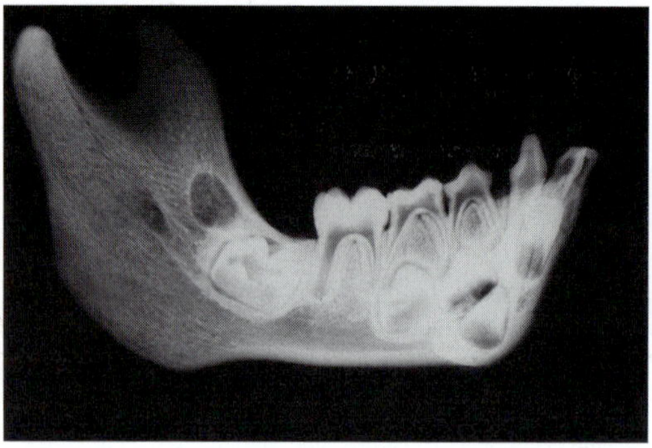

Figure 9.1b X-ray of just the hemi-mandible from the captive juvenile gorilla showing the permanent incisors and canines in crypt, as well as the permanent M_2 nearly crown complete in its crypt. Note the presence of a crypt for the M_3, but no evidence of crown initiation.

mesial and distal cusp tips and dentine horns of both the M_1 and M_2, passing through the protoconid/metaconid and the hypoconid/entoconid, respectively. For *Gorilla*, sections were prepared from the midline axial plane for anterior teeth and from the mesial and distal cusp planes for posterior teeth, such that each section traversed both cusp tips and dentine horns. All sections were mounted to microscope slides, lapped with 3 μm aluminum oxide powder to a final thickness of 90–110 μm, polished with a 0.1 μm diamond suspension paste, placed in an ultrasonic bath to remove surface debris, dehydrated through a graded series of alcohol baths, cleared in xylene, mounted with cover slips in DPX mounting medium and, finally, analyzed using polarized light microscopy (Olympus BX-52).

Short-period (i.e. daily cross striations) and long-period (i.e. striae of Retzius) lines were clearly visible throughout the enamel. Both types of incremental markings were used to measure daily enamel secretion rates (DSRs) and total crown formation times (CFTs) for each tooth. CFTs were determined by summing the time taken to form the cuspal (appositional) and lateral (imbricational) components of each tooth. The transition between cuspal and lateral enamel was defined as the point where successive domes of enamel formation are no longer completely buried within the cusp by subsequently formed enamel, but rather outcrop on the enamel surface of the tooth as perikymata. In most ape anterior teeth, Retzius lines often do not reach the surface as perikymata, due to the presence of a thin layer of aprismatic enamel. This is not problematic in histological studies, as Retzius lines are clearly visible; however, it does hamper attempts at determining CFTs by counting perikymata on the labial surface of most anterior teeth. Lateral enamel formation time in days was simply recorded as the total number of imbricational striae multiplied by the striae periodicity (number of days between adjacent striae). Determining CFTs in this manner was repeated for each tooth to calculate the rate and duration of growth, and the total amounts of pre- and postnatal tooth growth.

9.4 Results: creating a dental chronology

Reconstructing the entire schedule of dental growth requires three critical pieces of information: (1) the position of the neonatal line, (2) the developmental relationship of all teeth to one another (so-called "registering teeth"), and (3) the position of accentuated lines and total crown formation times to construct the dental chronology. Each is detailed below.

9.4.1 Finding the neonatal line

To create a chronology of dental development, the first molar must be registered in time-at-zero-days development (i.e. the day of birth). This was accomplished by charting the position of the neonatal line in the only permanent tooth to be forming at the time of birth: the M1 (Figure 9.2a). The neonatal line is thought to mark a brief period of disruption to enamel secretion (Beynon *et al.*, 1991b, 1998; Christensen and Kraus, 1965; Kraus and Jordan, 1965; Rushton, 1933; Schour, 1936; Schwartz *et al.*, 2002), and appears as a prominent accentuated line – even in long extinct taxa like the *c.* 18 mya *Proconsul* from Rusinga Island (Figure 9.2b). It is often easy to recognize in developing M1s, as prenatal enamel does not normally contain accentuated lines.

In the *Megaladapis edwardsi* specimen, the neonatal line is visible in the outer third of the M_1 cuspal enamel. By counting short-period lines in the enamel, it was determined that M_1 initiated 132 days prior to birth. A neonatal line was also present in the M_2 (see below for an explanation of how this was determined), indicating that crown development began 75 days before birth (Schwartz *et al.*, 2005). In the *Gorilla gorilla gorilla* specimen, a neonatal line is present only in the permanent M1s, indicating that crown formation began 70 days (maxillary) and 82 days (mandibular) prenatally (Schwartz *et al.*, 2006).

9.4.2 Registering teeth to one another

Accentuated striae of Retzius mark brief periods of disruption in enamel and dentine matrix secretion, and are often caused by physiological "insults" of one kind or another. As these events occur at a particular point in development, they are recorded in *all teeth* developing at that particular time. Thus, charting

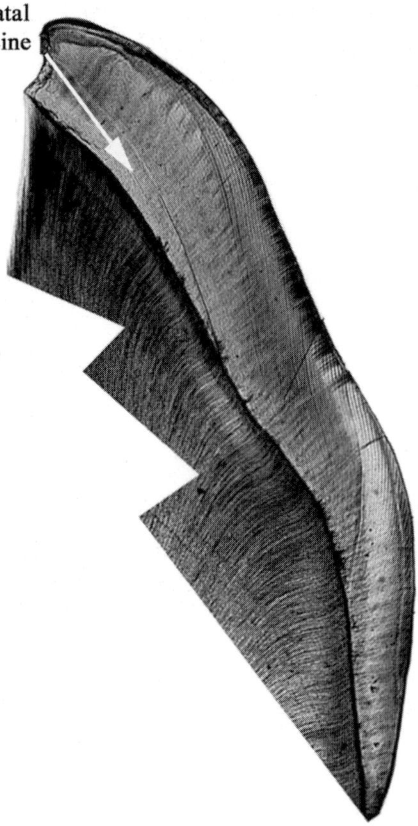

Figure 9.2a Left: Transmitted light montage of the LM^1 crown (lingual cusp) illustrating the position of the neonatal line (white arrow) associated with birth (i.e. day zero). Note: the major accentuated line occurring extremely close to the neonatal line was caused by a traumatic injury to the orbital region (see Schwartz *et al.*, 2006 for a more detailed discussion).

the relative position of accentuated striae facilitates the calibration of dental development across teeth; i.e. each striation provides a temporal benchmark for registering all teeth developing at the same point in time to one another.

As an example, Figure 9.3 depicts the process of temporally registering the developing M_1 to the M_2, using accentuated lines in the enamel of *Megaladapis edwardsi*. The gray bars indicate the duration of M_1 and M_2 crown formation, while the dotted lines represent time devoted to root formation. Within each molar, a set of three marked and closely spaced accentuated lines are apparent. It is clear that the first accentuated line apparent in the M_1 represents the neonatal line (see Schwartz *et al.*, 2005 for explanation). Thus, it was relatively

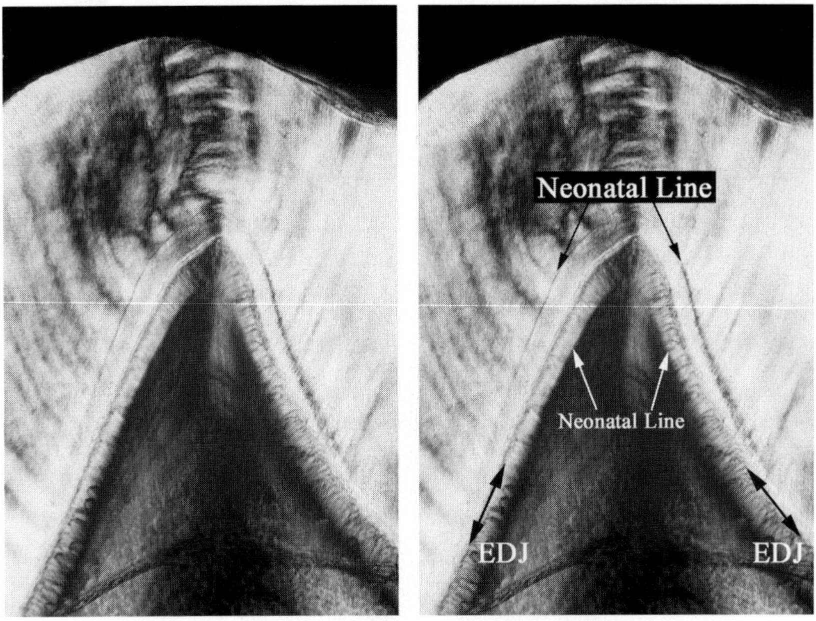

Figure 9.2b Polarized light micrograph of a section through the mesial cusps of an M_1 of *Proconsul heseloni* (Individual IV from the Kaswanga primate site on Rusinga Island) illustrating the position of a neonatal line in enamel just above the enamel dentine junction, as well as a neonatal line in dentine.

straightforward to determine the amount of pre- and postnatal M_1 crown formation, as well as the number of days between accentuated lines: 22 days and 17 days, respectively. For the M_1 then, the three accentuated lines (i.e. neonatal line, Line A, and Line B) were formed at 132, 154, and 171 days after initiation of the M_1 crown.

At this point, it is unknown whether the set of three lines in the M_2 represent the same secretion disturbances as seen in the M_1. For this to be so, the three lines *must* be the same number of days apart. Counting short-period cross striations in the enamel of the M_2 revealed that the lines were indeed 22 days and 17 days apart, and thus represent the same development disturbances. Since a disturbance in enamel secretion is recorded in all tooth crowns developing at that particular moment in time, the appearance of the same set of three accentuated lines allows us to register the amount of M_1 crown formed relative to that in the M_2. Thus, the event associated with the three accentuated lines occurred at 74, 99, and 116 days, respectively, after the initiation of the M_2. The lines can be clearly seen in a transmitted polarized light micrograph of the cuspal portion of the M_2.

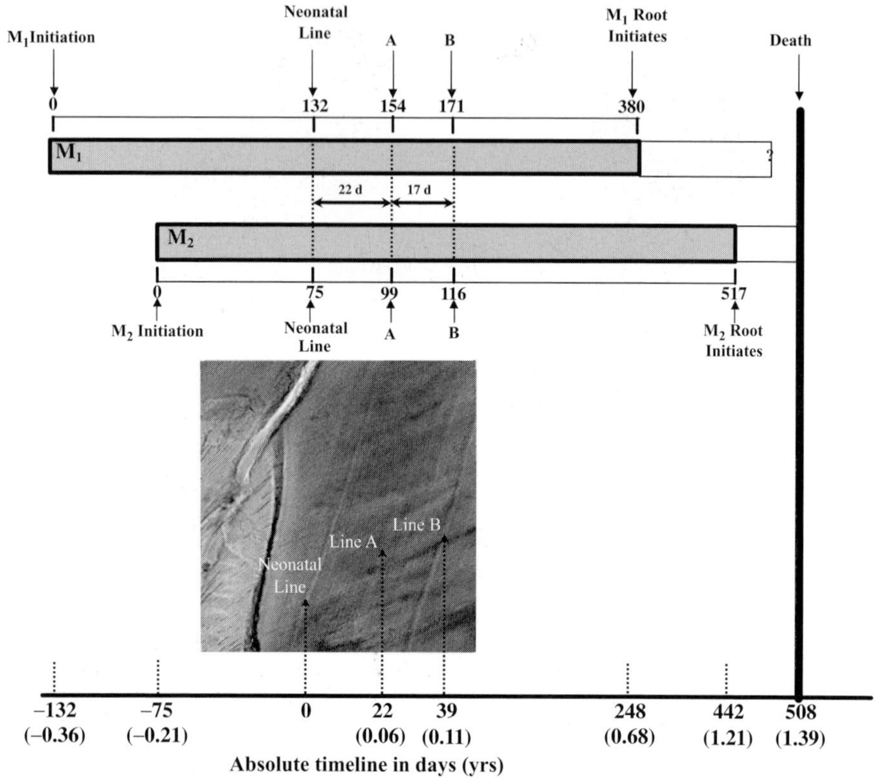

Figure 9.3 Diagram illustrating the process of registering in time the developing M_1 to the developing M_2, using accentuated lines in enamel. Gray bars represent crown formation times; dotted lines represent time devoted to root formation. The same set of three accentuated lines (the first being the neonatal line, the second, Line A, and the third, Line B) are apparent in the crowns of both molars. These lines were formed at 132, 154, and 171 days after initiation of the M_1 crown and at 74, 99, and 116 days after the initiation of the M_2, respectively. The separation of these two accentuated lines by 22 and 17 days in both of the developing molars demonstrates that they represent the same temporal events. The transmitted light micrograph of the cuspal portion of the M_2 illustrates the position of these three lines.

9.4.3 *Constructing the dental chronology*

Once the position of the neonatal line and accentuated striae are charted and cross-matched between developing teeth, it is necessary to determine the point at which crown formation terminates and root formation commences. From counts of daily cross striations and striae of Retzius, it was determined that the *Megaladapis* M_1 continued formation for *c*. 248 days after the position of the

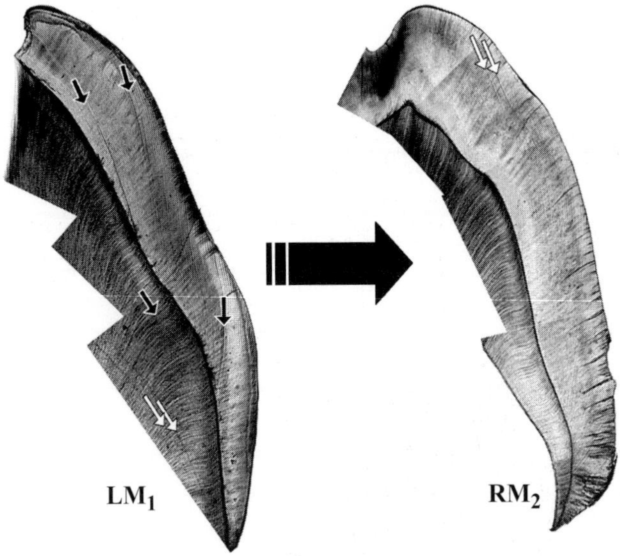

Figure 9.4 LM_1 and RM_2 of *G. g. gorilla* illustrating the technique of registering one tooth to another during development. Several accentuated lines appear throughout crown development (black arrows in enamel and dentine of the LM_1). A "doublet" (two white arrows), representing the two stress events close in time, is visible in both teeth and enables tying in the proportion of crown developed in the RM_2 with that in LM_1; nearly two-thirds of the RM_2 crown is completed at the same time that the entire LM_1 crown formed. The events associated with the white arrows are indicated as the final dashed horizontal line in the dental chronology presented in Figure 9.5.

neonatal line, yielding a total crown formation time of *c.* 380 days. Likewise, the M_2 crown continued forming for 508 days, at which point the individual died as evidenced by the incomplete M_2 crown (see Figure 9.3).

The gorilla specimen was quite interesting in that nearly a dozen marked accentuated lines were visible throughout the period of dental development (Figure 9.4). By correlating and cross-matching these lines across teeth, a chronology of dental development was produced (Figure 9.5).

9.5 Discussion and conclusion

To build a chronology of dental development from which life-history schedules can be inferred, it is necessary to document the position and timing of the neonatal line, any accentuated lines, and the total periods of crown and root formation (using short- and long-period incremental lines in enamel and dentine)

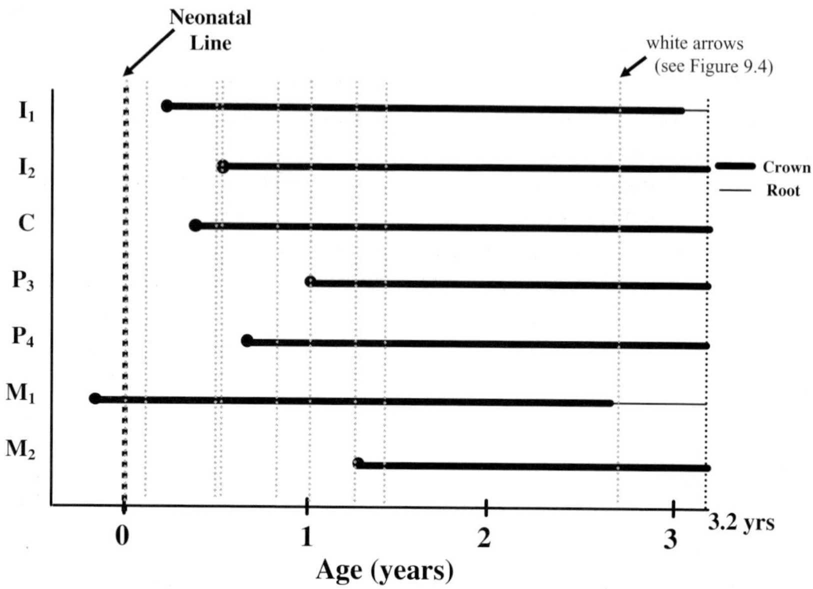

Figure 9.5 A composite dental chronology (averaging the intiation times of the mandibular and maxillary teeth within each tooth type) for the western lowland gorilla (*G. g. gorilla*) that also shows the timing of the major accentuated lines (vertical gray dotted lines) including the events shown by the doublet of white arrows in Figure 9.4; each gray line represents an episode of stress and cuts across all teeth developing at that particular point in time.

for each analyzed tooth. As accentuated lines usually correspond to "stressful events" they are simultaneously recorded in all developing teeth, and therefore can be used to register the relative degree of crown and root formation in each tooth to the same moment in time. In this chapter we have outlined the technique for utilizing all of these lines for building a dental chronology in extant and extinct primates.

Reconstructing a dental chronology should not be the goal of any particular histological investigation; rather, it should be used as a tool to aid in elucidating other aspects of an organism's maturational trajectory. For instance, this technique can be used to assess age at death of dentally immature individuals, thereby providing an "age for stage" of dental development. The chronology provided for *M. edwardsi* indicates that this individual died at 508 days, or 1.39 years of age, while that for the gorilla indicates death occurred at 1168 days, or 3.20 years (Figures 9.3 and 9.5).

Dental chronologies can also be used to compare the degrees of molar crown formation of different taxa at different life history "events," such as birth or weaning. For example, the position of the neonatal line can be used to calculate the proportional amounts of tooth crown formed pre- and postnatally, and to assess dental precocity at birth. Such comparisons have recently led to fascinating insights about the relative degree of dental precocity in certain Malagasy lemurs (Godfrey *et al.*, 2001; Schwartz *et al.*, 2005).

The time of emergence of the first molar (M1) is also of special interest, given its correlation with other life history variables for most primates. The best way in which to obtain age at M1 emergence is to target immature individuals, whose M1s are the process of erupting, or have just erupted (i.e. are relatively unworn). Lacking that, and assuming we can identify a neonatal line on M1, we can use postnatal CFT, plus information on root extension rates and the amount of root present at emergence to estimate age at M1 gingival eruption. Postnatal ages at crown completion, coupled with estimates for root extension, can be used to estimate emergence ages for second and third molars as well.

So, for example, we are able to infer that the age at M_1 eruption in *Megaladapis* occurred, at the very latest, at 1.39 years or 17 months; however, it was likely earlier, as the M_1 was in full occlusion and slightly worn when this individual died (Figure 9.1). Likewise, the age at M_1 crown completion provides a minimum age at M_1 eruption, which in this case occurred at 0.68 years, or 8.3 months. Allowing at least one or two months for root development prior to eruption, gingival emergence can be estimated to have occurred between 9–13 months; it most likely occurred at *c.* 11 months (0.9 yrs).

The gorilla specimen also died at a roughly similar stage of molar development, though the M_2 crown was not quite complete. The M_1 was in functional occlusion, indicating that the age at M_1 eruption must have occurred at <3.2 yrs (see. Figure 9.5) – this is slightly younger than the eruption age of 3.5 yrs widely reported in the literature (e.g. Smith, 1986, 1989a; Willoughby, 1978), and perhaps suggests the presence of a slightly faster life history schedule relative to chimpanzees (Schwartz *et al.*, 2006).

Minimum gestation lengths can also be determined from the dental chronologies of fossil taxa if they have a high percentage of M1 crown formation that occurred prenatally. If it is assumed that calcification of the permanent M1 cannot begin prior to the end of the first trimester (the normal transition from embryological to fetal growth phase), then the duration of prenatal M1 CFT (as determined by the position of the neonatal line) provides a minimum value for gestation length. More compelling estimates of gestation length in a fossil taxon can be made using gestation lengths for that taxon's closest living relatives, coupled with a knowledge of when within those gestation periods M1 crown mineralization begins. In anthropoid primates, mineralization of the permanent M1 crown normally begins late in the third trimester; in living lemurs, it can begin much earlier.

It is therefore possible to reconstruct gestation lengths using the data provided here for *Megaladapis*. A minimum gestation length is calculated as: [prenatal CFT + 0.5(prenatal CFT)], because M1 initiation cannot take place until, at the earliest, the end of the first trimester. In other words, the amount of prenatal M_1 CFT is equivalent to two-thirds of the total gestation period. Prenatal CFT is 132 days, generating a minimum gestation length of 198 days (0.54 years or 6.5 months); it is possible that gestation was slightly longer if the M1 initiated at a point in time within the second trimester. For comparison, gestation length is 6.0 months in *Papio cynocephalus* and 5.4 months in *Macaca mulatta*. A minimum gestation length was also calculated to be *c*. 9.0 months for another giant (albeit smaller than *Megaladapis*) lemur, *Palaeopropithecus ingens*, suggesting that gestation lengths in giant sub-fossil lemurs were not short by primate standards (Schwartz *et al.*, 2002, 2006).

Acknowledgments

The first author would like to thank Joel Irish and Greg Nelson for organizing the dental anthropology symposium, for inviting us to contribute this chapter, and for their patience in putting this volume together. This work was in part supported by an NSF grant (BCS-0503988) to GTS, and a Leverhulme Trust grant to MCD. We would also like to thank the many other researchers who have contributed greatly to the analyses summarized here, including Kierstin Catlett, Frank Cuozzo, Laurie Godfrey, Bill Jungers, Patrick Mahoney, Don Reid, and Adrienne Zihlman.

References

Anemone, R. L., Mooney, M. P., and Siegel, M. I. (1996). Longitudinal study of dental development in chimpanzees of known chronological age: implications for understanding the age at death of Plio-Pleistocene hominids. *American Journal of Physical Anthropology*, **99**, 119–33.

Beynon, A. D., and Dean, M. C. (1988). Distinct dental development patterns in early fossil hominids. *Nature*, **335**, 509–14.

Beynon, A. D., Dean, M. C., Leakey, M. G., Reid, D. J., and Walker, A. (1998). Comparative dental development and microstructure of *Proconsul* teeth from Rusinga Island, Kenya. *Journal of Human Evolution*, **35**, 163–209.

Beynon, A. D., Dean, M. C., and Reid, D. J. (1991a). On thick and thin enamel in hominoids. *American Journal of Physical Anthropology*, **86**, 295–309.

Beynon, A. D., Dean, M. C., and Reid, D. J. (1991b). Histological study on the chronology of the developing dentition in gorilla and orang. *American Journal of Physical Anthropology*, **86**, 189–203.

Christensen, G. J. and Kraus, B. S. (1965). Initial calcification of the human permanent first molar. *Journal of Dental Research*, **44**, 1338–3342.

Conroy, G. C., and Kuykendall, K. L. (1995). Paleopediatrics: or when did human infants really become human? *American Journal of Physical Anthropology*, 98, 121–31.

Conroy, G. C., and Vannier, M. W. (1991a). Dental development in South African australopithecines. Part I: problems of pattern and chronology. *American Journal of Physical Anthropology*, **86**, 121–36.

Conroy, G. C., and Vannier, M. W. (1991b). Dental development in South African australopithecines. Part II: dental stage assessment. *American Journal of Physical Anthropology*, **86**, 137–56.

Dean, M. C. (1987). Growth layers and incremental markings in hard tissues: a review of the literature and some preliminary observations about enamel structure in *Paranthropus boisei. Journal of Human Evolution*, **16**, 157–72.

Dean, M. C. (1998). A comparative study of cross striation spacings in cuspal enamel and of four methods of estimating the time taken to grow molar cuspal enamel in *Pan, Pongo* and *Homo. Journal of Human Evolution*, **35**, 449–62.

Dean, M. C., Beynon, A. D., Thackeray, J. F., and Macho, G. A. (1993). Histological reconstruction of dental development and age at death of a juvenile *Paranthropus robustus sp*ecimen, SK 63, from Swartkrans, South Africa. *American Journal of Physical Anthropology*, **91**, 401–19.

Dean, M. C., Leakey, M. G., Reid, D. J., Schrenk, F., Schwartz, G. T., Stringer, C., and Walker, A. C. (2001). Growth processes in teeth distinguish modern humans from *Homo erectus* and earlier hominins. *Nature*, **414**, 628–31.

Dean, M. C. and Reid, D. J. (2001). Perikymata spacing and distribution on hominid anterior teeth. *American Journal of Physical Anthropology*, **116**, 209–15.

Dirks, W. (1998). Histological reconstruction of dental development and age at death in a juvenile gibbon (*Hylobates lar*). *Journal of Human Evolution*, **35**, 411–26.

Dirks, W., Reid, D. J., Jolly, C. J., Phillips-Conroy, J. C., and Brett, F. L. (2002). Out of the mouths of baboons: stress, life history and dental development in the Awash National Park hybrid zone, Ethiopia. *American Journal of Physical Anthropology*, **118**, 239–52.

Godfrey, L. R., Samonds, K. E., Jungers, W. L., and Sutherland, M. R. (2001). Teeth, brains, and primate life histories. *American Journal of Physical Anthropology*, **114**, 192–214.

Godfrey, L. R., Petto, A. J., and Sutherland, M. R. (2002). Dental ontogeny and life history strategies: the case of the giant extinct indroids of Madagascar. In *Reconstructing Behavior in the Primate Fossil Record*, ed. J. M. Plavcan, R. F. Kay, W. L. Jungers, and C. P. van Schaik. New York: Kluwer Academic/Plenum Publishers, pp. 113–58.

Godfrey, L. R., Samonds, K. E., Jungers, W. L., Sutherland, M. R., and Irwin, M. T. (2004). Ontogenetic correlates of diet in Malagasy lemurs. *American Journal of Physical Anthropology*, **123**, 250–76.

Guatelli-Steinberg, D. (2001). What can developmental defects of enamel reveal about physiological stress in non-human primates. *Evolutionary Anthropology*, **10**, 138–51.

Kelley, J., and Smith, T. M. (2003). Age at first molar emergence in early Miocene *Afropithecus turkanensis* and life-history evolution in the Hominoidea. *Journal of Human Evolution*, **44**, 307–29.

Kraus, B. S., and Jordan, R. E. (1965). *The Human Dentition Before Birth.* Philadelphia: Lea and Febiger.

Kuykendall, K. L. (1996). Dental development in chimpanzees (*Pan troglodytes*): the timing of tooth calcification stages. *American Journal of Physical Anthropology*, **99**, 135–57.

Kuykendall, K. L., Mahoney, C. J., and Conroy, G. C. (1992). Probit and survival analysis of tooth emergence ages in a mixed-longitudinal sample of chimpanzees (*Pan troglodytes*). *American Journal of Physical Anthropology*, **89**, 379–99.

Liversidge, H. M., Speechly, T., and Hector, M. P. (1999). Dental maturation in British children: are Demirjian's standards applicable? *International Journal of Pediatric Dentistry*, **9**, 263–9.

Mann, A. E. 1974. *Some Paleodemographic Aspects of the South African Australopithecines*. Philadelphia: University of Pennsylvania Press.

Ramirez Rozzi, F. and Bermudez de Castro, J. M. (2004). Surprisingly rapid growth in Neanderthals. *Nature*, **428**, 936–9.

Reid, D. J., Schwartz, G. T., Chandrasekera, M. S., and Dean, M. C. (1998). A histological reconstruction of dental development in the common chimpanzee, *Pan troglodytes. Journal of Human Evolution*, **35**, 427–48.

Ross, C. (1998). Primate life histories. *Evolutionary Anthropology*, **6**, 54–63.

Rushton, M. A. (1933). Fine contour lines of enamel milk teeth. *Dental Record*, **53**, 170.

Schour, I. (1936). Neonatal line in enamel and dentin of human deciduous teeth and first permanent molar. *Journal of Dental Research*, **18**, 91–102.

Schultz, A. H. (1935). Eruption and decay of the permanent teeth in primates. *American Journal of Physical Anthropology*, **19**, 489–581.

Schultz, A. H. (1960). Age changes in primates and their modification in man. In *Human Growth*, ed. J. M. Tanner. New York: Pergamon Press, pp. 1–20.

Schwartz, G. T., Samonds, K. E., Godfrey, L. R., Jungers, W. L., and Simons, E. L. (2002). Dental microstructure and life history in subfossil Malagasy lemurs. *Proceedings of the National Academy of Sciences USA*, **99**, 6124–9.

Schwartz, G. T., Mahoney, P., Godfrey, L. R. *et al.* (2005). Dental development in *Megaladapis edwardsi* (Primates, Lemuriformes): Implications for understanding life history variation in subfossil lemurs. *Journal of Human Evolution*, **49**, 702–21.

Schwartz, G. T., Reid, D. J., Dean, M. C., and Zihlman, A. L. (2006). A faithful record of stressful life events preserved in the dental developmental record of a juvenile gorilla. *International Journal of Primatology*, **27**, 1201–19.

Smith, B. H. (1986). Dental development in *Australopithecus* and *Homo*. *Nature*, **323**, 327–30.

Smith, B. H. (1989a). Dental development as a measure of life history in primates. *Evolution*, **43**, 683–8.

Smith, B. H. (1989b). Growth and development and its significance for early hominid behaviour. *Ossa*, **14**, 63–96.

Smith, B. H. (1991). Standards of human tooth formation and dental age assessment. In *Advances in Dental Anthropology*, ed. M. Kelley and C. S. Larsen. New York: Alan R. Liss, pp. 143–68.
Smith, B. H. (1992). Life history and the evolution of human maturation. *Evolutionary Anthropology*, **1**, 134–42.
Smith, B. H. (2000). "Schultz's Rule" and the evolution of tooth replacement patterns in primates and ungulates. In *Development, Function and Evolution of Teeth*, ed. M. F. Teaford, M. M. Smith, and M. W. J. Ferguson. Cambridge: Cambridge University Press, pp. 212–27.
Smith, B. H., Crummett, T. L., and Brandt, K. L. (1994). Ages of eruption of primate teeth: a compendium for aging individuals and comparing life histories. *Yearbook of Physical Anthropology*, **37**, 177–231.
Smith, T. M., Martin, L. B., and Leakey, M. G. (2003a). Enamel thickness, microstructure and development in *Afropithecus turkanensis*. *Journal of Human Evolution*, **44**, 283–306.
Smith, T. M., Dean, M. C., Kelley, J. *et al.* (2003b). Molar crown formation in Miocene hominoids: A preliminary synthesis. *American Journal of Physical Anthropology,* Suppl. **36**, 196.
Willoughby, D. P. (1978). *All About Gorillas*. London: AS Barnes & Co.
Zihlman, A. L., Bolter, D., and Boesch, C. (2004). Wild chimpanzee dentition and its implications for assessing life history in immature hominin fossils. *Proceedings of the National Academy of Sciences USA*, **101**, 10541–3.

Endnote

1. Accentuated striae differ from "normal" striae in their optical properties when viewed under polarized light. Wilson bands are a special sub-set of accentuated striae that correspond to hypoplastic lesions on the external crown surface. Accentuated striae can occur between two successive, or be coincident with, "normal" striae.

RM-ID 384

10 *Dental age revisited*

HELEN LIVERSIDGE

10.1 Introduction

Tooth formation spans childhood, with hard tissue formation beginning during the first trimester in utero, continuing during infancy up to adulthood, and ends with maturation of the root apices of the third permanent molars. This long duration makes developing teeth a useful indicator of maturation in the clinical setting, and estimator of age of minors who lack official identification and/or seek asylum, forensic identification, and for immature skeletal remains obtained from archaeology contexts. Measuring tooth formation is complex and differs from other maturing body systems; as such, some knowledge of the difficulties and challenges of different methods is needed to estimate age. This chapter builds on work by Scheuer and Black (2000), and is divided into two sections: quantifying dental formation and estimating age. Each section includes definitions, descriptions of difficulties, how to measure growth and maturation of teeth and the dentition, how to estimate age from growth and maturation references, some comparison between methods, and finally, recommendations.

10.2 Quantifying dental formation

10.2.1 Definitions of dental growth and maturation

Although growth and maturation are intimately related, some definitions are needed to clarify the differences between these two processes and the techniques used to measure them. Two recent books review the principles and methodology of human growth and maturation (Cameron, 2002; Hauspie *et al.*, 2004) and are highly recommended. Growth represents an increase in the size/volume, and once dentine and enamel begin to form, growth of a tooth can be quantified by measuring crown height, root length/volume, root cone angle, apex width, or other dimensions. Growth of the dentition can be measured by counting the number of developing teeth within the jaws, or erupted teeth present in the oral cavity.

Technique and Application in Dental Anthropology ed. Joel D. Irish and Greg C. Nelson
Published by Cambridge University Press.

Maturation is the process of change from an immature to a mature state. A developing tooth will grow in size, volume, and length, but it also matures from cusp tips to a fully formed crown, full length root, and a mature root apex that appears closed radiographically. In multirooted teeth, the distal root usually matures later than the others. When assessing maturation of such teeth, the observer should base their estimate on the later-maturing distal root. During root formation, the tooth erupts into the oral cavity (a maturity event). Eruption occurs at the same time as alveolar bone resorption and formation, as well as development of the periodontium and gingivae. These latter processes continue until the tooth is fully erupted into a functionally occluding position with the tooth in the opposite jaw. Once the third molar root is complete, the dentition has reached full maturity. Maturation of individual teeth has been well documented, although there is considerable discrepancy between reference studies despite large samples, wide age ranges, and sound statistical methods. Dental maturity of the developing dentition has also been quantified using tooth formation and/or eruption, where scores convert to an age scale, expressing age up to full maturity.

10.2.2 Differences between the dentition and other body systems

Growth and maturation of individual teeth and the dentition as a whole differ from other maturing body systems in two important ways. First, dental maturation appears to be independent of both skeletal and secondary sexual maturation, and less influenced by nutritional and other environmental insults. A child's height and weight reflects health and nutrition. This is true on both individual and population levels. Differences between populations in these parameters (including age of puberty) are due to interaction between genetic and environmental factors, hence the reason for population-specific references. Substantial environmental influences have not been demonstrated for dental maturity. Rather, dental maturity appears to be largely genetically controlled on both individual and population levels (Pelsmaekers *et al.*, 1997), but clear genetic differences in maturation of the dentition have not, as yet, been documented.

The second difference between the dentition and other systems that mature is that tooth formation proceeds at a chronologically regular rate. An inherent problem of skeletal and secondary sexual maturation is that individuals exhibit considerably uneven maturation (see Cameron, 2002). There is marked variation in the "rate" or tempo of maturation with different bones or organs – each maturing at different speeds within an individual. This is different from the developing dentition, because once the process of dentinogenesis begins, the crown, root, and pulp continue development until the root apex and periodontal attachments are mature and the tooth is fully erupted.

10.2.3 How tooth formation differs between individuals/groups

Three factors can influence tooth formation that result in differences: (1) the time of initiation, (2) the rate of formation, and (3) the morphology, including root length. If the initial timing of cusp-tip mineralization differs, then individuals and groups differ in the timing of all subsequent crown and root stages. Radiographic verification of this is difficult because, with few exceptions, the minimum age of subjects is between two and three years of age, or in some cases considerably later.

Tooth formation can also differ in the rate of crown or root formation. Some knowledge of dental histology is necessary to appreciate that the most likely way in which the rate of amelogenesis and odontogenesis can differ, is a change in the number of differentiating cells that secrete hard tissue. Histological analysis of the entire dentition, and the few studies that document the timing and duration of individual teeth, reveal that the interval of molar crown development differs little between European, African, and North American groups (Reid and Dean, 2006). Some differences in the rate of anterior crown formation have been documented from this study, although it remains to be seen if these are apparent at the resolution seen on radiographs. The third difference relates to morphology of the crown and root, including root length. If a tooth, say a third molar, has a short root, the duration of root formation will be shorter and the age at full maturity of this individual will be earlier than someone with a long-rooted tooth.

10.3 Measuring dental growth and maturation

10.3.1 How do we measure dental growth?

Dental growth can be quantified in several ways, including tooth length or volume from either isolated teeth or radiographs, as well as combinations and ratios of crown, root, apex, pulp dimensions, or root cone angle for age (Cameriere, *et al.*, 2004, 2006; Dean, 1985; Deutsch *et al.*, 1985; Harris and Nortjé, 1984; Kullman *et al.*, 1995; Liversidge and Molleson, 1999; Liversidge *et al.*, 1993; Mörnstad *et al.*, 1994; Stack, 1960). Growth of the dentition can be measured by counting the number of teeth present in the mouth or the number of developing teeth in the jaws. This can be expressed as number of teeth erupted at specific ages or average age when a certain number of teeth are present, but only a handful report standard deviation. More recent studies do include a meta-analysis of the number of deciduous teeth in the mouth (Townsend and Hammell, 1990), including one from Finland (Nyström *et al.*, 2000, 2001), Sweden (Hägg and Taranger, 1985), two groups from Kenya (Hassanali and Odhiambo, 1982), Zambia (Gillett, 1997), and a report on Punjabi children from India (Kaul and Pathak, 1988).

10.3.2 Dental maturity indicators

Maturity of individual teeth is a continuous process. In order to measure this process, the continuum is arbitrarily divided into discrete maturity indicators or, in this case, crown and root stages. The number of stages should include a sufficient number to quantify variability, while maintaining adequate reliability. Too many stages decrease reliability, while too few compromise sensitivity. For this reason, the 14 stages developed by Moorrees and coworkers (1963), along with adaptations of this scheme, remain popular. Estimating fractions of crown height or root length are subjective. Measurement of root length relative to crown height partly overcomes this difficulty. The eight stages of Demirjian and co workers (1973) are clearly described and accompanied by a radiograph and line drawing for each stage and tooth type.

Choice of maturity indicators is determined by a number of factors (see Cameron, 2002). Among other things, these indicators should be reliable (good intra- and inter-observer agreement) and show a quality of completeness (increase in prevalence from 0 to 100 % in a short period of time). This last feature presents a challenge with regard to dental formation, and highlights the need for a large number of children within each age year cohort. This is illustrated in Figure 10.1a showing preliminary results of a radiographic investigation of the timing of initial mineralization (1a) and apex maturation (1b) of mandibular third molars. The proportion of two groups of children in London (Bangladeshi and white) at each stage is plotted by age group: N 807 and 946. These cumulative curves show the youngest age of each stage up to the age when all children have reached the stage. At age five, no child shows initial cusp tip formation; by age 14 all children do. Similarly, no 15-year-olds have reached apex closure, while 100 % of 24-year-olds have.

10.3.3 How is dental maturity measured?

Maturity can be measured in several ways. The three methods applicable for assessment of the developing dentition are the atlas, timing of crown and root stages of individual teeth, and a maturity scale using tooth-specific scores.

The atlas is by far the easiest method. With an atlas, maturity is compared to reference drawings of developing teeth at specific ages. This method suffers from several difficulties. The first is the problem of age, for not all children match the drawings. In fact, not all teeth will match the maturity levels. Another limitation is assessing eruption on a dry specimen. Alveolar eruption is not equivalent to clinical emergence into the mouth. To date, the variability and timing of eruption stages have not been incorporated into an updated atlas. A further difficulty is maturity overlap. This occurs when a tooth or group of teeth is not in synchrony with the rest of the developing dentition. In such cases, the researcher is forced to choose whatever drawing for age that fits most closely to the individual being assessed.

The second method measuring maturity involves calculation of the timing of maturity indicators for individual teeth. This can be done in two ways. The first involves calculation of the average age of entering the stage. This can be illustrated by plotting a cumulative frequency distribution or cumulative percentage curve of children who have reached a maturity indicator by age. This will demonstrate if the age range is appropriate (Figure 10.1). The average age at entry is best calculated using logistic or probit regression equivalent to the age when half the children (50th percentile) reach or have surpassed that maturity indicator/stage. Many maturity indicators show high variance, and children who mature early will enter a defined stage considerably earlier than a child who matures later. The appropriate way to compare groups is to contrast the average age for each maturity stage (again see Figure 10.1). The proportion of children with "Ci" increases with age until 100 % of the age group attained the stage. The average age of entering stage "Ci" (cusp initiation) and "Ac" (apex closure) is the age when 50 % of the whole sample attains these stages. If the third molar takes about 10 years to form, the extremes of formation time in the groups shown in Figure 10.1 will be 6 to 16 in an early maturing child, and 13 to 23 years of age in a later-maturing individual. The 50th percentile, as well as extremes (3rd and 97th percentile), are useful to describe maturity of this stage. One group (dotted line, Bangladeshi) appears to be earlier at the 50 % level, and for most of the age groups except for 7 and 13 for "Ci" and 17 and 22 year olds for "Ac."

Although a number of studies claim that population differences exist in tooth formation, scrutiny of their methodology and age distribution suggests that neither cumulative methods nor sufficient age ranges are used. One large study of children of European origin showed neither consistent nor systematic differences in the timing of mandibular permanent teeth (Liversidge *et al.*, in press). To date, comparison of tooth formation from different regions has not yet been documented; however, first results from a large worldwide study show that the

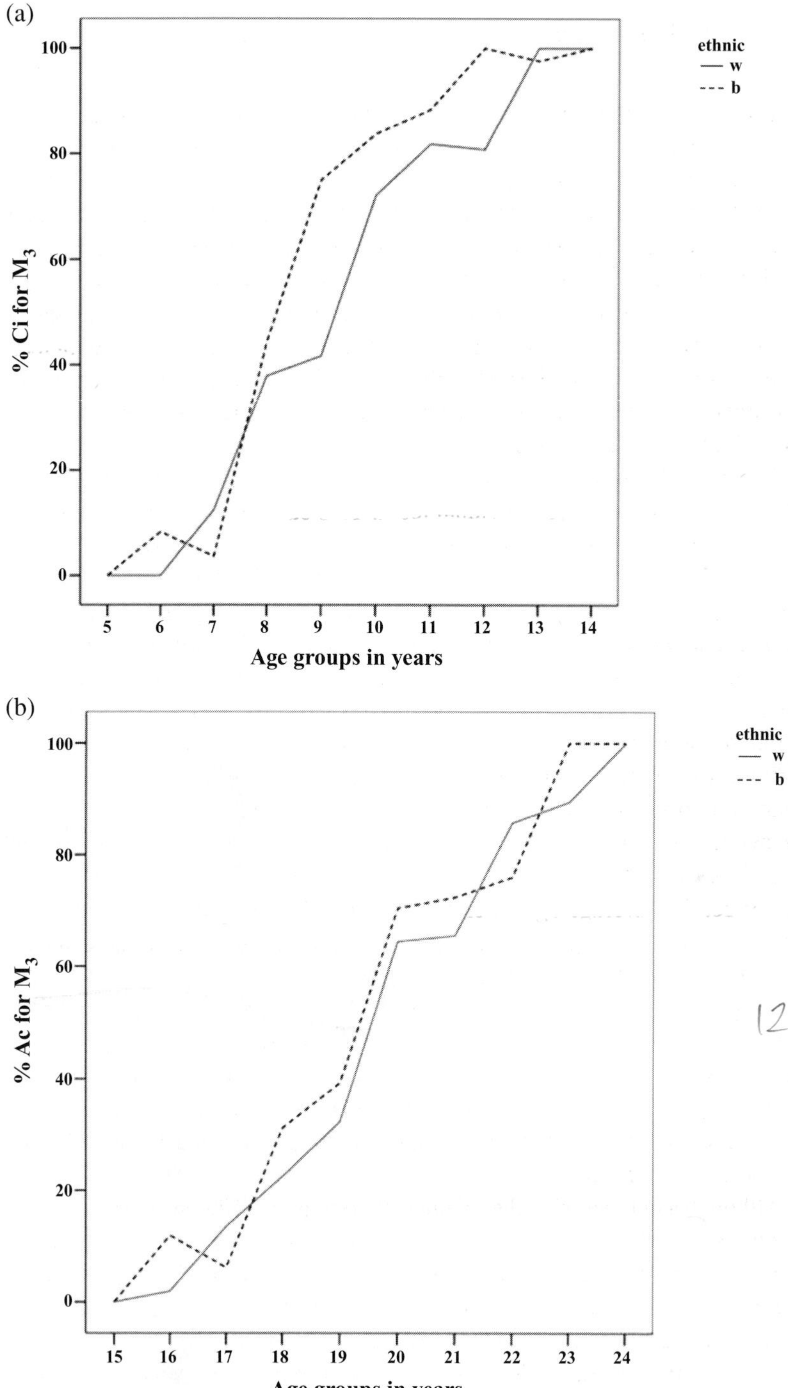

Figure 10.1 Cumulative percentage of children in London with ‘Ci’(a) and ‘Ac’(b) of M_3 plotted against the beginning of the age group. w = white (n = 946), b = Bangladeshi (n = 807).

third molar is significantly delayed in two London groups and one Cape group compared to Southern African black children (Liversidge, in press).

Timing of individual maturity indicators can also be determined, secondly, by calculating the average age of children who show the stage in question. The average is influenced by sample size and age distribution (ideally 3rd to 97th percentile should be included). This method is not suitable for the most mature stage of formation. Studies that report "population differences" (particularly of the third molar) using average age midstage rather than mean age at entry should be interpreted with this in mind.

The third method to quantify dental maturity employs tooth-specific scores that add up to dental age. The maturity of individual wrist bones does not coincide, and maturity can be expressed using a weighted score from a combination of bones (see Cameron, 2004. p. 117). This minimized disagreement thereby overcomes the problem of uneven maturity. The frequency of individuals in the sample increase for each bone (tooth) maturing from 0 to 100 %, and maturity of a child is compared to the reference study. Each developing left mandibular tooth is given a score, depending on the stage of crown or root formation. The sum of these scores converts to percentage mature and dental age. The most widely used application is by Demirjian and coworkers on a large French-Canadian sample (Demirjian *et al.*, 1973; Demirjian, 1986, 1994), where maturity of seven permanent mandibular teeth is assessed. Demirjian's method is appropriate from 2.5 to 16 years of age. The dental maturity minimum score is around 12 % and corresponds to age 2.5 at the 50th percentile; the maximum score is 100 % mature at age 16 (defined as the second molar distal root apex closed with a uniform width of the periodontal ligament).

10.3.4 *Difficulties with Demirjian's dental maturity score and its interpretation*

Demirjian's method is useful in assessing dental maturity, but it is compromised by several problems. The first is the difficulty in determining variation from the graphs. Variation is provided not in age, but in scores for 3rd, 10th, 50th, 90th and 97th percentiles. If a boy has a score of 54, the 50th percentile is seven years. If we look at the 3rd and 97th percentile scores for a seven-year-old boy they are 35 and the 74. These scores can be traced back on the graph to the 50th percentile of 5.4 to about 8.4 years. If we take the extremes, then a boy with a score of 35 at the 97th percentile could be aged 3.5 and, similarly, the 97th percentile of score 74 is a dental age of almost 10. If this was an average-maturing child, his dental age would correspond to known age, and when calculating dental age using this method it is reasonable to assume that the child is an average-maturing child at the 50th percentile. Another difficulty involves the weighted score, which is adjusted by a number of researchers using much smaller samples and one larger sample (Chaillet *et al.*, 2005). The easiest and most accurate (see below) gives scores that add up directly to give dental age (Willems *et al.*, 2001). The standard deviation peaks around eight years of age for both sexes (Chaillet *et al.*, 2005), while the difference in scores between boys and girls is greatest at 12 to 13 years. Such results reflect the weighted scoring, and do not mirror the biological variation of tooth formation. We know that the variation in the timing of dental formation stages increases with age (Moorrees *et al.*, 1963), and that the largest sex difference in timing are the canine late root stages (Thompson *et al.*, 1975). It is not surprising that those differences between individuals, and between groups, peak at the age when the standard deviation is highest. The majority of maturity indicators occur in girls during the fourth year. Figure 10.2a shows the timing of the 39 maturity indicators for girls and how these decrease with age. This means that a one stage difference in older children can result in a large jump in dental age. For example, if all mandibular teeth are in stage H (mature apices), except for the second molar, which is stage G (walls of distal root are parallel/open apex), dental age is 14.6 years. A one stage difference from stage G to H of M_2 results in a jump in dental age to 16 years.

Numerous dental maturity studies of groups in different parts of the world have demonstrated advancement compared to the Canadian reference, and have been interpreted as population differences or a secular trend; it is probable that neither is correct. A secular trend would need a comparative reference sample that antedates World War II, but all large dental radiographic studies are later than this (see Cole, 2003). Differences in maturity score between groups are difficult to interpret, are complicated by the scoring matrix, and may have no biological meaning (Prahl-Andersen *et al.*, 1979). This finding is supported by the lack of any consistent tooth differences in the timing of these stages between children from a large database from Australia, Belgium, Finland, France, Quebec, Korea, and Sweden (Liversidge *et al.*, in press). In fact, a curious finding in this large database was the late apical maturation of the first permanent molar in children from Quebec; might this account for the difference in dental maturity between the reference and other groups? Figure 10.2b shows differences in dental maturity for girls expressed in standard deviation or z scores. These are from studies that document difference in years or score by age group (Eid *et al.*, 2002; Farah *et al.*, 1999; Fatemi, personal communication; Hedge and Sood, 2002; Nyarady *et al.*, 2005; Nyström *et al.*, 1986; Zhao *et al.*, 1990). Differences of more than one z score are mostly between ages four and eight years, and tail off for later ages when few maturity indicators occur.

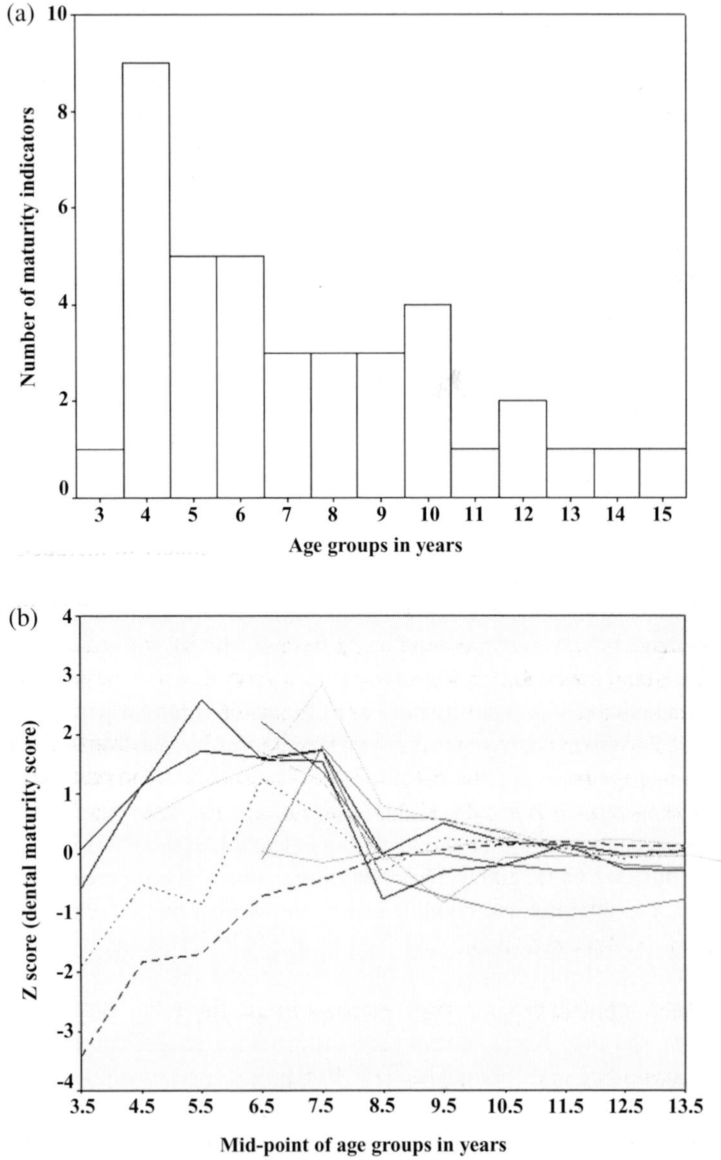

Figure 10.2 (a) Dot plot of the timing of maturity events in girls with Demirjian's dental maturity score. (b) Z scores of difference in Demirjian's dental maturity plotted against age groups.

10.3.5 Other difficulties with tooth formation/dental maturity data

A common and major misconception of any maturity grade/score is the fundamental principle that it is not per se a parameter; it is not a measurement, for it has no units and, therefore, parametric statistics using numerical maturity scores are flawed. The interval between different crown or root stages differs, and consecutive maturity indicators are not of equal duration, hence the choice of nominal or tooth formation stages (A to H from Demirjian, 1 to 10 from Nolla, 1960). Changing nominal maturity indicators to numerical values (stage A = 1, B = 2 . . .) and calculating the "average stage" goes against the basic principle of measuring maturation and is incorrect. Despite this, numerous studies of third molar formation show a lack of understanding of principles of dental growth and maturation. Further difficulties that complicate interpretation of comparisons of dental formation and maturity between groups include: small sample sizes, uneven age/sex distribution, and non-random selection. If the sample is large enough, outliers will not greatly alter the 50th percentile; further, if only a few individuals for a year of age are included, this is unlikely to include sufficient individuals who are "average."

The exact age at which a maturational event occurs in a child will only be observed if that child is followed longitudinally at frequent intervals. Assessing maturation of teeth is retrospective, as one can only see if the event has or has not occurred, i.e. if the tooth has erupted into the oral cavity or if the crown is complete. The duration of crown or root stages of individuals is best determined from longitudinal radiographic studies. Because of this, the precious historical collections from the middle of the last century represent a rich and precious source.

10.4 Estimating age

10.4.1 Definitions and how accuracy is measured

Accuracy is a measure of how close dental age can estimate known age. Hence, a method with high accuracy will provide an estimate of age that is close to known age, while an inaccurate method will over- or underestimate known age. The difference between dental age and known age is one way to express accuracy. Lovejoy *et al.* (1985) describe the difference between estimated and known age as bias, as it measures the amount of over- and underestimation. Another measure is the proportion of the test sample where estimated age is within ±0.5 years, ±1 year, etc. of known age or age class. This has an advantage that skewness, kurtosis, and rank distribution for each age class can be quantified. Some studies correlate estimated and known age or tooth stage and age; however, although this measures association, it is influenced by age range and gives little information of how close estimated age is to known age. Sensitivity (true positive), specificity (true negative), likelihood or odds ratio, and area under the receiver operating characteristic (ROC) curve are designed for diagnostic discrimination. Discriminating between age categories such as younger or older than 14 or 18 years is likely to prove useful in the legal context.

The continuous maturation process of the tooth, from crypt formation to apical maturation, is arbitrarily divided into stages. When one examines a developing tooth we recognize and classify it into a defined crown or root stage; however, if it entered this stage some time previously, it might be midstage or close to entering the next stage. Smith (1991) suggested that a midpoint between entering tooth stages would be more accurate than age at entry, and adapted data from Moorrees *et al.* (1963) for estimation. A sensible approach is to assume that the individual, for whom age is to be estimated, was an average child whose biological age reflects his/her chronological age.

10.4.2 Difficulties comparing published results

Several problems come to light when published results of accuracy tests of age-estimation methods using dental maturation are compared. These problems result from how accuracy is measured and the nature of the test sample. It is useful to report both accuracy (closeness to true age) and absolute accuracy. Comparing accuracy between different crown or root stages, different teeth, age groups, or methods is difficult when accuracy is measured in so many different ways. This is further complicated if a separate test sample is not used, or if the test sample is grouped or is small with a narrow or uneven age range. Test samples usually use autopsy collections, recent archaeological collections of known age, and larger groups of living children. Ideally a test sample should be of sufficiently large size, have an even age distribution (similar numbers in each year of age), and encompass an appropriate age range and a separate test to study sample. If a new method of age prediction is described, the accuracy should be tested on a different sample.

Similar difficulties that hamper dental maturity studies also affect test samples. For example, if the test sample age range is small and consists of fewer than ten children for a year of age, it will probably not include enough average maturers, and several advanced or delayed children may skew results. This also occurs if the age range of the test sample is inappropriate. With increasing age and maturation, the number of developing teeth decreases, so that by about age 14 only the third molar is usually incomplete. There is then another problem for tests of accuracy if individual teeth are used to estimate age. From the age of 13, a few children will have completed apical maturation of the second premolar and second molar, and so drop out of the test sample. This means that the later age groups are smaller, and these children are those that are slow to reach maturity (above the 90th percentiles). This is a reflection of maturity data being slightly skewed to the right. Even with a large test sample, it is not unusual to find a small number of children with delayed tooth formation and estimated age, for these individuals will be considerably underestimated.

10.4.3 The level of accuracy

An acceptable level of accuracy has not been clarified. Accuracy is more precise in younger children, where maturity indicators are more frequent and the rate of growth and maturation is most rapid. Calculating age of an individual who died prior to completion of tooth formation is possible by making histological sections of all teeth, and counting enamel cross striations from the neonatal line (see Boyde, 1963). The neonatal line allows calculation of the exact timing and duration of tooth formation in an individual (Dean and Beynon, 1991; Dean *et al.*, 1993; Reid *et al.*, 1998), but this method is complex and time consuming. The best deciduous tooth to view the neonatal line within the dentine and enamel is the second deciduous molar (W. Birch, personal communication). It is thought that the presence of this accentuated growth line in deciduous teeth (and mesiobuccal cusp of the first permanent molar) indicates that the individual survived birth by probably one or two weeks. Absence of this line does not rule out a live birth, as the neonatal line is visible in most, but not all histological sections of deciduous teeth; Schour could identify it in 90 of 100 sections (Schour, 1936). Factors that influence this presence include position of the section and the quality of preparation.

10.4.4 Which tooth formation method is most accurate?

Maber *et al.* (2006) compared the difference in estimated and known age using several dental maturity methods: Demirjian (1994), Willems *et al.* (2001), Nolla (1960), and individual teeth from Haavikko (1970) on a test sample of 946 children aged 3 to 16.99 years. These data were further analyzed for this chapter, with the addition of several methods and calculation of absolute accuracy.

Table 10.1 *Average difference and median of absolute difference between estimated and known age in years for different methods. Sample is 946 radiographs used in Maber* et al. *2006.*

Method	*N*	Difference mean	Absolute difference median
Demirjian 1994	946	0.23	0.59
Willems *et al.* 2001 scores	946	−0.12	0.52
Chaillet *et al.* 2005	946	−0.26	0.55
Nolla 1960	946	−1.02	0.93
Haavikko 1970	832	−0.67	0.64
Moorrees *et al.* 1963	833	−1.19	1.00
Smith 1991 (Moorrees adapted)	833	−0.67	0.64
Liversidge *et al.* 2006 (mean entering . . .)	812	−1.13	0.98
Liversidge *et al.* 2006 (adapted)	812	−0.20	0.56
Liversidge *et al.* 2006 (mean age midstage)	827	−0.12	0.78

Absolute accuracy does not consider whether estimated age is over- or underestimated, and reports only the time distance from true age. Results are shown in Table 10.1. Absolute accuracy was 0.65 years for Willems *et al.* (2001), followed by 0.70 years using Demirjian (1994) and updated scores (Chaillet *et al.*, 2005). Adapted data (cumulative mean age of attainment plus half the interval to the next stage) using Liversidge *et al.* (in press) had an absolute accuracy of 0.75. These values for Smith's adapted method (1991) and Haavikko (1970) were 0.86 and 0.90 years. Mean age of children in a stage (Liversidge *et al.* in press) was 0.95, while Nolla (1960) was 1.11 years. Mean age at entry used to estimate age showed absolute accuracy values greater than one year: Moorrees *et al.* (1963) and Liversidge *et al.* (in press) at 1.22 and 1.24 years, respectively.

These results suggest that estimated age using developing teeth will have an absolute accuracy between six months and a year, depending on which method is used to assess crown and root formation. The use of Demirjian's tooth stages and his method, or Willems *et al.*'s (2001) adapted scoring to calculate dental age will estimate age best. Individual developing mandibular teeth (using these stages) will estimate age to 0.75 years (see Table 10.3, adapted from Table 9 in Liversidge *et al.*, in press). Smith's adapted method (1991) is next best, followed by Haavikko (these stages exclude cusp outline complete, initial root, root cleft of molars, and apex half closed, although no mean age is given for initial root formation). Nolla (1960) and Moorrees *et al.* (1963) age at entry are not recommended, as they are the least accurate.

Inspection of the surrounding alveolar bone can help estimate age if the tooth is not in position. The shape of the tooth crypt at the depth of the developing root apex intimately mirrors the root shape; it will be broad and rounded if the root is still growing. Similarly, if the furcation shape of a molar crypt is visible, the roots will have matured past the cleft stage. A bony groove on the normally sharply defined alveolar bone crest may be seen around an erupting tooth, and this may be seen even if the tooth is not present. If a fractured root tip is *in situ*, it may be possible to see if the apical root canal is wide open, suggesting that the apex is not yet mature.

We have to make several assumptions about the individual for whom we are estimating age. The most important is that the child was average, and at the mean value or 50th percentile of growth and maturity. We assume that he/she entered this tooth stage at the average age, and is half way between this and the subsequent stage. We know that the standard deviation in timing of any tooth formation stage can be up to a year; for instance, the mean age and SD of M_1 stage E (includes initial root, cleft and quarter root) is 4.98 $\pm$1.02 years (pooled sex, Liversidge *et al.*, in press). It is possible that the child was advanced and in the 3rd percentile, having reached this stage at a considerably younger age than average. On the other hand, the child may have been dentally delayed (in the 97th percentile) and reached this stage at a much older age. Hence the need for documented measures of variation (3rd and 97th centiles or standard deviation). The 3rd and 97th centiles can be calculated as mean $\pm$ $kxSD$, where SD is standard deviation and k is the multiplier, in this case 1.88, provided the distribution is Gaussian (see Cole, 2002). These extreme values, and also the first and last stages of maturation, can provide one-sided age limits "at least" and "older than" categories. If a tooth reached apex closure, the individual might have reached this stage a considerable time earlier, so only a minimum age can be given; yet, the 50th or 97th percentile of entering that stage increases precision of an estimated minimum age.

The recommendations for age estimation are as follows.

(1) In early childhood, tooth length of developing deciduous teeth is an easy and accurate method.

(2) The timing of eruption stages of teeth, such as alveolar eruption, is also useful. Age of alveolar eruption, adapted for age estimation for mandibular deciduous and some permanent molars, is shown in Table 10.2 (boys and girls combined).

(3) Tooth formation stages with high reproducibility are more likely to have better accuracy than subjective crown or root fractions. Crown completion, especially of skeletal material, root length equal to crown height, and root apex open are useful stages. They are also useful cut-off points, and provide guidance that an individual is younger/older than the average age of the stage.

Table 10.2 *Average age in years of eruption stages for mandibular deciduous teeth and first two permanent molars (sexes pooled) adapted for estimating age. Alveolar eruption, cusp tip(s) at alveolar bone level; partial eruption, cusp tip(s) or occlusal level of tooth between alveolar bone level and occlusal level of fully erupted teeth.*

	Alveolar eruption	Partial eruption
i_1	0.46	0.78
i_2	0.84	1.15
c	1.18	1.62
m_1	1.05	1.43
m_2	1.72	2.28
M_1	5.25	6.24
M_2	10.78	12.01

(4) The average age of crown completion of the permanent first molar occurs at 3 to 3.3 years. The ages for anterior permanent crown completion are detailed in Reid and Dean (2006).

(5) Estimating age from individual developing teeth is best using adapted age at entry methods. These are detailed in Table 10.3 for mandibular permanent molars for tooth formation stages described by Moorrees *et al.* (1963) and Demirjian (1994) for boys and girls combined.

(6) Dental maturity calculated from seven mandibular teeth is marginally more accurate using scores from Willems *et al.* (2001) compared to Demirjian or updated scores (Chaillet *et al.* 2005).

10.5 Summary

Understanding the principles of growth and maturation is essential in order to compare maturation between groups of children, and appropriately use such reference studies to estimate age. The average age at entry (the age when half the sample has reached or passed the stage in question) is appropriate for comparison. Using such data will underestimate age by more than a year. Some knowledge of the average timing and variation of dental formation is a good background to the use of tooth formation reference studies to appropriately estimate age. There is a need for population-specific references of tooth formation from major regions and groups of the world, and several studies are underway. To date, the only clear difference between groups appears to be the

Table 10.3 *Average age in years of some tooth formation stages for some mandibular permanent molars adapted for estimating age. Demirjian (1994) stage D corresponds approximately to Moorrees* et al. *(1963) stage Cc, stage E includes Ri, Rcl and R1/4, stage F corresponds to R1/2 and R3/4, while G is similar to Rc. Timing of midstage and Liversidge adapted are from Liversidge* et al. *(2006). Data for Liversidge midstage are for sex pooled.*

	Moorrees stage	Smith (1991) Boys	Smith (1991) Girls	Demirjian stage	Liversidge adapted Boys	Liversidge adapted Girls	Liversidge midstage
M1	Cc	2.5	2.4	D	–	–	3.90 ± 1.18
	Ri	3.2	3.1				
	Rcl	4.1	4.0	E	4.80	4.58	4.98 ± 1.02
	R1/4	4.9	4.8				
	R1/2	5.5	5.4	F	6.20	5.81	6.25 ± 1.09
	R3/4	6.1	5.8				
	Rc	7.0	6.5	G	8.38	7.84	8.45 ± 1.36
	A12	8.5	7.9				
M2	Cc	6.8	6.6	D	7.78	7.45	7.81 ± 1.10
	Ri	7.6	7.3				
	Rcl	8.7	8.4	E	9.74	9.35	9.54 ± 1.14
	R1/4	9.8	9.5				
	R1/2	10.6	10.3	F	11.46	10.84	11.08 ± 1.15
	R3/4	11.4	11.0				
	Rc	12.3	11.8	G	13.74	12.92	13.16 ± 1.44
	A12	13.9	13.5				

age of initiation of the third molar. Assessing dental maturity of small regional groups of narrow age range is now of little interest, especially for children of European origin. The biological meaning of differences in Demirjian's dental maturity between groups is unclear.

Far more interesting questions concern differences in the timing of initiation and completion of teeth, the overlap between tooth types, and how root growth and length can differ between groups. Other questions include how morphologic differences occur between groups and how these relate to tooth formation, as well as jaw growth, space within the mandible, and interaction between crown/root morphology and formation.

References

Boyde, A. (1963). Estimation of age at death of young human skeletal remains from incremental lines in dental enamel. *Proceedings of Third International Meeting of Forensic Immunology, Medicine, Pathology and Toxicology*, London. Reprinted

(1990) in *Primate Life History and Evolution*, ed. C. Jean DeRousseow. New York: Wiley-Liss, pp. 260–7.

Cameriere, R., Ferrante, L., and Cingolani, M. (2004). Precision and reliability of pulp/tooth area ratio (RA) of second molar as indicator of adult age. *Journal of Forensic Sciences*, **49**, 1319–23.

Cameriere, R., Ferrante, L., and Cingolani, M. (2006). Age estimation in children by measurement of open apices in teeth. *International Journal of Legal Medicine*, **120**, 49–52.

Cameron, N. (2002). *Human Growth and Development*. San Diego, California: Academic Press.

Cameron, N. (2004). Measuring maturity. In *Methods in Human Growth Research*, ed. R. C. Hauspie, N. Cameron, and L. Molinari. Cambridge: Cambridge University Press, pp. 108–40.

Chaillet, N., Nyström, M., and Demirjian, A. (2005). Comparison of dental maturity in children of different ethnic origins: international maturity curves for clinicians. *Journal of Forensic Science*, **50**, 1164–74.

Cole, T. J. (2002). Growth references and standards. In *Human Growth and Development*, ed. N. Cameron. San Diego: Academic Press. pp. 383–413.

Cole, T. J. (2003). The secular trend in human physical growth: a biological view. *Economics and Human Biology*, **1**, 161–8.

Dean, M. C. (1985). Variation in the developing root cone angle of the permanent mandibular teeth of modern human man and certain fossil hominids. *American Journal of Physical Anthropology*, **68**, 233–8.

Dean, M. C. and Beynon, A. D. (1991). Histological reconstruction of crown formation time and initial root formation times in a modern human child. *American Journal of Physical Anthropology*, **86**, 215–28.

Dean, M. C., Beynon, A. D., Reid, D. J., and Whittaker, D. K. (1993). A longitudinal study of tooth growth in a single individual based on long and short period incremental markings in dentine and enamel. *International Journal of Osteoarchaeology*, **3**, 249–64.

Demirjian, A. (1986). Dentition. In *Human Growth: A Comprehensive Treatise, Postnatal Growth and Neurobiology*, ed. T. J. Falkner. New York: Plenum Press, pp. 269–98.

Demirjian, A. (1994). *Dental Development*. CD Rom. Norwood, MA: Silver Platter Education.

Demirjian, A., Goldstein, H., and Tanner, J. M. (1973). A new system of dental age assessment. *Human Biology*, **45**, 211–27.

Deutsch, D, Tam, O., and Stack, M. V. (1985). Postnatal changes in size, morphology and weight of developing postnatal deciduous anterior teeth. *Growth*, **49**, 202–17.

Eid, R. M., Simi, R., Friggi, M. N., and Fisberg, M. (2002). Assessment of dental maturity of Brazilian children aged 6 to 14 years using Demirjian's method. *International Journal of Paediatric Dentistry*, **12**, 423–8.

Farah, C. S., Booth, D. R., and Knott, S. C. (1999). Dental maturity of children in Perth, Western Australia, and its application in forensic age estimation. *Journal of Clinical Forensic Medicine*, **6**, 14–18.

Gillett, R. M. (1997). Dental emergence among urban Zambian school children: An assessment of the accuracy of three methods in assigning ages. *American Journal of Physical Anthropology*, **102**, 447–54.

Haavikko, K. (1970). The formation and the alveolar and clinical eruption of the permanent teeth. *Proceedings of the Finnish Dental Society*, **66**, 103–70.

Hägg, U. and Taranger J. (1985). Dental development, dental age and tooth counts. *The Angle Orthodontist*, **55**, 93–107.

Harris, M. J. and Nortjé, C. J. (1984). The mesial root of the third mandibular molar. A possible indicator of age. *The Journal of Odonto-Stomatology*, **2**, 39–43.

Hassanali, J. and Odhiambo, J. W. (1982). Estimation of calendar age from eruption times of permanent teeth in Kenyan Africans and Asians. *Annals of Human Biology*, **9**, 175–7.

Hauspie, R., Cameron, N., and Molinari, L. (2004). *Methods in Human Growth Research*. Cambridge: Cambridge University Press.

Hedge, R. J. and Sood, P. B. (2002). Dental maturity as an indicator of chronological age: radiographic evaluation of dental age in 6 to 13 years children in Belgium using Demirjian methods. *Journal of Indian Society of Preventative Dentistry*, **20**, 132–8.

Kaul, S. S. and Pathak, R. K. (1988). Estimation of calendar age from the emergence times of permanent teeth in Punjabi children in Chadigarh, India. *Annals of Human Biology*, **15**, 307–9.

Kullman, L, Martinsson, T., Zimmerman, M., and Welander, U. (1995). Computerized measurements of the lower third molar related to chronological age in young adults. *Acta Odontologica Scandinavica*, **53**, 211–16.

Liversidge, H. M. (in press). The timing of third molar formation in four groups. *American Journal of Physical Anthropology.*

Liversidge, H. M. and Molleson, T. (1999). Developing permanent tooth length as an estimate of age. *Journal of Forensic Science*, **44**, 917–920.

Liversidge, H. M., Dean, M. C., and Molleson, T. I. (1993). Increasing human tooth length between birth and 5.4 years. *American Journal of Physical Anthropology*, **90**, 307–13.

Liversidge, H. M., Chaillet, N., Mörnstad, H. *et al.* (in press). Timing of Demirjian tooth formation stages. *Annals of Human Biology*.

Lovejoy, C. O., Meindl, R. S., Mensforth, R. P. and Barton, T. J. (1985). Multifactorial determination of skeletal age at death: a method and blind tests of its accuracy. *American Journal of Physical Anthropology*, **68**, 1–14.

Maber, M, Liversidge, H. M., and Hector, P. (2006). Accuracy of age estimation of radiographic methods using developing teeth. *Forensic Science International*, **159**, 68–73.

Moorrees, C. F. A., Fanning E. A., and Hunt, E. E. (1963). Age variation of formation stages for ten permanent teeth. *Journal of Dental Research*, **42**, 1490–502.

Mörnstad, H., Staaf,.V., and Welander, U. (1994). Age estimation with the aid of tooth development: a new method based on objective measurements. *Scandinavian Journal of Dental Research*, **102**, 137–43.

Nolla, C. M. (1960). The development of the permanent teeth. *Journal of Dentistry for Children*, **27**, 254–66.

Nyarady, Z., Mörnstad, H., Olasz, L., and Szabo, G. (2005). Age estimation of children in south-western Hungary using the modified Demirjian method. *Fogorvosi Szemli*, **98**, 193–8. (in Hungarian.)

Nyström, M., Haataja, J., Kataja, M. *et al.* (1986). Dental maturity in Finnish children, estimated from the development of seven permanent mandibular teeth. *Acta Odontologica Scandinavica*, **44**, 193–8.

Nyström, M., Kleemola-Kujala, E., Evalahti, M., Peck, L. and Kataja, M. (2001). Emergence of permanent teeth and dental age in a series of Finns. *Acta Odontologica Scandinavica*, **59**, 49–56.

Nyström, M., Peck, L., Kleemola-Kujala, E., Evalahti, M., and Kataja, M. (2000). Age estimation in small children: Reference values based on counts of deciduous teeth in Finns. *Forensic Science International*, 110, 179–188.

Pelsmaekers, B., Loos, R., Carels, C., Derom, C., and Vlietinck, R. (1997). The genetic contribution to dental maturation. *Journal of Dental Research*, **76**, 1337–40.

Prahl-Andersen, B., Kowalski, C. J., and Heydendael, P. (1979). *A Mixed-Longitudinal, Interdisciplinary Study of Growth and Development*. San Francisco: Academic Press.

Reid, D. J., Beynon, A. D., and Ramirez Rozzi, F. (1998). Histological reconstruction of dental development in four individuals from a medieval site in Picardy, France. *Journal of Human Evolution*, **35**, 463–77.

Reid, D. J. and Dean, M. C. (2006). Variation in modern human enamel formation times. *Journal of Human Evolution*, **50**, 239–46.

Scheuer, L. and Black, S. (2000). *Developmental Juvenile Osteology*. San Diego: Academic Press.

Schour, I. (1936). The neonatal line in the enamel and dentin of the human deciduous teeth and first permanent molar. *Journal of the American Dental Association*, **23**, 1946–55.

Smith, B. H. (1991). Standards of human tooth formation and dental age assessment. In *Advances in Dental Anthropology*, ed. M. Kelley and C. S. Larsen. New York: Alan R. Liss, pp. 143–68.

Stack, M. V. (1960). Forensic estimation of age in infancy by gravimetric observations on the developing dentition. *Journal of Forensic Science*, **1**, 49–59.

Thompson, G. W., Anderson, D. L., and Popovich, F. (1975). Sexual dimorphism in dentition mineralization. *Growth*, **39**, 289–301.

Townsend, N. and Hammel, E. A. (1990). Age estimation from the number of teeth erupted in young children: an aid to demographic studies. *Demography*, **27**, 165–74.

Willems, G., Van Olmen, A., Spiessens, B. and Carels, C. (2001). Dental age estimation in Belgian children: Demirjian's technique revisited. *Journal of Forensic Science*, **46**, 893–5.

Zhao, J, Ding, L., and Li, R. (1990). Study of dental maturity in children aged 3–16 years in Chengdu. *Journal of West China University of Medical Sciences*, **21**, 242–6.

11 *Primate dental topographic analysis and functional morphology*

PETER S. UNGAR AND JONATHAN M. BUNN

11.1 Introduction

Researchers often use tooth form/function relationships in living primates to reconstruct the diets of early hominins and other fossil primates. One relatively new approach that has become an important tool for dental anthropologists is dental topographic analysis (see Teaford and Ungar, 2006; Ungar, 2006, 2007; Ungar and Daegling, 2007 for recent reviews). In this chapter, we summarize briefly this approach in the context of earlier studies of primate dental functional morphology, and present some new data to illustrate how dental topographic analysis works.

Here we present our first dental topographic analysis of Old World monkeys. Preliminary results for *Cercocebus torquatus atys* and *Procolobus badius badius* suggest that these primates: (1) follow the same patterns of decreasing occlusal slope and relief with wear evinced by apes, New World monkeys, and lemurs examined in previous studies, (2) differ from one another in occlusal slope and relief as expected, given dietary differences reported in the literature, and (3) have, on average, more occlusal slope and relief than do apes with similar diets at given stages of wear.

11.1.1 Historical background

Researchers have considered relationships between diet and tooth form in primates for a very long time. Gregory (1922), for example, suggested that molar shape evolved primarily to improve mechanical efficiency for chewing. Workers in the 1970s (e.g. Crompton and Sita-Lumsden, 1970; Kay and Hiiemae, 1974) built on this idea, viewing teeth as guides for masticatory movements. Insectivorous and folivorous primates, for example, were recognized to have steep-sloped cusps with blade-like crests for shearing tough insect chitin and cellulose, whereas frugivorous primates and bamboo specialists have blunter, flatter cusps, oriented for crushing and grinding (e.g. Kay and

Technique and Application in Dental Anthropology ed. Joel D. Irish and Greg C. Nelson
Published by Cambridge University Press.

Hiiemae, 1974; Kinzey, 1978; Rosenberger and Kinzey, 1976; Seligsohn and Szalay, 1978).

As the research focus on primate dental functional morphology developed, it became clear that some quantitative measure was needed for further progress. Kay's (1977) shearing quotient (SQ) quickly became the standard measure of molar shear potential. SQ reflects the combined lengths of the crests running mesially and distally from the major cusps on a primate molar tooth relative to the length of that tooth. The value is calculated as a residual from a regression line of summed crest length over tooth length for a group of closely related primates with a given type of diet, such as frugivorous Old World monkeys. In this case, a cercopithecoid with a high SQ would be deemed to have longer crests and more shear potential than expected of a fruit-eater.

Shearing quotients have been very effective for distinguishing primates on the basis of their diets. For example, folivorous and insectivorous species have relatively longer crests (higher SQs) than do frugivores. Further, among frugivores, those primates that consume harder, more brittle foods have the shortest crests (and lowest SQ values). These relationships between SQ and diet have been demonstrated for strepsirhines, platyrrhines, cercopithecoids, and hominoids (Anthony and Kay, 1993; Kay and Covert, 1984; Meldrum and Kay, 1997; Strait, 1993; Ungar, 1998). It is important to understand, however, that these relationships hold only when comparing closely related species. Cercopithecoids, for example, have relatively longer crests than hominoids independent of diet (Kay and Covert, 1984) – presumably because the first Old World monkey had longer crests than did the earliest apes. Thus, while SQ accurately tracks adaptation within higher-level taxa, phylogeny determines the starting point of the morphology (Kay and Ungar, 1997; Ungar, 2005).

11.1.2 Dental topographic analysis

Shearing quotient studies have been very valuable for assessing relationships between diet and the morphology of unworn molars, but not worn teeth. As the cusp tips used for crest length measurement become obliterated with wear, SQ values become impossible to determine. This is a problem because primate teeth begin to wear as soon as they come into occlusion, so most teeth available for study are worn. Further, the restriction of analyses to unworn teeth gives us only a limited view of dental functional morphology. Surely primate teeth have evolved to wear in a manner that keeps them efficient for fracturing the foods a species is adapted to eat.

Dental topographic analysis has been developed with this worn tooth conundrum in mind, providing a method for characterizing and comparing the shapes of variably worn teeth (Dennis *et al.*, 2004; King *et al.*, 2005; M'Kirera and

Ungar, 2003; Ungar, 2004; Ungar and M'Kirera, 2003; Ungar and Williamson, 2000). This approach uses a scanning device to obtain a point cloud representing the occlusal surface of a tooth, and geographic information systems (GIS) technology to generate a digital elevation model of that surface. Cusp slopes, occlusal relief, and other values are calculated from the model, and specimens are compared by taxon and degree of wear.

Dental topographic analyses have, to this point, been published for living hominoids (M'Kirera and Ungar, 2003; Merceron *et al.*, 2006; Ungar, 2006; Ungar and M'Kirera, 2003), platyrrhines (Dennis *et al.*, 2004), and strepsirhines (King *et al.*, 2005). These data offer some important insights. First, occlusal slope and relief values for all species tend to be lower in more worn specimens. This is not "rocket science;" teeth become flatter as they wear down. Second, differences in occlusal topography reflect differences in diet. Gorillas, for example, have steeper sloped surfaces and more occlusal relief than do chimpanzees. Orangutans are intermediate. This corresponds to expected differences given assumed fracture properties, especially toughness, of the diets of these apes – gorillas consume more leaves and stems than the other species, and chimpanzees consume the least. Finally, differences observed between these ape species are consistent when individuals with similar degrees of tooth wear are considered, suggesting that occlusal topography of worn molars can be compared between taxa, so long as we can identify and control for wear stage.

11.2 Dental topography of *Cercocebus torquatus* and *Procolobus badius*

The dental topographic analysis approach can best be described by example. Here we present some new data on two Old World monkey species, *Cercocebus torquatus* and *Procolobus badius*. These are, to the best of our knowledge, the first dental topography data published for Old World monkeys. Results allow us to begin to consider some new and interesting questions. First, do cercopithecoids follow the same general pattern of changing dental topography with tooth wear already identified for other primates? Second, do cercopithecoids show the same general relationships between diet and dental topography demonstrated for hominoids? Finally, does occlusal topography differ between cercopithecoids and other higher-level taxa, independent of diet?

11.2.1 Materials and methods

This study included only undamaged lower second molars (M_2s) of *Cercocebus torquatus atys* ($n = 48$) and *Procolobus badius badius* ($n = 50$) in the collections of the Stattliches Museum für Naturkunde in Karlsruhe, Germany. Kingdon (1997) considers these sooty mangabeys to be a distinct species, *Cercocebus atys*, and Napier (1985) places the red colobus in the genus *Piliocolobus*. The Karlsruhe samples are well-provenienced, with all specimens collected in the wild during the late 1950s. The *C. torquatus* individuals were recovered from what had, at the time, been northeastern Central Province in Liberia. The *P. badius* specimens came from southeastern Sierra Leone near the Liberian border.

The M_2 was chosen for analysis because this is the tooth type used in previous dental topographic analyses and most SQ studies. The taxa were selected because of their contrasting diets. The two taxa are often found sympatric, with *P. badius badius* more arboreal, and *C. torquatus atys* more terrestrial (McGraw and Bshary, 2002). *Cercocebus torquatus atys* prefers fruit flesh and seeds, supplemented with small invertebrates (e.g. Bergmüller, 1998). By contrast, leaves make up more than half of the *P. badius badius* diet, with seeds and flowers contributing most of the rest (e.g. Davies *et al.*, 1999).

High-resolution molar replicas were prepared following conventional procedures (see Ungar and M'Kirera, 2003 for details). Molds were made using President's Jet (Coltène-Whaledent Corp., Mawah, NJ) regular-body polyvinylsiloxane dental impression material, and casts were poured using Epotek 301 (Epoxy Technologies, Inc., Billerica, MA) epoxy colored with a pale tan pigment. Resulting replicas were coated with a thin layer of Magniflux SKD-S2 developer (Illinois Tool Works, Inc., Glenview, IL) to mitigate specimen translucency.

Specimens were then examined using an XSM multi-sensor scanning machine (Xystum Corp., Turino, Italy) with an integrated OTM3 laser head (Dr. Wolf & Beck GmbH, Wangen, Germany). Replicas were oriented on the laser scanner stage to maximize the buccolingual and mesiodistal dimensions of occlusal surface in top view as is usual for dental topographic analyses (Ungar *et al.*, 2002). Elevation data were collected for the occlusal surface of each specimen at 25 μm intervals in the *x,y* plane, with a vertical resolution of 25 μm. This resulted in a matrix of 1600 evenly spaced *z* values for each 1 mm^2.

Each point cloud was rendered and processed using the laser scanner, and resultant data were opened as a table in ArcView 3.2 (ESRI Corp., Redlands, CA) with Spatial Analyst and 3D Analyst extensions. Tooth surfaces were interpolated using inverse distance weighting, and cropped to include only the surface above a horizontal plane intersecting the lowest point on the central basin (Ungar and Williamson, 2000).

Average slope (in degrees) between adjacent elevations and an occlusal surface relief index were then calculated for each specimen. Relief is defined as the 3D surface area of the occlusal table (calculated from a triangulated irregular network model generated in ArcView) divided by the projected horizontal or 2D planimetric area multiplied by 100.

Finally, molar replicas were scored for gross wear using a variant of Scott's (1979) method. Individual cusps were scored for degree of faceting or dentine exposure, and scores for all four cusps were summed. Specimens were then arranged into seven wear stages based on their Scott score values: (1) ≤ 10, (2) 11–15, (3) 16–20, (4) 21–25, (5) 26–30, (6) 31–35, and (7) 36–40. These Scott scores are not equivalent to (and should not be compared directly with) those published for extant hominoids. Cercopithecoid M_2s lack hypoconulids, so scores for the Old World monkeys are based on four cusps rather than five.

Statistical analyses were conducted separately on average slope and relief index data. First, these data were rank-transformed to mitigate violation of assumptions inherent to parametric statistical analyses (Conover and Iman, 1981). Two-way ANOVAs with taxon and wear stage as the factors were then run for slope and relief index to assess the effects of species and degree of wear on each variable. These models also allowed us to assess possible interactions between the two factors. Wear stage 1 was excluded from statistical analyses because of insufficient sample size (only one *C. torquatus* and two *P. badius* M_2s were unworn or nearly unworn).

The null hypotheses, based on results of dental topographic analyses for other primates and on feeding ecology observations reported in the literature, were: (1) less-worn M_2s should have higher mean slope values and relief indices than more worn specimens, (2) *P. badius* should have steeper sloped cusps and more occlusal relief than *C. torquatus*, and (3) there should be no interaction between taxon and wear-stage factors. The first two tests are one-tailed, and assessed for significance using a $p \leq 0.1$ criterion (Sokal and Rohlf, 1994).

11.2.2 Results

Descriptive statistics are presented in Table 11.1 and sample digital elevation models (triangulated irregular networks) are illustrated in Figure 11.1. Results are presented in Table 11.2 and depicted graphically in Figure 11.2. Three distinct patterns are apparent. First, both occlusal slope and relief index decline through successive wear stages, except for the most worn specimens. By implication, molar teeth of both taxa tend to become flatter as they wear, at least until they become extremely worn. Second, *Procolobus badius* tends to show higher average occlusal relief and slope values at given stages of wear than does *Cercocebus torquatus*. Finally, the differences between the two species seem to be of about the same order of magnitude at most stages of wear.

Table 11.1 *Summary statistics for the dental topographic analysis*

	Cercocebus torquatus			*Procolobus badius*		
Wear	Mean	*SD*	*N*	Mean	*SD*	*N*
A. Slope						
1	49.63		1	43.031	1.888	2
2	41.71	3.953	8	40.923	5.038	6
3	30.80	7.936	21	39.142	5.420	25
4	27.75	7.299	9	35.694	4.362	7
5	25.00	4.054	4	30.537	2.335	4
6	19.24	2.944	2	27.901	6.088	2
7	27.81	8.888	3	28.981	9.137	4
B. Relief						
1	193.43		1	225.156	46.652	2
2	161.68	8.279	8	187.793	13.157	6
3	141.92	16.537	21	185.546	17.231	25
4	141.51	22.540	9	175.424	15.268	7
5	137.82	16.365	4	157.100	22.230	4
6	124.70	16.622	2	157.656	18.754	2
7	151.34	39.139	3	165.559	26.402	4

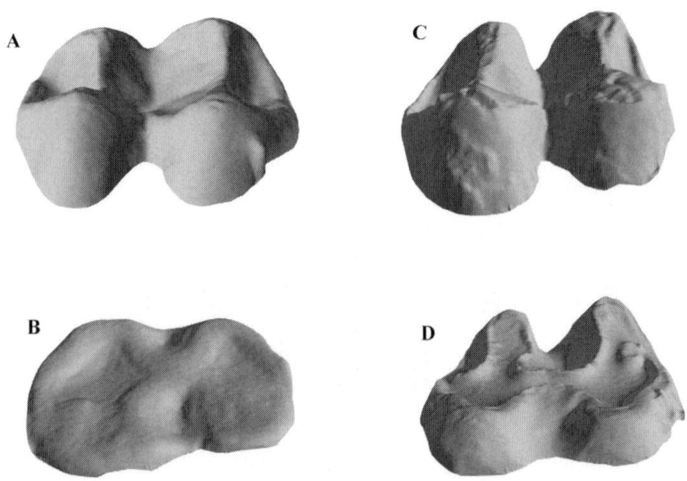

Figure 11.1 Triangulated irregular network representations of surface data for M_2s of *Cercocebus torquatus atys* (A, B) and *Procolobus badius badius* (C, D) at wear stages 2 (A, C) and 5 (B, D). These models depict data for (A) SMNK 712, (B) SMNK 372, (C) SMNK 3102, and (D) SMNK 422. Specimens are scaled to the same size for illustration.

Table 11.2 *Analytical statistical analyses: individual ANOVAs*

Effect	Species	Wear	Interaction
Slope	2.936[a]	37.247[b]	0.055
Relief	32.972[b]	12.130[b]	2.415
df	2, 90	2, 90	1, 91

[a] $p < 0.1$
[b] $p < 0.05$

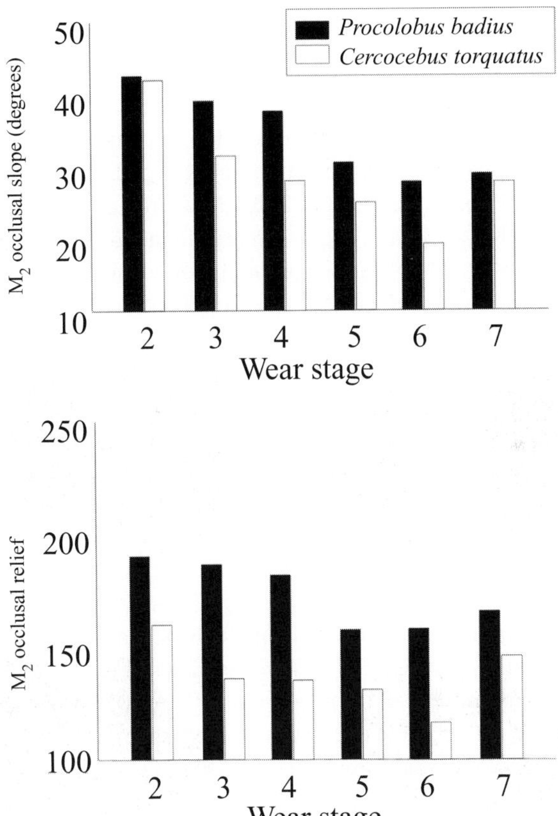

Figure 11.2 Comparisons of mean slope (above) and relief index (below) values for *Cercocebus torquatus atys* and *Procolobus badius badius* at given wear stages (see text for details).

Statistical analyses bear out these observations. Two-way ANOVA results for both mean slope and relief index showed significant variation between the wear stages and between the taxa. Less worn teeth have more occlusal slope and relief than do more worn teeth. Further, *P. badius* has steeper-sloping surfaces and more occlusal relief than *C. torquatus*. Neither slope nor relief models showed a significant interaction between the factors. This means that the differences between taxa are not dependent on wear for those specimens included in the statistical analyses. In other words, the colobus monkeys show steeper slopes and more occlusal relief than do the mangabeys, independent of wear stage examined.

11.2.3 Discussion

These results can be interpreted in light of studies documenting dental topography in apes, New World monkeys, and lemurs (e.g. Dennis *et al.*, 2004; King *et al.*, 2005; M'Kirera and Ungar, 2003; Merceron *et al.*, 2006; Ungar, 2006; Ungar and M'Kirera, 2003), and differences in diet between *Cercocebus torquatus atys* and *Procolobus badius badius* reported in the literature (e.g. Bergmüller, 1998; Davies *et al.*, 1999). First, both species showed a pattern of decreasing occlusal slope and relief in progressively more worn specimens until the last wear stage. Mangabey and colobus monkey teeth evidently become flatter as they wear down. This same general pattern has been documented for samples of extant apes (M'Kirera and Ungar, 2003; Ungar and M'Kirera, 2003) and fossil hominins (Ungar, 2004, 2007). Decreasing molar slope and relief have also been observed in longitudinal studies of individual howling monkeys (Dennis *et al.*, 2004) and lemurs (King *et al.*, 2005) in the wild.

It also follows that once much of the occlusal surface is obliterated by wear, slope and relief values may actually increase slightly as the softer dentin wears more quickly than the remaining enamel rim. This is again the same pattern observed for apes, and is explained by M'Kirera and Ungar (2003) as a function of the unworn convex surfaces of cusps becoming flatter with wear, then more concave as the exposed dentin is excavated. Indeed, the point at which slope and relief begin to increase may correspond roughly to that identified by King and coauthors (2005) as dental senescence (see also Dennis *et al.*, 2004).

The differences observed between the two cercopithecoid species are as expected, given the presumed material properties of the foods they eat. The fracture properties of plant foods vary depending on the part of the fruit or leaf examined, and its state of development (e.g. Lucas, 2004; Teaford *et al.*, 2006). Nevertheless, leaves, especially the veins of mature leaves, can be very tough compared with fruit flesh comprised of larger cells (Lucas, personal communication). The fact that folivorous primates tend to have teeth with longer, sharper shearing crests than do closely related frugivores makes sense in this context (e.g. Anthony and Kay, 1993; Kay and Covert, 1984; Meldrum and Kay, 1997; Strait, 1993; Ungar, 1998).

The *P. badius* diet is dominated by leaves, nearly 40 % of which are mature (Davies *et al.*, 1999). *Cercocebus torquatus*, in contrast, consumes more fruit flesh than does the red colobus monkey (Bergmüller, 1998). As one would expect, unworn *P. badius* M_2s have longer shearing crests than do those of *C. torquatus* (Kay, 1978). This is consistent with dental topographic analysis results presented here, which is not surprising given that relative shearing crest lengths can be viewed as 2D measures of relief (M'Kirera and Ungar, 2003). Indeed, *P. badius* had higher values than *C. torquatus* for both attributes at all stages of wear for which there were sufficient samples to evaluate them.

These results are similar to those reported for apes (M'Kirera and Ungar, 2003; Merceron *et al.*, 2006; Ungar and M'Kirera, 2003). More folivorous gorillas show higher slope and relief values for M_2s at each stage of wear than do more frugivous chimpanzees. Orangutans, which are intermediate in their dietary proclivities, are intermediate in mean slope and occlusal relief. Data for the cercopithecoids and hominoids are unfortunately not directly comparable, however, because their wear score values are not directly comparable (Old World monkey Scott scores are based on four cusps while those for the apes are based on five).

Nevertheless, both slope and relief index values for *P. badius* tend to be greater than those for *Gorilla gorilla*, and those for *C. torquatus* tend to be greater than those for *Pan troglodytes*. In fact, we expect that cercopithecoids as a group probably have, on average, higher slopes and more occlusal relief than do hominoids. As Kay and Covert (1984) have noted, Old World monkeys have longer shearing crests than apes independent of diet. This raises the specter of phylogenetic effects on the interpretation of adaptation, and reinforces the importance of comparing species within and not between higher-level taxa (see Kay and Ungar, 1997).

11.3 Conclusions

Researchers have demonstrated repeatedly relationships between tooth form and function in living primates. The lengths of shearing crests on unworn molar teeth, for example, reflect adaptations to the fracture properties of foods. Folivores have the longest crests for shearing tough leaf parts, whereas frugivores have shorter crests and blunter molars for crushing and grinding the fruits to which they are adapted.

Dental topographic analysis provides a technique for comparing functionally relevant aspects of occlusal morphology of worn teeth. Studies published to date have demonstrated that molars become flatter as they wear, but that similarly worn teeth can be compared between species. More folivorous gorillas, for example, tend to have more sloping cusps and more occlusal surface relief at a given stage of wear than do more frugivorous orangutans and especially chimpanzees. These patterns hold for the Old World monkey taxa *Cercocebus torquatus atys* and *Procolobus badius badius*. Again, the more folivorous taxon has more sloping cusps and more occlusal relief than does the more frugivorous one at given stages of wear. Apparent differences between these cercopithecoids and hominoids with similar diets underscore the importance of limiting comparisons to closely related species.

In sum, dental topographic analysis is a valuable tool for functional morphologists interested in understanding dental/dietary adaptations. Work is progressing to expand our comparative database to include more primate taxa and human bioarcheological samples. The primary goals of this research are to provide new insights into the relationships between dental form and function, and to better understand the effects of tooth wear on these relationships.

Acknowledgments

The molar replicas used for this project were prepared from molds collected for another study. We are most grateful to Mark Teaford, Fred Grine, and Gildas Merceron for their help in collecting these dental impressions, and to Hans-Walter Mittmann for access to specimens in his care and for his hospitality in Karlsruhe. We also thank Joel Irish and Greg Nelson for inviting us to contribute this "minichapter," and to Peter Lucas for discussions related to aspects of this work. This research was funded in part by the National Science Foundation and the University of Arkansas.

References

Anthony, M. R. L. and Kay, R. F. (1993). Tooth form and diet in ateline and alouattine primates: reflections on the comparative method. *American Journal of Science*, **293A**, 356–82.

Bergmüller, R. (1998). Nahrungsökologie der Rauchgrauen Mangabe (*Cercocebus torquatus atys*): Ein Schlüssel zur sozialen Organisation? Thesis, Nürnberg: University of Erlangen-Nürnberg.

Conover, W. J. and Iman, R. L. (1981). Rank transformations as a bridge between parametric and nonparametric statistics. *American Statistician*, **35**, 124–9.

Crompton, A. W. and Sita-Lumsden, A. G. (1970). Functional significance of therian molar pattern. *Nature*, **227**, 197–9.

Davies, A. G., Oates, J. F., and Dasilva, G. L. (1999). Patterns of frugivory in three West African colobine monkeys. *International Journal of Primatology*, **20**, 327–57.

Dennis, J. C., Ungar, P. S., Teaford, M. F., and Glander, K. E. (2004). Dental topography and molar wear in *Alouatta palliata* from Costa Rica. *American Journal of Physical Anthropology*, **125**, 152–61.

Gregory, W. K. (1922). *The Origin and Evolution of Human Dentition*. Baltimore: Williams and Wilkins.

Kay, R. F. (1977). Evolution of molar occlusion in Cercopithecidae and early catarrhines. *American Journal of Physical Anthropology*, **46**, 327–52.

Kay, R. F. (1978). Molar structure and diet in extant Cercopithecidae. In *Development, Function, and Evolution of Teeth*, ed. P. M. Butler and K. A. Joysey, pp. 309–339. New York: Academic Press.

Kay, R. F. and Covert, H. H. (1984). Anatomy and behavior of extinct primates. In *Food Acquisition and Processing in Primates*, ed. D. J. Chivers, B. A. Wood, and A. Bilsborough. New York: Plenum Press, pp. 467–508.

Kay, R. F. and Hiiemae, K. M. (1974). Jaw movement and tooth use in recent and fossil primates. *American Journal of Physical Anthropology*, **40**, 227–56.

Kay, R. F. and Ungar, P. S. (1997). Dental evidence for diet in some Miocene catarrhines with comments on the effects of phylogeny on the interpretation of adaptation. In *Function, Phylogeny and Fossils: Miocene Hominoids and Great Ape and Human Origins*, ed. D. R. Begun, C. Ward, and M. Rose. New York: Plenum Press, pp. 131–51.

King, S. J., Arrigo-Nelson, S. J., Pochron, S. T. *et al.* (2005). Dental senescence in a long-lived primate links infant survival to rainfall. *Proceedings of the National Academy of Sciences, USA*, **102**, 16579–83.

Kingdon, J. (1997). *The Kingdon Field Guide to African Mammals*. San Diego: Academic Press.

Kinzey, W. G. (1978). Feeding behavior and molar features in two species of titi monkey. In *Recent Advances in Primatology, Volume 1, Behavior*, ed. D. J. Chivers and J. Herbert. New York: Academic Press, pp. 373–85.

Lucas, P. W. (2004). *Dental Functional Morphology: How Teeth Work*. New York: Cambridge University Press.

M'Kirera, F. and Ungar, P. S. (2003). Occlusal relief changes with molar wear in *Pan troglodytes troglodytes* and *Gorilla gorilla gorilla*. *American Journal of Primatology*, **60**, 31–41.

McGraw, W. S. and Bshary, R. (2002). Association of terrestrial mangabeys (*Cercocebus atys*) with arboreal monkeys: experimental evidence for the effects of reduced ground predator pressure on habitat use. *International Journal of Primatology*, **23**, 311–25.

Meldrum, D. J. and Kay, R. F. (1997). *Nuciruptor rubricae*, a new pitheciin seed predator from the Miocene of Colombia. *American Journal of Physical Anthropology*, **102**, 407–27.

Merceron, G., Taylor, S., Scott, R., Chaimanee, Y., and Jaeger, J. J. (2006). Dietary characterization of the hominoid *Khoratpithecus* (Miocene of Thailand): evidence from dental topographic and microwear texture analyses. *Naturwissenschaften*, **93**, 329–33.

Napier, P. H. (1985). *Catalogue of Primates in the British Museum (Natural History) and Elsewhere in the British Isles, Part 3: Family Cercopitehcidae, Subfamily Colobinae*. London: British Museum of Natural History.

Rosenberger, A. L. and Kinzey, W. G. (1976). Functional patterns of molar occlusion in platyrrhine primates. *American Journal of Physical Anthropology*, **45**, 281–97.

Scott, E. C. (1979). Dental wear scoring technique. *American Journal of Physical Anthropology*, **51**, 213–17.

Seligsohn, D. and Szalay, F. S. (1978). Relationship between natural selection and dental morphology: tooth function and diet in *Lepilemur* and *Hapalemur*. In *Development, Function and Evolution of Teeth*, ed. P. M. Butler and K. A. Joysey. New York: Academic Press, pp. 289–307.

Sokal, R. R. and Rohlf, F. J. (1994). *Biometry: The Principles and Practice of Statistics in Biolgical Research*. New York: W. H. Freeman and Company.

Strait, S. G. (1993). Molar morphology and food texture among small bodied insectivorous mammals. *Journal of Mammalogy*, **74**, 391–402.

Teaford, M. F., Lucas, P. W., Ungar, P. S., and Glander, K. E. (2006). Mechanical defenses in leaves eaten by Costa Rican howling monkeys (*Alouatta palliata*). *American Journal of Physical Anthropology*, **129**, 99–104.

Teaford, M. F. and Ungar, P. S. (2006). Dental adaptations of African apes. To be published in *Handbook of Paleoanthropology. Volume1: Principles, Methods, and Approaches*, ed. W. Kenke, W. Rothe, and I. Tattersall. Heidelberg: Springer Verlag, in press.

Ungar, P. S. (1998). Dental allometry, morphology, and wear as evidence for diet in fossil primates. *Evolutionary Anthropology*, **6**, 205–17.

Ungar, P. S. (2004). Dental topography and diets of *Australopithecus afarensis* and early *Homo*. *Journal of Human Evolution*, **46**, 605–22.

Ungar, P. S. (2005). Dental evidence for the diets of fossil primates from Rudabánya, northeastern Hungary with comments on extant primate analogs and "noncompetitive" sympatry. *Palaeontographica Italica*, **90**, 97–111.

Ungar, P. S. (2006). Dental functional morphology: the known, the unknown and the unknowable. In *Evolution of the Human Diet: The Known, the Unknown and the Unknowable*, ed. P. S. Ungar. Oxford: Oxford University Press, pp. 39–55.

Ungar, P. S. (2007). Dental topography and human evolution: with comments on the diets of *Australopithecus africanus* and *Paranthropus robustus*. To be published in *Dental Perspectives on Human Evolution: State of the Art Research in Dental Anthropology*, ed. S. Bailey, and J. J. Hublin, New York: Springer-Verlag.

Ungar, P. S. and Daegling, D. (2007). The functional morphology of jaws and teeth, and their implications for understanding early hominin dietary adaptations. To be published in *Early hominin paleoecology*, ed. M. Sponheimer, P. Ungar, K. Reed, and J. Lee-Thorp. Boulder: University of Colorado Press.

Ungar, P. S. and M'Kirera, F. (2003). A solution to the worn tooth conundrum in primate functional anatomy. *Proceedings of the National Academy of Sciences of the United States of America*, **100**, 3874–7.

Ungar, P. S. and Williamson, M. (2000). Exploring the effects of tooth wear on functional morphology: a preliminary study using dental topographic analysis. *Paleontologica Electronica*, **3**, 18.

Ungar, P. S., Dennis, J., Kirera, F., Wilson, J., and Grine, F. (2002). Quantification of tooth crown shape by dental topographic analysis. *American Journal of Physical Anthropology*, **Supplement 34**, 158–9.

12 *Forensic dental anthropology: issues and guidelines*

CHRISTOPHER W. SCHMIDT

12.1 Introduction

There is no doubt that over the years dentists around the world have positively identified a large percentage of the victims found at death scenes. They have done so by employing many tried-and-true dental procedures, including dissecting/resecting jaws from disfigured and decomposed victims, comparing ante- and postmortem dental radiographs, and studying bite marks inflicted on one person by another (Bowers, 2004; Bowers and Bell, 1995; Sopher, 1993; Stimson and Mertz, 1997). These and other procedures have been used for decades to positively identify recently deceased people. It would seem, then, that odontology is one area of forensic analysis that would not be in particular need of assistance from non-clinical personnel, i.e. biological anthropologists. However, forensic odontological studies proceed more efficiently when identifications are made on more or less complete dentitions. There are, of course, instances where teeth are significantly fragmented and commingled. With their training in the recovery and reconstruction of human remains, forensic dental anthropologists (odontoanthropologists in Wagner, 1997) are able to locate and rebuild dentitions and make them more amenable to study by the forensic dentist. Are forensic dentists capable of working in the absence of forensic dental anthropologists, even when confronted with commingled remains? Certainly, and many have (see Bowers and Bell, 1995; Morlang, 1997 for guidelines regarding forensic odontological mass disaster management). But, as I talk with forensic dentists, I have learned that most are willing to obtain assistance from dental anthropologists in difficult circumstances.

12.2 Spatial context

Forensic anthropologists in general, and forensic dental anthropologists in particular, assist those in the medicolegal community wanting to know the circumstances surrounding the deposition of a body and its identification. With their

Technique and Application in Dental Anthropology ed. Joel D. Irish and Greg C. Nelson
Published by Cambridge University Press.

archeological training, forensic dental anthropologists are able to establish the spatial context of dental remains before investigators gather them. They can also document the physical environment and the precise placement of remains, as well as any associated material culture, to determine the agents that brought forth the condition in which the remains were found. Moreover, the spatial context provided by forensic dental anthropologists yields data available only at the time of recovery, much of which aids law enforcement and expedites the process of positive identification.

12.2.1 Human vs. non-human

With a few exceptions, especially cervid incisors, a complete non-human tooth is almost impossible to confuse with that of a human. However, small root and crown fragments can be confounding, and may require intensive study to make a determination. Human enamel is relatively thick, especially on the molars and generally ranges from 1–2 mm (Grine, 2005). Human cusps are low, rounded, and dissimilar from most North American mammals, with the possible exception of bears. In my experience, however, the only bear tooth that appears human-like is the third molar of a polar bear. Though similar, one can usually distinguish between bear third molars and human molars, as the former tend to have more occlusal crenulations, relatively longer mesiodistal diameters, more conical roots, and shorter crowns relative to root length. Domesticated pigs also have low, rounded cusps, but their crenulated occlusal surfaces readily distinguish them.

At the microscopic level, human enamel has a keyhole pattern. In cross section (Figure 12.1), enamel rods have distinct margins superiorly, while their inferior aspects are poorly defined and the crystallites look as if they are spilling into the surrounding inter-rod material (Ten Cate, 1994). Many animals with teeth similar in size to those of humans do not have this pattern; their rod margins are distinct and/or are arranged more linearly (Hillson, 1986, 1996). Possible exceptions to this are carnivores like large canids and bears. Thus, one must look at as many morphological variables as possible to make a determination.

12.2.2 Tooth taphonomy

A sizeable percentage of a forensic dental anthropologist's value to the forensic dentist comes in the area of tooth taphonomy. Bowers (2004), for example, includes a discussion of taphonomy in his volume, *Forensic Dental Evidence*. It

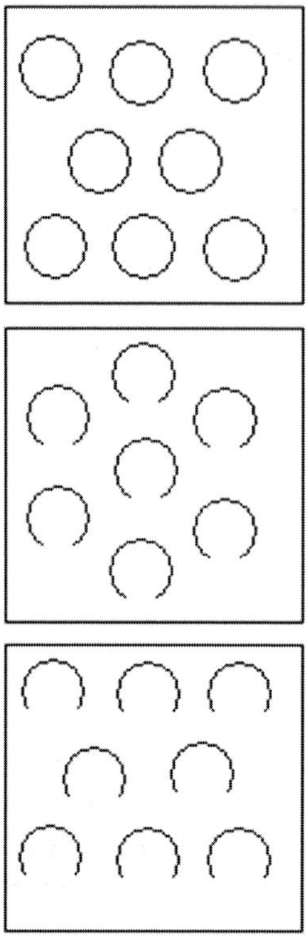

Figure 12.1 Schematic of enamel cross sections. The bottom pattern is found in humans (modified from Hillson, 1996).

takes a great deal of time and training to understand the gamut of agents that can alter human hard tissues, both biological and non-biological (Bonnichsen and Sorg, 1989; Haglund and Sorg, 1997, 2002). The following information outlines a number of the taphonomic factors germane to the recovery and reconstruction of teeth.

Biological taphonomic processes

Plant roots can "etch" their way across dental remains that have been buried or left on the surface. These marks usually manifest as lightly colored striae that are branching or reticulated in appearance (Hall, 1997). Given enough time, the actions of roots can completely fragment a dentition. Plants that take up residence on surface-deposited remains are capable of staining them or creating a mottled appearance. Likewise, mosses and lichens are capable of discoloring exposed human tooth roots.

Insects and herbivorous burrowing animals can damage human hard tissues (Catts and Haskell, 1990; Haglund, 1997a). Rodents can be especially destructive, gnawing the edges of almost any bone they can get their jaws around and leaving a distinctive scalloped appearance (Haglund, 1997a). Carnivorous animals like coyotes and domesticated dogs have been known to eat much of the face of deceased humans, including the dentition. At the very least, they are capable of dragging the skull a great distance, dislodging anterior teeth along the way (Haglund, 1997b; Schmidt and Greene, 1998). Teeth that are swallowed and subsequently excreted from an animal may evidence exposure to digestive juices, usually manifest as pitting and edge rounding created during the mechanical and chemical processes of digestion (Butler and Schroeder, 1998; Rensberger and Krentz, 1988). Dentin is more likely to show pitting than the enamel; pits are usually small, focal, and not discolored.

Non-biological taphonomic factors

There are numerous non-biological processes that can affect human teeth, such as wind, water, solar energy, and the Earth itself. Wind can affect surface-deposited remains by abrading them with particles of sand, silt, and clay. In arid environments, wind driven sand can significantly erode hard tissues, as well as bury them. If a tooth is washed into a rapidly moving stream it can become "water-worn" or smoothed by the action of water and suspended particles. Water also can lead to a darkening of dental tissues as it percolates through enamel and dentin, depositing various minerals. Crowns that have been submerged for a long period of time may turn brown, dark gray, or they may not change color at all (Schmidt *et al.*, 1998).

Local geologic and hydrologic events can displace and fracture teeth. Colluvium may cover human remains at the bottom of a cliff or rock overhang, while alluvium can bury human elements in a floodplain. Of course, moving water can easily displace remains (Nawrocki, *et al.*, 1997). Posterior teeth may remain in their crypts as the body moves through water, but the anterior teeth will dislodge as soon as the mechanical trauma exceeds the adherence capabilities of the soft tissues. It is possible for anterior teeth to fall out before the body is washed away, marking the spot of initial deposition (e.g. Nawrocki *et al.*, 1998). If a body is buried, the surrounding sediment will likely stain exposed dentin, making it light brown or soft orange, but often will not affect enamel color.

Soil staining creates a veneer of discoloration that rarely penetrates the dentin beyond 1 mm or so. Breaks in dentin long after the body was buried have nearly white "cortices" beneath the stained exterior. By contrast, teeth broken at the time of burial will have fracture-exposed surfaces stained in a manner like that of the external surfaces, as both were in direct soil contact.

Solar energy can bleach and crack dental tissues, although enamel's nearly complete absence of organic material and water makes it much less susceptible to such breakdown. Solar bleaching can be of particular help when interpreting the disturbance history of the remains. If a tooth is found with its solar bleached side down, it clearly was moved from a previous position.

Teeth are primarily comprised of hydroxyapatite (Ten Cate, 1994), a calcium-rich inorganic material that maintains its integrity in a neutral to slightly basic environment. Acids, like those produced by certain organic soil constituents (including some peats), or even those created by oral bacteria, can rapidly break down bones and teeth (Pindborg, 1970; Ten Cate, 1994). For example, bodies in acidic peat bogs of northern Europe are famous for their remarkable soft tissue preservation despite being thousands of years old; yet their hard tissues are poorly preserved (Coles and Coles, 1989; Glob, 1988; Painter, 1995). Further, in a relevant case, Indiana's Department of Natural Resources requested that Dr. Stephen Nawrocki and I recover disturbed human remains from a homestead cemetery in southern Indiana that was impacted by heavy machinery. Some skeletal material was exposed on the surface, but we also investigated a burial shaft revealed by the machinery. At the bottom of the shaft we found a bead necklace and organic stain in the shape of a coffin. Although the burial was only 100 to 150 years old, soil acidity completely eliminated the skeleton and teeth.

Acids can leach into a burial from many sources, including agricultural and industrial runoff, adjacent refuse pits, and building foundations. Acids create pits and broad, shallow areas of eroded tissue on teeth, especially the dentin. The damaged area may be outlined in black, and the exposed area may be gray and flaky. Erosive pits on enamel are often brown, and tend to occur on the labial aspect of the crown near the cervical line – where enamel can be quite thin (especially in incompletely developed crowns). The teeth degrade as damaged areas coalesce, first in the dentin and later in the enamel.

The presence of alkaline materials near the body, such as lime, limestone, and invertebrate shells, can mitigate soil acidity. Shell middens over prehistoric burials have actually aided in the preservation of skeletons in several cemeteries throughout North America, but particularly in the valleys of the Ohio and Green Rivers in Indiana and Kentucky; in these cases, excellent bone preservation has been noted in burials that are 3000 to 5000 years old (Schmidt, *et al.*, in press; Webb, 1974). It seems that if neutral to slightly basic soil pH is maintained, bones can last almost indefinitely. For example, in the alkaline environment of a limestone sinkhole in central Indiana, unfossilized Pleistocene animal bones and teeth (ranging from frogs to a type of rhinoceros) were found in perfect condition despite being approximately five million years old (Farlow *et al.*, 2001).

Taphonomic cultural processes

There are cultural practices that directly impact tooth color and quality. In antiquity, it was not uncommon for copper artifacts to accompany the dead; these items can result in green stains if in contact with the body. Similar staining can result today in forensic contexts. For example, degraded dental appliances have been known to stain teeth (e.g. Sopher, 1993).

Bodies that are covered before burial (e.g. placed in a coffin or tarp) will preserve longer than those placed directly into the ground. Coffin wood often stains bone dark brown, but rarely affects the teeth. Things that confine the body help keep the dentition intact, even as the body slumps after soft tissue decay. I have seen forensic cases where assailants used tarps, sleeping bags, plastic bags, concrete blocks, and other materials to cover their victims; as a result, the teeth were generally preserved in or near their proper anatomical orientation (Schmidt, *et al.*, 2006).

Antemortem vs. taphonomic tooth modification

When studying tooth taphonomy, it is important to keep in mind that teeth are the only hard tissues designed to interact with the outside environment. Thus, not all tooth stains, cracks, and pits are created taphonomically. Dietary and recreational resources like tea, coffee, tobacco, and even betelnut can leave dark stains on the dentition. Tobacco can cause brown stains especially interproximally and along the gum line (Sopher, 1993); chewing betelnut, a tradition in Southeast Asia, can turn the entire anterior dentition black.

Antemortem tooth fractures can be distinguished from those occurring postmortem, in that the former often exhibit polishing and wear. Perimortem and postmortem breaks are stark and jagged, and lack any signs of rounding on their margins. Perimortem damage from high-speed projectiles (i.e. bullets and buckshot) can significantly fracture teeth, hindering dental identification. However, proper excavation of the remains, including screening the area around the head with 1/8″ (or finer) wire mesh can recover tiny dental fragments necessary to reconstruct teeth.

In instances where the teeth are forced into the head, by projectiles or blunt instruments, a careful examination of the endocranial vault may yield fragments. When soft tissues are present, radiographs can be used to locate imbedded tooth fragments. For example, fire investigators and I recovered the body of a woman killed in a blaze that completely destroyed her house. Her body was found in the basement. The distal aspects of the limbs had fallen off, and the skull was markedly reduced in size – apparently because much of the cranial vault was fractured and had fallen away. The orbits were the only landmarks clearly visible; the rest was either charred or missing. At the time of recovery there was no evidence of the dentition. Her body was radiographed at the office of the medical examiner, and several teeth were found in what remained of her brain. From these teeth a positive identification was made. It is surmised that the woman was asleep on the second floor of the home during the fire, and fell into the basement as the house collapsed. The impact of the fall forced her dentition back into her head.

Antemortem pits caused by heavy occlusal wear or dental caries are most readily distinguished from taphonomic pitting by their location and shape. Carious lesions tend to be circular, deep (i.e. extending into the dentin), and occur along the occlusal grooves and fissures, or are adjacent to the interproximal contact facets. Taphonomic pitting is more random, and the eroded patches are usually shallow and amorphous. Particularly in the enamel, taphonomically created pits are accompanied by yellow-brown staining, probably caused by enamel thinning through which the underlying dentin is visible. In a relevant case study, construction workers renovating a late nineteenth/early twentieth century Indianapolis home found what they believed to be human teeth. I was part of a forensic team that eventually recovered several human teeth, many of which exhibited caries and fillings. Roots were darkly stained, and some discoloration was noted near the cervix. No bones were recovered. Under the microscope, I observed that the discolorations were actually indentations on the labial and lingual aspects; they were caused by a compressive force, and appeared on nearly every tooth and in virtually the same locations. I realized that the damage was not taphonomic; it occurred antemortem. The indentations were caused during dental extraction. Further evidence of extraction was evident in the molars, most of which had fractured and missing roots – a condition not seen in the anterior teeth. Research into the history of the house revealed that a dentist resided there during the early 1900s (Nawrocki *et al.*, 1996).

Burned teeth

High temperatures can drastically affect the appearance and quality of teeth. As temperatures and/or duration of exposure increase, teeth char by turning a deep black or brown color; then they turn blue-gray and finally white (calcined) (Buikstra and Swegle, 1989; Shipman *et al.*, 1984). Since thermally induced color changes in teeth are related to loss of the organic component (mostly collagen), dentin will start to change color quite readily. Immature enamel has a higher organic component and will darken to a blue-gray, but mature enamel will resist color changes.

As teeth begin to calcinize the enamel fractures and falls away, leaving behind the shrunken discolored dentin. Erupted teeth that remain in their crypts during burning tend to have their roots protected, at least until the surrounding bone fractures. In instances where the maxilla and mandible remain intact, the enamel and dentin component of the crown will be calcined and fractured, while the root will have only darkened. Should such a tooth fall out after the fire, it will retain evidence of its dual exposure – giving the analyst an opportunity to reconstruct the burning event (Schmidt, in press). In general, anterior teeth fall out more frequently than molars, as the latter are multirooted. Molars can become dislodged, however, especially if they fracture at the root furcations. In these instances, it can be difficult to distinguish anterior tooth roots from isolated molar roots. Fortunately, there is a telltale identifier of molar roots if enough of the cervical area remains intact. Individual molar roots (radicals) will have a spur or notch at the point where they were conjoined with the other radicals prior to the thermal exposure (Schmidt, in press).

Teeth that have yet to erupt usually show less thermal damage than those that have erupted. This is an important consideration, especially if the teeth are commingled. When it comes time to assemble dentitions, one must consider the possibilities of tooth association based on age, and not necessarily degree of burning. For example, a heavily burned adult central incisor and a nearly unburned second molar crown could easily be from the same person, despite the marked difference in heat related damage.

Identifying burned teeth can be trying, and it is likely that in a collection of hundreds of dental fragments, only a small percentage will be identified with confidence. When enamel is missing, the analyst can use the morphology of the coronal dentin since it has the same general shape as the complete crown. Isolated roots of anterior teeth are often more difficult to identify than crown fragments, as fracturing and shrinking obscures many diagnostic landmarks. Fortunately, roots tend to keep their general shape, i.e. upper roots still appear rounded and lower roots compressed. To illustrate, I was called upon to help in the investigation of a man, married with children, who murdered at least 11 men after having sexual relations with them in his north Indianapolis home. The disarticulated bodies of most victims were found along and within a small creek near the property; a few others were found, heavily burned, in an adjacent wooded area. The burned bone fragments were rarely more than a few cm in length and had been distributed down slope by rain. Several thousand bone fragments and approximately 100 burned and unburned dental fragments were archaeologically excavated.

Using dental morphology and expressions of dental pathology and restoration, I reconstructed three dentitions, each of which contained maxillary and mandibular components. Adjacent teeth were aligned using the orientation of inter-proximal contact facets, while maxillary and mandibular teeth were matched by aligning incisal wear facets. Despite having been commingled and heavily damaged, two of these three dentitions were subsequently, positively identified by the forensic dentist.

12.3 Biological context

Once the analyst has established the spatial context of the teeth, it is time to consider the biological context. Specifically, the focus is to address a separate suite of questions, usually pursued in the lab, concerning characterization of the teeth and the individuals from which they derive.

12.3.1 Minimum number of individuals

In the laboratory, the teeth are cleaned with toothbrushes and tap water and reconstructed with a household glue designed for ceramics such as Duco® cement. Teeth are identified using standard anatomical features (e.g. Bass, 1995; Hillson, 1996; Jordan and Abrams, 1992; Steele and Bramblett, 1988; Taylor, 1978; White, 2000) and counted. Next, the analyst determines how many individuals are represented by noting duplicate elements. For example, if the final tally yields six lower left third molars, four upper right first molars, and three upper central incisors, the minimum number of individuals (MNI) is six. However, there is a challenge with this procedure that is particularly acute in the study of teeth.

Human polyphyodonty renders two separate dentitions, both of which are present throughout much of childhood. When performing the MNI, therefore, the developmental age of each tooth must be considered. Going back to the last example, let us say that one of the four upper right first molars is an unerupted, incompletely formed crown. The adult MNI remains at six, because of the six third molars; however, now there is also evidence for at least one sub-adult – moving the overall MNI to seven. Failing to establish a proper age-inclusive MNI may result in a significant error of underestimation.

12.3.2 Biological profile

The biological profile involves reconstructions of each decedent's age, sex, ancestry, and anatomical idiosyncrasies. Dental-based profiles can be used to either supplement profiles generated from the osseous material, or the teeth can be used independently if they are found in isolation or the skeleton is badly damaged.

Age: sub-adults

Perhaps the most reliable system of aging sub-adults involves scoring the developmental stage of each tooth and comparing the scores, either as individual teeth or as composite maturity scores, to published standards of human tooth development (e.g. Demirjian *et al.*, 1973; Demirjian and Goldstein, 1976; Haavikko, 1970; Massler and Schour, 1958; Moorrees *et al.*, 1963a, 1963b; Smith, 1991). These systems are generally seen as quite good, because they take into account both dental formation and eruption (Bowers, 1995). However, dental development can be impacted by such variables as sex, health, and biological ancestry (Liversidge *et al.*, 1998). Moreover, aging based upon dental development is only of value until such a time when the adult third molar roots complete formation – generally in an individual's early 20s.

Saunders *et al.* (1993) studied a large sample of nineteenth-century sub-adult skeletons ($n = 282$) to address the efficacy of the Moorrees *et al.* (1963a, 1963b) aging standards; overall they found the standards to provide accurate estimates of age. Maber *et al.* (2006) applied each of the aforementioned dental age standards (as well as some variations) to radiographs of sub-adult dentitions in an effort to find the best means of sub-adult aging; they found that all methods were capable of producing sound age estimates.

Recent updates to the Demirjian method incorporated multiple regression analysis so that age can be predicted from the maturity score in a more statistically appropriate manner (Chaillet and Demirjian, 2004; Chaillet *et al.*, 2004a; Chaillet *et al.*, 2004b). New standards have been produced specifically for French, Finnish, and Belgian children, and they clearly demonstrate the benefits of population-specific formulae. When compared to age estimates using Demirjian's original standards, the overall accuracies of the polynomial regressions are similar, yet the likelihood of misclassification is dramatically improved (Chaillet, *et al*, 2004a).

Software designed to assist analysts making dental-based age estimates in children is currently being developed. Reichs and Demirjian (1998) describe "The Electronic Encyclopedia on Maxillo-Facial, Dental and Skeletal Development," which is a CD-ROM database comprised of radiographs taken of 263 children aged 0–6 and 79 children aged 6–17 years, all from Canada. Dental age estimates for each individual, however, are only available for children from the older age group (similar software is mentioned in Chaillet *et al.*, 2004a).

Because individuals with nearly complete third molars can be confused with people who have completed molar development, much effort has gone into the study of third molar formation and its efficacy in age estimation (e.g. De Salvia *et al.*, 2004; Dhanjal *et al.*, 2006; Mincer *et al.*, 1993; Solari and Abramovitch, 2002). Third molar age is calculated in the same manner as other teeth, by comparing the developmental stage of the tooth to standards of dental development, like Moorrees *et al.* (1963a, 1963b) and Demirjian *et al.* (1973). Although third molar development can be quite varied from individual to individual (Mincer *et al.*, 1993) third molar-based age estimates can be accurate to within three years (Solari and Abramovitch, 2002).

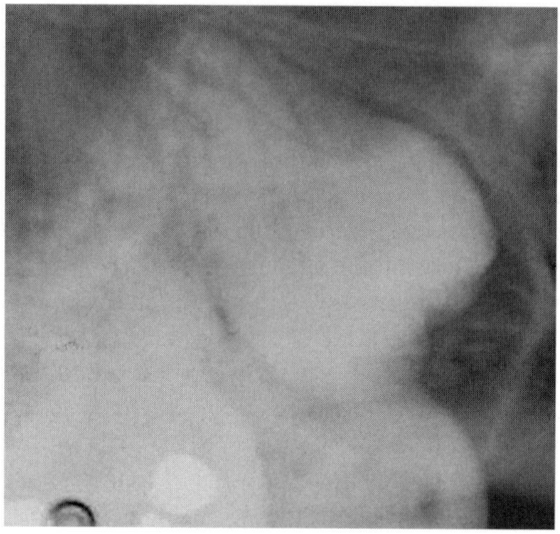

Figure 12.2 Radiograph of impacted third molar. Notice the incomplete formation of the root apex near the top of the image (photo courtesy of Matthew Williamson).

In a relevant case study, a colleague in the lab where I was working at in 1993 received the bones of an unidentified, recently deceased female. Another anthropologist had already studied the remains and estimated her age to be less than 18 years based on unerupted third molars. My colleague, however, took radiographs of the mandible and realized that these teeth were almost fully developed, with the root apices in the process of closing. The third molars had not erupted because they were impacted (Figure 12.2). His age estimate was 20–24 years, and the woman was soon positively identified (Williamson and Larsen, 1993).

Age: adults

Aging older individuals is far more difficult and many approaches have been developed to address this dilemma. Rösing and Kvaal (1998) note that teeth show signs of aging in at least 11 discernible ways, including: (1) the number of teeth, (2) their color and fluorescence, (3) attrition, (4) periodontal recession, (5) cementum apposition to the root, (6) root resorption, (7) secondary dentin in the pulp, (8) root translucency, (9) peritubular dentin, (10) racemization, and (11) cementum annulation (Rösing and Kvaal, 1998, p. 444). Space does not permit a detailed discussion of all these signs, but many are described below.

Teeth wear down as a normal result of mastication; therefore, older people tend to have more occlusal macrowear than younger people. For decades, bio-archaeologists used this phenomenon to provide relative ages of people within a particular population (e.g. Lev-Tov Chattah and Smith, 2006; Lovejoy, 1985; Schmidt, 1998; Smith, 1972; Walker *et al.*, 1991). For the most part, macrowear is scored using an ordinal scale based upon dentin exposure (e.g. Lovejoy, 1985; Molnar, 1971; Scott, 1979; Smith, 1984). In forensic contexts, macrowear is of value when trying to match dentitions in commingled assemblages, i.e. placing similarly worn teeth together. However, there is no universal standard that helps to accurately estimate a person's age because diets and extramasticatory tooth uses vary greatly from population to population.

More complex means of aging include the study of root transparency and cementum annulation. Root transparency, or sclerosis, is a result of dentinal tubules filling with translucent peritubular dentin crystals over a person's lifetime (Hillson, 1996). Older individuals have more translucent roots, a phenomenon that can be viewed macroscopically by placing a tooth in front of a light source; the sclerosity begins at the root apex and expands cervically with age (Hillson, 1996). Regression formulae are used to determine the approximate age for an individual based upon the relative amount of sclerotic root (Bang and Ramm, 1970; Harms, 2004; Lamendin *et al.*, 1992). Age estimates based upon root transparency have standard error ranges from ±9–14 years – values that are comparable to error ranges reported for ectocranial suture closure and auricular surface aging (Brooks and Suchey, 1990; Drusini, 1991; Drusini, *et al.*, 1989; Harms, 2004; Lamendin *et al.*, 1992; Lorentsen and Solheim, 1989; Nawrocki, 1998).

Study of tooth cementum annulations (TCA) requires thin sectioning of a tooth root and viewing it under a light microscope (for discussions on making dental thin sections see Charles *et al.* (1986) for TCA and Marks *et al.* (1996) for sectioning teeth in general). Age estimation is usually accomplished by viewing the root in cross section and adding the total number of cementum rings to the estimated age at which the tooth erupted (Charles *et al.*, 1986; Condon *et al.*, 1986; Wittwer-Backofen *et al.*, 2004). Wittwer-Backofen *et al.* (2004) conducted a blind study on a sample of 363 teeth designed specifically to assess the accuracy of TCA via the development of 95% confidence intervals. Their results suggest that TCA can predict age to within ±2.5 years. Pilloud (2004) compared the efficacy of TCA in a group of older adults (age 57–90 years) to a group of younger adults (age 21–45); the disparity between predicted and actual age was greater in the older group.

New efforts are being made to automate TCA and improve replicability. In their study, Czermak and colleagues (2006) describe software that uses Fourier analysis and algorithms as a means of image analysis. The program scans the image and counts gray-scale peaks within specific areas. The hope is that taking a more automated approach will reduce inter-observer error when counting annulations. The future of TCA seems promising, but there remains some concern regarding how certain variables, like health, sex, and extreme age, can affect cementum deposition (Olze *et al.*, 2004; Pilloud, 2004).

Age can be assessed by looking at a number of aging techniques simultaneously. Forensic dentists and dental anthropologists are familiar with Gustafson (1950) who developed a system that combines scores from six dental traits: tooth wear, expression of periodontosis, cementum apposition, root transparency, secondary dentin deposition, and root resorption at the apex. Johanson (1971) altered this method by making changes in the scoring system and using the new scores in a multiple-regression analysis. But, there have been criticisms of Johanson's method because its accuracy was determined using the original study sample (Maples and Rice, 1979). Burns and Maples (1976) and Maples (1978) further refined the Gustafson approach on a larger sample of teeth (357 from 267 individuals) and "improved the multiple regression analysis" (Bowers, 1995, p. 91). Periodic updates to the Gustafson method are important because it has been revealed that certain variables used by Gustafson, such as attrition, are relatively weak indicators of age and can be excluded from multivariate age estimates (Maples, 1978).

Sex

Sex is more difficult to determine than age from teeth, short of extracting DNA from the pulp cavity (e.g. Pillay and Kramer, 1997). While teeth are somewhat dimorphic, they are not extraordinary indicators of sex. Males tend to have larger teeth than females (e.g. Garn, *et al.*, 1979; Harris *et al*, 2001; Hill, 2003; Keiser, 1990; Lund and Mörnstad, 1999; Perzigian, 1976; Sciulli, 1979). Most comparisons of tooth size employ crown measurements, but some researchers have measured maximum cervical diameters to avoid problems with teeth that are heavily worn (e.g. Alt, *et al.*, 1998a; Goose, 1963; Hillson, 1996, 2005).

The means by which many dental anthropologists may sex teeth is through the use of discriminant functions that place individuals into a male or female category based upon crown measurements (e.g. DeVito and Saunders, 1990; Ditch and Rose, 1972; Owsley, 1982; and Scott and Parham, 1979). In general, the formulae developed by the aforementioned authors tend to produce sex estimates that are around 80% accurate when applied to the sample from which the functions were derived (Teschler-Nicola and Prossinger, 1998). Accuracy of estimates drop when teeth from other populations are used (Owsley and Webb, 1983). In addition, care needs to be taken to ensure that any given dentition is complete enough for discriminant analysis, and is devoid of pathological conditions that could affect overall tooth size (such as tooth fusions, megadontia, microdontia, etc.).

Schwartz and Dean (2005) describe an approach for sexing that accounts for the entire tooth, not just the crown. They have found statistically significant differences between male and female permanent first molars and canines by making gravitimetric comparisons; males have heavier teeth.

Harris *et al.* (2001) found that larger male tooth sizes are related to greater amounts of dentin and larger pulp cavities; the thickness of male and female enamel is generally similar. Garn *et al.* (1979) reported that canine root lengths were as good as or better than crown measurements in determining sex, although Alt *et al.* (1998a) found contradictory results. Alt and colleagues also report that neck diameters are more useful than crown diameters; in these cases the most dimorphic teeth are the first molar, maxillary first premolar, and canines. Yadav *et al.* (2002) was able to find sex-based differences in a modern population from India by comparing both canine and inter-canine arch measurements. Kondo *et al.* (2005) report that first and second molar cusp sizes are dimorphic, with the cusps of the M2 being more so.

Sex determination is often hampered by extreme taphonomic degradation (i.e. cremation). The best procedure for sexing fragmented and incomplete dentitions involves sorting the teeth by shape, color, and idiosyncratic traits into clusters that likely came from the same individual. From these clusters, lower and upper canines, which are most dimorphic, are used to determine sex (Alt *et al.*, 1998b; Lund and Mörnstad, 1999; Pettenati-Soubayroux *et al.*, 2002). If canines are not available, one can resort to less dimorphic teeth (i.e. first molar and upper first premolar).

In osteology, one can seriate elements and assume that the larger bones are from males. While this approach is tempting, and may be satisfactory in archaeological contexts where the question of identity is not an issue, it is not efficacious in forensic studies. Forensic dentitions need to be reconstructed as completely as possible – an endeavor that may or may not combine teeth of the same general size. For example, a collection of commingled teeth may produce two distinct dentitions – one with larger and one with smaller canines. However, the individual with small canines may have large incisors. If one makes a decision to cluster the large incisors with the large canines, a positive identification could be hampered as neither reconstructed set of teeth would represent an actual person. If reconstructed dentitions are complete, it is not necessary to rely on representative teeth. In such cases, the discriminant formulae mentioned above can be used.

For the most part in osteology, sex determination is reserved for adults, since children tend to be less dimorphic. However, researchers are reporting success with discriminating male and female children using dental metrics (Anderson, 2005; DeVito and Saunders, 1990; Kondo and Townsend, 2004;

Tsutsumi *et al.*, 1993). They are reporting successful sex determination rates approaching 80%.

As for DNA extraction, it is a promising area of forensic dental study, especially as DNA amplification methods improve and because teeth harbor DNA very well (Pillay and Kramer, 1997), even if a body has been exposed to high temperatures (e.g. Walker *et al.*, in press). The downside, of course, is the time and expense involved in the extraction and laboratory work. It is also modestly destructive and there is a risk of contamination from lab personnel. Despite these concerns, it is foreseeable in the not-too-distant future that tooth-derived DNA analysis will become a standard practice in dental anthropological study.

Ancestry

Over the years, understanding the relationship between ancestry and teeth has perhaps received the greatest amount of attention from dental anthropologists, and these studies are ongoing with great vigor (e.g. Edgar, 2005; Haeussler, 1998; Hanihara and Ishida, 2005; Harris and McKee, 1995; Harris and Rathbun, 1991; Hemphill *et al.*, 1998; Irish, 1997,1998, 2006; Lease and Sciulli, 2005; Lukacs, 1998; Lukacs and Hemphill, 1991; Lukacs *et al.*, 1998; Schnutenhaus and Rösing, 1998; Scott and Turner, 1997; Stamfelj *et al.*, 2006; Tasa and Lukacs, 2001; Ullinger, *et al.* 2005). In fact, the discipline known as dental anthropology today, in many ways, arose from early studies of population-based dental morphological variation (e.g. Dahlberg, 1949, 1963, 1971; Hrdlicka, 1920, 1921; see Alt *et al.*, 1998a for a detailed discussion of the history of dental anthropology). Studies of morphology focus on crown and root traits that occur in varying frequencies, depending upon the population. Morphological traits are thought of as quasi-continuous rather than truly discrete in nature, because quantitative differences in expression can be measured (e.g. Griffin, 1993). For example, Carabelli's trait ranges in expression from a small pit to a very large cusp. It is possible to measure the size of the cusp. However, the standard procedure is to use the Arizona State University coding system developed by Turner and colleagues, which places trait expression into an ordinal scale (Turner *et al.*, 1991).

Ancestral differences also are demonstrated metrically (e.g. Keiser, 1990; Sciulli, 1998). In general, people of African ancestry tend to have relatively large teeth (especially cheek teeth) while people of European ancestry tend to have small cheek teeth and more pronounced anterior teeth. People of Asian ancestry have metric values that are somewhat intermediate (Keiser, 1990).

One approach to determine dental ancestry starts with the help of Scott and Turner (1997). Their text, *The Anthropology of Modern Human Teeth*, provides a detailed description of non-metric traits used for study and a guideline for traits that are more or less likely to appear in various groups (e.g. European,

African, and Asian). Their approach is qualitative, but generally reliable if the analyst exercises proper caution. Simply assuming that, for example, shovel-shaped incisors indicate that a person is of Asian ancestry is hazardous. The key is to include many dental non-metric (and metric) traits in the analysis so that the determination of ancestry is broadly based.

Additional approaches to the question of ancestry are more quantitative; they compare metric and non-metric traits using multivariate statistics, such as logistic regression, to place dentitions into specific ancestral groups (e.g. Edgar, 2005; Lease and Sciulli, 2005). Edgar (2005) found eight dental characteristics that successfully classify 90% of a sample of 40 individuals as African American or European American. Likewise, discriminant functions have been developed to determine ancestry for particular groups; Matis and Zwemer (1971) were able to dentally distinguish American Indians and Eskimos.

Sub-adult teeth can also provide indications of ancestry. This is due to the fact that an individual's deciduous teeth express roughly the same morphological traits as do their adult teeth (Saunders and Mayhall, 1982). Several recent studies found statistically significant differences between sub-adults of different ancestral groups, often combining metric and non-metric data (e.g. Anderson, 2005; Harris and Lease, 2005; Harris *et al.*, 2001; Lease and Scuilli, 2005; Liu *et al.*, 2001). Such studies are helping the forensic dental anthropologist to garner more information regarding ancestry from fragmented dentitions than one is likely to ascertain from much of the rest of the sub-adult skeleton.

Dental idiosyncrasies

A final component of the biological profile concerns traits that are particular to the individual in question. Age, sex, and ancestry are general characteristics that help narrow the search when attempting a positive identification. However, it is a person's unique traits that get him or her identified (Reichs and Craig, 1998; Rogers, 1988; Wagner, 1997) (Figure 12.3). Idiosyncratic traits include inherited polymorphisms, as well as those acquired during life (Weedn, 1997). Inherited idiosyncrasies include unique crown and root forms, developmental and degenerative pathological conditions, and patterns of formation/eruption. Examples of acquired traits include dental traumata, unique patterns of wear due to pipe smoking or some other extramasticatory use of the teeth (Sopher, 1993), and cultural practices such as dental cosmetics, restorations, and prosthetics.

Of course, in the context of fragmented or commingled dentitions, the evidence for some of these cultural traits may be indirect. Fillings can melt in a fire, and it may be the etchings on the tooth rather than the filling itself that confirms the identity (e.g. Fairgrieve, 1994). Some metal (from bridges, dentures, or implants) may stain enamel, or leave behind evidence on other teeth in the form of diagnostic attachment points or calculus deposits.

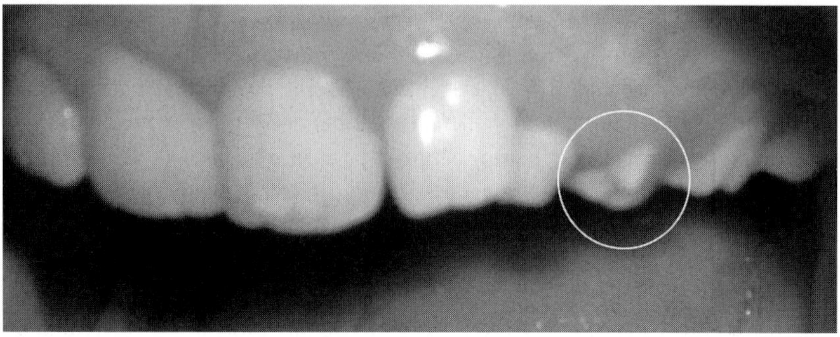

Figure 12.3 Idiosyncratic extra cusp on a deciduous maxillary molar.

Pathological conditions can leave behind idiosyncratic features. The most obvious are patterns of carious lesions. Frequent vomiting associated with bulimia nervosa can create marked enamel loss, particularly on the labial aspects of anterior teeth (Pindborg, 1970). Other conditions that can lead to similar enamel loss include "asthma, caffeine addiction, diabetes mellitus, exercise dehydration, functional depression, gastroesophageal reflux associated with alcoholism, hypertension and other conditions that lead to salivary hypofunction" (Young, 2005, p. 68). In fact, the expression of almost any pathological condition is going to be idiosyncratic; some common conditions that may help with identifying isolated teeth include malformations (i.e. severe hypoplasia or amelogenesis imperfecta), dens invaginatus, enamel pearls, taurodont teeth, tooth twinning/fusion, mega- or microdontism, calculus deposits, and antemortem fractures (Pindborg, 1970).

To illustrate, in the aforementioned forensic case, where several men were murdered and their bodies burned, some skeletal elements remained unburned. The latter included three mandibles: one with major dental restorations, one with a few restorations, and one with none at all. In all instances, the anterior teeth were largely absent since they were recovered from a creek bed where they had lain for approximately three years. The forensic dentist and I quickly realized that we could identify the individual with just a few restorations because radiographs provided by local law enforcement included a man with an identical pattern of dental work. The individual with no restorations had all of his teeth fully erupted and bore no significant pathological conditions. He did, however, have a subtle mesial rotation to his canines, and his third molars were mesially tilted. The radiographs we had included a panoramic image with the same canine and third molar orientations, as well as other anatomical points of concordance. Thus, the first victim was positively identified via his acquired traits (i.e. restorations) while the latter was identified solely with inherited idiosyncrasies.

12.4 Conclusion

Forensic dental anthropologists are especially valuable when the teeth to be studied have been dramatically altered from their original state. There is a synergism between the dental anthropologist's experience with archaeology and human variation and the forensic odontologist's expertise in dentistry. Proper study starts in the field and with the recovery of teeth and any associated cultural materials. The dentition(s) are reconstructed in the laboratory and an MNI is established. From the dentitions, biological profiles are generated and the teeth are made available for positive identification – usually by a forensic dentist. Given the challenges of a complex forensic scene, the forensic dental anthropologist is most able to hasten the recovery, reconstruction, and analysis of highly fragmented dentitions, leading to quicker positive identifications and assistance with the interpretations of the circumstances of death.

Acknowledgments

I want to thank Stephen Nawrocki, Gregory Reinhardt, and Matthew Williamson for their support of my desire to apply dental anthropology to forensic contexts. I thank Molly Hill for commenting on early drafts. I also thank the anonymous reviewer, Joel Irish, and Greg Nelson for their much-appreciated guidance on this chapter.

References

Alt, K. W., Brace, C. L., and Türp, J. C. (1998a). The history of dental anthropology. In *Dental Anthropology, Fundamentals, Limits, and Prospects*, ed. K. W. Alt, F. W. Rösing, and M. Teschler-Nicola. New York: Springer, pp. 15–40.

Alt, K. W., Riemensperger, B., Vach, W., and Krekeler, G. (1998b). Tooth root length and tooth neck diameter as indicators in sex determination of human teeth. *Anthropologischer Anzeiger*, **56**, 131–44.

Anderson, A. A. (2005). Dentition and occlusion development in African American children: mesiodistal crown diameters and tooth-size ratios of primary teeth. *Pediatric Dentistry*, **27**, 121–8.

Bang, G., and Ramm, E. (1970). Determination of age in humans from root dentin transparency. *Acta Odontologica Scandinavica*, **28**, 3–35.

Bass, W. H. (1995). *Human Osteology: A Laboratory and Field Manual of the Human Skeleton*, 4th edn. Columbia: Missouri Archaeological Society.

Bonnichsen, R. and Sorg, M. H. (1989). *Bone Modification*. Orono, ME: Center for the Study of the First Americans.

Bowers, C. M. (1995). Maples aging method review. In *Manual of Forensic Odontology*, 3rd edn., ed. C. M. Bowers and G. L. Bell. Saratoga Springs, NY: American Society of Forensic Odontology, pp. 91–2.
Bowers, C. M. (2004). *Forensic Dental Evidence*. Oxford: Elsevier.
Bowers, C. M. and Bell, G. L. (1995). *Manual of Forensic Odontology*, 3rd edn. Saratoga Springs, NY: American Society of Forensic Odontology.
Brooks, S. T., and Suchey, J. M. (1990). Skeletal age determination based on the Os Pubis: a comparison of the Acsádi-Nemeskéri and Suchey-Brooks methods. *Human Evolution*, **5**, 227–38.
Buikstra, J. E. and Swegle, M. (1989). Bone modification due to burning: Experimental evidence. In *Bone Modification*, ed. R. Bonnichsen and M. H. Sorg. Orono: Center for the Study of the First Americans, University of Maine, pp. 247–58.
Burns, K. R. and Maples, W. R. (1976). Estimation of age from individual adult teeth. *Journal of Forensic Sciences*, **21**, 343–56.
Butler V. L. and Schroeder, R. A. (1998). Do digestive processes leave diagnostic traces on fish bones? *Journal of Archaeological Science*, **25**, 957–71.
Catts, E. P. and Haskell, N. H. (1990). *Entomology and Death*. Clemson, S C: Joyce Print Shop.
Chaillet, N., and Demirjian, A. (2004). Dental maturity in South France: a comparison between Demirjian's method and polynomial functions. *Journal of Forensic Sciences*, **49**, 1059–66.
Chaillet, N., Nystrom, M., Kataja, M., and Demirjian, A. (2004a). Dental maturity curves in Finnish children: Demirjian's method revisited and polynomial function for age estimation. *Journal of Forensic Sciences*, **49**, 1–8.
Chaillet, N., Willems, G., and Demirjian, A. (2004b). Dental maturity in Belgian children using Demirjian's method and polynomial functions: New standard curves for forensic and clinical use. *Journal of Forensic Odontostomatology*, **22**, 18–27.
Charles, D. K., Condon, K., Cheverud, J. M., and Buikstra, J. E. (1986). Cementum annulation and age determination in *Homo sapiens* I. Tooth variability and observer error. *American Journal of Physical Anthropology*, **71**, 311–20.
Coles, B. and Coles J. (1989). *People of the Wetlands: Bogs, Bodies, and Lake Dwellers*. New York: Thames and Hudson.
Condon, K., Charkes, D. K., Cheverud, J. M., and Buikstra, J. E. (1986). Cementum annulation and age determination in *Homo sapiens* II. Estimates and accuracy. *American Journal of Physical Anthropology*, **71**, 321–30.
Czermak, A., Ernst, H., and Grupe, G. (2006). A new method for the automated age-at-death evaluation by tooth-cementum annulation (TCA). *Anthropologischer Anzeiger*, **64**, 25–40.
Dahlberg, A. A. (1949). The dentition of the American Indian. In *The Physical Anthropology of the American Indian*, ed. W. S. Laughlin. New York: The Viking Fund, Inc., pp. 138–74.
Dahlberg, A. A. (1963). Analysis of the American Indian dentition. In *Dental Anthropology*, ed. D. R. Brothwell. Oxford: Pergamon Press, pp. 147–77.
Dahlberg, A. A. (1971). *Dental Morphology and Evolution*. Chicago: University of Chicago Press.

Demirjian, A., Goldstein, H., and Tanner, J. M. (1973). A new system of dental age assessment. *Human Biology*, **45**, 211–27.
Demirjian, A., and Goldstein, H. (1976). New systems for dental maturity based on seven and four teeth. *Annals of Human Biology*, **3**, 411–21.
De Salvia, A., Calzetta, C., Orrico, M., and De Leo, D. (2004). Third mandibular development as an indicator of chronological age in a European population. *Forensic Science International*, **146**, S9–12.
DeVito, C. and Saunders S. R. (1990). A discriminant function analysis of deciduous teeth to determine sex. *Journal of Forensic Sciences*, **35**, 845–58.
Dhanjal, K. S., Bhardwaj, M. K., and Liversidge, H. M. (2006). Reproducibility of radiographic stage assessment of third molars. *Forensic Science International*, **159**, S74–7.
Ditch L. E., and Rose J. C. (1972). A multivariate dental sexing technique. *American Journal of Physical Anthropology*, **37**, 64–7.
Drusini, A. (1991). Age-related changes in root transparency of teeth in males and females. *American Journal of Human Biology*, **3**, 629–37.
Drusini, A., Businaro, F., and Volpe, A. (1989). Age determination from root dentin transparency of intact human teeth. *Cahiers d'Anthropologie et Biometrie Humaine*, **7**, 109–27.
Edgar, H. J. (2005). Prediction of race using characteristics of dental morphology. *Journal of Forensic Sciences*, **50**, 269–73.
Fairgrieve, S. I. (1994). SEM analysis of incinerated teeth as an aid to positive identification. *Journal of Forensic Sciences*, **39**, 557–65.
Farlow, J. O., Sunderman, J. A., Havens, J. J. *et al.* (2001). The Pipe Creek sinkhole biota, a diverse late Tertiary continental fossil assemblage from Grant County, Indiana. *American Midland Naturalist*, **145**, 367–78.
Garn, S. M., Cole, P. E., and van Alstine, W. L. (1979). Sex discriminatory effectiveness using combitions of root length and crown diameters. *American Journal of Physical Anthropology*, **50**, 115–18.
Glob, P. V. (1988). *The Bog People: Iron Age Man Preserved*. Ithaca, NY: Cornell University Press.
Goose, D. H. (1963). Dental measurements: an assessment of its value in anthropological studies. In *Dental Anthropology*, ed. D. R. Brothwell. London: Pergamon Press, pp. 125–48.
Griffin, M. C. 1993. *Morphological variation of the late precontact and contact period guale*. Ph.D. dissertation, Purdue University.
Grine, F. E. (2005). Enamel thickness of deciduous and permanent molars in modern *Homo sapiens*. *American Journal of Physical Anthropology*, **126**, 14–31.
Gustafson, G. (1950). Age determination at death. *Journal of the American Dental Association*, **41**, 45–54.
Haavikko, K. (1970). The formation and the alveolar and clinical eruption of the permanent teeth. An orthopantomographic study. *Proceedings of the Finnish Dental Society*, **66**, 103–70.
Haeussler, A. (1998). Origins and relationships of peoples buried in large Ukrainian Mesolithic era cemeteries: the evidence from dental morphology. In *Human Dental Development, Morphology, and Pathology, a Tribute to Albert A.*

Dahlberg, ed. J. R. Lukacs. Eugene: University of Oregon Anthropological papers, No. 54, pp. 79–118.
Haglund, W. D. (1997a). Rodents and human remains. In *Forensic Taphonomy*. ed. W. D. Haglund and M. H. Sorg. Boca Raton: CRC Press, pp. 405–14.
Haglund, W. D. (1997b). Dogs and coyotes: postmortem involvement with human remains. In *Forensic Taphonomy*, ed. W. D. Haglund and M. H. Sorg. Boca Raton: CRC Press, pp. 367–82.
Haglund, W. D. and Sorg. M. H. (1997). *Forensic Taphonomy*. Boca Raton: CRC Press.
Haglund, W. D. and Sorg. M. H. (2002). *Advances in Forensic Taphonomy*. Boca Raton: CRC Press.
Hall, D. W. (1997). Forensic Botany. In *Forensic Taphonomy*. ed. W. D. Haglund and M. H. Sorg. Boca Raton: CRC Press, pp. 353–66.
Hanihara, T. and Ishida, H. (2005). Metric variation of major human populations. *American Journal of Physical Anthropology*, **128**, 287–98.
Harms, J. (2004). *The determination of age-at-death through the examination of root transparency*. Unpublished M.S. Thesis, University of Indianapolis, Indianapolis, Indiana.
Harris, E. F. and Lease, L. R. (2005). Mesiodistal tooth crown dimensions of the primary dentition: a worldwide survey. *American Journal of Physical Anthropology*, **128**, 593–607.
Harris, E. F. and McKee, J. H. (1995). Tooth mineralization standards for blacks and whites from the midsouth United States. In *Manual of Forensic Odontology*, 3rd edn., ed. C. M. Bowers and G. L. Bell. American Society of Forensic Odontology, pp. 92–8.
Harris, E. F. and Rathbun, T. A. (1991). Ethnic differences in the apportionment of tooth sizes. In *Advances in Dental Anthropology*, ed. M. A. Kelley and C. S. Larsen. New York: Wiley-Liss, pp. 121–42.
Harris, E. F., Hicks, J. D., and Barcraft, B. D. (2001). Tissue contributions to sex and race: differences in tooth crown size of deciduous molars. *American Journal of Physical Anthropology*, **115**, 223–37.
Hemphill, B. E., Christensen, A. F., and Mustafakulov, S. I. (1998). Biological adaptations and affinities of Bronze Age Bactrians: II. dental morphology. In *Human Dental Development, Morphology, and Pathology, a Tribute to Albert A. Dahlberg*, ed. J. R. Lukacs. Eugene: University of Oregon Anthropological papers, No. 54, pp. 51–78.
Hill, M. K. (2003). *Dental reduction and diet in the prehistoric Ohio River Valley*. Unpublished M.S. Thesis. University of Indianapolis, Indianapolis, IN.
Hillson, S. W. (1986). *Teeth*. Cambridge: Cambridge University Press.
Hillson, S. W. (1996). *Dental Anthropology*. Cambridge: Cambridge University Press.
Hillson, S. W. (2005). Alternative dental measurements: proposals and relationships with other measurements. *American Journal of Physical Anthropology*, **126**, 413–26.
Hrdlicka, A. (1920). Shovel-shaped teeth. *American Journal of Physical Anthropology*, **3**, 429–65.
Hrdlicka, A. (1921). Further studies of tooth morphology. *American Journal of Physical Anthropology*, **4**, 141–76.

Irish. J. D. (1997). Characteristic high- and low-frequency dental traits in Sub Saharan African populations. *American Journal of Physical Anthropology*, **102**, 455–67.

Irish, J. D. (1998). Dental morphological indicators of population discontinuity and Egyptian gene flow in past-Paleolithic Nubia. In *Human Dental Development, Morphology, and Pathology, a Tribute to Albert A. Dahlberg*, ed. J. R. Lukacs. Eugene: University of Oregon Anthropological papers, No. 54, pp. 155–72.

Irish, J. D. (2006). Who were the ancient Egyptians? Dental affinities among Neolithic through Postdynastic Peoples. *American Journal of Physical Anthropology*, **129**, 529–43.

Johanson, G. (1971). Age determinations in human teeth. *Odontologisk Revy*, **22** (supplement 21), 1–126.

Jordan, R. E., and Abrams L. (1992). *Kraus' Dental Anatomy and Occlusion*, 2nd edn. St. Louis: Mosby.

Keiser, K. A. (1990). *Human Adult Odontometrics*. Cambridge: Cambridge University Press.

Kondo S., and Townsend G. C. (2004). Sexual dimorphism in crown units of mandibular deciduous and permanent molars in Australian Aborigines. *Homo*, **55**, 53–64.

Kondo, S., Townsend, G. C., and Yamada, H. (2005). Sexual dimorphism of cusp imensions in human maxillary molars. *American Journal of Physical Anthropology*, **128**, 870–7.

Lamendin, H., Caccino, E., and Humber, J. F. (1992). A simple technique for age estimation in adult corpses: the two criteria dental method. *Journal of Forensic Sciences*, **37**, 1373–9.

Lease, L., and Sciulli, P. W. (2005). Brief communication: discrimination between European-American and African American children based on deciduous dental metrics and morphology. *American Journal of Physical Anthropology*, **126**, 56–60.

Lev-Tov Chattah, N. and Smith, P. (2006). Variation in occlusal dental wear of two Chalcolithic populations in the southern Levant. *American Journal of Physical Anthropology*, **130**, 471–9.

Liu, H. H., Dung, S. Z., and Yang, Y. H. (2001). Crown diameters of the deciduous teeth of Taiwanese. *Kaohsiung Journal of Medical Sciences*, **16**, 299–307.

Liversidge, H. M., Herdeg, B., and Rösing, F. W. (1998). Dental age estimation of non-adults. A review of methods and principles. In *Dental Anthropology, Fundamentals, Limits, and Prospects*, ed. K. W. Alt, F. W. Rösing, and M. Teschler-Nicola. New York: Springer, pp. 419–42.

Lorentsen, M. and Solheim, T. (1989). Age assessement based on translucent dentine. *Journal of Forensic Odontostomatology*, **7**, 3–9.

Lovejoy, C. O. (1985). Dental wear in the Libben population: its functional pattern and role in the determination of adult skeletal age at death. *American Journal of Physical Anthropology*, **68**, 47–56.

Lukacs, J. R., ed. (1998). *Human Dental Development, Morphology, and Pathology, a Tribute to Albert A. Dahlberg*. Eugene: University of Oregon Anthropological papers, No. 54.

Lukacs, J. R. and Hemphill, B. E. (1991). The dental anthropology of prehistoric Baluchistan: a morphometric approach to the peopling of South Asia. In *Advances in Dental Anthropology*, ed. M. A. Kelley and C. S. Larsen. New York: Wiley-Liss, pp. 77–120.

Lukacs, J. R., Hemphill, B. E., and Walimbe, S. R. (1998). Are Mahars autochthones of Maharashtra?: dental morphology and population history in South Asia. In *Human Dental Development, Morphology, and Pathology, a Tribute to Albert A. Dahlberg*, ed. J. R. Lukacs. Eugene: University of Oregon Anthropological papers, No, 54, pp. 119–54.

Lund, H. and Mörnstad, H. (1999). Gender determination by odontometrics in a Swedish population. *Journal of Forensic Odontostomatology*, **17**, 30–4.

Maber, M., Liversidge, H. M., and Hector, M. P. (2006). Accuracy of age estimation of radiographic methods using developing teeth. *Forensic Science International*, **159**, 568–73.

Maples, W. R. (1978). An improved technique using dental histology for estimation of adult age. *Journal of Forensic Sciences*, **23**, 764–70.

Maples, W. R. and Rice, P. M. (1979). Some difficulties in the Gustafson dental age estimations. *Journal of Forensic Sciences*, **23**, 747–70.

Marks, M. K., Rose, J. C., and Davenport, W. D. Jr. (1996). Technical note: thin section procedure for enamel histology. *American Journal of Physical Anthropology*, **99**, 493–8.

Massler, M. and Schour, I. (1958). *Atlas of the Mouth in Health and Disease*. Chicago: American Dental Assocation.

Matis, J. A., and Zwemer, T. J. (1971). Odontognathic discrimination of United States Indian and Eskimo groups. *Journal of Dental Research*, **50**, 1245–8.

Mincer, H. H., Harris, E. F., and Berryman, H. E. (1993). The A.B.F.O. study of third molar development and its use as an estimator of chronological age. *Journal of Forensic Sciences*, **38**, 379–90.

Molnar, S. (1971). Human tooth wear, tooth function and cultural variability. *American Journal of Physical Anthropology*, **34**, 175–90.

Moorrees, C. F. A., Fanning, E. A., and Hunt, E. E. (1963a). Age variation of formation stages for ten permanent teeth. *Journal of Dental Research*, **42**, 1490–502.

Moorrees, C. F. A., Fanning, E. A., and Hunt, E. E. (1963b). Formation and resorption of three deciduous teeth in children. *American Journal of Physical Anthropology*, **21**, 205–13.

Morlang, W. M. II. (1997). Mass disaster management. In *Forensic Dentistry*, ed. P. G. Stimson and C. A. Mertz. New York: CRC Press, pp. 185–236.

Nawrocki, S. P., (1998). Regression formulae for estimating age at death from cranial suture closure. In *Forensic Osteology*, 2nd edn., ed. K. J. Reichs. Springfield, IL: CC Thomas, pp. 276–92.

Nawrocki, S. P., Schmidt, C. W. and Baumann, K. (1996). *Analysis of human teeth from a possible dental waste pit recovered in Indianapolis, Marion County, Indiana (12-Ma-776)*. Report submitted to the Indian Department of Natural Resources, Division of Historic Preservation and Archaeology, Indianapolis, IN.

Nawrocki, S. P., Pless, J. E., Hawley, D. E. and Wagner, S. A. (1997). Fluvial transport of human crania. In *Forensic Taphonomy*, ed. W. D. Haglund and M. H. Sorg. Boca Raton: CRC Press, pp. 529–52.

Nawrocki, S. P., Schmidt, C. W., Williamson, M. A., and Reinhardt, G. A. (1998). *Excavation and analysis of human remains from the Fox Hollow serial homicide site in Hamilton County, Indiana.* Paper presented at the Annual Meeting of the American Academy of Forensic Sciences, San Francisco, CA.

Olze, A., Geserick, G., and Schmeling, A. (2004). Age estimation of unidentified corpses by measurement of root translucency. *Journal of Forensic Odontostomatology*, **22**, 28–33.

Owsley, D. W. (1982). Dental discriminant sexing of Arikara skeletons. *Plains Anthropologist*, **27**, 165–9.

Owsley, D. W. and Webb, R. S. (1983). Misclassification probability of dental discrimination functions for sex determination. *Journal of Forensic Sciences*, **28**, 181–5.

Painter, T. J. (1995). Chemical and microbiological aspects of the preservation process in Sphagnum peat. In *Bog Bodies, New Discoveries and New Perspectives*, ed. R. C. Turner and R. G. Scaife. London: British Museum Press, pp. 88–99.

Perzigian, A. J. (1976). The dentition of the Indian Knoll skeletal population: odontometrics and cusp number. *American Journal of Physical Anthropology*, **44**, 113–22.

Pettenati-Soubayroux, I., Signoli, M., and Dotour, O. (2002). Sexual dimorphism in teeth: discriminatory effectiveness of permanent lower canine size observed in a XVIIIth century osteological series. *Forensic Science International*, **126**, 227–32.

Pillay, U. and Kramer B. (1997). A simple method for the determination of sex from the pulp of freshly extracted human teeth utilizing the polymerase chain reaction. *Journal of the Dental Association of South Africa*, **52**, 673–7.

Pilloud, S. (2004). Can there be age determination on the basis of the dental cementum also in older individuals as a significant context between histological and real age determination? *Anthropologischer Anzeiger*, **62**, 231–9.

Pindborg, J. J. (1970). *Pathology of the Dental Hard Tissues*. Copenhagen: Munksgaard.

Reichs, K. J. and Craig, E. (1998). Facial approximation: procedures and pitfalls. In *Forensic Osteology*, 2nd edn., ed. K. J. Reichs. Springfield, IL: CC Thomas, pp. 491–513.

Reichs, K. J. and Demirjian, A. (1998). A multimedia tool for the assessment of age in immature remains: the electronic encyclopedia for maxillo-facial, dental and skeletal development. In *Forensic Osteology*, 2nd edn., ed. K. J. Reichs. Springfield, IL: CC Thomas, pp. 253–75.

Rensberger, J. M. and Krentz, H. B. (1988). Microscopic effects of predator digestion on the surfaces of bones and teeth. *Scanning Microscopy*, **2**, 1541–51.

Rogers, S. L. (1988). *The Testimony of Teeth: Anthropologic and Forensic Aspects of Human Dentition*. Springfield, IL: C. C. Thomas.

Rösing, F. W. and Kvaal, S. I. (1998). Dental age in adults – a review of estimation methods. In *Dental Anthropology, Fundamentals, Limits, and Prospects*, ed. K. W. Alt, F. W. Rösing, and M. Teschler-Nicola. New York: Springer, pp. 443–68.

Saunders, S. and Mayhall, J. T. (1982). Developmental patterns of human dental morphological traits. *Archives of Oral Biology*, **27**, 45–9.

Saunders, S. R., DeVito, C., Herring, A., Southern, R. and Hoppa, R. (1993). Accuracy tests of tooth formation age estimations for human skeletal remains. *American Journal of Physical Anthropology*, **92**, 173–88.

Schmidt, C. W. 1998. *Dietary reconstruction in prehistoric humans from Indiana: an analysis of dental macrowear, dental pathology, and dental microwear*. Ph.D. dissertation, Purdue University.

Schmidt, C. W. (in press). The recovery and study of burned human teeth. In *The Analysis of Burned Human Remains*, ed. C. W. Schmidt and S. Symes. Oxford: Elsevier.

Schmidt, C. W., and Greene, T. R. (1998). *Excavation of Human Remains*. Report submitted to the Morgan County Coroner's Office and the Morgan County Sheriff's Department, Mooresville, IN.

Schmidt, C. W., Greene, T. R., and Megyesi, M. (1998). *Analysis of an Isolated Human Mandible Recovered on the Lake Michigan National Lakeshore*. Report submitted to the National Park Service, Indiana Dunes National Lakeshore, Porter, IN.

Schmidt, C. W., Schiel, M., Kiley, S., and Gore, T. (2006). *Excavation of human remains from Kokomo, Howard County, Indiana (UI-28–06)*. Report submitted to the Howard County Coroner's Office, Kokomo, IN.

Schmidt, C. W., Smith, M. O., Moore, C. R., Hill, M. K., and Rhodes, J. (in press). Late Archaic limb burials: trophies or mortuary ritual? In *War and Violence in the prehistoric Southeast*, ed. M. O. Smith. Tuscaloosa: University of Alabama Press.

Schnutenhaus, S. and Rösing, F. W. (1998). World variation in tooth size. In *Dental Anthropology, Fundamentals, Limits, and Prospects*, ed. K. W. Alt, F. W. Rösing, and M. Teschler-Nicola. New York: Springer, pp. 521–36.

Schwartz, G. T. and Dean, M. C. (2005). Sexual dimorphism in modern human permanent teeth. *American Journal of Physical Anthropology*, **128**, 312–17.

Sciulli, P. W. (1979). Size and morphology of the permanent dentition in prehistoric Ohio Valley Amerindians. *American Journal of Physical Anthropology*, **50**, 615–28.

Sciulli, P. W. (1998). Evolution of the dentition in prehistoric Ohio Valley Native Americans: II. Morphology of the deciduous dentition. *American Journal of Physical Anthropology*, **106**, 189–205.

Scott, E. C. (1979). Dental wear scoring technique. *American Journal of Physical Anthropology*, **51**, 213–18.

Scott, G. R., and Turner, C. G. (1997). *The Anthropology of Modern Human Teeth*. Cambridge: Cambridge University Press.

Scott, G. T., and Parham, K. R. (1979). Multivariate dental sexing: discrimination of the sexes within an East Tennessee Mississippian skeletal sample. *Tennessee Anthropologist*, **4**, 189–98.

Shipman, P., Foster, G., and Schoeninger, M. (1984). Burnt bones and teeth: an experimental study of color, morphology, crystal structure and shrinkage. *Journal of Archaeological Science*, **11**, 307–25.

Smith, B. H. (1984). Patterns of molar wear in hunter-gatherers and agriculturalists. *American Journal of Physical Anthropology*, **63**, 39–56.

Smith, B. H. (1991). Standards of human tooth formation and dental age assessment. In *Advances in Dental Anthropology*, ed. M. A. Kelley and C. S. Larsen. New York: Wiley-Liss, pp. 143–68.
Smith, P. 1972. Diet and attrition in the Natufians. *American Journal of Physical Anthropology*, 37, 233–8.
Solari, A. C., and Abramovitch, K. (2002). The accuracy and precision of third molar development as an indicator of chronological age in Hispanics. *Journal of Forensic Sciences*, **47**, 531–5.
Sopher, I. M. (1993). Forensic Odontology. In *Spitz and Fisher's Medicolegal Investigation of Death*, 3rd edn., ed. W. U. Spitz. Springfield, IL: C. C. Thomas, pp. 118–36.
Stamfelj, I., Stefancic, M., Gaspersic, D., and Cvetko, E. (2006). Carabelli's trait in the contemporary Slovenes and inhabitants of a medieval settlement (Sredisce by the Drava River). *Collegium Antropologicum*, **30**, 421–8.
Steele, D. G., and Bramblett, C. A. (1988). *The Anatomy and Biology of the Human Skeleton*. College Station: Texas A&M University Press.
Stimson, P. G. and Mertz, C. A. (1997). *Forensic Dentistry*. New York: CRC Press.
Tasa, G. L. and Lukacs, J. R. (2001). The prevalence and expression of primary double teeth in western India. *ASCD Journal of Dentistry for Children*, **68**, 196–200.
Taylor, R. M. S. (1978). *Variation in Morphology of Teeth: Anthropologic and Forensic Aspects*. Springfield, IL: C. C. Thomas.
Ten Cate, A. R. (1994). *Oral Histology, Development, Structure and Function*, 4th edn. St. Louis: Mosby.
Teschler-Nicola, M. and Prossinger, H. (1998). Sex determination using tooth dimensions. In *Dental Anthropology, Fundamentals, Limits, and Prospects*, ed. K. W. Alt, F. W. Rösing, and M. Teschler-Nicola. New York: Springer, pp. 521–36.
Tsutsumi, H., Matsui, N., Morita, Y. *et al.* (1993). Sex determination with a discriminant function analysis of deciduous teeth in plaster models. *Nippon Hoigaku Zasshi*, **47**, 466–80.
Turner, C. G., Nichol, C. R., and Scott, G. R. (1991). Scoring procedures for key morphological traits of the permanent dentition: the Arizona State University Dental Anthropology System. In *Advances in Dental Anthropology*, ed. M. A. Kelley and C. S. Larsen. New York: Wiley-Liss, pp. 13–32.
Ullinger, J. M., Sheridan, S. G., Hawkey, D. E., Turner II, C. G., and Cooley, R. (2005). Bioarchaeological analysis of cultural transition in the southern Levant using dental nonmetric traits. *American Journal of Physical Anthropology*, **128**, 466–76.
Wagner, G. N. (1997). Scientific methods of identification. In *Forensic Dentistry*, ed. P. G. Stimson and C. A. Mertz. New York: CRC Press, pp. 1–36.
Walker, P. L., Dean, G., Shapiro, P. (1991). Estimating age from tooth wear in archaeological populations. In *Advances in Dental Anthropology*, ed. M. A. Kelley and C. S. Larsen. New York: Wiley-Liss, pp. 169–78.
Walker, P. L., Miller, K. W. P., and Richman, R. (in press). Time, temperature and oxygen availability: an experimental study of the effects of environmental conditions on the color and organic content of cremated bone. In *The Analysis of Burned Human Remains*, ed. C. W. Schmidt and S. Symes. Oxford: Elsevier.
Webb, W. S. (1974). *Indian Knoll*. Knoxville: The University of Tennessee Press.

Weedn, V. W. (1997). DNA identification. In *Forensic Dentistry*, ed. P. G. Stimson and C. A. Mertz. New York: CRC Press, pp. 37–46.
White, T. D. (2000). *Human Osteology*, 2nd edn. New York: Academic Press.
Williamson, M. A., and Larsen, C. S. (1993). *Analysis of human skeletal remains recovered in Lake County, Indiana, Case Number A-40–93/ PUF/5*. Report submitted to the Lake County Coroner's Office, Crown Point, Indiana.
Wittwer-Backofen, U., Gampe, J., and Vaupel, J. W. (2004). Tooth cementum annulation for age estimation: results from a large known-age validation study. *American Journal of Physical Anthropology*, **123**, 119–29.
Yadav S., Nagabhushana, D., Rao, B. B., and Mamatha, G. P. (2002). Mandibular canine index in establishing sex identity. *Indian Journal of Dental Research*, **13**, 143–6.
Young, W. G. (2005). Tooth wear: diet analysis and advice. *International Dental Journal*, **55**, 68–72.

13 *Inter- and intra-specific variation in* Pan *tooth crown morphology: implications for Neandertal taxonomy*

SHARA E. BAILEY

13.1 Introduction

The taxonomic position of Neandertals plays a central role in the debate over modern human origins. In the past decade, the focus of this debate has shifted from strict interpretations of the two polarized sides (e.g. out of Africa vs. multiregional evolution) to interpretations that incorporate more (substantial) or less (trivial) gene flow between modern humans and their archaic predecessors. Nonetheless, paleoanthropologists from the two "camps" are still divided on whether or not Neandertals should be considered their own species, *Homo neanderthalensis*. Generally speaking, supporters of the replacement model (i.e. out of Africa) view Neandertals as a distinct species (Harvati, 2003; Rak, 1986; Schwartz and Tattersall, 1996; Stringer, 1996), whereas supporters of continuity models (i.e. multiregional evolution, assimilation, etc.) view Neandertals as a racial variant or sub-species of *Homo sapiens* (Frayer *et al.*, 1993; Smith *et al.*, 1989; Wolpoff *et al.*, 1994). Whether or not Neandertals and modern humans were distinct species (*Homo neanderthalensis* and *Homo sapiens*, respectively) has implications regarding the significance of gene flow and continuity between archaic and modern Europeans.

Recent genetic research has provided new insight into this problem. Studies of mitochondrial DNA (mtDNA) have shown that: (1) substantial differences distinguish Neandertal from contemporary human mtDNA (Krings *et al.*, 1997, 1999, 2000; Ovchinnikov *et al.*, 2000), (2) regional affiliation between Neandertal mtDNA and that of living Europeans is lacking (Krings *et al.*, 2000; Ovchinnikov *et al.*, 2000), and (3) Neandertal mtDNA cannot be found in modern humans (Serre *et al.*, 2004). Although this provides strong evidence for the distinct specific status of Neandertals, not all agree that it is the only explanation for the findings (Gutiérrez *et al.*, 2002; Hawkes and Wolpoff, 2001; Relethford, 2001).

Technique and Application in Dental Anthropology ed. Joel D. Irish and Greg C. Nelson
Published by Cambridge University Press.

With regard to the fossil evidence, cranial differences are among the most obvious features differentiating Neandertals and modern humans; cranial metrics and morphology have traditionally played important roles in the species question. The focus has been on whether or not Neandertals present uniquely derived features (autapomorphies) – which would suggest specific status, whether or not homologous features can be found in modern humans (especially early Upper Paleolithic modern humans) – which would suggest gene flow between Neandertals and Upper Paleolithic moderns, and whether or not Neandertal metric variation lies outside the variation of modern humans. One thing that complicates interpretations of cranial morphology is the influence of environmental factors. While moderately heritable (Sjøvold, 1984), cranial metric and non-metric variables are also under the influence of environmental factors (e.g. diet and tooth use – Lieberman *et al.*, 2004).

In this regard, teeth may be particularly useful. While environmental factors may have some effect on tooth size (Perzigian, 1977, 1984), discrete dental crown traits appear to be much less plastic than cranial metrics. Inasmuch as heritability estimates accurately reflect underlying genetic influence on traits, the heritability of dental crown traits appears to be high. Depending on the traits studied and the method used to score them, heritability ranges from 0.19 to 0.92, with an average of around 0.5 (0.456, 0.34 and 0.59 in three different studies (Mizoguchi, 1977; Scott and Potter, 1984; Scott and Turner, 1997)). Twin studies suggest that environmental factors may influence individual trait expression to some extent (Townsend and Martin, 1992), but the extent to which they affect population trait frequencies is unknown. Moreover, the standard scoring method for assessing dental morphology (Arizona State University Dental Anthropology System (ASUDAS) (Turner *et al.*, 1991)) utilizes traits that have been well established to be the most genetically and evolutionarily stable (Scott and Turner, 1997). Thus, when the appropriate traits are used, tooth crown morphology can be an excellent tool for assessing biological relationships among both contemporary and fossil humans.

Recent studies of Neandertals and modern human dentitions show that there are significant differences between these groups in both trait frequencies and trait expression. In a study of ancestral dental traits, Irish (1998) found a large divergence between Krapina Neandertals and certain contemporary human groups using the ASUDAS (see below). Using a larger set of tooth crown characters, Bailey (2002b, 2006) estimated measures of divergence between a larger sample of Neandertals and contemporary and fossil modern populations. Significant differences based on the mean measure of divergence (MMD) were obtained for Neandertal and modern human comparisons regardless of their geographic and/or temporal position. Based on post-canine dental morphology (Bailey, 2002b), Neandertals were found to be at least three times as different from contemporary modern humans as were the most different contemporary modern humans from one another. The marked divergence between Neandertals and both contemporary and Upper Paleolithic Europeans suggested to Bailey (2002b, 2006) that Neandertals did not contribute significantly to the modern human gene pool. However, until now, no attempt has been made to determine the taxonomic significance of these MMD values.

13.2 The present study

The goal of this study was to test whether the dental morphological differences between Neandertals and modern humans were typical of sub-specific or closely related specific taxa. Teeth preserve better than other parts of the body and for that reason make up a large portion of the fossil and archaeological records. While the exact genetic basis for dental traits has not yet been fully demonstrated, they remain one of the best ways in which to identify biological relationships among archaeologically derived human samples (Bailey *et al.*, 1998; Dahlberg, 1951, 1963, 1965; Haeussler, 1985, 1996; Haeussler and Turner, 1992; Hanihara, 1977; Hanihara *et al.*, 1975; Hanihara, 1989; Harris and Bailit, 1980; Hawkey, 1998; Irish, 1993, 1997; Irish and Turner, 1990; Lipschultz, 1997; Lukacs, 1983, 1986; Lukacs and Walimbe, 1984; Scott *et al.*, 1986; Sofaer *et al.*, 1986; Turner, 1969, 1983, 1987, 1990, 1993, 1995; Zubov, 1973). Moreover, reconstructions of population relationships based on dental morphological variation largely agree with those based on genetic variation (Cavalli-Sforza *et al.*, 1994; Sofaer *et al.*, 1986), which suggests that it is reflecting true genetic relationships among humans.

There is a general consensus that in order to interpret the meaning of the differences observed between Neandertals and modern humans, comparisons must be made with extant primate taxa (see Kimbel and Martin, 1993). Recently, researchers have begun to do this for craniofacial and basicranium form (Harvati, 2002, 2003; Schillaci and Froehlich, 2001). Their research, whether focused on phylogenetically appropriate (*Pan*, *Homo sapiens*) or ecologically appropriate (Papionins) models, showed that the variation between Neandertals and modern humans exceed both intra- and inter-specific variation observed in nearly all non-human primate taxa. And they concluded that Neandertals were not members of the species *Homo sapiens*, and did not contribute substantially to the evolution of modern humans.

Despite the fact that most genetic diversity occurs within rather than between human populations (Lewontin, 1972), certain phenotypic variation (e.g. skin color and dental morphology) shows distinct geographic patterning in contemporary modern humans (Relethford, 2002; Scott and Turner, 1997). It is

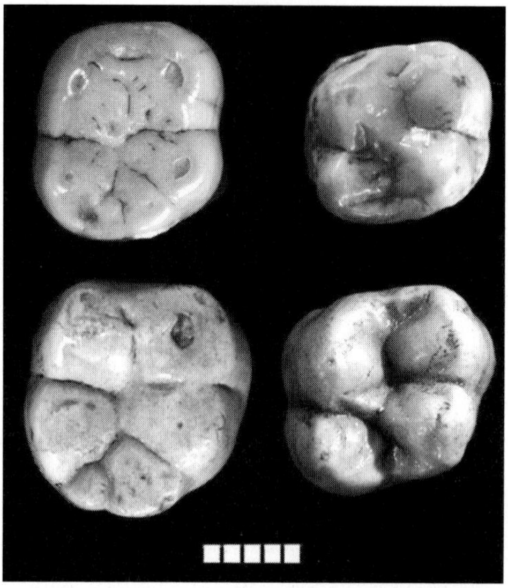

Figure 13.1 Morphological similarities between Pan and *Homo sapiens* molars. Upper row *Pan* lower first molar (left) and upper first molar (right). Lower row: *Homo sapiens* lower first molar (left) and upper first molar (right). Both lower molars present a supplementary *tuberculum sextum* (Cusp 6). Both upper molars show four cusps with moderate Carabelli's trait.

generally agreed that dental morphological variation is the result of genetic drift, although some degree of selection cannot be ruled out (Mizoguchi, 1985). By virtue of their marked intra-specific dental morphological differences, contemporary human groups make an appropriate model for comparing the morphological differences observed between Neandertals and modern humans, especially if more temporally appropriate (Upper and Middle Paleolithic/Middle Stone Age) modern human samples are included.

Pan, by virtue of it being a sister taxon to the genus *Homo*, and the only genus within the extant family Hominidae that is generally accepted to comprise more than one living species, provides an appropriate yardstick against which to assess variation. Pilbrow (2003) has shown that dental morphometric variables accurately reflect known species and sub-species differences in *Pan*. Conveniently, the human dentition is evolutionarily conservative (Scott and Turner, 1988), and in many respects crown morphology of *Pan* and *Homo* is similar (Figure 13.1). This suggests that one could apply a human-based system to scoring chimpanzee variation, at least as a baseline.

While it may also be informative to assess inter- and intra-specific dental variation in other non-human primates, specifically ecologically appropriate species such as Papionins, it is difficult to use human-based scoring methods on more distantly related non-human primates like monkeys. Although attempts have been made to establish new traits and devise scoring criteria for non-human higher primates (Hlusko, 2002; Pilbrow, 2003), to date few of these new traits have been standardized as they have for modern humans. In addition, it is not clear to what degree these traits can be found in humans, and whether or not they are homologous to those in humans and apes.

Assuming that *Pan* is an appropriate "yardstick" against which to judge the significance of the differences observed between modern humans and Neandertal dental morphology, it is predicted that if Neandertals represent a different species from modern humans, the morphological divergence between Neandertals and modern humans would be greater than the morphological divergence between the most different modern human populations. It would also be greater than that between the two chimpanzee sub-species, and would be equivalent to (or greater than) that between the two chimpanzee species. In addition, it is predicted that Neandertals would not show morphological similarities to the Upper Paleolithic European specimens, which may be expected under models involving extensive gene flow between the two. If instead Neandertals represent a sub-species of *Homo sapiens*, it is predicted that the morphological distance between Neanderthals and modern humans would be equivalent to that between any two modern human populations or between the two chimpanzee sub-species. Under this hypothesis, Neandertals may not show affinities to recent Europeans, but they would show similarities to the Upper Paleolithic European samples.

13.3 Materials

The samples included in the study are presented in Table 13.1. The *Homo* sample includes European and Asian Neandertals, Middle and Upper Paleolithic modern humans, and contemporary modern humans sampled from eight geographic regions. The *Pan* sample includes approximately equal numbers of male and female *P. troglodytes troglodytes, P.t. schweinfurthi*, and *P. paniscus*. The subspecies *P.t. verus* was not used in this study because its sub-specific status has been questioned (Morin *et al.*, 1994).

All data were collected directly from fossil and skeletal remains. The contemporary human data were collected at the American Museum of Natural History and the Natural History Museum, London. Fossil data were collected from a number of museums and institutions (see Acknowledgements). *Pan* data were gathered from skeletal collections at the Powell Cotton Museum, Birchington, Kent (*P.t. troglodytes, P.t. schwenfurthi*) and the Royal Museum of Central Africa, Turveren (*P. paniscus*).

Table 13.1 *Samples used in the present study*

Sample	Site/Region	No.[a]
Homo		
Neandertals	Krapina, Malarnaud, Ehringsdorf, Pontnewydd, Monsempron, Regourdou, Arcy-sur-Cure, St. Césaire, Devil's Tower, Ochoz, Kulna, Petit Puymoyen, Hortus, Taubauch, La Fate, Roc de Marsal, Ciota Ciara, Ciutarun, Grotte Taddeo, Grotte Poggio, Guattari, Saccopastore, Vindija, Spy, Le Moustier, La Quina, Montgaudier, Combe Grenal, Chateauneuf, Marillac, Le Ferrassie, Obi Rakhmat, Amud, Kebara, Shanidar, Tabun	40
Modern humans		
Middle Paleolithic/ Middle Stone Age	Qafzeh, Skhul, Die Kelders, Equus Cave, Klasies River Mouth, Hoedies Punt, Sea Harvest	12
Upper Paleolithic	Vachons, Pech de la Boissiere, Roc de Combe, Laugerie Basse, La Gravette, Dolní Vestonici, Pavlov, Abri Pataud, Abri Labatut, Abri Blanchard, Miesslingtal, Farincourt, Fontechevade, Arcy-sur-Cure, Oase, La Ferrassie, Mladeč, Grotte de Rois, Grotte de Abeilles, La Madeleine, St. Germaine la Rivière, Oberkassel, Isturitz, Solutre, La Chaud, Gough's Cave	28
Contemporary	North Africa, Southern Africa, West Africa, West Asia, Europe, India, Northeast Asia, Australasia	185
Pan		
P. troglodytes troglodytes		37
P. troglodytes schweinfurthi		44
P. paniscus		33

[a] Maximum number of individuals for a particular trait. Number of individuals for each trait varies.

For any particular trait, samples sizes varied (see Table 13.2). Trait sample sizes in the Upper Paleolithic group ranged from 4 to 28 individuals, while those in the Neandertal group ranged from 15 to 40, depending on the trait. The Middle Paleolithic modern human sample was considerably smaller, with samples for some traits including only two individuals.

13.4 Methods

13.4.1 Data collection

Although the ASUDAS is a commonly (and successfully) used standard for scoring dental variation on contemporary human teeth, Bailey (2002a, 2002b, 2006; Bailey and Lynch, 2005) has shown that there are several additional traits

Table 13.2 *List of traits used in the two analyses (see text), their breakpoints and their frequencies (and number of individuals) in the groups of interest*

Trait	NEAND	MPM	UPM	WAF	NAF	SAF	IND	EUR	NEAS	WAS	AUS	PTT	PTS	PP
Shoveling (UI1)[1HP,2HP]	95.8	33.3	50.0	33.3	66.7	81.8	27.3	6.3	66.7	0.0	0.0	37.5	21.7	33.3
+ = ASU 2–7	(25)	(6)	(12)	(3)	(9)	(11)	(11)	(16)	(9)	(5)	(8)	(24)	(23)	(18)
Labial convexity (UI1)[1HP,2HP]	100	50.0	18.8	0.0	22.2	16.7	46.7	11.8	12.5	20.0	0.0	62.5	68.8	72.7
+ = ASU 2–4	(24)	(8)	(16)	(4)	(9)	(12)	(15)	(17)	(8)	(5)	(8)	(32)	(32)	(22)
Double shoveling (UI1)[2H]	4.3	0.0	0.0	0.0	44.4	0.0	6.7	35.3	62.5	0.0	14.3	*	*	*
+ = ASU 2–5	(23)	(7)	(16)	(4)	(9)	(12)	(15)	(17)	(8)	(5)	(7)			
Tuberculum dentale (UI2)[1HP,2HP]	96.0	66.7	0.0	50.0	31.3	41.7	36.4	33.3	0.0	33.3	21.4	73.9	95.5	100.0
+ = ASU 2–7	(25)	(6)	(7)	(4)	(16)	(12)	(11)	(18)	(10)	(3)	(14)	(23)	(22)	(17)
Interruption groove (UI2)[2H]	42.9	14.3	12.5	50.0	0.0	0.0	21.1	38.5	0.0	33.3	0.0	*	*	*
+ = ASU +	(28)	(7)	(8)	(4)	(12)	(13)	(19)	(13)	(8)	(3)	(15)			
Canine mesial ridge (Bushman's canine) (UC)[2H]	42.9	0.0	14.3	0.0	0.0	75.0	0.0	0.0	0.0	25.0	0.0	*	*	*
+ = ASU 1–3	(21)	(5)	(7)	(7)	(13)	(12)	(12)	(16)	(9)	(4)	(11)			
Distal accessory ridge (UC)[2H]	46.7	50.0	100	71.4	00	30.0	25.0	30.0	42.9	25.0	75.0	*	*	*
+ = ASU 2–5	(15)	(2)	(4)	(7)	(8)	(10)	(4)	(10)	(7)	(4)	(4)			
Carabelli's cusp (UM1)[1HP,2HP]	68.0	33.3	40.0	63.2	69.2	57.1	46.2	59.1	43.8	50.0	35.1	71.4	81.4	62.5
+ = ASU 3–7	(25)	(6)	(20)	(19)	(26)	(21)	(13)	(44)	(16)	(4)	(37)	(35)	(43)	(24)
Cusp 5 (UM1)[1HP,2HP]	63.6	40.0	52.9	88.9	50.0	15.4	30.0	30.6	42.9	75.0	90.6	12.1	16.3	6.7
+ = ASU 1–5	(22)	(5)	(17)	(9)	(22)	(13)	(10)	(36)	(14)	(4)	(32)	(33)	(43)	(30)
Hypocone reduction (UM2)[1HP,2HP]	18.2	14.3	45.0	30.0	28.6	14.3	26.3	23.4	18.8	40.0	13.9	0.0	2.9	16.7
+ = ASU 0–3.5	(33)	(7)	(20)	(20)	(21)	(21)	(19)	(47)	(16)	(5)	(36)	(23)	(35)	(24)

(cont.)

Table 13.2 (*cont.*)

Trait	NEAND	MPM	UPM	WAF	NAF	SAF	IND	EUR	NEAS	WAS	AUS	PTT	PTS	PP
Metaconid placement (LP3)[1HP,2HP]	6.3	50.0	20.0	47.4	4.8	21.1	15.0	42.9	18.2	43.8	72.2	0.0	0.0	3.6
+ = mesial (Bailey, 2002b)	(32)	(4)	(15)	(19)	(21)	(19)	(20)	(35)	(11)	(16)	(18)	(27)	(28)	(28)
Metaconid placement (LP4)[1HP,2HP]	96.9	50.0	66.7	78.9	72.2	87.5	60.0	67.6	60.0	80.0	75.0	50.0	63.9	53.6
+ = mesial (Bailey, 2002b)	(32)	(6)	(12)	(19)	(18)	(16)	(20)	(34)	(10)	(15)	(16)	(30)	(36)	(28)
Distal accessory ridge	90.0	50.0	100	55.6	56.3	61.5	50.0	31.0	63.6	50.0	68.8	30.4	17.9	37.0
(LP3)[1HP,2HP]	(20)	(2)	(9)	(18)	(16)	(13)	(14)	(29)	(11)	(14)	(16)	(23)	(28)	(27)
+ = 1–3 (Bailey, 2002b)														
Mesial Accessory ridge (LP3)[2]	23.5	0.0	12.5	21.1	0.0	6.7	0.0	9.1	0.0	0.0	31.3	29.2	21.4	25.0
+ = 1–3 (Bailey, 2002b)	(17)	(2)	(8)	(19)	(17)	(15)	(17)	(33)	(11)	(13)	(16)	(24)	(28)	(28)
Lingual cusp number (LP4)[1,2]	93.5	66.7	38.5	63.2	58.8	37.5	20.0	55.9	50.0	40.0	87.5	16.7	13.9	75.0
+ = ASU 2–9	(31)	(6)	(13)	(19)	(17)	(16)	(20)	(34)	(10)	(15)	(16)	(30)	(36)	(28)
Metaconid individuation (LP4)[1HP]	42.3	80.0	61.5	89.5	87.5	75.0	90.0	100	80.0	66.7	64.7	10.0	36.1	100.0
+ = 2–3 (Bailey, 2002b)	(26)	(5)	(13)	(19)	(16)	(16)	(20)	(34)	(10)	(15)	(16)	(30)	(36)	(27)
Transverse Crest (LP4)[2H]	93.5	16.7	28.6	15.8	18.8	7.7	20.0	17.6	20.0	0.0	44.4	93.3	80.6	38.5
+ = 1–3 (Bailey, 2002b)	(31)	(6)	(14)	(19)	(16)	(13)	(20)	(34)	(10)	(15)	(18)	(30)	(36)	(26)
Cusp 6 (LM1)[1HP,2HP]	36.4	0.0	19.0	18.8	7.4	25.0	0.0	8.3	44.4	9.1	42.9	16.2	2.3	0.0
+ = ASU 1–5	(22)	(7)	(21)	(16)	(27)	(12)	(11)	(24)	(9)	(11)	(21)	(37)	(43)	(33)
Cusp 7 (LM1)[1HP,2HP]	16.7	41.7	3.6	61.1	10.0	36.8	5.6	3.3	9.1	8.3	6.9	0.0	0.0	9.1
+ = ASU 2–4	(36)	(12)	(28)	(18)	(30)	(19)	(18)	(30)	(11)	(12)	(29)	(37)	(44)	(33)
Mid-trigonid crest (LM1)[1HP,2HP]	93.5	20.0	0.0	0.0	0.0	16.7	0.0	0.0	0.0	14.3	0.0	8.3	18.2	28.1
+ = ASU 1–3	(31)	(5)	(23)	(18)	(22)	(18)	(14)	(21)	(10)	(7)	(26)	(36)	(44)	(32)
Deflecting wrinkle (LM1)[2H]	3.8	75.0	16.7	28.	33.3	16.7	50.0	8.3	14.3	20.0	7.7	*	*	*
+ = ASU 2–3	(26)	(4)	(18)	(7)	(9)	(12)	(4)	(12)	(7)	(5)	(13)			

Table 13.2 (*cont.*)

Trait	NEAND	MPM	UPM	WAF	NAF	SAF	IND	EUR	NEAS	WAS	AUS	PTT	PTS	PP
Anterior fovea (LM1)[1HP,2HP]	88.6	83.3	55.6	27.8	14.3	56.3	11.1	25.0	33.3	37.5	29.4	97.2	92.7	96.3
+ = ASU 2–3	(35)	(6)	(18)	(18)	(21)	(16)	(9)	(16)	(9)	(8)	(17)	(36)	(41)	(27)
Protostylid (LM1)[1HP,2HP]	0.0	10.0	3.6	0.0	0.0	5.0	0.0	0.0	00	0.0	3.3	5.6	11.6	12.5
+ = ASU 3–7	(40)	(10)	(28)	(18)	(30)	(20)	(19)	(19)	(10)	(12)	(30)	(36)	(43)	(32)
Cusp number (LM2)[2H]	0.0	10.0	35.0	17.6	54.5	18.2	100.0	81.3	33.3	72.2	20.7	*	*	*
+ = 4 cusps	(39)	(10)	(20)	(17)	(22)	(22)	(16)	(32)	(12)	(11)	(29)			
Cusp pattern (LM2)[2H]	75.0	100	44.0	31.8	13.6	40.9	40.0	28.1	7.7	9.1	25.8	*	*	*
+ = Y	(36)	(6)	(25)	(22)	(22)	(22)	(20)	(32)	(13)	(11)	(31)			
Cusp pattern (LM3)[1HP, 2P]	41.2	50.0	52.9	41.2	0.0	33.3	25.0	10.5	16.7	50.0	17.4	100	66.7	92.3
+ = Y	(17)	(6)	(17)	(17)	(10)	(15)	(16)	(19)	(12)	(8)	(23)	918)	(12)	(13)
Anterior fovea (UM2)[2P]	*	*	*	*	*	*	*	*	*	*	*	11.5	25.0	52.6
+ = any expression												(26)	(28)	(19)
Cusp 6 (UM2)[2P]	*	*	*	*	*	*	*	*	*	*	*	3.7	5.9	0.0
+ = any expression												(27)	(34)	(25)
Distobuccal cusp (LP4)[2P]	*	*	*	*	*	*	*	*	*	*	*	41.2	76.7	29.2
+ = any expression												(17)	(30)	(24)
Buccal cingulum (LP3)[2P]	*	*	*	*	*	*	*	*	*	*	*	34.6	46.4	22.2
+ = any expression												(26)	(28)	(27)
Posterior fovea (LM1)[2P]	*	*	*	*	*	*	*	*	*	*	*	84.4	100	89.3
+ = any expression												(32)	(40)	(28)

[1] traits used in the first analysis
[2] traits used in the second analysis
[H] = *Homo* analysis, [P] = *Pan* analysis
* trait not present or invariable in this group

of interest in fossil hominin teeth that are not included in the system, but which may have phylogenetic value (e.g. P_4 asymmetry, P_4 transverse crest, M_1 cusp placement). In addition, a recent study of *Pan* and Pliocene hominin teeth, indicated that even an extended system (such as that used on Neandertals) does not account for the variation observed in chimpanzees and Pliocene hominins (Bailey and Wood, in press). Although up to 135 dental traits were collected on each individual, most could not be used in this analysis for reasons outlined below.

The analysis was undertaken in two steps. For both, the trait had to show at least 5% difference between at least one pair in a comparative sample to be included. In addition, because of the potential for inter-trait correlation to confound results (Scott and Turner, 1997), traits included in this study were not duplicated on different teeth (e.g., Carabelli's cusp was used on M_1 only) unless trait independence was relatively certain (e.g. lingual cusp number in P_3 and P_4 in *Pan*, second analysis).

In order to compare divergence values directly (Analysis 1) it was important that each group be represented by the same traits. The decision to include a trait in the first analysis was dictated by the requirement that they: (1) could be scored in both the *Pan* and the *Homo* samples, and (2) were variable among groups (see above). In the first analysis the trait list was weighted more heavily toward those that are important in discriminating among contemporary human groups; it did not include several traits that may be important in discriminating among *Pan* groups, as they were not present or were invariable in the humans. A possible consequence of this bias is that divergence values among *Pan* species/sub-species may be lower, making *Pan* species/sub-species appear more similar to each other than they would if the analysis was based on traits particular to *Pan*. In the end, 17 traits were used in the first analysis. Description of the traits and their presence/absence breakpoints can be found in Table 13.2. Thirteen traits were scored according to standards outlined by the ASUDAS (Turner *et al.*, 1991); the remaining four (P_3 and P_4 metaconid placement, P_3 distal accessory ridge, P_4 metaconid individuation), were based on standards outlined by Bailey (2002b) and Suwa (1990).

Because it was of interest to investigate whether trait choice (e.g. the abbreviated trait list necessary for direct comparison of divergence between *Pan* and *Homo*) affected divergence estimates, a second analysis was undertaken. This analysis utilized different trait sets for *Pan* and for *Homo* (Table 13.2). For *Homo*, nearly all standard ASUDAS traits were used in addition to non-ASUDAS traits identified as useful in discriminating among fossil and recent humans by Bailey (2002b). For *Pan*, many of the same traits were used – the exceptions being those that were absent (e.g. double shoveling) or invariable (e.g. P_4 transverse crest). Additional traits observed to be variable among *Pan* species/sub-species were added to this list (e.g. M_2 anterior fovea). Although direct comparison of divergence values could not be made in this analysis, it is relevant to examine the relative distances between species and sub-species of *Pan*, and compare that to what is observed between Neandertals and modern humans.

13.4.2 Analysis

The MMD statistic was used to assess dental phenetic similarity through estimation of the dental divergence among groups. This multivariate statistic utilizes multiple traits to provide a relative dissimilarity among groups. The resulting divergence values are particular to the traits used, and adding or excluding traits in the analysis may affect the results (e.g. 26- vs. 12-trait study in Bailey, 2002b). While sample sizes for most groups in this analysis are "respectable," there are certain traits for which sample sizes are quite low. One of the risks in using small samples involves the chance that an MMD value will be zero or negative because the correction factor is larger than the MMD (see Harris, 2004 for a review); the smaller the sample size, the larger the correction factor. In addition, although the MMD program utilizes the Freeman and Tukey angular transformation to correct for small samples (Berry and Berry, 1967; Green and Suchey, 1976; Sjøvold, 1973), sample sizes for some traits in the Middle Paleolithic group are likely too small even for this correction. Therefore, the statistical significance of the pair-wise differences between the Middle Paleolithic moderns and other groups should be interpreted cautiously.

Clustering analyses using Ward's (1963) method was used to visualize the phenetic distances among samples. Ward's clustering algorithm is generally preferred by dental anthropologists because it has been shown that the clusters produced conform to known population relationships based on other (e.g. genetic) data. This method bases cluster membership on the total sum of squared deviations from the mean of the cluster. It joins the two clusters that will result in the smallest increase in the pooled within-cluster variation.

13.5 Results

The results of the two MMD analyses are presented in Tables 13.3 and 13.4. These findings are summarized below.

Table 13.3 *Mean measure of divergence values (with standard deviations) for Analysis 1 (see text)*

	NEAND	MPM	UPM	WAF	NAF	SAF	IND	EUR	NEAS	WAS	AUS
NEAND		0.565	1.100 [a]	1.046	1.015	0.647	1.195	1.496	1.080	0.959	1.487
		0 (0.07)[a]	(0.04)[a]	(0.05)[a]	(0.03)[a]	(0.04)[a]	(0.04)[a]	(0.03)[a]	(0.04)[a]	(0.06)[a]	(0.03)[a]
MPM			0.237	0.074	0.250	0.013	0.101	0.195	0.197	−0.012	0.328
			0 (0.08)[a]	(0.09) NS	(0.08)[a]	(0.08) NS	(0.08) NS	(0.07)[a]	(0.09)[a]	(1.05) NS	(0.08)[a]
UPM				0.239	0.224	0.178	0.188	0.367	0.001	0.051	0.318
				0 (0.06)[a]	(0.04)[a]	(0.05)[a]	(0.05)[a]	(0.04)[a]	(0.05) NS	(0.07) NS	(0.04)[a]
WAFRICA					0.151	0.162	0.206	0.173	0.140	−0.0645	0.128
					0 (0.06)[a]	(0.06)[a]	(0.06)[a]	(0.05)[a]	(0.07)[a]	(0.09) NS	(0.06)[a]
NAFRICA						0.142	0.027	0.119	0.018	0.112	0.383
						0 (0.04)[a]	(0.04) NS	(0.04)[a]	(0.05) NS	(0.07) NS	(0.04)[a]
SAFRICA							0.166	0.298	0.054	0.073	0.503
							0 (0.05)[a]	(0.04)[a]	(0.06) NS	(0.07) NS	(0.04)[a]
INDIA								0.044	0.094	0.040	0.421
								0 (0.04) NS	(0.06) NS	(0.07) NS	(0.04)[a]
EUROPE									0.158	0.061	0.234
									0 (0.05)[a]	(0.06) NS	(0.04)[a]
NEASIA										0.037	0.221
										0 (0.08) NS	(0.05)[a]
WASIA											0.069
											0 (0.062) NS
AUSTR											0

NEAND: Neandertal, MPM: Middle Paleolithic/Middle Stone Age modern, UPM: Upper Paleolithic modern, WAF: West Africa, NAF: North Africa, SAF: Southern Africa, IND: India, EUR: Europe, NEAS: Northeast Asia, WAS: West Asia, AUS: Australasia.

	PTT	PTS	PP
PTT	0	0.148 (0.02)[a]	0.463 (0.03)[a]
PTS		0	0.302 (0.03)[a]
PP			0

PTT: *Pan troglodytes troglodytes*, PTS: *Pan troglodytes schweinfurthi*, PP: *Pan paniscus*

[a] Significant at $p < 0.05$

Table 13.4 *Mean measure of divergence values (with standard deviations) for Analysis 2 (see text)*

	NEAND	EMHS	UPMOD	WAF	NAF	SAF	IND	EUR	NEA	WAS	AUS
Neandertal		0.608	0.959	0.905	1.134	0.688	1.345	1.343	1.131	1.100	1.247
		0 (0.07)[a]	(0.04)[a]	(0.05)[a]	(0.03)[a]	(0.03)[a]	(0.04)[a]	(0.03)[a]	(0.04)[a]	(0.06)[a]	(0.03)[a]
EMHS			0.274	0.180	0.374	0.183	0.258	0.320	0.374	0.208	0.374
			0 (0.08)[a]	(0.06)[a]	(0.08)[a]	(0.08)[a]	(0.08)[a]	(0.07)[a]	(0.08)[a]	(0.10)[a]	(0.08)[a]
UPMOD				0.160	0.393	0.264	0.312	0.352	0.144	0.183	0.226
				0 (0.06)[a]	(0.04)[a]	(0.05)[a]	(0.05)[a]	(0.04)[a]	(0.05)[a]	(0.07)[a]	(.05)[a]
WAFRICA					0.271	0.275	0.310	0.174	0.219	0.005	0.110
					0 (0.06)[a]	(0.05)[a]	(0.06)[a]	(0.05)[a]	(0.06)[a]	(0.08) NS	(0.06) NS
NAFRICA						0.290	0.101	0.142	0.011	0.106	0.414
						0 (0.04)[a]	(0.05)[a]	(0.03)[a]	(0.05) NS	(0.06) NS	(0.04)[a]
SAFRICA							0.407	0.433	0.264	0.135	0.520
							0 (0.05)[a]	(0.03)[a]	(0.05)[a]	(0.06)[a]	(0.04)[a]
INDIA								0.05	0.231	0.045	0.522
								0 (0.04) NS	(0.05)[a]	(0.07) NS	(0.05)[a]
EUROPE									0.145	0-0.0007	0.244
									0 (0.04)[a]	(0.05) NS	(0.04)[a]
NEASIA										0.119	0.199
										0 (0.07) NS	(0.05)[a]
WASIA											0.216
											0 (0.07)[a]
AUSTR											0

NEAND: Neandertal, EMHS: Early Modern *Homo sapiens*, UPMOD: Upper Paleolithic modern, WAF: West Africa, NAF: North Africa, SAF: Southern Africa, IND: India, EUR: Europe, NEAS: Northeast Asia, WAS: West Asia, AUS: Australasia.

	PTT	PTS	PP
PTT	0	0.095 (0.02)[a]	0.218 (0.02)[a]
PTS		0	0.189 (0.02)[a]
PP			0

PTT: *Pan troglodytes troglodytes*, PTS: *Pan troglodytes schweinfurthi*, PP: *Pan paniscus*

[a] Significant at $p < 0.05$

13.5.1 Analysis 1

This analysis allows for direct comparison of MMD values. All pair-wise comparisons between Neandertals and modern humans are high and significant. Thus, the dental pattern of Neandertals is quite different from all modern humans, regardless of temporal or geographical space. Neandertals are least divergent from Middle Paleolithic moderns and most divergent from contemporary Europeans. The high MMD value between Neandertals and Upper Paleolithic modern humans (which is higher than five Neandertal/contemporary human comparisons) suggests no particularly close phenetic relationship between these groups.

Among the fossil modern humans, Middle Paleolithic moderns show the least divergence from West Asia and the most divergence from Australasia. They are surprisingly distant from the Upper Paleolithic group, considering the close relationship found previously based on post-canine data (Bailey, 2002b). Upper Paleolithic moderns show the smallest divergence from Northeast Asia and the largest divergence from contemporary Europeans. Among the modern human pair-wise comparisons, the West Asian group shows the least divergence from all modern human groups (fossil and contemporary) with an average MMD value of 0.049.

The MMD value between *Pan* subspecies (*P.t. schweinfurthi* and *P.t. troglodytes*) is 0.148. This value is comparable to that observed between modern human populations from North and West Africa. The MMD value between *Pan troglodytes* subspecies and *Pan paniscus* is 0.463 (*P.t. troglodytes*) and 0.302 (*P.t. schweinfurthi*). Compared to *Pan*, Neandertals are between 3.8 and 10 times more divergent from fossil and recent modern humans than the two sub-species of *Pan* are from each other. They are also between 1.2 and 3.3 times more divergent from recent and fossil modern humans than species of *Pan* are from each other. However, six of the 45 pair-wise comparisons among modern humans also resulted in MMD values that are higher than that between the two *Pan* species.

13.5.2 Analysis 2

In order to determine the effect of trait choice, the second analysis involved tailoring the trait lists specifically to *Homo* and *Pan*. Because different traits were used, the MMD values cannot be compared directly as they were in Analysis 1. However, the relative distance between Neandertals and modern humans can be compared to that between *Pan* species and sub-species. In the second analysis the *Pan* species are approximately twice as dentally divergent as are the two *Pan* sub-species. The relative divergence between *P. paniscus* and *P.t. troglodytes* is slightly higher (2.3 times that of sub-species) than that between *P. paniscus* and *P.t. schweinfurthi* (2.0 times that of sub-species). In contrast, the average pair-wise distance among Neandertals and modern humans is 1.046, but the average pair-wise distances among modern humans, fossils included, is 0.211. Therefore, the average pair-wise distance between Neandertals and modern human groups is nearly five times (4.96) the distance observed among the modern human groups.

However, it should be noted that distances among modern humans vary widely, and range from 0.0 (West Asia–Europe) to 0.522 (India–Australia). When distances between Neandertals and modern humans are compared on a pair-by-pair basis, Neandertals are between 1.2 and 2.6 times more divergent from modern humans than the *most divergent* modern human groups are from each other.

13.5.3 Comparing analysis 1 and analysis 2

The choice of traits appears to have a larger effect on the modern/modern than it does on the Neandertal/modern analyses (compare dendrograms for the two analyses in Figure 13.2). The average distance between Neandertals and modern humans does not change much in the two analyses; it is slightly less in the second analysis than in the first (1.046 vs. 1.059). The average distance among modern humans, however, changes more dramatically; the average distance is lower in the first than in the second analysis (0.145 vs. 0.211). This is not unexpected, since many important traits had to be eliminated from the first analysis to make comparisons with *Pan* (e.g. double shoveling). Regardless of which analysis is used, the Neandertal group remains a clear outlier in both instances.

As for *Pan*, in the first analysis the average difference between species is greater than in the second analysis (2.58 vs. 2.15 times the difference between sub-species). This is somewhat surprising, since the second analysis included traits specific to *Pan*, and were thought to separate the species/sub-species better. Nonetheless, the overall pattern of divergence between *Pan* species/sub-species holds. Of the sub-species of *P. troglodytes*, *P.t. troglodytes* is slightly more divergent from *P. paniscus* than is *P.t. schweinfurthi*.

13.6 Conclusions and discussion

The specific status of Neandertals has long been debated in anthropology. In this regard, the results of the present investigation are somewhat mixed. On

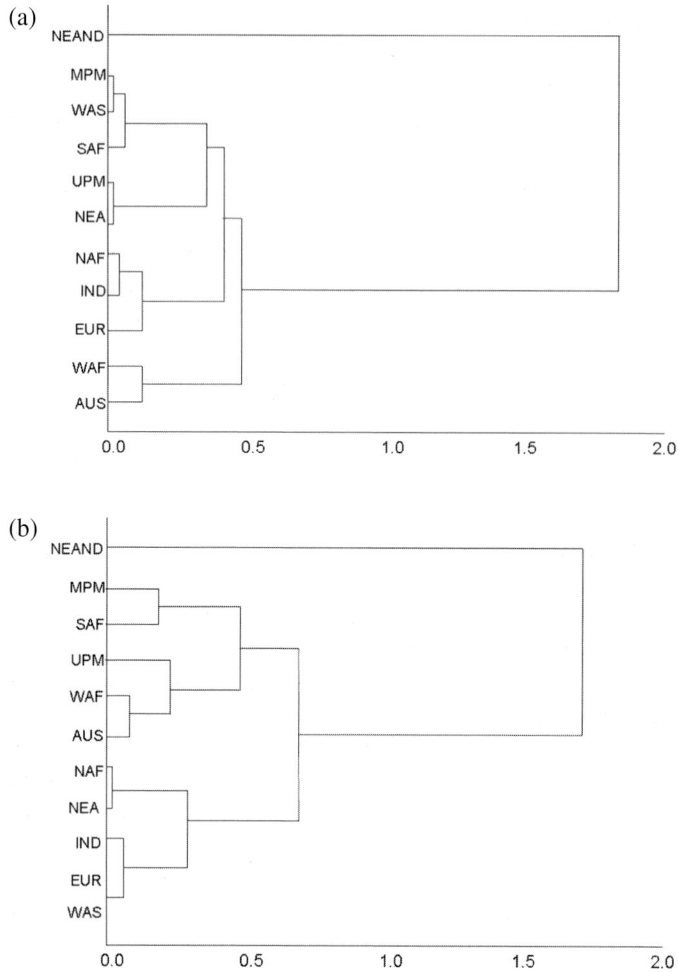

Figure 13.2 Dendrograms of MMD values using Ward's method (a) based on 17 traits; (b) based on 22 traits. The position of the modern human groups changes based on which trait list is used, however the position of Neandertals as an outlier remains the same.

the one hand, dental morphology of Neandertals is more divergent from that of modern humans than it is between the two species of *Pan*. In addition the average Neandertal/modern human MMD value is nearly five times larger than the average MMD among modern humans, and 1.2 times that of the most divergent modern humans. Finally, where MMD values could be compared directly, the smallest Neandertal/modern human comparison (Southern Africa = 0.647) exceeded the average inter-specific MMD value between *Pan troglodytes* and *Pan paniscus* (0.258) by more than 2.5 times. Thus, based on the predictions outlined in the introduction, there appears to be some support for distinguishing Neandertals as a distinct species from *Homo sapiens* based on their dental morphology.

On the other hand, an examination of the divergence values among modern human groups shows that many MMDs between modern human groups are equal to, or greater than, that between two sub-species of *Pan*. Moreover, there are six pair-wise comparisons resulting in MMD values that exceed that *between* species of *Pan*. (e.g. Australia and contemporary Southern Africa, India, and Europe).

Interestingly, similar results were found by Harvati (2003) based on craniometric data. Like here, the average Neandertal/modern human distance (D^2) exceeded the average inter-specific distance between non-human primates. However, in one case (Australia/Andaman Islander comparison) the D^2 value of 36.03 substantially exceeded the average between *Pan* species ($D^2 = 25.29$).

Harvati (2003) concluded that the high level of divergence in modern humans may indicate that humans follow a different pattern of variation than chimpanzees. This may not be surprising given the wide geographic distribution of modern humans. In this regard, it may be worth noting that the largest differences in contemporary modern humans are found between agricultural and non-agricultural groups and between those with the largest and smallest teeth (e.g. Australia/West Africa and other groups). Although dental morphological differences among contemporary humans is usually considered to be largely the result of genetic drift (e.g. Scott and Turner, 1997), this finding may suggest that natural selection is acting on dental morphology more than previously assumed. Future researchers may want to reconsider examining correlations between trait patterns and environmental, cultural, and/or climatic factors.

The specific status of Neandertals is relevant to the question of whether or not (and if so how much) they and early modern humans inter-bred. Given some early studies on "hybridization" in contemporary humans (Baume and Crawford, 1978; Hanihara, 1963) one would predict that if there was significant inter-breeding between Neandertals and Upper Paleolithic modern humans, it would be observable in the latter's dental trait frequencies. However, whether or not the dental data support the specific status of Neandertals, there is very little indication in this dataset for substantial contribution of Neandertal dental genes to the modern human gene pool. This supports earlier suggestions based on dental morphology that inter-breeding between Neandertals and modern humans was trivial at best (Bailey, 2002b, 2006).

The choice of characters certainly has an effect on MMD values, and direct comparisons between *Pan* and *Homo* species will always be difficult because some variation in one group is missing or invariable in the other. It is certain that comparisons with other non-human primates will suffer from the same problem. However, the comparisons among human groups are still quite compelling. That the intra-modern human comparisons are fairly accurate is suggested by the fact that the average contemporary human MMD value obtained here (0.141) is only slightly less than the value of 0.177 obtained by Turner (1992), which was based on a much larger sampling of world populations.

Beyond the question of the specific status of Neandertals, there are some interesting patterns in the modern human data that are worthy of mention. The similarity between Upper Paleolithic moderns and Northeast Asia is curious, given that other research found Asian-derived populations (e.g. Sinodonts) to be among the most divergent of modern human groups (Irish, 1998; Turner, 1992). This may be a sampling artifact, but it may also be worthy of further study with a larger sample size of Northeast Asian groups. The distance between Upper Paleolithic moderns and Middle Paleolithic/Middle Stone Age moderns is larger in this analysis than in a previous one (Bailey, 2002b). This is most likely attributable to differences in the traits used (i.e. post-canines only in the earlier study) and the expansion of this study to include African Middle Stone Age individuals. Still, the number of individuals for certain traits is quite small ($n = 2$) and the results should not be over interpreted.

That the Middle Paleolithic/Middle Stone Age sample shows the greatest biological affinities to West Asia and to Southern Africa may be of interest since it is composed of Southern African and West Asian samples. Thus, small sample size considered, this may indicate continuity in this area, which is in marked contrast to the discontinuity observed in Europe between Neandertals and Upper Paleolithic Europeans and between Upper Paleolithic Europeans and contemporary Europeans.

Finally, the relatively low distances between the West Asians and all other groups may be of interest and worthy of additional study. The mean MMD for West Asia (0.102, second analysis) was only slightly higher than that found by Turner (1992) for early Southeast Asia (mean MMD = 0.098). Of course, samples here were smaller than those used by Turner (1992) and the trait set differed somewhat. Nonetheless, it may be of interest to expand the samples from this area to help clarify West Asia's phenetic relationships with the rest of the world.

13.7 Summary

This study attempted to interpret the large divergence values obtained from dental non-metric data between Neandertals and modern humans in terms of sub-specific/specific variation. The analysis of dental morphological variation in Neandertals, modern humans, and *Pan* species/sub-species supports all the predictions for Neandertals to be considered a distinct species from modern humans. First, the smallest Neandertal/modern human divergence value (Neandertal/Middle Paleolithic modern) is greater than the largest divergence value among all modern human groups (Australasia/India). Second, this distance it is not only greater than that found between the two subspecies of *Pan*, but also greater than that of the two *Pan* species. Finally, there is no indication of any special dental morphological relationship between Neandertals and Upper Paleolithic Europeans as may be predicted if there were significant gene flow between the two groups. In fact, the divergence between these two groups is greater than five of the eight Neandertal/contemporary human comparisons.

Although every one of the above predictions for the specific status of Neandertals is supported here, the conclusion that Neandertals should be considered their own species, *Homo neanderthalensis*, is hampered by the large divergence values found between certain contemporary human groups. It was found that contemporary modern humans show surprisingly high levels of divergence when compared to that between sub-species of *Pan*. Several modern/modern comparisons were more divergent than that between sub-species of *Pan*, and three were larger than the divergence between *Pan* species.

At minimum the results of this study support little or no admixture between Neandertals and Upper Paleolithic Europeans. They also provide tentative (but not unequivocal) support for the specific status of Neandertals. In this regard, the results of dental morphological patterns agree with those based on craniofacial morphometrics and mtDNA.

References

Bailey, S. E. (2002a). A closer look at Neanderthal postcanine dental morphology. I. The mandibular dentition. *Anatomical Record (New Anatomist)*, **269**, 148–56.

Bailey, S. E. (2002b). *Neandertal dental morphology: implications for modern human origins.* Ph.D. Dissertation, Arizona State University.

Bailey, S. E. (2006). Beyond shovel shaped incisors: Neandertal dental morphology in a comparative context. *Periodicum Biologorum*, **108**, 253–67.

Bailey, S. E. and Lynch, J. M. (2005). Diagnostic differences in mandibular P4 shape between Neandertals and anatomically modern humans. *American Journal of Physical Anthropology*, **126**, 268–77.

Bailey, S. E., Turner, C. G., II, and du Souich, P. (1998). Dental morphological evidence for population affinities of the Iberian Peninsula (100 BC–1300 AD) and Western Balearic Islands. *American Journal of Physical Anthropology*, **25**, 65 (abstract).

Bailey, S. E. and Wood, B. A. (in press). The evolution of premolar and molar crown morphology within the hominin clade. In *Dental Perspectives on Human Evolution: State of the Art Research in Dental Paleoanthropology*, ed. S. E. Bailey and J.-J. Hublin. New York: Springer.

Baume, R. M. and Crawford, M. H. (1978). Discrete dental traits in four Tlaxcaltecan Mexican populations. *American Journal of Physical Anthropology*, **49**, 351–60.

Berry, A. and Berry, R. (1967). Epigenetic variation in the human cranium. *Journal of Anatomy*, **101**, 361–79.

Cavalli-Sforza, L., Menozzi, P., and Piazza, A. (1994). *The History and Geography of Human Genes*. Princeton: Princeton University Press.

Dahlberg, A. (1951). The dentition of the American Indian. In *Papers on the Physical Anthropology of the American Indian*, ed. W. S. Laughlin. New York: Viking Fund, pp. 138–76.

Dahlberg, A. (1963). Analysis of the American Indian dentition. In *Dental Anthropology*, ed. D. Brothwell. New York: Pergamon, pp. 149–77.

Dahlberg, A. (1965). Geographic distribution and origin of dentitions. *International Dental Journal*, **15**, 348–55.

Frayer, D., Wolpoff, M., Thorne, A., Smith, F., and Pope, G. (1993). Theories of modern human origins: the paleontological test. *American Anthropologist*, **95**, 14–50.

Green, R. F. and Suchey, J. M. (1976). The use of inverse sign transformations in the analysis of non-metric cranial data. *American Journal of Physical Anthropology*, **50**, 629–34.

Gutiérrez, G., Sánchez, D., and Marín, A. (2002). A reanalysis of the ancient mitochondrial DNA sequences recovered from Neandertal bones. *Molecular Biology and Evolution*, **19**, 1359–66.

Haeussler, A. (1985). *Dental morphology of New World Eastern Siberia and Soviet Central Asia Populations.* Master's Thesis, Arizona State University.

Haeussler, A. (1996). *Biological relationships of Late Pleistocene and Holocene Eurasian and American Peoples: the dental anthropological evidence.* Ph.D. Dissertation, Arizona State University.

Haeussler, A. M. and Turner, C. G., II (1992). The dentition of Soviet Central Asians and the quest for New World ancestors. *Journal of Human Ecology, Special Issue*, **2**, 273–97.

Hanihara, K. (1963). Crown characters of the deciduous dentition of the Japanese-American hybrids. In *Dental Anthropology*, ed. D. R. Brothwell. New York: Pergamon Press, pp. 105–24.

Hanihara, K. (1977). Dentition of the Ainu and the Australian aborigines. In *Orofacial Growth and Develoment*, ed. A. Dahlberg and T. Graber. The Hague: Mouton Publishers, pp. 195–200.

Hanihara, K., Masuda, T., and Tanaka, T. (1975). Affinities of dental characteristics in the Okinawa Islanders. *Journal of the Anthropological Society of Nippon*, **82**, 75–82.

Hanihara, T. (1989). Affinities of the Philippine Negritos as viewed from dental characters: a preliminary report. *Journal of the Anthropological Society of Nippon*, **97**, 327–39.

Harris, E. (2004). Calculation of Smith's mean measure of divergence for intergroup comparisons using nonmetric data. *Dental Anthropology*, **17**, 83–93.

Harris, E. and Bailit, H. (1980). The metaconule: a morphologic and familial analysis of a molar cusp in humans. *American Journal of Physical Anthropology*, **53**, 349–58.

Harvati, K. (2002). Models of shape variation between and within species and the Neanderthal's taxonomic position: a 3D geometric morphometrics approach based on temporal bone morphology. *BAR International Series*, **1049**, 25–30.

Harvati, K. (2003). The Neanderthal taxonomic position: models of intra- and inter-specific craniofacial variation. *Journal of Human Evolution*, **44**, 107–32.

Hawkes, J. and Wolpoff, M. H. (2001). Paleoanthropology and the population genetics of ancient genes. *American Journal of Physical Anthropology*, **114**, 269–72.

Hawkey, D. (1998). *Out of Asia: dental evidence for affinities and microevolution of early populations from India/Sri Lanka.* Ph.D. Dissertation, Arizona State University.

Hlusko, L. J. (2002). Expression types for two cercopithecoid dental traits (interconulus and interconulid) and their variation in a modern baboon population. *International Journal of Primatology*, **23**, 1309–18.

Irish, J. D. (1993). *Biological affinities of Late Pleistocene through modern African Aboriginal populations: the dental evidence.* Ph.D. Dissertation, Arizona State University.

Irish, J. D. (1997). Characteristic high and low frequency dental traits in sub-Saharan African populations. *American Journal of Physical Anthropology*, **102**, 455–67.

Irish, J. D. (1998). Ancestral dental traits in recent sub-Saharan Africans and the origins of modern humans. *Journal of Human Evolution*, **34**, 81–98.

Irish, J. D. and Turner, C. G., II (1990). West African dental affinity of Late Pleistocene Nubians: peopling of the Eurafrican-South Asian triangle II. *Homo*, **41**, 42–53.

Kimbel, W. H. and Martin, L. B. (1993). *Species, Species Concepts and Primate Evolution.* New York: Plenum Press.

Krings, M., Capelli, C., Tschentscher, F. *et al.* (2000). A view of Neandertal genetic diversity. *Nature Genetics*, **26**, 144–6.

Krings, M., Geisert, H., Schmitz, R., Krainitzki, H., and Pääbo, S. (1999). DNA sequence of the mitochondrial hypervariable region II from the Neandertal type specimen. *Proceedings of the National Academy of Sciences, USA.*, **96**, 5581–5.

Krings, M., Stone, A., Schmitz, R. W. *et al.* (1997). Neandertal DNA sequences and the origin of modern humans. *Cell*, **90**, 19–30.

Lewontin, R. C. (1972). The apportionment of human diversity. *Evolutionary Biology*, **6**, 381–98.

Lieberman, D. E., Krovitz, G. E., Yates, F. W., Devlin, M., and St Claire, M. (2004). Effects of food processing on masticatory strain and craniofacial growth in a retrognathic face. *Journal of Human Evolution*, **46**, 655–77.

Lipschultz, J. G. (1997). *Who were the Natufians? a dental assessment of their population affinities.* Master's Thesis, Arizona State University.

Lukacs, J. R. (1983). Dental anthropology and the origins of two Iron Age populations from northern Pakistan. *Homo*, **34**, 1–15.

Lukacs, J. R. (1986). Dental morphology and odontometrics of early agriculturalists from Neolithic Mehrgarh, Pakistan. In *Teeth Revisited: Proceedings of the VIIth International Symposium*, ed. D. Russell, J.-P. Santoro, and D. Sigogneau-Russell. Paris: Mémoires de la Museé national Histoire naturelle (série C), pp. 285–303.

Lukacs, J. R. and Walimbe, S. (1984). Deciduous dental morphology and the biological affinities of a late Chalcolithic skeletal series from western India. *American Journal of Physical Anthropology*, **65**, 23–30.

Mizoguchi, Y. (1977). Genetic variability in tooth crown characters: analysis by the tetrachoric correlation method. *Bulletin of the National Science Museum*, **3**, 37–62.

Mizoguchi, Y. (1985). *Shovelling: A statistical analysis of its morphology*. Tokyo: University of Tokyo Press.

Morin, P., Moore, J., Chakraborty, R. *et al.* (1994). Kin selection, social structure, gene flow and the evolution of chimpanzees. *Science*, **265**, 1193–201.

Ovchinnikov, I. V., Götherström, A., Romanova, G. P. *et al.* (2000). Comparison of modern human and Neanderthal DNA. *Nature*, **404**, 490–3.

Perzigian, A. J. (1977). Fluctuating dental asymmetry variation among skeletal populations. *American Journal of Physical Anthropology*, **47**, 81–8.

Perzigian, A. J. (1984). Human odontometric variation: an evolutionary and taxonomic assessment. *Anthropologie*, **22**, 193–8.

Pilbrow, V. (2003). *Dental variation in African apes with implications for understanding patterns of variation in species of fossil apes.* Ph.D. dissertation, New York University.

Rak, Y. (1986). The Neandertal: a new look at an old face. *Journal of Human Evolution*, **15**, 151–64.

Relethford, J. H. (2001). Absence of regional affinities of Neandertal DNA with living humans does not reject multiregional evolution. *American Journal of Physical Anthropology*, **115**, 95–8.

Relethford, J. H. (2002). Apportionment of global human genetic diversity based on craniometrics and skin color. *American Journal of Physical Anthropology*, **118**, 393–8.

Schillaci, M. A. and Froehlich, J. W. (2001). Nonhuman primate hybridization and the taxonomic status of Neanderthals. *American Journal of Physical Anthropology*, **115**, 157–66.

Schwartz, J. and Tattersall, I. (1996). Significance of some previously unrecognized apomorphies in the nasal region of *Homo neanderthalensis*. *Proceedings of the National Academy of Sciences, USA*, **93**, 10852–4.

Scott, G., Street, S., and Dahlberg, A. (1986). The dental variation of Yuman speaking groups in an American Southwest context. In *Teeth Revisited: Proceedings of the VIIth International Symposium on Dental Morphology*, ed. D. Russell, J.-P. Santoro, and D. Sigogneau-Russel. Paris: Mémoires de la Museé national Histoire naturelle (série C), 305–19.

Scott, G. R. and Potter, R. H. Y. (1984). The analysis of tooth crown morphology in American white twins. *Anthropologie*, **22**, 223–31.

Scott, G. R. and Turner, C. G., II (1988). Dental anthropology. *Annual Review of Anthropology*, **17**, 99–126.

Scott, G. R. and Turner, C. G., II (1997). *The Anthropology of Modern Human Teeth. Dental Morphology and its Variation in Recent Human Populations*. Cambridge: Cambridge University Press.

Serre, D., Langaney, A., Chech, M. *et al.* (2004). No evidence of Neandertal mtDNA contribution to early modern humans. *Plos Biology*, **2**, 313–17.

Sjøvold, T. (1973). The occurrence of minor non-metrical variants in the skeleton and their quantitative treatment for population comparisons. *Homo*, **24**, 204–33.

Sjøvold, T. (1984). A report on the heritability of some cranial measurements and non-metric traits. In *Multivariate Statistical Methods in Physical Anthropology*, ed. G. Van Ark & W. W. Howells, pp. 223–46. Dordrecht: D. Reidel Publishing.

Smith, F., Falsetti, A., and Donnelly, S. (1989). Modern human origins. *Yearbook of Physical Anthropology*, **32**, 35–68.

Sofaer, J., Smith, P., and Kaye, E. (1986). Affinities between contemporary and skeletal Jewish and non-Jewish groups based on tooth morphology. *American Journal of Physical Anthropology*, **70**, 265–75.

Stringer, C. (1996). Current issues in modern human origins. In *Contemporary Issues in Human Evolution*, ed. W. Meikle, F. C. Howell, and N. Jablonski. San Francisco: California Academy of Sciences, pp. 116–34.

Suwa, G. (1990). *A comparative analysis of hominid dental remains from the Shungura and Usno Formations, Omo Valley, Ethiopia.* Ph.D. Dissertation, University of California at Berkeley.

Townsend, G. and Martin, N. G. (1992). Fitting genetic models to Carabelli trait data in South Australian twins. *Journal of Dental Research*, **71**, 403–9.

Turner, C. G., II. (1969). Microevolutionary interpretations from the dentition. *American Journal of Physical Anthropology*, **30**, 421–6.

Turner, C. G., II (1983). Sinodonty and Sundadonty: a dental anthropological view of Mongoloid microevolution, origin, and dispersal into the Pacific basin, Siberia, and the Americas. In *Late Pleistocene and Early Holocene Cultural Connections of Asia and America*, ed. R. Vasilievsky. Novosibirsk: USSR Academy of Science, Siberian Branch, pp. 72–6.

Turner, C. G., II (1987). Late Pleistocene and Holocene population history of east Asia based on dental variation. *American Journal of Physical Anthropology*, **73**, 305–21.

Turner, C. G., II (1990). Origin and affinity of the prehistoric people of Guam: a dental anthropological assessment. In *Recent Advances in Micronesian Archaeology, Micronesia Supplement No. 2*, ed. R. Hunter-Anderson. Mangilao: University of Guam Press, 403–16.

Turner, C. G., II (1992). Microevolution of East Asian and European populations: a dental perspective. In *The Evolution and Dispersal of Modern Humans in Asia*, ed. T. Akazawa, K. Aoki and T. Kimura. Tokyo: Hokusen-Sha Pub. Co, pp. 415–38.

Turner, C. G., II (1993). Southwest Indians: prehistory through dentition. *National Geographic Research & Exploration*, **9**, 32–53.

Turner, C. G., II (1995). Shifting continuity: modern human origin. In *The Origin and Past of Modern Humans as Viewed from DNA*, ed. S. Brenner and K. Hanihara. Singapore: World Scientific Publishing Company, pp. 216–43.

Turner, C. G., II, Nichol, C. R., and Scott, G. R. (1991). Scoring procedures for key morphological traits of the permanent dentition: the Arizona State University Dental Anthropology System. In *Advances in Dental Anthropology*, ed. M. Kelley and C. S. Larsen. New York: Wiley Liss, pp. 13–31.

Ward, J. (1963). Hierarchical groupings to optimize an objective function. *Journal of the American Statistical Association*, **58**, 236–44.

Wolpoff, M., Thorne, A., Smith, F., Frayer, D., and Pope, G. (1994). Multiregional evolution: a world-wide source for modern human populations. In *Origins of Anatomically Modern Humans*, ed. M. Nitecki and D. Nitecki. New York: Plenum Press, pp. 176–99.

Zubov, A. A. (1973). *Ethnic Odontology*. Moscow: Nauka.

14 *The quantitative genetic analysis of primate dental variation: history of the approach and prospects for the future*

OLIVER T. RIZK, SARAH K. AMUGONGO, MICHAEL C. MAHANEY, AND LESLEA J. HLUSKO

14.1 Introduction

From the size and shape of teeth we can learn much about an animal's diet, gain some insight as to how it interacted with its conspecifics and environment, and draw conclusions about its phylogenetic placement. Consequently, primate dental variation has been the focus of an immense amount of research (as evidenced by this volume). These adaptive and phylogenetic scenarios rely on the assumption that variation in the dental phenotype is heritable, or rather, that this variation can be passed on from generation to generation as selection filters through the available phenotypic variance.

In this chapter, we discuss the history of research that tests this hypothesis through quantitative genetic analyses. We will focus attention on analyses of crown morphology with the aim of summarizing what is currently known and unknown about the extent to which dental variation is influenced by genetic factors. And last, we discuss two directions through which quantitative genetics will further enhance our understanding of the evolution of our ancestors and closest relatives.

14.2 Quantitative genetics

Quantitative genetics is concerned with the inheritance of those differences between individuals that are of degree rather than of kind, quantitative rather than qualitative. These are the individual differences which, as Darwin wrote, "afford materials for natural selection to act on and accumulate . . ." An understanding of the inheritance

Technique and Application in Dental Anthropology ed. Joel D. Irish and Greg C. Nelson
Published by Cambridge University Press.

> of these differences is thus of fundamental significance in the study of evolution and in the application of genetics to animal and plant breeding. (Falconer, 1989, p. 1)

The theories and methods of quantitative genetics extended Gregor Mendel's principles of inheritance – originally adduced from the study of the transmission of qualitative traits – to the analysis of quantitative, or continuously varying, traits in populations. This extension took advantage of theoretical developments in two nascent fields of scientific inquiry: the inheritance of measurements, or biometry, introduced by Francis Galton in the late 1800s, and the genetics of populations, introduced by a number of scientists following the rediscovery of Mendel's work in the early 1900s (Falconer, 1989; Lynch and Walsh, 1998; Provine, 1971). The theoretical basis for quantitative genetics was advanced, coincident with much of inferential statistics, by the early 1920s in the works of Fisher (1918), Haldane (reviewed in 1932), and Wright (1921). Since its formulation, the theory of quantitative genetics primarily has been applied to predicting the genetic properties of populations conditional on the properties of genes, predicting the quantitative outcomes of breeding strategies, and predicting evolutionary change in quantitative traits: conditional, real, or hypothesized genetic properties in agricultural and experimental populations of animals and plants (Falconer, 1989). In the last few decades, it has been extended to the detection, characterization, localization, and identification of genes influencing quantitative variation in traits of basic, evolutionary, and biomedical importance in humans and non-human primates as well (Rogers *et al.*, 1999).

At least three general premises are fundamental to much of the quantitative genetics work currently underway. The first is that the inheritance of quantitative differences (and, similarities) is mediated by the Mendelian segregation of genes at many loci. The second premise is the common observation of a greater similarity in measurements for quantitative traits in samples of closely related individuals than in samples of more distantly related individuals. This is explained, in part, by the fact that the former share more genes than the latter. The third premise is that environmental (i.e. non-inherited) factors also contribute to the pattern of observed quantitative differences in traits within a population. Consequently, a common goal of genetic analyses is to assess the relative importance of genotype versus environment to the observed variation in the trait of interest. According to basic quantitative genetic theory, the overall phenotypic, or anatomical variance (σ_P^2) may be decomposed into variance due to the effects of genes (σ_G^2) and variance due to "environment" (σ_E^2), such that:

$$\sigma_P^2 = \sigma_G^2 + \sigma_E^2 \tag{14.1}$$

Given this relationship, an estimate of the *heritability* (h^2), or the proportion of the total phenotypic variance accounted for by genetic effects, is:

$$h^2 = \frac{\sigma_G^2}{\sigma_P^2} \quad (14.2)$$

Dental anthropologists and researchers from other disciplines have employed a variety of quantitative genetic approaches and study designs (sampling and analytical strategies) to determine the relative importance of genes and environmental factors to quantitative variation in dental traits; all of them require quantitative data from samples of related individuals, e.g. twins, sibling pairs, sibships, nuclear families, and extended families, etc. All other things being equal, the greater the number and variety of relative pairs in a sample, the greater the statistical power to detect and estimate the effects of genes and environmental factors on quantitative variation in a trait. This is simply a matter of information available for analysis, i.e. sibships provide more information than sibling pairs, and extended families provide more than nuclear families, etc. However, in quantitative genetics, different research questions/hypotheses may require different study designs, and different study designs may require different analytical approaches (Blangero, 2004). Further, the genealogical structure of anthropologically relevant samples (or of samples typically available to dental anthropologists) can influence the kinds of questions that can be addressed and, consequently, the analytical approaches employed.

We will briefly summarize the history of the use of some of these techniques to address questions of interest to dental anthropologists. Although we categorize these studies into "early," "middle," and "later" years, the reader should realize that the breaks between these categories are somewhat arbitrary.

14.3 The early years (1920s–1950s)

The earliest studies exploring genetic contributions to dental variation utilized twin, sibling, and parent–offspring relationships, and were concerned primarily with patterns of resemblance and inheritance for dental caries and orthodontic disorders (e.g. Bachrach and Young, 1927; Moore and Hughes, 1942). With the exception of studies exploring the susceptibility to dental caries in inbred rat populations (Hunt *et al.*, 1944; Rosen *et al.*, 1961), dental quantitative genetics research in the 1940s and 1950s was dominated by the human monozygotic (MZ) and dizygotic (DZ) twin study model. Investigations of tooth size and occlusion (Lundström, 1948), date of eruption (Hatton, 1955), and molar cusp variation (Ludwig, 1957) from this period established the practice of variance comparison between the two twin types, consistently demonstrating greater variability for dental traits of DZ twins relative to that of MZ twins. The greater concordance between MZ twins and, in general, the high degree of resemblance between related individuals reported in these studies, provides some of the earliest evidence for genetic inheritance of dental variation and the foundation for all subsequent work.

14.4 The middle years (1950s–1970s)

During the 1950s, 1960s, and 1970s, genetic contributions to dental variation were inferred mainly through studies of inter-populational differences, familial aggregation, and relative pair correlations. Results and observations from the first two classes of study provided circumstantial evidence for heritability, while those from the third category – e.g. comparison of intra-pair variance ratios between twin types, simple measurements of concordance and correlation in twins, the regression and correlation of parents and offspring, and the correlations between full and half siblings – provided improved estimates of the magnitude of the effects of genes on the traits under study. We discuss this research by phenotype, i.e. caries, tooth size, Carabelli's cusp, etc. It is important to note that, as seen in the early years, work from this period focused almost completely on humans. The non-human primate studies by Sirianni and Swindler (1973, 1974) (discussed below) are the few exceptions to this trend.

14.4.1 Caries and occlusion

Our review focuses on crown size and shape; however, it is important to note that quantitative genetic analyses of dental variation continued to demonstrate a genetic contribution to dental caries susceptibility (e.g. Finn and Caldwell, 1963; Horowitz *et al.*, 1958b). Assessing the degree to which intra-pair variance in DZ twins exceeded the variance in MZ twins provided a heritability estimate of 0.85 (Goodman *et al.*, 1959). However, the observation that both twin types had a higher concordance compared to the controls indicated a significant environmental influence on caries experience (Mansbridge, 1959).

Research on occlusion suggested that despite observed genetic variability, environmental factors are more important among families for traits such as overjet, overbite, molar relationship, crowding, and rotations, and as such, occlusal/dental arch variation has lower heritability estimates than does tooth crown size (Bowden and Goose, 1968; Harris and Smith 1980; Lee and Goose, 1982, but see the latter for contrasting estimation for overjet). This importance of environmental contributions to the phenotypic variance will be addressed in detail later.

14.4.2 Tooth and cusp dimensions

Numerous researchers reported evidence for a genetic contribution to tooth size, i.e. linear measurements of crown mesiodistal and buccolingual lengths. Studies of tooth size incorporating familial relationships in the house mouse (Bader, 1965; Bader and Lehmann, 1965) preceded human research for this trait, introducing the calculation of heritability from coefficients of variance derived from population and sibling comparisons. Numerous human family studies that followed demonstrated that most of the tooth size dimensions could be attributed to additive genetic effects (Bowden and Goose, 1969; El-Nofely and Tawfik, 1995; Goose, 1968; Niswander and Chung, 1965; Townsend and Brown, 1978a, 1978b). Correlations between family members, including twin, sibling, parent–child and cousin, showed a significant genetic basis for crown size, with heritability estimates falling between 0.80 and 0.90 (Garn *et al.*, 1968). Data for deciduous teeth from an Aboriginal population agreed with these high estimates of genetic variability in tooth size (Townsend, 1980).

Interestingly though, researchers detected patterned differences in heritability among linear metric phenotypes. A full sib correlation comparison estimated higher heritabilities for labiolingual compared to mesiodistal dimensions in 13 of 16 possible comparisons, suggesting a greater genetic factor for the former set of dimensions (Alvesalo and Tigerstedt, 1974). Additionally, heritability of inter-cuspal distances was found to be less than that for crown diameters of maxillary premolar teeth (Townsend, 1985). Another study found that variation in molar cusp size suggested little difference between MZ and DZ cusp area variance, and hence, a relatively low heritability (Biggerstaff, 1975, 1976). These differences in heritability were thought to possibly represent differing genetic control, with implications for the evolution of the primate dentition.

Multivariate analyses of linear metrics provided additional insight to the genetic contributions to tooth size. Factor analysis demonstrated that three common factors could collectively describe the 56 dimensions of 28 permanent teeth and account for more than one half of total variance of these measurements (Potter *et al.*, 1968).

Analyses of size variation in the anterior dentition suggested that genetic control in the various tooth categories differs. In a sibling study that explored the genetic involvement in specific components of occlusion characteristics, the highest degree of correlation was found in incisor width, which suggests stronger genetic involvement for this tooth dimension (Chung and Niswander, 1975). The presence of a genetic component for overall tooth size was indicated in an analysis of variance and concordance in a study of three sets of triplets (Menezes *et al.*, 1974). A study of the maxillary and mandibular permanent anterior teeth in MZ and DZ twins demonstrated a greater genetic influence for the incisors than the canines (Horowitz *et al.*, 1958a; Osborne *et al.*, 1958). Cross twin analysis also indicated that the anterior dentition might be under genetic control in terms of both general tooth size and adjacent tooth size (Osborne *et al.*, 1958). Interestingly, intra-pair variances of mesiodistal crown diameters of deciduous anterior teeth showed high genetic variability in canines and, to a lesser degree, central incisors (Di Salvo *et al.*, 1972).

A variety of dental traits other than tooth and cusp dimensions were also explored using quantitative genetic analyses. For example, tooth width of the anterior teeth (Lundström, 1964), mesial ridge counts (although only at a significant level in the maxillary second premolar) (Gilmore, 1968), and intra-alveolar development of the crown and root of permanent mandibular canines, premolars, and first and second molars (Green and Aszkler, 1970).

14.4.3 Morphological traits

The standardization of scoring for morphological traits (Dahlberg, 1956) provided a significant number of dental phenotypes that were also analyzed using quantitative genetic approaches during this time period. Heritability estimates were generally found to be lower for these phenotypes compared to linear metrics. The dichotomization of continuously variable traits inherent in the standardized scoring procedure typically employed in these analyses results in the loss of a significant amount of descriptive power, and therefore may account for these lower heritability estimates.

Carabelli's cusp is perhaps the most "famous" of these morphologies (Figure 14.1), and it was the subject of considerable genetic analysis. Population studies used genetic frequencies of Carabelli's trait to test hereditary models (Turner, 1967) and describe inter-group variation (Scott, 1980). In sibling studies, the frequency of Carabelli's trait in the deciduous and permanent dentition was found to be higher for the siblings of individuals with the character than for siblings from the general population, suggesting some evidence for a genetic basis (Garn *et al.*, 1966). Twin research found that concordance of the Carabelli's trait is generally higher in MZ than DZ twins, with heritability estimates as high as 0.91 (Skrinjaric *et al.*, 1985). However, this was not a ubiquitous conclusion. A separate study found relatively low MZ concordance, and that concordance sometimes differed enough between antimeres to suggest separate genetic factors for each side of the dentition (Biggerstaff, 1973). Quantitative analysis by tetrachoric correlation of 14 non-metric characters, including Carabelli's trait, also indicated low genetic variability (Mizoguchi, 1977).

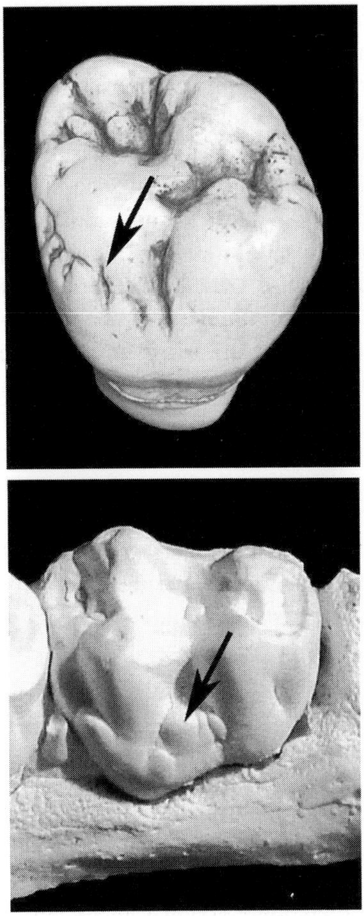

Figure 14.1 Top panel shows expression of the cingular remnant Carabelli's cusp on an upper left third molar of a 2.5 million year old hominid from the Omo, Ethiopia (specimen number L 50–2). The bottom panel shows expression of the cingular remnant in the maxillary molar of an extant baboon (*Papio hamadryas*).

Family studies employed in an attempt to establish the mode of inheritance of Carabelli's trait, shoveling of incisors, maxillary molar cusp number, mandibular cusp number, and fissure patterns suggested that these traits are continuous and not discrete; they are, therefore, likely to be inherited in a multifactorial way (Goose and Lee, 1971; Lee and Goose, 1972). However, reducing Carabelli's trait into fewer categories, typically employed by dental anthropologists (Turner *et al.*, 1991), resulted in high sibling similarity with values of the coefficient of contingency approximating 0.50 (Garn *et al.*, 1966). A separate analysis of variation in expression of Carabelli's trait in sib pairs reported no correlation, suggesting that it is not due to genetic factors (Alvesalo *et al.*, 1975). In addition to Carabelli's cusp, other phenotypes such as shovel form, molar cusp number, and groove pattern were shown to generally have low but positive within-individual correlations with one another, possibly attributable to a general effect of tooth size (Sofaer *et al.*, 1972). Also, despite higher MZ values, 100% concordance in MZ twins was rarely reached in an examination of 26 minor variants of the dental crown (Kaul *et al.*, 1985). Parent–offspring and sib correlations demonstrated genetic control over the frequency of expression of 20 tooth crown traits (Scott, 1973).

Heritability estimated from parent–offspring correlation showed that about 68% of maxillary incisor shovel shape variation could be explained by additive genetic effects (Blanco and Chakraborty, 1976). A sibship analysis found the frequency of shoveling to be higher among the sibs of affected persons than among randomly sampled sibs from the study population, also showing that the character is heritable (Portin and Alvesalo, 1974).

The genetic contributions to metaconule expression were also explored; estimates of the additive genetic component were found to be 65% for the first molar, but only 15% for the second (Harris and Bailit, 1980).

14.4.4 Asymmetry

Biggerstaff, in his analysis of Carabelli's cusp (1973) and concordance of mandibular molar cusp size between twins (1970), noted that concordance differed enough between antimeres to suggest separate genetic factors for each side of the dentition. This observation and conclusion is remarkable in that it contradicts the bilateral symmetry commonly assumed to be inherent to the dentition (and vertebrate bodies in general).

During the 1950s–1970s considerable research was designed to test whether or not genetic influences could explain dental asymmetry. The results from these studies were mixed. Support for a genetic influence was found when comparing individual teeth and tooth-width sums, although a greater non-genetic influence was observed in the former (Lundström, 1967). An investigation of permanent mandibular first molar and first and second premolars in MZ and DZ twins and non-twins found greater bilateral asymmetry in MZ twins for the seventh cusp of the first molar, but equal asymmetry in MZ and DZ twins for hypoconulid occurrence and premolar cusp number; this suggests a mixed amount of genetic influence (Staley and Green, 1971). Additional work, in which a distinction was made between measurements of discordance, bilateral asymmetry, and mirror imaging in comparing variance ratios for dimensions of the permanent dentition, showed no sign of a genetic component (Potter and Nance, 1976). A population study of Mexican and Belizean groups found little asymmetry and high correlations between each side of the dentition for a set of discrete dental traits; these findings lead to the conclusion that similar genetic factors may exist for both sides, and that environmental factors may play a significant role in asymmetry (Baume and Crawford, 1980). In a study done to establish dental asymmetry as an indicator of genetic and environmental conditions of human populations, non-significant heritability estimates that ranged between 2–5% suggested a low component of additive genetic variance for fluctuating asymmetry (Bailit *et al.*, 1970).

Although genetic factors have not been ruled out in the case of asymmetry, the twin and population data from this period are inconclusive and suggest, if anything, a large environmental influence. For the current status of this debate see Leamy *et al.* (2000, 2005).

14.4.5 Development

During this time, several studies also looked at genetic control of tooth development. Family line analysis (Garn *et al.*, 1960) and sibling correlation studies (Garn *et al.*, 1965a; Merwin and Harris, 1998) assessed the genetic influence on the tempo of tooth growth and mineralization. Strong genetic control was indicated by a heritability of 0.82 calculated from intra-class correlations between full siblings (Merwin and Harris, 1998).

14.4.6 Sex effects

Sex effects on tooth size were also reported. In comparing the size of the permanent teeth in like- and unlike-sexed siblings, X-chromosomal linkage was suggested by sister–sister correlations that exceeded brother–brother correlations, which in turn exceeded sister–brother correlations (Garn *et al.*, 1965b; Lewis and Grainger, 1967). Other sibling correlation studies also suggested genetic control over sexual dimorphism in tooth size (Garn *et al.*, 1967). However, several population studies comparing sib correlations for tooth size did not show evidence for the presence of sex-linked genes (Niswander and Chung, 1965; Townsend and Brown, 1978a). Investigations of tooth size inheritance in non-human primates used sib correlations from a captive macaque population to test the hypothesis of X-chromosome mediation, but instead found support for involvement of the Y-chromosome (Sirianni and Swindler, 1973, 1974).

14.4.7 Maternal effects

Both maternal and gestational factors were found to influence crown dimensions. Relatively high mother–offspring correlations were interpreted as a sign of environmental effects associated with the mother (Goose, 1967). Prolonged gestation, high birth weight and length, and maternal hypothyroidism and diabetes were associated with an increase in tooth size, while short gestation, lower birth weight and length, and maternal hypertension were associated with decreased crown dimensions (Garn *et al.*, 1980). An analysis of covariance done to determine whether maternal effects influence the development of the permanent dentition showed that dental development is significantly different between families after adjustment for maternal age, birth order, and birth weight (Bailit and Sung, 1968). A cross-fostering experiment between inbred strains of the house mouse that analyzed the prenatal and postnatal maternal environmental effects on molar size variation indicated a non-genetic prenatal factor, as well as strain-specific genetic determinants for the second molar; however, there was little prenatal environment intra-strain influence on the third molar (Tenczar and Bader, 1966).

14.4.8 Dental variation diagnosis of twin zygosity

The high degree of concordance between MZ twins in crown morphology, presence of Carabelli's trait, and molar cusp number proved to be useful for diagnosing zygosity (Townsend *et al.*, 1988; Wood and Green, 1969), comparable to that of other phenotypes such as fingerprints and blood grouping (Kraus *et al.*, 1959). One twin study showed that concordance comparisons across the entire dentition were able to diagnose zygosity accurately approximately 94% of the time (Lundström, 1963).

14.5 The later years (1970s–1980s)

In the late 1970s, statistical analyses of twin and familial data progressed beyond the simple concordance and correlation techniques employed in the previous decades, as exemplified by the multivariate work by Potter *et al.* (1976). Using this method, within-pair difference covariance matrices were created for each twin type, suggesting that a greater number of genetic factors were influencing mandibular tooth size. In addition to a supposed independence of the mandibular and maxillary dentition, separate factors were indicated for mesiodistal and buccolingual dimensions, in contrast to what appeared to be shared genetic determinants for antimeres (Potter *et al.*, 1976, 1978).

The early 1980s saw the introduction of complex segregation analysis into dental genetics, facilitating the identification of genetic and common environmental influences on Carabelli's trait (Kolakowski *et al.*, 1980) and tooth dimensions (Kolakowski and Bailit, 1981) from sibling and parent-offspring data. Path analysis was first utilized to investigate the influence of small crown characters on tooth dimension and shoveling (Mizoguchi, 1978). In a later study, path analysis modeling detected environmental variance components responsible for sibling correlation in mesiodistal measurements of the upper left permanent first molar and lateral incisor (Potter *et al.*, 1983). A study combining complex segregation analysis of morphological traits and path analysis of tooth size measurements identified roles for both genetic and environmental factors (Nichol, 1990).

In 1979, an attempt to find any association of twin zygosity with tooth size indicated that an important assumption of the twin model, environmental variance equality, had been violated, prompting a refinement of the statistical testing used in later studies (Potter *et al.*, 1979). The finding that variances were not necessarily homogenous across twin types suggested the existence of unequal environmental influences, and bias in previous estimates of variance and heritability from studies in which heterogeneity had not been assessed (reviewed in the previous section). Additionally, Potter *et al.*'s (1979) study indicated that among-pair sex differences existed for MZ and DZ mean squares, a confounding factor for variance heterogeneity.

The direct result of this restatement of the twin model and its assumptions was the incorporation of sex differences, mean equality, variance heterogeneity, and environmental equality tests into subsequent studies of occlusal variation using multivariate and principal component analyses to investigate trait interactions. After environmental inequalities and MZ–DZ mean differences were accounted for, an overall average heritability for occlusal traits was estimated as 0.25, reflecting biases that had gone undetected in prior studies of occlusion and the large environmental influence on variance (Corruccini and Potter, 1980). A subsequent analysis of size, asymmetry, and occlusion in the permanent first molar found heritable components for only the lower molars, averaging 0.62 (in contrast to 0.09 for the upper molars) and non-significant genetic components for asymmetry and occlusal discrepancy (although the latter tended to be higher) (Corruccini and Potter, 1981). A general conclusion from the occlusal variance studies from this period indicated a greater environmental than genetic influence on the traits examined (Corruccini and Potter, 1980, 1981; Potter *et al.*, 1981).

Investigators of tooth dimension also adopted the refined twin study protocol. A comparison of American and Punjabi MZ and DZ twin pairs yielded an average heritability estimate of 0.73 for tooth size, and when not invalidated by environmental covariance inequality, mesiodistal and buccolingual dimensions of individual teeth in the Punjabi twin population were used to derive heritability estimates that ranged from 0.26 to 0.72 after correction for variance heterogeneity (Corruccini and Sharma, 1985; Sharma, *et al.*, 1985). The size of the maxillary right lateral incisor was found to have a significant heritability estimate of 0.42 (Townsend *et al.*, 1986), and heritabilities of mesiodistal tooth dimensions ranged from 0.64 to 0.88, and 0.10 to 0.60 for buccolingual dimensions when calculated using multiple estimation methods (Harzer, 1987). In addition to the more informative narrow-sense heritability estimates provided in these studies, the use of more sophisticated statistical analyses elucidated specific patterns of heritability within the dentition. Summation of dimensions for tooth groups yielded the highest estimates, which was interpreted as an indicator of greater genetic control over tooth groups compared to individual teeth (Harzer, 1987, 1995). Also demonstrated was a general decrease in heritability from anterior to posterior teeth in the upper jaw, a pattern not observed in the mandible (Harzer, 1987, 1995).

14.6 Today (1990s–present)

Following the revisions and elaborations of statistical methods in the 1970s and 1980s, several novel study designs were introduced. A new dimension to dental twin studies was added by the use of twins reared apart in an investigation of caries experience, occlusion, and tooth morphology (Boraas *et al.*, 1988). Another original approach to estimating environmental and genetic effects used the offspring of MZ twins and their spouses to perform analyses of variance only possible in half-sib design studies, allowing for detection of common environmental influences, maternal effects, and assortative mating (Potter, 1990).

Studies in the 1990s also introduced the use of statistical software to generate various models representing the genetic and environmental factors involved in the dentition. Once generated, the best fitting model was determined using maximum-likelihood methods and chi-square testing. Using the LISREL software package and PRELIS pre-processor, it was determined that the best model for explaining variation in the Carabelli trait on the permanent maxillary first molar was comprised of additive genetic effects, a general environmental factor, and an environmental component specific to each side; this produced a heritability estimate of 0.94 for the left molar and 0.86 for the right (Townsend and Martin, 1992). More conservative estimates for the Carabelli trait, 0.51 for the right and 0.37 for the left, and for tooth size, 0.60, were calculated after observing possible non-additive genetic effects and overall variance heterogeneity in 11 of 56 variables (Townsend *et al.*, 1992).

Multivariate model-fitting analyses (in which progressively more complicated models were fit to data, beginning with a model incorporating unique environmental influences only, followed by a model including unique environmental and additive genetic factors, and eventually non-additive and common environmental factors) showed that the majority of the variation observed in incisor crown size could be accounted for by unique environmental and additive genetic effects alone (Dempsey *et al.*, 1995). Also noted was a general genetic factor influencing all incisors, specific genetic factors for each pair of antimeric teeth, and unique environmental factors specific to each tooth, as well as the entire group of incisors. An average heritability estimate of 0.86 was in agreement with the large amount of additive genetic variance illustrated in this model (Dempsey *et al.*, 1995). Using similar statistical analyses, the best fitting model describing variance components of dental maturation in twins was found to incorporate additive genetic, and both unique and common environmental factors. The additive genetic component accounted for 43% of the total variance, while approximately half was attributed to the common environment, a reflection of the twins' shared prenatal, natal and postnatal circumstances of tooth maturation (Pelsmaekers *et al.*, 1997).

The more recent quantitative genetic dental research has investigated the covariance structure of dimensions of the deciduous teeth for signs of genotype by environment interaction or directional dominance, and found evidence for neither; the conclusion was that a model incorporating only additive genetic (ranging from 62–91%) and unique environmental components of variance sufficiently explains the total variance in all teeth except for the lower central incisor in females (Hughes *et al.*, 2000). When similar methods were applied to crown size of permanent teeth, in the absence of genotype by environmental interaction or assortative mating, a model incorporating additive genetic and unique environmental factors was adequate for all but two teeth: the maxillary left central incisor and right canine, for which introducing non-additive genetic or common environmental factors into the model provided a better fit. The lowest heritability estimates were associated with the mesiodistal length of the maxillary first molar, 0.50–0.60, and the highest with the buccolingual breadth of the maxillary premolars, 0.90, illustrating that no consistent pattern could be assigned to the observed heritabilities (Dempsey and Townsend, 2001). Additive genetic and unique environmental models were also fitted to crown measurements with inter-cuspal dimensions, producing higher heritability estimates for crown size than for inter-cuspal distances (Townsend *et al.*, 2003).

14.7 From heritability estimation to redefining the phenotype

All of the quantitative genetics research on primate dental variation to date demonstrates that the size and shape of teeth are influenced significantly by the additive effects of genes. Therefore, the assumptions inherent to the adaptive and phylogenetic interpretations noted at the beginning of this chapter are merited. However, it is probably clear to the reader at this point that heritability estimates by themselves, once demonstrated, are rather limited in what they can tell us about the genetic architecture of the dentition. Each estimate is specific to the population studied, and given the variety of analytical approaches, direct comparisons of heritability point estimates are somewhat meaningless. Have we hit a brick wall with quantitative genetic approaches? Is this all that we can learn from these types of analyses?

We argue that the answer to both questions is a resounding "no." The future for quantitative genetic analyses of dental variation will witness significant new insights into primate tooth biology primarily through two directions: quantitative trait locus (QTL)/linkage analyses and the estimation of genetic correlations.

14.7.1 Quantitative genetics and "evo-devo"

Advances in developmental genetics over the last 20 years have shown that genes operate through a series of complex spatial and temporal interactions to form the phenotype, and patterned phenotypes often reflect spatial and temporal relationships between functioning genomic regions. For example, the number and morphology of vertebrae in an organism correspond to the patterned expression of members of the *Hox* gene family, a pattern that is highly conserved across vertebrate taxa (Carroll *et al.*, 2005; Galis, 1999).

Another example is the paired vertebrate appendages (i.e. limbs) that result from a different cascade of patterned and overlapping *Hox* gene expressions (Carroll *et al.*, 2005; Shubin, 2002). Shubin *et al.* (1997) and Shubin (2002) argue that the origin of digits in tetrapods during the Devonian may well correspond to a duplication event of part of the *Hox* gene family to form a third phase of expression during limb development. The fossil record, therefore, provides significant insight into when, and in what types of environments and selective regimes, novel morphologies (such as digits) arose – providing the proverbial "evo" to studies of "devo" (evolutionary developmental genetics).

The dentition provides a similar opportunity to understand morphological evolution from an integrated geno- and phenotypic perspective. Teeth preserve well in the fossil record due to a largely inorganic content that makes them very hard. As is seen in most vertebrate lineages, the mammalian fossil record is dominated by teeth, with many taxa known only by their dentitions. These fossils record information about the evolving genotype as selection operated on the phenotype. A significant barrier, however, is deciphering what these morphological changes represent in terms of the underlying genetics.

Quantitative genetics provides an important opportunity for unlocking this information. Our current understanding of tooth developmental genetics derives almost exclusively from rodent models, and addresses two fundamental questions – how is the overall dental pattern determined (i.e. incisors vs. molars), and how is the morphology of an individual tooth determined. Tooth developmental genetics is beyond the scope of this chapter and we refer the reader to several excellent reviews for more information (Jernvall and Thesleff, 2000; Stock, 2001; Tucker and Sharpe, 2004; Weiss, *et al.*, 1998).

As is commonly recognized, the genes necessary to form an organ are not necessarily the same ones that code for its minor phenotypic variation. From the perspective of a mammalian paleontologist, the mechanisms that underlie the variation upon which natural selection typically operates (population level variation) are of more critical concern. One way to obtain genetic information about minor phenotypic variation is to work from the phenotype back toward the genome. Quantitative genetic analyses provide such an approach.

14.7.2 QTL analyses

Gene-mapping techniques have been extremely useful in identifying genes that underlie genetic disorders, such as hemophilia (Lawn, 1985) and cystic fibrosis (Drumm and Collins, 1993). It is now possible to use these same techniques to study the genetic basis of polygenic traits, such as tooth size. There are two techniques that fall under the umbrella of QTL analyses. The first is a candidate gene approach, in which genetic variation at or near a known gene is tested for association with particular phenotypic variants. The second, and perhaps more relevant, approach to this discussion are quantitative trait loci (QTL) analyses, in which individual genes of small phenotypic effect are identified. This latter approach does not require a priori knowledge of gene function, and enables the identification of previously unknown genes that influence the phenotype of interest. Cheverud and Routman (1993) provide a nice overview.

Cheverud, Routman, and colleagues have also performed the majority of published QTL analyses on dental variation to date. By crossing two inbred strains of mice, one large and one small, and comparing the association of genetic marker alleles with morphological variation in the F2 generation, they identified more QTL for molar shape than size, as well as dominance effects for both (Workman *et al.*, 2002). This may indicate that the genetic basis for molar size is simpler than that for shape. Additionally, they did not find any differences in the effects of the shape QTL between the three molars, suggesting that these are not distinct developmental structures (Workman *et al.*, 2002). A similar study analyzed mandibular size and shape, through which 12 QTL were identified as significantly influencing size and 25 QTL affecting shape (Klingenberg *et al.*, 2001).

14.7.3 Morphological integration and modularity

Aside from providing information about the chromosomal locations of genes that influence mouse molar variation, these analyses also yield information about the inter-relatedness of various teeth. The lack of difference in the associated QTL for the first, second, and third molars indicates that variation in the size and shape of these structures is influenced by the same genetic effects, or rather, that these three molars are affected by complete pleiotropy. Pleiotropy underlies much of the rationale for the concept of morphological integration.

This concept was first introduced by Olson and Miller (1959) and revived by Cheverud (1982, 1989, 1995, 1996; Cheverud *et al.*, 1983; Marroig *et al.*, 2004). Morphological integration is the idea that phenotypic traits will be tightly correlated when they share a common developmental pathway and/or ultimate function. As such, individual morphological traits can be conceptualized as parts of sets. Identification of these integrated units is based on phenotypic correlations that have been shown to correspond to genetic correlations (Cheverud, 1988; Cheverud *et al.*, 1997; Ehrich, *et al.*, 2003; Klingenberg *et al.*, 2001; Leamy *et al.*, 1999; Mezey *et al.*, 2000). Quantitative genetic models argue that these heritable patterns of variation may be stable over reasonably long periods of evolutionary time (Lande, 1979, 1980).

Morphological integration is thought to reflect developmental and molecular modularity. Developmental genetics shows that organisms have morphological and developmental modularity that results from modules at the genomic level, such as gene families (Carroll *et al.*, 2005; Stern 2000; von Dassow *et al.*, 2000; Weiss, 1990), and from modules in embryogenesis (Raff, 1996). This modularity has been defined as "a genotype-phenotypic map in which there are a few pleiotropic effects among characters serving different functions, with pleiotropic effects falling mainly among characters that are part of a single functional complex" (Wagner and Altenberg, 1996, p. 967). This modularity is critical since it enables an organism to be "evolvable" (Wagner and Altenberg, 1996).

Integration is, of course, a matter of degree (Lewontin, 2001; Magwene, 2001). An organism is itself an integrated unit, otherwise it could not function properly. However, it is obvious that an organism is comprised of sub-units that work together to form a whole. Therefore, morphological integration and modularity are hierarchical, though somewhat arbitrary, and can be investigated at multiple levels.

Although the dentition is in a sense its own module, given the hierarchical nature of its development (Bateson, 1892; Stock, 2001), there is also modularity within the dentition. Quantitative genetic analyses, through the estimation of genetic correlations, are further elucidating such modules. This is the level of modularity often thought to be represented by characters in paleontological analyses, especially those at the sub-family level or below (Hlusko, 2004; Peyer, 1968; Swindler, 2002).

14.7.4 Redefining dental phenotypes

We are using quantitative genetic analyses to identify shared genetic effects on the dental variation of a captive pedigreed baboon colony (Hlusko *et al.*, 2002, 2004a, 2004b, in press a, in press b; Hlusko and Mahaney, 2003). Our goal is to reveal the genetic architecture that underlies primate dental variation. This is a meticulous process, as we first test for genetic correlations between all possible dental phenotype pairs. When a genetic correlation is estimated, we then test the extent of this correlation – is it 100%, indicating complete pleiotropy? Or is it lower, indicative of incomplete pleiotropy? Through this process, we are identifying phenotypes that represent the same genetic effects, phenotypes that have overlapping, but not identical, genetic effects, and phenotypes that are genetically independent. This knowledge enables the redefinition of the dentition based on the underlying genetic architecture.

For example, we have found complete pleiotropy for antimeres of all phenotypes studied to date, including linear metrics (Hlusko, 2000), morphological traits (Hlusko and Mahaney, 2003), loph/lophid orientation (Hlusko *et al.*, 2004b), and 2D areas (Hlusko *et al.*, in press b). There is evidence for incomplete pleiotropy between the maxillary and mandibular arches (Hlusko, 2000; Hlusko and Mahaney, 2003). We have also found significant genetic correlations between molar crown size and crown–rump length (body size) (Hlusko *et al.*, in press a).

As evidence for genetic correlations improves our understanding of morphological evolution, estimates of no genetic correlation can also be informative, although this must be done with caution. For example, we have performed a quantitative genetic analysis of enamel thickness in baboons as a model for understanding the genetic architecture of this phenotype in other primates, including humans (Hlusko *et al.*, 2004b). Hominid paleontologists have emphasized the importance of enamel thickness for decades, starting with "*Ramapithecus*" (Simons and Pilbeam, 1972), and more recently in the identification of newly recovered late Miocene hominids (Andrews, 1995; Brunet *et al.*, 2002; Leakey *et al.*, 1995; Senut *et al.*, 2001; White *et al.*, 1995). Genetic analyses of linear measurements of radial molar enamel thickness in this population of pedigreed baboons indicate that enamel thickness is heritable. However, interestingly, it is not genetically correlated with either sex or tooth size. This result suggests that enamel thickness could evolve rapidly through evolutionary time, tracking dietary shifts, and increasing the likelihood for homoplasy in this character.

We are also using these tests of genetic correlation to redefine the dental phenotype. Although much of this work is still in progress, we have reported results that demonstrate a genetic modularity that does not correspond with developmental modules. The orientation of mesial molar lophids is affected by complete pleiotropy along the tooth row, as is the orientation of the distal lophids. However, the mesial and distal lophids are found to be genetically independent (represented in Figure 14.2). As Workman *et al.* (2002) interpreted the mouse molar series to be indicative of the same genetic factors, baboon molars are similarly reflexive of the same genetic effects. However, the mesial and distal portions of the molar crown are independent of each other in terms of the orientation of the lophids, suggesting a level of modularity that cuts across the developmental module of a tooth.

Another dental phenotype studied in this population of pedigreed baboons also contributes new information about modularity, although the results are more difficult to reconcile with developmental genetics at this point in time. 2D molar cusp area appears to vary taxonomically in primates, although the majority of research to date has focused on extant and extinct hominoids (e.g. Bailey 2004; Corruccini, 1977; Erdbrink 1967; Hills *et al.* 1983; Kondo and Townsend, 2006; Macho, 1994; Sperber, 1974; Suwa *et al.*, 1994, 1996; Uchida 1998a, 1998b; Wood and Engleman 1988; Wood *et al.*, 1983). We undertook a quantitative genetic analysis of variation in this phenotype in this pedigreed population of baboons (Hlusko *et al.*, in press b). Our results show that while variation in cusp size is heritable and sexually dimorphic, there are interesting patterns of genetic correlation between the various cusps. For the first, second, and third mandibular molars the metaconid-hypoconid correlation is consistently estimated as 0.0, whereas the entoconid-protoconid correlation is estimated as 1.0. The other cusp pairs demonstrate incomplete pleiotropy. This diagonal pattern of complete and no genetic correlation counters what we currently know about tooth development and mineralization. We are now collecting data on maxillary molars in baboons and molar cusp area, in general, for mice in an attempt to clarify this conundrum.

Considerably more research is needed to determine whether or not the modularity identified through quantitative genetic analyses of mouse and baboon dental variation is also present in other primates. However, the approach looks promising. A similar analysis of cranial variation in New World monkeys has

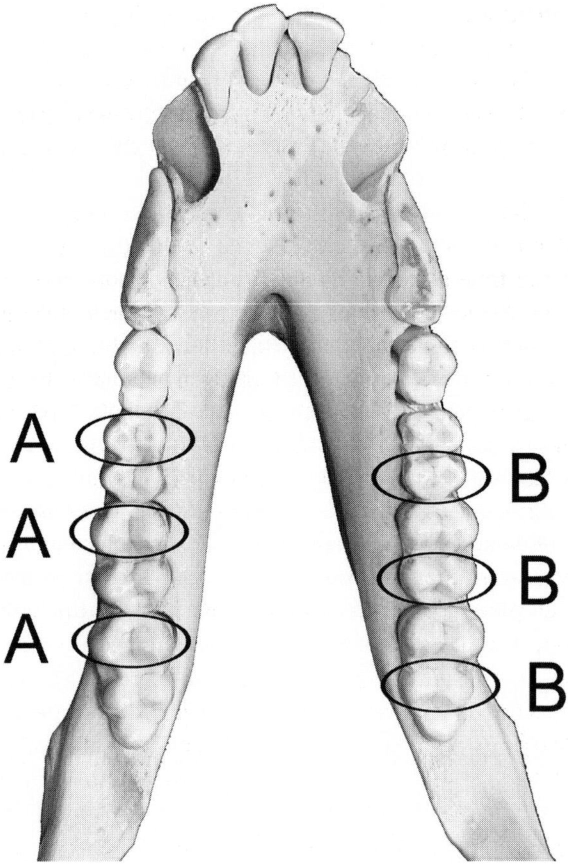

Figure 14.2 Baboon mandible in occlusal view. Quantitative genetic analyses have shown that first, second and third molar mesial lophid orientation (A) along the tooth row is determined by the same genetic effects, as is distal lophid orientation (B). However, the orientations of A and B on the same crown are genetically independent (Hlusko *et al.*, 2004a). See text for more details.

found that the genetic architecture appears to be conserved across taxa that diverged 30 million years ago (Marroig and Cheverud, 2005). Given that this cranial study relied on phenotypes with lower heritabilities than those of the dentition, we feel confident that the approach described herein for the dentition will yield informative results. If our initial results are bolstered through further analyses, these newly defined phenotypes will enable us to study dental variation in fossil taxa with a better understanding of what those morphological changes represent in terms of the evolving genotype, enabling us to reconstruct a genetic evolutionary history of the primate dentition (Hlusko, 2004).

14.8 Conclusions

The past 80 years have witnessed a revolution in quantitative genetic approaches to primate dental variation. What started out as a simple question concerning the presence or absence of a genetic contribution to population-level variation has diversified into fairly detailed questions of genetic correlation and gene mapping. Through all of this we have gained tremendous insight to the genetic architecture of primate dental variation. Virtually all tooth size and shape variation is heritable, with most estimates attributing a large portion of the variance to the additive effects of genes. Variation in occlusion, arch shape, and crowding appears to result primarily from non-genetic influences. Dominance, sex, and maternal effects have also been identified. Researchers have found evidence for differing genetic factors for anterior vs. posterior tooth types, and future research estimating genetic correlations promise to refine these propositions. We find two research directions particularly compelling at this point: (1) QTL analyses that are identifying specific chromosomal loci that have phenotypic effects, and (2) estimation of genetic correlations that are elucidating evolutionary modularity. The application of quantitative genetics to dental anthropology may just now be entering its heyday with much promise for the future.

Acknowledgments

MCM and LJH's research cited herein has been supported by the National Science Foundation under Grants No. 0500179 and 0130277. National Institutes of Health, National Center for Research Resources P51 RR013986 supports the Southwest National Primate Research Center. OTR is supported by a Chancellor's Fellowship, University of California Berkeley. SKA is supported in part by a Professional Development International Fellowship from the Wenner-Gren Foundation.

References

Alvesalo, L. and Tigerstedt, P. M. A. (1974). Heritabilities of human tooth dimensions. *Hereditas*, **77**, 311–18.

Alvesalo, L., Nuutila, M. and Portin, P. (1975). The cusp of Carabelli: occurrence in first upper molars and evaluation of its heritability. *Acta Odontologica Scandinavica*, **33**, 191–7.

Andrews, P. (1995). Ecological apes and ancestors (comment). *Nature*, **376**, 555–6.

Bachrach, F. H. and Young, M. (1927). A comparison of the degree of resemblance in dental characters shown in pairs of twins of identical and fraternal types. *British Dental Journal*, **48**, 1293–304.

Bader, R. S. (1965). Heritability of dental characters in the house mouse. *Evolution*, **19**, 378–84.

Bader, R. S. and Lehmann, W. H. (1965). Phenotypic and genotypic variation in odontometric traits of the house mouse. *American Midland Naturalist*, **74**, 28–38.

Bailey, S. E. (2004). A morphometric analysis of maxillary molar crowns of Middle-Late Pleistocene hominins. *Journal of Human Evolution*, **47**, 183–98.

Bailit, H. L. and Sung, B. (1968). Maternal effects on the developing dentition. *Archives of Oral Biology*, **13**, 155–61.

Bailit, H. L., Workman, P. L., Niswander, J. D., and MacLean, C. J. (1970). Dental asymmetry as an indicator of genetic and environmental conditions in human populations. *Human Biology*, **42**, 626–38.

Bateson, W. (1892). On numerical variation in teeth, with a discussion of the conception of homology. *Zoological Society of London, Proceedings*, pp. 102–5.

Baume, R. M. and Crawford, M. H. (1980). Discrete dental trait asymmetry in Mexican and Belizean groups. *American Journal of Physical Anthropology*, **52**, 315–21.

Biggerstaff, R. H. (1970). Morphological variations for the permanent mandibular first molars in human monozygotic and dizygotic twins. *Archives of Oral Biology*, **15**, 721–30.

Biggerstaff, R. H. (1973). Heritability of the Carabelli cusp in twins. *Journal of Dental Research*, **52**, 40–4.

Biggerstaff, R. H. (1975). Cusp size, sexual dimorphism, and heritability of cusp size in twins. *American Journal of Physical Anthropology*, **42**, 127–40.

Biggerstaff, R. H. (1976). Cusp size, sexual dimorphism, and the heritability of maxillary molar cusp size in twins. *Journal of Dental Research*, **55**, 189–95.

Blanco, R. and Chakraborty, R. (1976). The genetics of shovel shape in maxillary central incisors in man. *American Journal of Physical Anthropology*, **44**, 233–6.

Blangero, J. (2004). Localization and identification of human quantitative trait loci: king harvest has surely come. *Current Opinion in Genetics and Development*, **14**, 233–40.

Boraas, J. C., Messer, L. B., and Till, M. J. (1988). A genetic contribution to dental caries, occlusion, and morphology as demonstrated by twins reared apart. *Journal of Dental Research*, **67**, 1150–5.

Bowden, D. E. J. and Goose, D. H. (1968). The inheritance of palatal arch width in human families. *Archives of Oral Biology*, **13**, 1293–5.

Bowden, D. E. J. and Goose, D. H. (1969). Inheritance of tooth size in Liverpool families. *Journal of Medical Genetics*, **6**, 55–8.

Brunet, M., Guy, F., Pilbeam, D. *et al.* (2002). A new hominid from the Upper Miocene of Chad, Central Africa. *Nature*, **418**, 145–51.

Carroll, S. B., Grenier, J. K., and Weatherbee, S. D. (2005). *From DNA to Diversity*, 2nd edn. Malden: Blackwell Publishing.

Cheverud, J. M. (1982). Phenotypic, genetic, and environmental morphological integration in the cranium. *Evolution*, **36**, 499–516.

Cheverud, J. M. (1988). A comparison of genetic and phenotypic correlations. *Evolution*, **42**, 958–68.

Cheverud, J. M. (1989). A comparative analysis of morphological variation patterns in the papionins. *Evolution*, **43**, 1737–47.

Cheverud, J. M. (1995). Morphological integration in the saddle-back tamarin (*Saguinus fuscicollis*) cranium. *American Naturalist*, **145**, 63–89.
Cheverud, J. M. (1996). Developmental integration and the evolution of pleiotropy. *American Zoologist*, **36**, 44–50.
Cheverud, J. M. and Routman, E. (1993). Quantitative trait loci: individual gene effects on quantitative characters. *Journal of Evolutionary Biology*, **6**, 463–80.
Cheverud, J. M., Rutledge, J. J., and Atchley, W. R. (1983). Quantitative genetics of development: genetic correlations among age-specific trait values and the evolution of ontogeny. *Evolution*, **37**, 895–905.
Cheverud, J. M., Routman, E. J., and Irschick, D. K. (1997). Pleiotropic effects of individual gene loci on mandibular morphology. *Evolution*, **51**, 2004–14.
Chung, C. S. and Niswander, J. D. (1975). Genetic and epidemiologic studies of oral characteristics in Hawaii's schoolchildren: V. Sibling correlations in occlusion traits. *Journal of Dental Research*, **54**, 324–9.
Corruccini, R. S. (1977). Crown component variation in hominoid lower third molars. *Zeitschrift für Morphologie und Anthropologie*, **68**, 14–25.
Corruccini, R. S. and Potter, R. H. Y. (1980). Genetic analysis of occlusal variation in twins. *American Journal of Orthodontics*, **75**, 140–54.
Corruccini, R. S. and Potter, R. H. Y. (1981). Developmental correlates of crown component asymmetry and occlusal discrepancy. *American Journal of Physical Anthropology*, **55**, 21–31.
Corruccini, R. S. and Sharma, K. (1985). Within- and between-zygosity variance in oral traits among US and Punjabi twins. *Human Heredity*, **35**, 314–18.
Dahlberg, A. A. (1956). *Materials for the Establishment of Standards for Classification of Tooth Characteristics, Attributes, and Techniques in Morphological Studies of the Dentition*. Chicago: Zoller Laboratory of Dental Anthropology, University of Chicago.
Dempsey, P. J., Townsend, G. C., Martin, N. G., and Neale, M. C. (1995). Genetic covariance structure of incisor crown size in twins. *Journal of Dental Research*, **74**, 1389–98.
Dempsey, P. J. and Townsend, G. C. (2001). Genetic and environmental contributions to variation in human tooth size. *Heredity*, **86**, 685–93.
Di Salvo, N. A., Alumbaugh, C. E., Kwochka, W., Pilvelis, A. A., and Willcox, J. R. (1972). Genetic influence on mesiodistal width of deciduous anterior teeth. *American Journal of Orthodontics*, **61**, 473–8.
Drumm, M. L. and Collins, F. S. (1993). Molecular biology of cystic fibrosis. *Molecular Genetic Medicine*, **3**, 33–68.
Ehrich, T. H., Vaughn, T. T., Koreishi, S. F. *et al.* (2003). Pleiotropic effects on mandibular morphology I. Developmental morphological integration and differential dominance. *Journal of Experimental Zoology. Part B. Molecular Developmental Evolution*, **296**, 58–79.
El-Nofely, A. and Tawfik, W. A. (1995). On inheritance of permanent teeth crown size in a Middle Eastern population. *Homo*, **46**, 51–62.
Erdbrink, D. P. (1967). A quantification of lower molar patterns in deutero-Malayans. *Zeitschrift für Morphologia und Anthropologie*, **59**, 40–56.

Falconer, D. S. (1989). *Introduction to Quantitative Genetics*, 3rd edn. New York: Longman Scientific & Technical.

Finn, S. B. and Caldwell, R. C. (1963). Dental caries in twins – I. A comparison of the caries experience of monozygotic twins, dizygotic twins and unrelated children. *Archives of Oral Biology*, **8**, 571–85.

Fisher, R. A. (1918). The correlation between relatives on the supposition of Mendelian inheritance. *Transactions of the Royal Society of Edinburgh*, **52**, 399–433.

Galis, F. (1999). On the homology of structures and *Hox* genes: the vertebral column. *Novartis Foundation Symposium*, **222**, 80–91.

Garn, S. M., Lewis, A. B., and Polacheck, D. L. (1960). Sibling similarities in dental development. *Journal of Dental Research*, **39**, 170–5.

Garn, S. M., Lewis, A. B., and Kerewsky, R. S. (1965a). Genetic, nutritional, and maturational correlates of dental development. *Journal of Dental Research*, **44**, 228–42.

Garn, S. M., Lewis, A. B., and Kerewsky, R. S. (1965b). X-linked inheritance of tooth size. *Journal of Dental Research*, **44**, 439–41.

Garn, S. M., Lewis, A. B., and Kerewsky, R. S. (1966). Genetic independence of Carabelli's trait from tooth size or crown morphology. *Archives of Oral Biology*, **11**, 745–7.

Garn, S. M., Lewis, A. B., Swindler, D. R., and Kerewsky, R. S. (1967). Genetic control of sexual dimorphism in tooth size. *Journal of Dental Research*, Supplement to No. 5, **46**, 963–72.

Garn, S. M., Lewis, A. B. and Walenga, A. J. (1968). Genetic basis of the crown-size profile pattern. *Journal of Dental Research*, **47**, 1190.

Garn, S. M., Osborne, R. H., Alvesalo, L. and Horowitz, S. L. (1980). Maternal and gestational influences on deciduous and permanent tooth size. *Journal of Dental Research*, **59**, 142–3.

Gilmore, R. W. (1968). Epidemiology and heredity of accessory occlusal ridges on the buccal cusps of human premolar teeth. *Archives of Oral Biology*, **13**, 1035–46.

Goodman, H. O., Luke, J. E., Rosen, S. and Hackel, E. (1959). Heritability in dental caries, certain oral microflora and salivary components. *American Journal of Human Genetics*, **11**, 263–73.

Goose, D. H. (1967). Preliminary study of tooth size in families. *Journal of Dental Research*, **46**, 959–62.

Goose, D. H. (1968). The inheritance of tooth size in British families. In *Dental Morphology and Evolution*, ed. A. A. Dahlberg. Chicago: University of Chicago Press, pp. 263–70.

Goose, D. H. and Lee, G. T. R. (1971). The mode of inheritance of Carabelli's trait. *Human Biology*, **43**, 64–9.

Green, L. J. and Aszkler, S. E. (1970). Intra-alveolar dental development in twins. *Journal of Dental Research*, **49**, 631–4.

Haldane, J. B. S. (1932). *The Causes of Evolution*. London: Longmans, Green.

Harris, E. F. and Bailit, H. L. (1980). The metaconule: a morphologic and familial analysis of a molar cusp in humans. *American Journal of Physical Anthropology*, **53**, 349–58.

Harris, E. F. and Smith, R. J. (1980). A study of occlusion and arch widths in families. *American Journal of Orthodontics*, **78**, 155–63.

Harzer, W. (1987). A hypothetical model of genetic control of tooth-crown growth in man. *Archives of Oral Biology*, **32**, 159–62.

Harzer, W. (1995). Size relationships and interactions between crown diameters in twins and family members. In *Proceedings of the Tenth International Symposium on Dental Morphology*, ed. R. Radlanski and H. Renz. Berlin: "M" Marketing Services, pp. 124–35.

Hatton, M. E. (1955). A measure of the effects of heredity and environment on eruption of the deciduous teeth. *Journal of Dental Research*, **34**, 397–401.

Hills, M., Graham, S. H., and Wood, B. A. (1983). The allometry of relative cusp size in hominoid mandibular molars. *American Journal of Physical Anthropology*, **62**, 311–16.

Hlusko, L. J. (2000). *Identifying the genetic mechanisms of dental variation in cercopithecoid primates.* Ph.D. Dissertation, The Pennsylvania State University, UMI 9982340.

Hlusko, L. J. (2004). Perspective: integrating the genotype and phenotype in hominid paleontology. *Proceedings of the National Academy of Sciences USA*, **101**, 2653–7.

Hlusko, L. J., Mahaney, M. C., and Weiss, K. M. (2002). A statistical genetic comparison of two techniques for assessing molar crown size in pedigreed baboons. *American Journal of Physical Anthropology*, **117**, 182–9.

Hlusko, L. J. and Mahaney, M. C. (2003). Genetic contributions to expression of the baboon cingular remnant. *Archives of Oral Biology*, **48**, 663–72.

Hlusko, L. J., Maas, M. L., and Mahaney, M. C. (2004a). Statistical genetics of molar cusp patterning in pedigreed baboons: implications for primate dental development and evolution. *Journal of Experimental Zoology. Part B. Molecular Developmental Evolution*, **302**, 268–83.

Hlusko, L. J., Suwa, G., Kono, R., and Mahaney, M. C. (2004b). Genetics and the evolution of primate enamel thickness: a baboon model. *American Journal of Physical Anthropology*, **124**, 223–33.

Hlusko, L. J., Lease, L. R., and Mahaney M. C. (in press a). Evolution of genetically correlated traits: tooth size and body size in baboons. *American Journal of Physical Anthropology*.

Hlusko, L. J., Do, N., and Mahaney, M. C. (in press b). Genetic correlations between mandibular molar cusp areas in baboons. *American Journal of Physical Anthropology*.

Horowitz, S. L., Osborne, R. H., and DeGeorge, F. V. (1958a). Hereditary factors in tooth dimensions, a study of the anterior teeth of twins. *Angle Orthodontist*, **28**, 87–93.

Horowitz, S. L., Osborne, R. H., and DeGeorge, F. V. (1958b). Caries experience in twins. *Science*, **128**, 300–1.

Hughes, T., Dempsey, P., Richards, L., and Townsend, G. (2000). Genetic analysis of deciduous tooth size in Australian twins. *Archives of Oral Biology*, **45**, 997–1004.

Hunt, H. R., Hoppert, C. A., and Erwin, W. G. (1944). Inheritance of susceptibility to caries in albino rats (*Mus norvegicus*). *Journal of Dental Research*, **23**, 385–401.

Jernvall, J. and Thesleff, I. (2000). Reiterative signaling and patterning during mammalian tooth morphogenesis. *Mechanisms of Development*, **92**, 19–29.

Kaul, S. S., Sharma, K., Sharma, J. C., and Corruccini, R. S. (1985). Non-metric variants of the permanent dental crown in human monozygous and dizygous twins. In: *Dental Anthropology: Application and Methods*, ed. V. Rami Reddy. New Delhi: Inter-India Publications, pp. 187–93.

Klingenberg, C. P., Leamy, L. J., Routman, E. J., and Cheverud, J. M. (2001). Genetic architecture of mandible shape in mice: effects of quantitative trait loci analyzed by geometric morphometrics. *Genetics*, **157**, 785–802.

Kolakowski, D. and Bailit, H. L. (1981). A differential environmental effect on human anterior tooth size. *American Journal of Physical Anthropology*, **54**, 377–81.

Kolakowski, D., Harris, E. F., and Bailit, H. L. (1980). Complex segregation analysis of Carabelli's Trait in a Melanesian population. *American Journal of Physical Anthropology*, **53**, 301–8.

Kondo, S. and Townsend, G. C. (2006). Associations between Carabelli trait and cusp areas in human permanent maxillary first molars. *American Journal of Physical Anthropology*, **129**, 196–203.

Kraus, B. S., Wise, W. J., and Frei, R. H. (1959). Heredity and the craniofacial complex. *American Journal of Orthodontics*, **45**, 172–217.

Lande, R. (1979). Quantitative genetic analysis of multivariate evolution, applied to brain:body size allometry. *Evolution*, **33**, 402–16.

Lande, R. (1980). Genetic variation and phenotypic evolution during allopatric speciation. *American Naturalist*, **116**, 463–79.

Lawn, R. M. (1985). The molecular genetics of hemophilia: blood clotting factors VIII and IX. *Cell*, **42**, 405–6.

Leakey, M. G., Feibel, C. S., McDougall, I. and Walker, A. (1995). New four-million-year-old hominid species from Kanapoi and Allia Bay, Kenya. *Nature*, **376**, 565–71.

Leamy, L., Routman, E., and Cheverud, J. M. (1999). Quantitative trait loci for early and late developing skull characters in mice: a test of the genetic independence model of morphological integration. *American Naturalist*, **153**, 201–14.

Leamy, L. J., Pomp, D., Eisen, E. J., and Cheverud, J. M. (2000). Quantitative trait loci for directional but not fluctuating asymmetry of mandible characters in mice. *Genetical Research*, **76**, 27–44.

Leamy, L. J., Workman, M. S., Routman, E. J., and Cheverud, J. M. (2005). An epistatic genetic basis for fluctuating asymmetry of tooth size and shape in mice. *Heredity*, **94**, 316–25.

Lee, G. T. R. and Goose, D. H. (1972). The inheritance of dental traits in a Chinese population in the United Kingdom. *Journal of Medical Genetics*, **9**, 336–9.

Lee, G. T. R. and Goose, D. H. (1982). Heritability of dental occlusal variables in a family study in Liverpool, UK. *Archives of Oral Biology*, **27**, 987–9.

Lewis, D. W. and Grainger, R. M. (1967). Sex-linked inheritance of tooth size: a family study. *Archives of Oral Biology*, **12**, 539–44.

Lewontin, R. (2001). Foreword. In *The Character Concept in Evolutionary Biology*, ed. G. P. Wagner. New York: Academic Press, pp. xvii–xxiii.

Ludwig, F. J. (1957). The mandibular second premolars: morphologic variations and inheritance. *Journal of Dental Research*, **36**, 263–73.
Lundström, A. (1948). *Tooth Size and Occlusion in Twins*, 2nd edn. Basel: S. Karger.
Lundström, A. (1963). Tooth morphology as a basis for distinguishing monozygotic and dizygotic twins. *American Journal of Human Genetics*, **15**, 34–43.
Lundström, A. (1964). Size of teeth and jaws in twins. *British Dental Journal*, **117**, 321–6.
Lundström, A. (1967). Genetic aspects of variation in tooth width based on asymmetry and twin studies. *Hereditas*, **57**, 403–9.
Lynch, M. and Walsh, B. (1998). *Genetics and Analysis of Quantitative Traits.* Sunderland: Sinauer Associates, Inc.
Macho, G. A. (1994). Variation in enamel thickness and cusp area within human maxillary molars and its bearing on scaling techniques used for studies of enamel thickness between species. *Archives of Oral Biology*, **39**, 783–92.
Magwene, P. M. (2001). New tools for studying integration and modularity. *Evolution*, **55**, 1734–45.
Mansbridge, J. N. (1959). Heredity and dental caries. *Journal of Dental Research*, **38**, 337–47.
Marroig, G., DeVivo, M., and Cheverud, J. M. (2004). Cranial evolution in sakis (*Pithecia*, Platyrrhini) II: evolutionary processes and morphological integration. *Journal of Evolutionary Biology*, **17**, 144–55.
Marroig, G. and Cheverud, J. M. (2005). Size as a line of least evolutionary resistance: diet and adaptive morphological radiation in New World monkeys. *Evolution*, **59**, 1128–42.
Menezes, D. M., Foster, T. D., and Lavelle, C. L. B. (1974). Genetic influences on dentition and dental arch dimensions: a study of monozygotic and dizygotic triplets. *American Journal of Physical Anthropology*, **40**, 213–20.
Merwin, D. R. and Harris, E. F. (1998). Sibling similarities in the tempo of human tooth mineralization. *Archives of Oral Biology*, **43**, 205–10.
Mezey, J., Cheverud, J. M., and Wagner, G. (2000). Is the genotype-phenotype map modular? A statistical approach using mouse QTL data. *Genetics*, **156**, 305–11.
Mizoguchi, Y. (1977). Genetic variability in tooth crown characters: analysis by the tetrachoric correlation method. *Bulletin of the National Science Museum. Series D, Anthropology*, **3**, 37–62.
Mizoguchi, Y. (1978). Tooth crown characters on the lingual surfaces of the maxillary anterior teeth: analysis of the correlations by the method of path coefficients. *Bulletin of the National Science Museum. Series D, Anthropology*, **4**, 24–57.
Moore, G. R. and Hughes, B. O. (1942). Familial factors in diagnosis, treatment, and prognosis of dentofacial disturbances. *American Journal of Orthodontics and Oral Surgery*, **28**, 603–39.
Nichol, C. R. (1990). *Dental genetics and biological relationships of the Pima Indians of Arizona.* Ph.D. Dissertation, Arizona State University.
Niswander, J. D. and Chung, C. S. (1965). The effects of inbreeding on tooth size in Japanese children. *American Journal of Human Genetics*, **17**, 390–8.
Olson, E. C. and Miller, R. L. (1958). *Morphological Integration.* Chicago, University of Chicago Press.

Osborne, R. H., Horowitz, S. L., and De George, F. V. (1958). Genetic variation in tooth dimensions: a twin study of the permanent anterior teeth. *American Journal of Human Genetics*, **10**, 350–6.

Pelsmaekers, B., Loos, R., Carels, C., Derom, C., and Vlietinck, R. (1997). The genetic contribution to dental maturation. *Journal of Dental Research*, **76**, 1337–40.

Peyer, B. (1968). *Comparative Odontology*. Chicago: The University of Chicago Press.

Portin, P. and Alvesalo, L. (1974). The inheritance of shovel shape in maxillary central incisors. *American Journal of Physical Anthropology*, **41**, 59–62.

Potter, R. H. (1990). Twin half-sibs: a research design for genetic epidemiology of common dental disorders. *Journal of Dental Research*, **69**, 1527–30.

Potter, R. H. and Nance, W. E. (1976). A twin study of dental dimension. I: Discordance, asymmetry, and mirror imagery. *American Journal of Physical Anthropology*, **44**, 391–6.

Potter, R. H. Y., Yu, P. L., Dahlberg, A. A., Merritt, A. D., and Conneally, P. M. (1968). Genetic studies of tooth size factors in Pima Indian families. *American Journal of Human Genetics*, **20**, 89–99.

Potter, R. H., Nance, W. E., Yu, P. L., and Davis, W. B. (1976). A twin study of dental dimension II: independent genetic determinants. *American Journal of Physical Anthropology*, **44**, 397–412.

Potter, R. H. Y., Nance, W. E., and Yu, P. L. (1978). Genetic determinants of dental dimension: a twin study. *Progress in Clinical and Biological Research*, **24**, 235–40.

Potter, R. H. Y., Yu, P. L., and Christian, J. C. (1979). Association of twin zygosity with the mean and variance of tooth size. *Acta Geneticae Medicae et Gemellologiae*, **28**, 211–23.

Potter, R. H. Y., Corruccini, R. S., and Green, L. J. (1981). Variance of occlusion traits in twins. *Journal of Craniofacial Genetics and Developmental Biology*, **1**, 217–27.

Potter, R. H. Y., Rice, J. P., Dahlberg, A. A., and Dahlberg, T. (1983). Dental size traits within families: path analysis for first molar and lateral incisor. *American Journal of Physical Anthropology*, **61**, 3–289.

Provine, W. B. (1971). *The Origins of Theoretical Population Genetics*. Chicago: University of Chicago Press.

Raff, R. A. (1996). *The Shape of Life*. Chicago: The University of Chicago Press.

Rogers, J., Mahaney, M. C., Almasy L., Comuzzie, A. and Blangero, J. (1999). Quantitative trait linkage mapping in anthropology. *Yearbook of Physical Anthropology*, **42**, 127–51.

Rosen, S., Hunt, H. R., and Hoppert, C. A. (1961). The importance of the genotype on susceptibility to dental caries in the rat. *Journal of Dental Research*, **40**, 352–4.

Scott, G. R. (1973). *Dental morphology: a genetic study of American white families and variation in living southwest Indians*. Ph.D. Dissertation, Arizona State University.

Scott, G. R. (1980). Population variation of Carabelli's trait. *Human Biology*, **52**, 63–78.

Senut, B., Pickford, M., Gommery, D. *et al.* (2001). First hominid from the Miocene (Lukeino Formation, Kenya). *Comptes Rendue de l'Academie des Sciences. Série II. Fascicule A – Sciences de la Terre et des Planetes*, **332**, 137–44.

Sharma, K., Corruccini, R. S., and Henderson, A. M. (1985). Genetic variance in dental dimensions of Punjabi twins. *Journal of Dental Research*, **64**, 1389–91.

Shubin, N. (2002). Origin of evolutionary novelty: examples from limbs. *Journal of Morphology*, **252**, 15–28.

Shubin, N., Tabin, C., and Carroll, S. (1997). Fossils, genes, and the evolution of animal limbs. *Nature*, **388**, 639–48.

Simons, E. L. and Pilbeam, D. R. (1972). Hominoid paleoprimatology. In *The Functional and Evolutionary Biology of Primates*, ed. R. Tuttle. Chicago: Aldine, pp. 36–62.

Sirianni, J. E. and Swindler, D. R. (1973). Inheritance of deciduous tooth size in *Macaca nemestrina. Journal of Dental Research*, **52**, 179.

Sirianni, J. E. and Swindler, D. R. (1974). Tooth size inheritance in *Macaca nemestrina. Symposium Volume of the Fifth International Congress of Primatology*. Basel: S. Karger, pp. 12–19.

Skrinjaric, I., Slaj, M., Lapter, V., and Muretic, Z. (1985). Heritability of Carabelli's trait in twins. *Collegium Antropologicum*, **2**, 177–81.

Sofaer, J. A., MacLean, C. J., and Bailit, H. L. (1972). Heredity and morphological variation in early and late developing human teeth of the same morphological class. *Archives of Oral Biology*, **17**, 811–16.

Sperber, G. (1974). *Morphology of the cheek teeth of early South African hominids.* Ph.D. Thesis, University of the Witwatersrand.

Staley, R. N. and Green, L. J. (1971). Bilateral asymmetry in tooth cusp occurrence in human monozygotic twins, dizygotic twins, and nontwins. *Journal of Dental Research*, **50**, 83–9.

Stern, D. L. (2000). Perspective: evolutionary developmental biology and the problem of variation. *Evolution*, **54**, 1079–91.

Stock, D. W. (2001). The genetic basis of modularity in the development and evolution of the vertebrate dentition. *Philosophical Transactions of the Royal Society of London. Series B, Biological Sciences*, **356**, 1633–53.

Suwa, G., Wood, B. A., and White, T. W. (1994). Further analysis of mandibular molar crown and cusp areas in Pliocene and early Pleistocene hominids. *American Journal of Physical Anthropology*, **93**, 407–26.

Suwa, G., White, T. D., and Howell, F. C. (1996). Mandibular postcanine dentition from the Shungura formation, Ethiopia: crown morphology, taxonomic allocations, and Plio-Pleistocene hominid evolution. *American Journal of Physical Anthropology*, **101**, 247–82.

Swindler, D. R. (2002). *Primate Dentition*. New York: Cambridge University Press.

Tenczar, P. and Bader, R. S. (1966). Maternal effect in dental traits of the house mouse. *Science*, **152**, 1398–400.

Townsend, G. C. (1980). Heritability of deciduous tooth size in Australian Aboriginals. *American Journal of Physical Anthropology*, **53**, 297–300.

Townsend, G. C. (1985). Intercuspal distance of maxillary pre-molar teeth in Australian Aboriginals. *Journal of Dental Research*, **64**, 443–6.

Townsend, G. C. and Brown, T. (1978a). Inheritance of tooth size in Australian Aboriginals. *American Journal of Physical Anthropology*, **48**, 305–14.

Townsend, G. C. and Brown, T. (1978b). Heritability of permanent tooth size. *American Journal of Physical Anthropology*, **49**, 497–504.

Townsend, G. C. and Martin, N. G. (1992). Fitting genetic models to Carabelli trait data in South Australian twins. *Journal of Dental Research*, **71**, 403–9.

Townsend, G. C., Brown, T., Richards, L. C. *et al.* (1986). Metric analyses of the teeth and faces of South Australian twins. *Acta Geneticae Medicae et Gemellologiae*, **35**, 179–92.

Townsend, G. C., Richards, L. C., Brown, T. and Burgess, (V. B.) (1988). Twin zygosity determination on the basis of dental morphology. *Journal of Forensic Odonto-Stomatology*, **6**, 1–15.

Townsend, G. C., Richards, L. C., Brown, T., Burgess, V. B., Travan, G. R. and Rogers, J. R. (1992). Genetic studies of dental morphology in South Australian twins. In *Structure, Function and Evolution of Teeth*, ed. P. Smith & E. Tchernov, pp. 501–18. London: Freund Publishing House.

Townsend, G., Richards, L., and Hughes, T. (2003). Molar intercuspal dimensions: genetic input to phenotypic variations. *Journal of Dental Research*, **82**, 350–5.

Tucker, A. and Sharpe, T. (2004). The cutting-edge of mammalian development; how the embryo makes teeth. *Nature Review Genetics*, **5**, 499–508.

Turner, C. G. II (1967). Dental genetics and microevolution in prehistoric and living Koniag Eskimo. *Journal of Dental Research*, **46**, 911–17.

Turner, C. G., II, Nichol, C. R., and Scott, G. R. (1991). Scoring procedures for key morphological traits of the permanent dentition: the Arizona State University Dental Anthropology System. In *Advances in Dental Anthropology*, ed. M. A. Kelley and C. S. Larsen. New York: Wiley-Liss, pp. 13–31.

Uchida, A. (1998a). Variation in tooth morphology of *Gorilla gorilla. Journal of Human Evolution*, **34**, 55–70.

Uchida, A. (1998b). Variation in tooth morphology of *Pongo pygmaeus. Journal of Human Evolution*, **34**, 71–9.

von Dassow, G., Meir, E., Munro, E. M. and Odell, G. M. (2000). The segment polarity network is a robust developmental module. *Nature*, **406**, 188–92.

Wagner, G. P. and Altenberg, L. (1996). Complex adaptations and the evolution of evolvability. *Evolution*, **50**, 967–76.

Weiss, K. M. (1990). Duplication with variation: metameric logic in evolution from genes to morphology. *Yearbook of Physical Anthropology*, **33**, 1–23.

Weiss, K. M., Stock, D. W., and Zhao, Z. (1998). Dynamic interactions and the evolutionary genetics of dental patterning. *Critical Reviews in Oral Biology and Medicine*, **9**, 369–98.

White, T. D., Suwa, G., and Asfaw, B. (1995). *Australopithecus ramidus*, a new species of early hominid from Aramis, Ethiopia. *Nature*, **375**, 88.

Wood, B. A. and Engleman, C. A. (1988). Analysis of the dental morphology of Plio-Pleistocene hominds. V. Maxillary postcanine tooth morphology. *Journal of Anatomy*, **161**, 1–35.

Wood, B. A., Abbott, S. A., and Graham, S. H. (1983). Analysis of the dental morphology of Plio-Pleistocene hominds. II. Mandibular molars – study of cusp areas, fissure pattern and cross sectional shape of the crown. *Journal of Anatomy*, **137**, 287–314.

Wood, B. F. and Green, L. J. (1969). Second premolar morphologic trait similarities in twins. *Journal of Dental Research*, **48**, 74–8.
Workman, M. S., Leamy, L. J., Routman, E. J., and Cheverud, J. M. (2002). Analysis of quantitative trait locus effects on the size and shape of mandibular molars in mice. *Genetics*, **160**, 1573–86.
Wright, S. (1921). Systems of mating. I. The biometric relations between parents and offspring. *Genetics*, **6**, 111–23.

Section IV

Forefront of technique

15 *Methods of ingestion and incisal designs*

KALPANA R. AGRAWAL, KAIYANG ANG, ZHONGQUAN SUI, HUGH T. W. TAN, AND PETER W. LUCAS

15.1 Introduction

Those who research in food texture have long known that the first bite is a critical element of the feeding process. It is probable that many sensory decisions about the nature of the food mechanical properties that control particle fracture are made at this point (Bourne, 2002; Vincent *et al.*, 2002). At least this is likely to be true for homogeneous foods that do not change much in texture as they are chewed (but is much less valid for industrially processed foods that melt or dissolve in the mouth). This "fact" appears to be recognized culturally, and is often imbued with social importance, such as when someone is expected or encouraged to express his or her appreciation of a dish at a social occasion immediately after "trying" something by biting into it (Visser, 1991). Taste is, of course, involved in such assessments, but texture nearly always has a role too.

Despite this interest, the first bite has not been the subject of much mechanical investigation. What happens when humans bite into food particles with their incisors? Is there simply flow of the food particle as the upper and/or lower teeth ease their way through it so as to eventually contact? It might be felt that the name "incision" implies that this is what happens. However, is fracture of the food particle involved? Why should the incisors of anthropoid primates be spatulate (when this is otherwise rare in mammals), and why is incisal shape generally very different from that of the postcanines? The answers are not trivial, just as they are not for the analysis of hand tools, things that Atkins and Mai (1985) have, for example, pointed out with respect to the explanation of the use of utensils for processing foods. Yet, little can be found in the literature on this point prior to the pioneering study of Osborn *et al.* (1986), and nothing systematic in the field prior to Ungar (1994) and Yamashita (2003).

Technique and Application in Dental Anthropology ed. Joel D. Irish and Greg C. Nelson
Published by Cambridge University Press.

15.2 Is incision a flow process or does it involve fracture?

Solids always have a significant elastic resistance to load because it is via this characteristic that they can maintain their shape. On unloading, they may return to their original shape immediately or, instead, take their time. The latter time-dependent elasticity is called "viscoelasticity" and is typical of biological tissues. Beyond a certain stress, i.e. the yield stress, all solids start to distort plastically and flow. However, even if some part of a solid object is flowing, it may also be developing cracks or fractures nearby. Does incision involve flow or fracture?

Firstly, the distinction between flow and fracture in solids is not necessarily the chasm that it can appear. Both processes create new surfaces, and fracture is often accompanied by flow. The closer that a true solid gets to its melting point, the more likely it is that there will be some flow close to the crack tip. Secondly, whatever the temperature, the smaller the particle, the more probable it is that a considerable amount of flow will accompany its fracture. If foods behave like real solids (and it must be remembered that foods are structured "solids" that also contain fluid and sometimes also air (Gibson and Ashby, 1997)), then there will be a critical particle size at which their behavior will change from fracturing at all, to instead start flowing under load. This size threshold is often called a "brittle–ductile" or "deformation" transition (Atkins and Mai, 1985). In any group of homogeneous solids with stress–strain behaviors that are linear almost to failure, a combination of material properties governs this change. The governing group of properties can be symbolized as $(ER)/Y^2$, where E is the elastic modulus, R the toughness (in terms of the energy required to make unit area of crack surface) and Y the yield stress. In some studies, instead of the yield stress, hardness (H) is used (Lawn, 1993) because it can be measured much more easily. Lawn gives $(ER)/H^2$ as the functional property group, for which there is lots of evidence from investigations on ceramics (Rhee *et al.*, 2001). In many materials, $H \approx 3Y$ (Ashby and Jones, 1996), but this relationship has to be viewed with reservation in any generalized sense because $H \approx Y$ in foams (Wilsea *et al.*, 1975). The latter probably has great relevance for foods since most of them are cellular in some way or other, and cellularity is a structural form that is effectively synonymous with the foams (Gibson and Ashby, 1997).

The particle size at which a deformation transition is observed depends not just on the above material property groups, but also on a constant that is very sensitive to the geometry of the load. Under compression, this constant is nearly equal to 10 (Kendall, 1978), while under indentation it may be 100 times that value (Atkins and Mai, 1985; Lawn, 1993).

It is unclear how far such indices can be translated to foods. Thus, all that this section of our chapter can really say is that the characteristics of the load, the mechanical properties of the food, and food particle size all influence whether food fractures or flows. However, it is certainly not true that flow is a pure function of tooth form. Although this is an undoubted influence, incision cannot always be categorized like this. The fact is not lost on the designers of modern foods. Thin chocolate bars flow when they are bitten into with the incisors, while fat ones may shatter – this being an important feature of chocolate texture. In short, we argue that rheology (the study of deformation and flow) is insufficient to understand incision, and that fracture mechanics is vital.

15.3 The evolution of spatulate incisors in primates

Most mammals have pointed incisors, and this was certainly a feature of the earliest forms (Hopson, 2001). Simian primates are different though, having a broad "spatulate" edge to their incisors (Martin, 1990). Anthropoids probably evolved in the Eocene into diurnal frugivores (Ross and Kay, 2004), and it has been suggested that spatulate incisors could have evolved in relation to fruit eating (Lucas, 1989, 2004; Lucas and Corlett, 1991). This argument rests on the characteristic covering of fruits that primates eat as a minority of their diets in tropical rain forests.

Generally, the flesh of fruits is the main constituent that plants construct with the intention that it be eaten (Vincent, 1990). The flesh has to be removed from around the enclosed seed(s), or else they are unlikely to germinate, instead being killed by fungal infections. Over the past 65 million years or more, as judged from angiosperm diversity data (Eriksson *et al.*, 2000), plants evolved an array of fruit characteristics in order to target guilds of fruit consumers that would favor the dispersal of their contained seed(s). These characteristics are many and include fruit color, size, shape, the number and form of the contained seeds, fruit flesh composition (in both chemical and physical senses), and the physical form of the outer covering.

Several "seed dispersal" syndromes have been suggested that associate a target guild of dispersers like birds, bats, or other mammals with particular fruit characteristics; however, confirmation of these relationships from field studies is generally lacking (Jordano, 1995). Fruits eaten almost exclusively by anthropoid primates are often quite large, sugar-fleshed, single-seeded fruits, with an orange, brown, or yellow coloration, and with a protective covering (Leighton, 1993) that is called a rind (Janson, 1983; Whitten, 1982) or a peel (Lucas, 1989). Anthropoid primates are one of a very few groups of extant animals that consume fruits with such coverings, which tend to peel cleanly from their underlying flesh. In this feature, they contrast with thinner fruit skins (Janson, 1983) that are difficult to remove without damaging the flesh. Yet, if a peel is not removed, digestion of the underlying flesh is obstructed.

Fruits with peels are rarely, if ever, the majority of fruits that modern simians consume (Gautier-Hion *et al.*, 1985, Janson, 1983; Lucas and Corlett, 1991); however, such fruits are difficult to consume at all unless animals have broad blade-like ingestive devices such as spatulate incisors. This is because any fracture created in the peel will easily divert from the peel-flesh interface unless the crack is fairly precisely controlled. Such a situation is commonly investigated in materials science where it has been realized that the difficulty in separating two adhering layers, such as those of a fruit peel and its underlying flesh, can be measured as the "work of peeling." The work of peeling is measured as the work required to separate a unit area of peel, with extensive investigations by Kendall (2001) proving that this is a fundamental physical quantity. This "work done per unit area" measure is an exact parallel of the toughness parameter R, described above, in that the integrity of the interface depends entirely on the energy required to cleave unit area of interfacial surface.

The work of peeling can be measured in a number of ways, but a common one involves the use of a wedge (Kendall, 2001). In such experiments (Figure 15.1a), a wedge is placed into a pre-arranged notch directed along the interface. The included angle of the wedge must be sufficiently large to impart enough strain energy, via bending one or both of the two layers, so as to extend the interfacial crack by a measurable amount. The tip of the wedge does not contact the crack tip, and so does not need to be particularly sharp. The use of wedges like this to measure interfacial toughness dates back to Obreimoff's investigation of mica in the 1930s – one of the earliest studies in fracture mechanics (Lawn, 1993). If the peel is tough enough, then it can also be lifted away from the underlying tissue directly (Figure 15.1b),with the work required per unit area of exposed undersurface being the same via the two methods of measurement, provided that friction is accounted for and that all work done in bending goes into crack growth.

Can spatulate incisors be compared to wedges? As will be discussed a little later, it has recently been argued that their tips can indeed be modeled in this way (Ang *et al.*, 2006). However, incisors are not experimental tools, and a primate needs first to penetrate the fruit peel before the incisors can be manipulated along the peel–flesh interface. The essential difference in form for this purpose between an incisor and a wedge involves the need for a sharp enough tip to pierce the peel in a controlled fashion. The work (again, per unit of fractured area) depends on peel toughness.

The design of the peel has to be organized by a plant so that it can be removed without fracturing. Accordingly, its thickness is likely to be restricted to below a

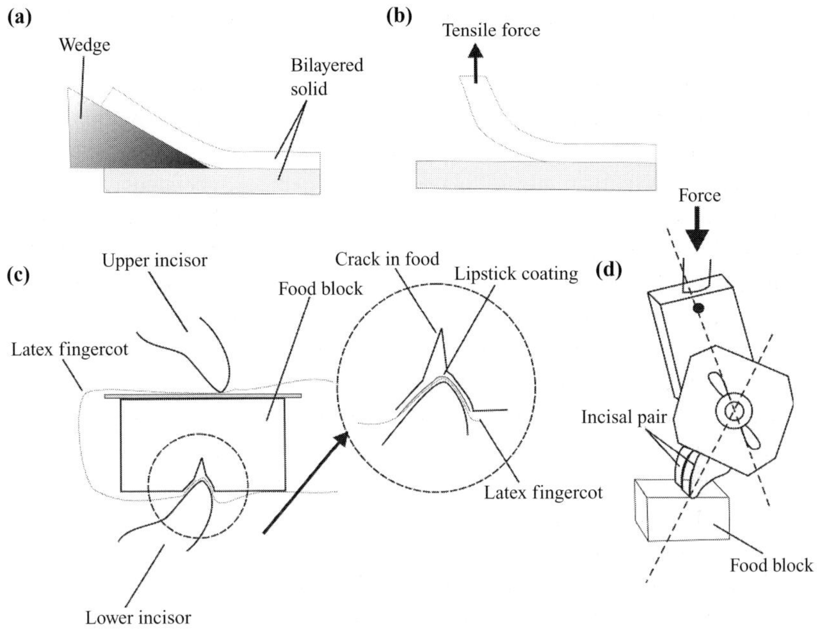

Figure 15.1 (a) and (b) show different ways in which the work of peeling can be measured. The resistance to peeling is given by the work per unit area of peeled surface and is independent of stress (Kendall, 2001). Provided that friction is taken into account in wedging, the two methods should give identical results. (c) shows the basis of the in vivo experimental setup of Agrawal and Lucas (2003); (d) that of the in vitro experiments of Sui *et al.* (2006).

deformation transition threshold in order that the target guild of fruit dispersers can remove it without fracturing. Birds have great difficulty attacking fruits with peels using their beaks, because any cracks they produce tend to divert into the flesh, leaving the peel essentially intact. The same appears true for mammals with pointed incisors.

The properties of fruit peels have nothing to do with that of the fruit flesh. Thus, the shapes of the incisors of simian primates need not have any relation to those of their postcanines.

15.4 Incisal orientation

In this section, we record our own initial investigations into how spatulate incisors work and how crown orientation affects this. We have concentrated on humans, who use their incisors in a wide variety of ways.

15.4.1 In vivo testing

Agrawal and Lucas (2003) investigated the use of the incisors in human subjects to fracture supra-threshold-sized particles of nuts and cheeses, using a well-known relationship between the energetic and stress-based methods of analyzing fracture. Brittle materials do not simply break when any given stress is exceeded; they break only when a given multiple of the stress and the square root of the length of the largest flaw within them occur, where this length is measured in the direction of the force. If the length of the initial flaw, usually introduced experimentally in the form of a thin notch, is denoted as a, and the stress at which this notch starts to grow under load as σ_F, then $\sigma_F.a^{1/2}$ gives the core of the definition of K – the "critical stress intensity factor" (also called "toughness" in some countries). The formal definition is:

$$K_{IC} = c_1 \sigma_F a^{1/2}, \tag{15.1}$$

where c_1 is a constant that depends again on the circumstances of loading. Of the subscripts of K, the Roman numeral "I" means fracture due to tensile stresses, while "C" means the "critical" value of K when the crack extends.

As shown in textbooks (e.g. Atkins and Mai, 1985), $K_{IC} \approx (ER)^{1/2}$, which means that:

$$(ER)^{1/2} = c_2 \sigma_F a^{1/2}, \tag{15.2}$$

where c_2 is a constant. This constant differs from c_1 because of approximations made in assuming $K_{IC} \approx (ER)^{1/2}$. Agrawal and Lucas (2003) offered a variety of foods to subjects for biting. They measured the food mechanical properties, E and R, on the left-hand side of Equation (15.2) by in vitro mechanical testing, and attempted to assess the variables, σ_F and a, on the right-hand side of the same equation by in vivo techniques. Then, for the different foods, the in vivo group $\sigma_F a^{1/2}$ was plotted against the in vitro property group $(ER)^{1/2}$ to establish if the relationship was linear as predicted and, if so, to calculate c_2.

The in vivo portion of the work involved trying to estimate the remote stress (equivalent to σ_F at failure) using a stress-sensitive film and the depth of incisal indentation (penetration) into a food particle prior to crack growth via marking the incisal tip with lipstick (denoting this as a Figure 15.1c). The problems with this study were the unknown accuracy of judging the stress, and the fact that the stress-sensitive film prevented the indentation of either upper or lower incisors. The uppers are impeded in Figure 15.1c, but the film can be switched to the lower side of the food specimen to investigate the bite of the uppers.

Agrawal and Lucas (2003) found that their plots were indeed linear, but that the high value of c_2 implied considerable inefficiency of the bite compared to theoretical predictions. Further, there was a lot of variation between subjects, which they speculated was connected to variability in incisal orientation.

15.4.2 In vitro tests on incisal replicas

In a search for more information on the effect of incisal orientation, Sui *et al.* (2006) mounted pairs of lower incisal replicas (cut from dental study models) on a testing machine. As shown in Figure 15.1d, only one pair of incisors, upper or lower, could be tested at a time. These replicas were oriented at varying angles to a force that their tips could apply to the surface of a (supra-threshold-sized) food specimen placed below them (Figure 15.1d). The experiments involved penetrating the food particles in a linearly vertical path, and recording the work done divided by the apparent area of new (fractured) surface they created. This quantity was termed the "work to fracture," and could be compared to values obtained from mechanical tests on the foods to check the relative efficiency of the bite. The results showed clearly again that bites are far from optimally efficient (at this particular task anyway), and that their orientation had a very strong effect on the work to fracture. The most efficient orientations were with incisors oriented close to vertical (i.e. with the axis bisecting the included angle of the tip being parallel to the direction of loading), with perhaps a slight proclination (procumbency) being optimal (although this lacked statistical support).

15.4.3 Theoretical modeling

The results of the above investigations need theoretical help, and Ang *et al.* (2006) supplied this by modeling the incisal tips (which were all that penetrated the food particles in Sui *et al.*'s study) as wedges. Obviously, this is an approximation, but it is necessary to allow equations to be constructed. The model was built on the solutions of Williams (1998) for a wedge oriented with one face parallel to the direction of the force (as in Figure 15.1a), impressing it into a food particle of given toughness, R. Since the equations do not take plastic flow into account, toughness is denoted as G, which is the "strain energy release rate" for a linearly elastic solid. The value of G is identical to R when there is a linear stress–strain gradient to fracture without any plastic contribution. Ang *et al.* (2006) furthered this result by considering a wedge inclined at various angles to the direction of loading. In all cases, the total work expended to create a unit length crack depended on the coefficient of friction between the wedge and food particle, the thickness of the wedge (its included angle), and the angle of inclination of the wedge. For a wedge of the thickness of a human incisor and coefficients of friction similar to those measured by Sui *et al.* (2006), curves similar to (but not matching) those of Sui *et al.*'s on incisal models were obtained. Orientations close to the vertical were more efficient than large inclinations. However, the lower the coefficient of friction, the more efficient inclinations of up to 30° off the vertical would be compared to 0° (vertical). The difference was marginal, but if the thickness (included angle) of the wedge was reduced, then theory definitely predicts the potential for an inclined wedge to be more efficient than a vertical one. The prediction is yet to be tested on wedges or, if this analogy is correct, on incisors. The work may be of major importance in explaining a number of features of tools that are currently discussed in an empirical way – in particular, the concepts of rake and relief (Ang *et al.*, 2006).

15.4.4 Measuring incisal proclination

There is no generally accepted method of measuring incisal orientation in primate skulls. We suggest that it could be achieved by measuring the position of four points on a skull or mandible very accurately. In Figure 15.2a, point 1 lies at the apex of the inter-alveolar crest between central incisors. Point 2 is the point of contact between the tips of the central incisors. Point 3 is at the apex of the inter-alveolar crest between canine and anterior premolar, while point 4 is at the apex of the inter-alveolar crest between this premolar and the one distal to it. The occlusal plane could be considered parallel to a plane including points 1, 3 and 4. The sagittal plane is normal to it and is defined relative to the occlusal plane by the inclusion of points 1 and 2 (Figure 15.2b). From this, the angle of incisal proclination or retroclination can be calculated, as in Figure 15.2c.

15.5 Incisal relationships

Many primates that feed predominantly on leaves have an incisal underbite (called an incisal underjet by dentists, a terminology followed here) in which the tips of the lower incisors lie anterior to those of the uppers (Sirianni, 1979; Swindler, 2002; Zingeser, 1970). Most other primates have an edge-to-edge incisal relationship or a slight incisal overjet instead. The exact function of an underjet in consuming leaves is not yet known, but it is believed to aid in stripping leaves (Ungar, 1992, 1994). This is an activity in which the incisors are used to grip leaves or branches rather than to fracture them. Here, we offer

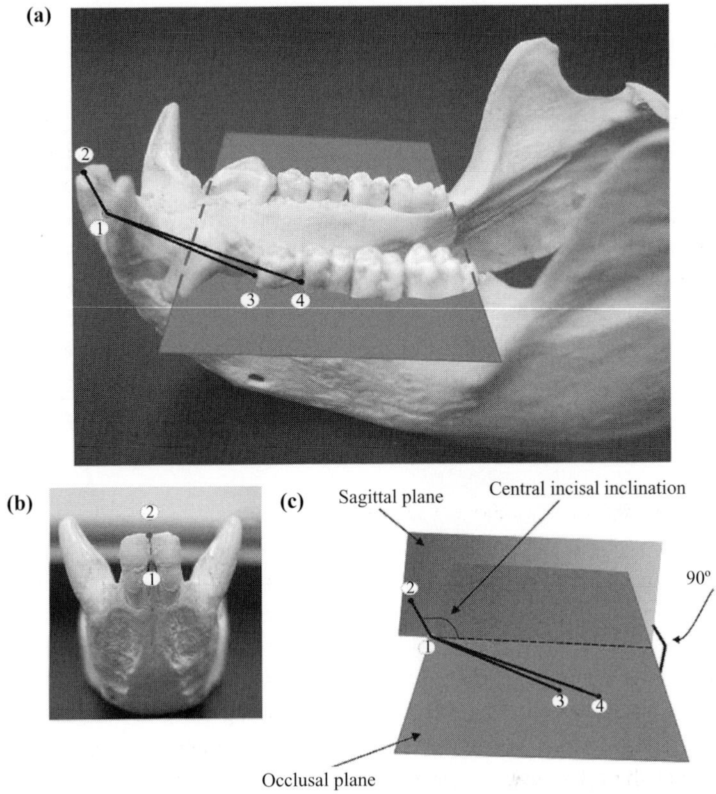

Figure 15.2 Four points that can be used to define angle of incisal proclination in primates. A male *Macaca nemestrina* mandible is illustrated. The points are defined in the text. (a) Points 1, 3 and 4 lie in the occlusal plane. (b) Points 1 and 2 lie in the sagittal plane. (c) shows the calculation of the angle of proclination.

an analysis of the relative ability of upper and lower incisors, arranged either as edge-to-edge, or with an overjet or underjet, for this gripping function. It is based on the assumption that when primates feed on leaves, they will use their hand(s) to hold a branch and then grip the leaves or branch using their incisors. Since the upper limbs are attached to the trunk below the jaw, the motion of the hand in stripping the leaves off a branch is downward and forward.

Figure 15.3a shows upper and lower central incisors gripping onto a branch or piece of leaf material in an edge-to-edge relationship. The gripping force is produced by pressing the lower incisors onto the upper incisors, and has a magnitude of $2\mu F$, where F is the normal contact force during mandibular elevation and μ is the coefficient of friction. In this case, the amount of grip may depend rather significantly on the area of contact between the incisal edge and

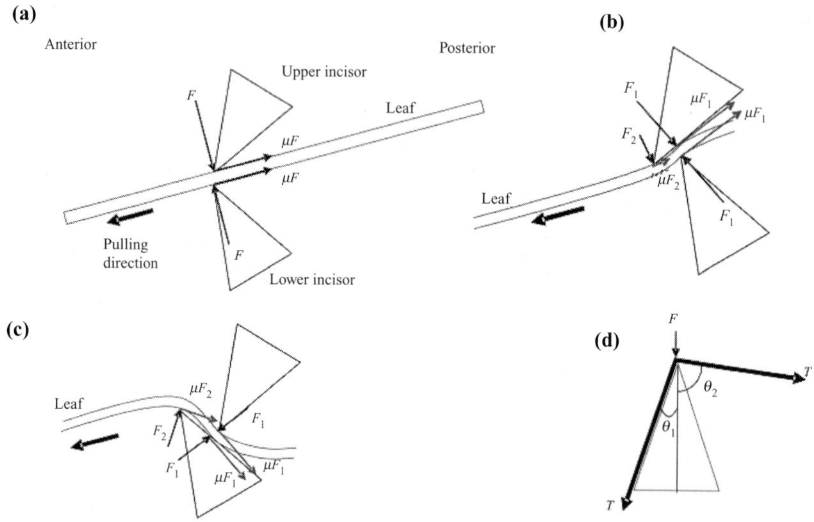

Figure 15.3 Factors that may favor an underjet in primates that strip leaves from branches (see text).

the leaf, because the area of contact may be tiny. Although macroscopically, friction is independent of surface area, microscopically, as surface area reduces, the friction coefficient can decrease, so reducing grip. Unless significant wear is present on the incisors, the contact area is likely to be very small, and hence friction is likely to be small too. The situation will be made worse if the upper and lower incisal edges do not contact fully.

In Figure 15.3b, an overjet incisal relationship is shown; here the direction of pulling, as well as the orientation of the incisors, remains unchanged from Figure 15.3a, except for a lateral translation of the lower incisors toward the posterior. As can be observed, there is an additional source of friction near the tip of the upper incisors, due to the bending of the leaf at the upper incisal edge. This additional frictional force only exists at certain angles of leaf pulling, and if the direction of pulling is directed too downward in the figure, there will no longer be any friction at the upper incisal edge; however, the friction at the lower incisal edge will increase. When a material is designed to move in a bending manner, the friction at the bends can be rather high. At the bends, the moving leaf will be pressed against the bending point (the upper incisal edge), and conform to the surface contours of the bending point. Therefore, even if the incisal edge is uneven, the leaf material will still deform to fit the surface contour, ensuring good contact between the incisal edge and the leaf surface. However, in overjet, the bending is not that severe, so the friction is not that great. Yet, with the slight bends and the addition of a frictional force at the upper incisal edge, the friction available in the overjet incisal relationship seems to be greater than for the edge-to-edge incisal relationship.

Finally in Figure 15.3c, we consider an underjet incisal relationship in which the direction of pulling, as well as the orientation of the incisors, remains unchanged – except for a lateral translation of the lower incisors toward the anterior. Similar to overjet, there exists a third frictional force – this time at the lower incisal edge. The magnitude of this third frictional force will be greater than the one in the overjet incisal relationship, due to the greater curvature of the leaf at the incisal edge. Such an underjet will function particularly well for gripping objects being pulled forward and downward. The greater the pulling force is directed downward, the greater will be the grip of the incisors. This kind of incisal relationship works in a way similar to the strap and buckle used in clothing. By bending a strap through a buckle, the friction between the strap and the buckle can be very great, and will increase as the strap is made to bend more. Figure 15.3d illustrates this point, where the force F acting at the equivalent of a lower incisal tip is given in terms of a pulling force T, and is equal to $T\cos\theta_1 + T\cos\theta_2$. As the strap is bent more, θ_1 will decrease due to the downward motion of the hand, and θ_2 may decrease depending on the action of the tongue. However, for any given value of μ, this increases the gripping force, which presumably increases success in stripping.

15.6 Deformation transitions

To go back to our first question, is incision a flow or a fracture process? The answer depends on the size of a food particle and its mechanical properties. Agrawal (unpublished) has attempted to define deformation transitions for seven foods: five cheeses and two nuts. All were picked because they are reasonably homogenous and have relatively linear stress–strain behaviors. Four human subjects made bites, as naturally as possible, on particles of these foods of differing thicknesses. Many particle thicknesses were made for these experiments, the other dimensions being, and kept, larger and constant. Fracture surfaces of foods are, in general, difficult to image because they are highly reflective; however, as far as possible, such images were inspected for the particle thickness above which fractures could be seen, and below which surfaces looked smooth (or "smeared") implying flow. In addition to E and R (measured without any plastic contribution; thus as G), H was also measured using Vickers macroindenters – allowing about 1 mm of indenter penetration. In Figure 15.4, the preliminary results are shown without error bars. The slope of the plot is ~3.1. Supposing $H = kY$, with k being a constant that for a Vickers indenter lies around 3, this

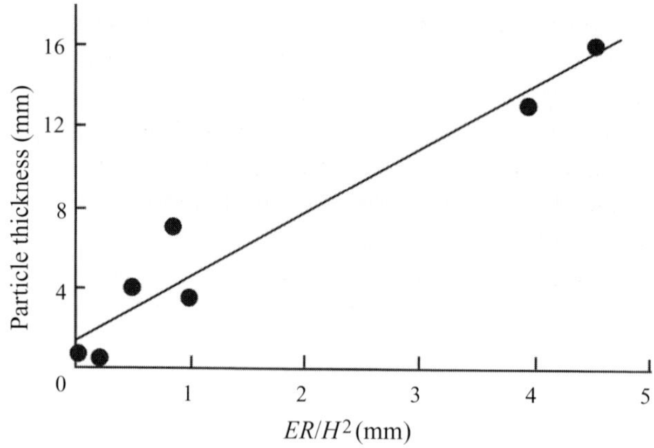

Figure 15.4 The relationship between the particle thickness of two types of nut (the two points lying at bottom left) and five cheeses above which particles fracture between the incisors and a group of mechanical properties that control this deformation transition in materials (see text).

result (graph slope multiplied by *k*) is consistent with Kendall's (1978) value for a deformation transition constant around 10 with a compressive loading.

If correct, this study has ramifications way beyond the modeling of incision. The whole diet of a primate or other mammal may be characterized for dental purposes by this property group. Lucas (2004) has suggested that if food particles propagate fractures, then the molars will have cusps and basins as their prominent features. In contrast, if foods will not crack, blades or crests are necessary. These features could in fact be predicted by measuring $(ER)/H^2$, the characteristic particle size that the incisors bite on, and the sizes that are typically ingested.

15.7 Conclusions

Incision is a far more complicated process than most people seem to think, and the work reported here actually only scratches the surface. All current work on incision seems to be focused on the investigation of the incisal bite force direction (Hylander, 1978; Paphangkorakit and Osborn, 1997) or biting efficiency (Agrawal and Lucas, 2003; Ang *et al.*, 2006; Osborn *et al.*, 1986; Sui *et al.*, 2006) in relation to movements that only involve the lowering and raising of the lower jaw. Undoubtedly, there are good reasons for doing so, because this simple movement is the most basic way to effect incision, and is possibly the easiest to study. However in real life, incision is often not just solely effected by the simple act of lowering and raising the lower jaw, but could also be accompanied by the movement of the head, neck, or both. Such additional movements may be especially necessary if the food is not ideally positioned for taking a bite, like the apples in a "bobbing for apples" game. Osborn *et al.* (1986) recognized this very clearly. However, while incision involving this additional maneuvering is difficult to study, it would probably reflect a truer picture of incision than those that require subjects to sit upright in a forward-facing position. Such studies, if undertaken, would probably require the extensive use of opto-electronic devices to record the movements and relate them to readings from force transducers placed intra-orally.

References

Agrawal, K. R. and Lucas, P. W. (2003). Mechanics of the first bite. *Proceedings of the Royal Society London series B*, **270**, 1277–82.

Ang, K. Y., Lucas, P. W., and Tan, H. T. W. (2006). Incisal orientation and biting efficiency. *Journal of Human Evolution*, **50**, 663–72.

Ashby, M. F. and Jones, D. R. H. (1996). *Engineering Materials 1*, 2nd edn. Oxford: Butterworth Heineman.

Atkins, A. G. and Mai, Y.-W. (1985). *Elastic and Plastic Fracture*. Chichester: Ellis Horwood.

Bourne, M. C. (2002). *Food Texture and Viscosity*. 2nd edn. New York: Academic Press.

Eriksson, O., Friis, E. M., and Löfgren, P. (2000). Seed size, fruit size, and dispersal systems in angiosperms from the early Cretaceous to the late Tertiary. *The American Naturalist*, **156**, 47–58.

Gautier-Hion, A., Duplantier, J. M., Quris, R. *et al.* (1985). Fruit characters as a basis of fruit choice and seed dispersal in a tropical forest vertebrate community. *Oecologia*, **65**, 324–37.

Gibson, L. J. and Ashby, M. F. (1997). *Cellular Solids: Structure and Properties*, 2nd edn. Cambridge: Cambridge University Press.

Hopson, J. A. (2001). Origin of mammals. In *Palaeobiology II*, ed. D. E. G. Briggs and P. R. Crowther. London: Blackwell, pp. 88–94.

Hylander, W. L. (1978). Incisal bite force direction in humans and the functional significance of mammalian mandibular translation. *American Journal of Physical Anthropology*, **48**, 1–7.

Janson, C. H. (1983). Adaptation of fruit morphology to dispersal agents in a neotropical forest. *Science*, **219**, 187–9.

Jordano, P. (1995). Angiosperm fleshy fruits and seed dispersers – a comparative analysis of adaptation and constraints in plant-animal interactions. *The American Naturalist*, **145**, 163–91.

Kendall, K. (1978). Complexities of compression failure. *Proceedings of the Royal Society of London series A*, **361**, 245–63.

Kendall, K. (2001). *Molecular Adhesion*. New York: Kluwer/Plenum Press.

Lawn, B. R. (1993). *Fracture of Brittle Solids*, 2nd edn. Cambridge: Cambridge University Press.

Leighton, M. (1993). Modeling dietary selectivity by Bornean orangutans: evidence for integration of multiple criteria in fruit selection. *International Journal of Primatology*, **14**, 257–313.

Lucas, P. W. (1989). A new theory relating seed processing by primates to their relative tooth sizes. In *The Growing Scope of Human Biology*, ed. L. H. Schmitt, L. Freedman and N. W. Bruce. Perth, Australia: Centre for Human Biology, University of Western Australia, pp. 37–49.

Lucas, P. W. (2004). *Dental Functional Morphology: How Teeth Work*. Cambridge: Cambridge University Press.

Lucas, P. W. and Corlett, R. T. (1991). The relationship between the diet of *Macaca fascicularis* and forest phenology. *Folia Primatologica*, **57**, 201–15.

Martin, R. D. (1990). *Primate Origins and Evolution*. Princeton: Princeton University Press.

Osborn, J. W., Baragar, F. A., and Grey P. E. (1986). The functional advantage of proclined incisors in man. In *Teeth Revisited: Proceedings of VII International Symposium on Dental Morphology*, ed. D. E. Russell, J. P. Santoro and D. Sigognean-Russell. *Memoirs du Musee National d'Histoire Naturelle, Paris (Serie C)*, **53**, 445–58.

Paphangkorakit, J. and Osborn, J. W. (1997). Effect of jaw opening on the direction and magnitude of human incisal bite forces. *Journal of Dental Research*, **76**, 561–7.

Rhee, Y.-W., Kim, H.-W., Deng, Y., and Lawn, B. R. (2001). Brittle fracture versus quasi plasticity in ceramics: a simple predictive index. *Journal of the American Ceramic Society*, **84**, 561–5.

Ross, C. F. and Kay, R. F. (2004). *Anthropoid Origins: New Visions*. New York: Kluwer Academic.

Sirianni, J. E. (1979). Craniofacial morphology of the underbite trait in *Presbytis*. *Journal of Dental Research*, **58**, 1655.

Sui, Z. Q., Agrawal, K. R., Corke, H., and Lucas, P. W. (2006). Biting efficiency in relation to incisal angulation. *Archives of Oral Biology*, **51**, 491–7.

Swindler, D. R. (2002). *Primate Dentition*. Cambridge: Cambridge University Press.

Ungar, P. S. (1992). *Incisal microwear and feeding behavior of four Sumatran anthropoids*. Ph.D. Dissertation, State University of New York at Stony Brook.

Ungar, P. S. (1994). Patterns of ingestive behavior and anterior tooth use differences in sympatric anthropoid primates. *American Journal of Physical Anthropology*, **95**, 197–219.

Vincent, J. F. V. (1990). Fracture properties of plants. *Advances in Botanical Research*, **17**, 235–87.

Vincent, J. F. V., Saunders, D. E. J., and Beyts, P. (2002). The use of stress intensity factor to quantify "hardness" and "crunchiness" objectively. *Journal of Texture Studies*, **33**, 149–59.

Visser, M. (1991). *The Rituals of Dinner*. Canada: HarperCollins.

Whitten, A. J. (1982). Diet and feeding behaviour of kloss gibbons on Siberut Island, Indonesia. *Folia Primatologica*, **37**, 177–208.

Williams, J. G. (1998). Friction and plasticity effects in wedge splitting and cutting fracture tests. *Journal of Materials Science*, **33**, 5351–7.
Wilsea, M., Johnson, K. L., and Ashby, M. F. (1975). Indentation of foamed plastics. *International Journal of Mechanical Sciences*, **17**, 457–60.
Yamashita, N. (2003). Food procurement and tooth use in the sympatric lemur species. *American Journal of Physical Anthropology*, **121**, 125–33.
Zingeser, M. R. (1970). The morphological basis of the underbite trait in langurs (*P. melalophos* and *T. cristatus*) with an analysis of adaptive and evolutionary implications. *American Journal of Physical Anthropology*, **32**, 179–86.

16 *Alternative methods of assessing tooth size in Late Pleistocene and Early Holocene hominids*

CHARLES M. FITZGERALD AND SIMON HILLSON

16.1 Introduction

Contemporary humans have, on average, the smallest teeth of any hominid throughout the evolutionary history of the family. Within the genus *Homo*, the trend over the past two million years has been one of dental reduction; however, many anthropologists believe that this has been especially marked over the last 100 000 years or so (the Late Pleistocene and Holocene periods), both in Neandertals and so-called anatomically modern *Homo sapiens* (Brace, 1964, 1967, 2000; Brace *et al.*, 1987; Calcagno, 1989; Calcagno and Gibson, 1991; Carlson and van Gerven, 1977; Frayer, 1978, 1984; y'Edynak, 1989, 1992). The way in which this reduction of tooth size came about is one of the key issues in the evolution of modern humans; yet, in order to understand this process, it is necessary to confront the issue of how tooth size should be assessed. It is clear that with rapidly advancing technology (some examples of which can be found in this volume), it may someday be possible to employ precise volumetric and morphometric methods of tooth assessment that can be easily applied in an "in vivo" field/collection situation. At present, however, it is more practical to use simple caliper measurements.

In this chapter we assess the traditional methods of determining tooth dimensions and discuss an alternative approach adopted for a study of dental reduction in hominids of the Late Pleistocene and Holocene. We then evaluate the effectiveness of the conventional methods vs. our proposed alternative. Our study lasted three years and collected data on 6650 teeth in institutions from Europe, the Middle East, and North America. As such, it provided an excellent opportunity to assess the merits of both approaches, and to see whether our alternative methodology met the objectives that we had set.

Technique and Application in Dental Anthropology ed. Joel D. Irish and Greg C. Nelson
Published by Cambridge University Press.

16.2 "Conventional" tooth size assessment

Methods of assessing tooth size by mensuration are deeply rooted in biological anthropology and have, surprisingly perhaps, been in continuous use with few major changes for more than a century (Kieser, 1990). Tooth size is customarily reckoned by measuring the two crown diameters: the "length,"[1] or mesiodistal diameter, and the "width," or buccolingual diameter. Although there are other dimensions that might seem to have explanatory power, such as root length or tooth height, tooth size has customarily been summed up by the crown length and width measures (and several indices based on them) (Mayhall, 2000). It might be assumed that with this extensive pedigree the diameters would be models of clarity and consistency; however, many investigators over the years have offered different definitions and approaches. Probably the method with widest current acceptance is that of Moorrees and Reed (1954). According to these authors, the mesiodistal crown diameter is taken to be: (1) the largest mesial to distal dimension, which is at the same time, (2) parallel to the occlusal surface (see Figure 16.1). Consistent with this, the buccolingual crown diameter is the greatest distance between the buccal (or labial) and lingual (or palatal) surfaces, in a plane that is perpendicular to the mesiodistal diameter.

These definitions, however, are not without their problems, as we have pointed out elsewhere (Hillson *et al.*, 2005). A significant concern centers on the axis of the mesiodistal crown diameter, which is critical to the system of measurements, but which is also unfortunately not clearly defined. Goose (1963) suggested that the mesiodistal diameter axis should run between the contact points of the tooth crown with its neighbors. In teeth such as unworn incisors and canines, the two definitions of mesiodistal crown diameter are, in effect, the same. The same is not necessarily true, however, of premolars and molars, in which the contact points may not be at the maximum bulge of the mesial and distal crown sides.

In theory, any change in the axis of the mesiodistal crown diameter would also change the measurement axis of the buccolingual crown diameter, which should be perpendicular to it, but in practice, there is no means by which the angle can be checked. This is usually overcome by relaxing the strict rule of measurement by rotating the tooth crown slightly until a maximum is found, resulting in a diameter that may not actually be perpendicular to the mesiodistal diameter, or to the occlusal plane.

The buccolingual crown diameter of molars is much more worrisome; it is often possible to take more than one maximum measurement between their buccal and lingual crown sides, since there are usually two bulges on the buccal side and a single bulge on the lingual side. Therefore, based on the earlier definitions, a buccolingual measurement axis perpendicular to the mesiodistal

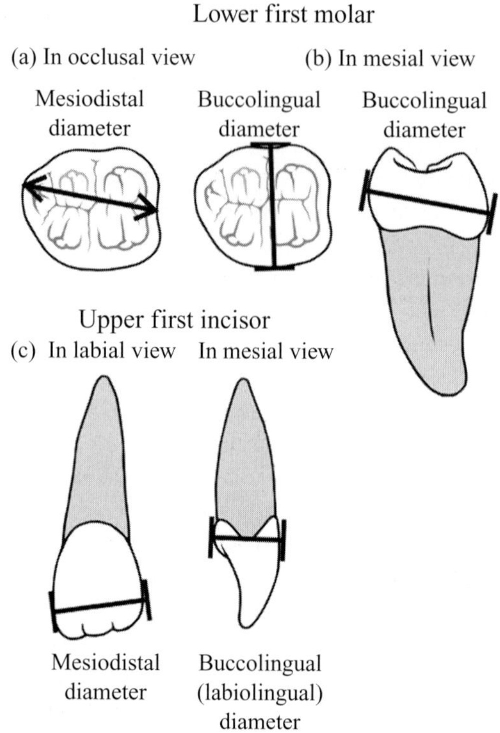

Figure 16.1 Maximum crown diameter measurements in (a) occlusal views of lower first molar, (b) mesial view of lower first molar, and (c) labial and mesial views of upper first incisor.

axis should, presumably, start from this single lingual bulge. If it does, then the other end of the axis falls between the twin bulges of the buccal crown side; thus, it does not record the maximum diameter. The only way to achieve a maximum is to rotate the crown so that the measurement is between the lingual bulge and the larger of the two buccal bulges (usually the most mesial); yet, in that case, the axis is no longer perpendicular to the mesiodistal diameter (Tobias, 1967). In addition, for both upper and lower molars, the main bulge of the lingual crown side is at about mid-crown height, whereas the buccal bulges are lower down toward the cervix. The maximum measurement is, therefore, achieved along a line that is not parallel to the occlusal surface – a fact that Tobias (1967) explicitly recognizes in his modifications to the definition.

When the teeth are present in the jaw, it is difficult to take the mesiodistal crown diameter because they fit tightly against their neighbors; the caliper points, thus, cannot be placed on the maximum convexity of the mesial and distal crown sides. In practice, calipers with needlepoints are used, and in some cases the teeth can be moved slightly in the jaw to allow a little access for measurement. Still, it is rarely possible to push the points far enough in. It is also all too easy to damage a delicate specimen.

However, to someone interested in studying dental reduction in earlier human populations, the most serious problem associated with dimensions that must be measured at the widest crown points is their ineffectiveness in the face of tooth attrition. Wear degrades the value of both traditional maximum measures, particularly the mesiodistal – which is strongly affected even at very early stages of approximal (inter-proximal or interstitial) attrition. Figure 16.2 demonstrates this fact in a simple example that reconstructs the worn portion of a molar. Approximal attrition proceeds by wearing away the rounded profile of the crown, producing flattened wear facets that can represent a significant proportion of the unworn diameter (approximately 10% of the tooth in this example). Incisors and canines are even more sensitive to wear (Frayer, 1978), since their maximum diameters occur close to their occlusal edges.

Given that crowns are measured to 0.1 mm, it is readily apparent that little wear is needed to reduce, by a measurable amount, mesiodistal dimensions taken along the line of the jaw. We believe that the error inherent in measuring worn teeth is significant enough to warrant concern, even in little-worn specimens. More significant amounts of wear can also jeopardize maximum buccolingual measures. All of this is most regrettable since, in the past, progressive occlusal attrition in agricultural, proto-agricultural, and gatherer–hunter peoples was an inevitable concomitant of normal aging. Wear cannot be seen as pathological in these societies since it was the normal condition of most dentitions. Often, by adulthood, crowns were significantly or even totally abraded (see the example in Figure 16.3); sometimes all that remains of these teeth are stumps of worn roots.

It is also unfortunate that the commonest overall pattern of wear seen in Paleolithic, Mesolithic, and Neolithic jaws is for anterior teeth to exhibit relatively more occlusal attrition than cheek teeth and, as pointed out, it is the mesiodistal diameters of anterior teeth that are most sensitive to wear. This is potentially a major problem, because it is anterior teeth that are claimed to have undergone the greatest degree of reduction. In sum, the attrition that is usual in ancient dentitions places severe constraints on those studies that use maximum measures to assess tooth size.

Most studies do not include measurements of teeth that are deemed too worn. The problem created by using maximum diameters is that if teeth too worn to measure are rigorously rejected (as they should be, although "too worn" is

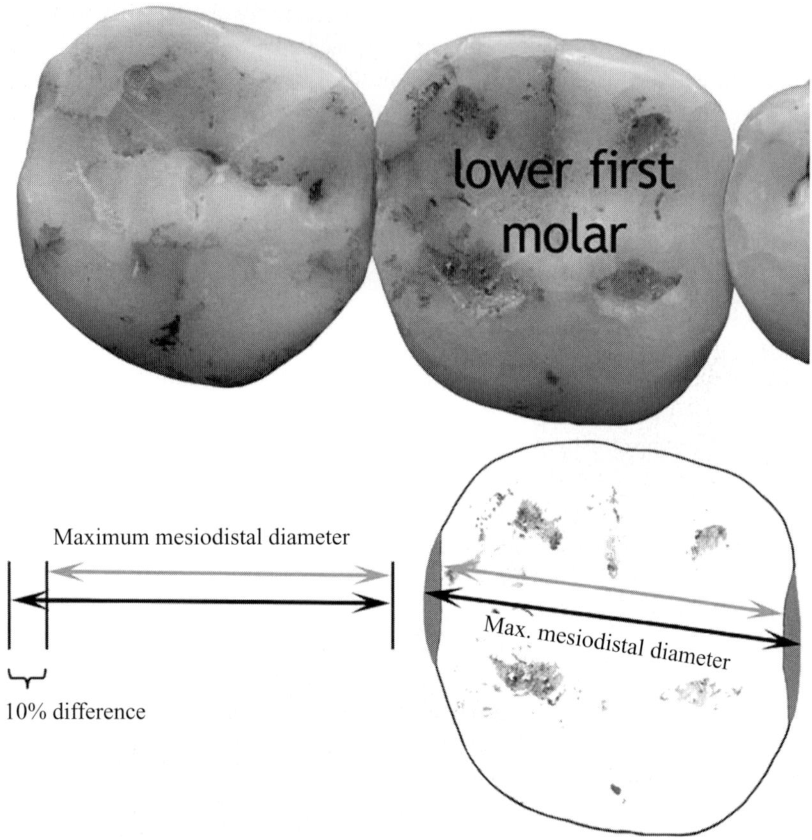

Figure 16.2 Demonstration of the significance of wear on the maximum mesiodistal diameter. A shows a lower first molar with moderate inter-proximal wear. B shows the outline of the first molar traced from the photograph with the inter-proximal wear reconstructed in dark gray. The black line with arrows indicates the maximal mesiodistal diameter of the estimated unworn occlusal profile of this tooth, and the light gray line marks the maximum mesiodistal diameter of the worn tooth. C compares the difference between the two diameters, and when measured this is just over 10% of the length of the unworn profile.

not precisely defined in most studies), then sample sizes for already small and often poorly preserved assemblages are further reduced. The alternative to rejection, i.e. inclusion, is a worse option since the validity of the measurements is questionable. In practice, however, almost all teeth in an assemblage show at least some wear and, because fossil hominin material is so scarce, most measurements included in any study have been affected to a greater or lesser extent.

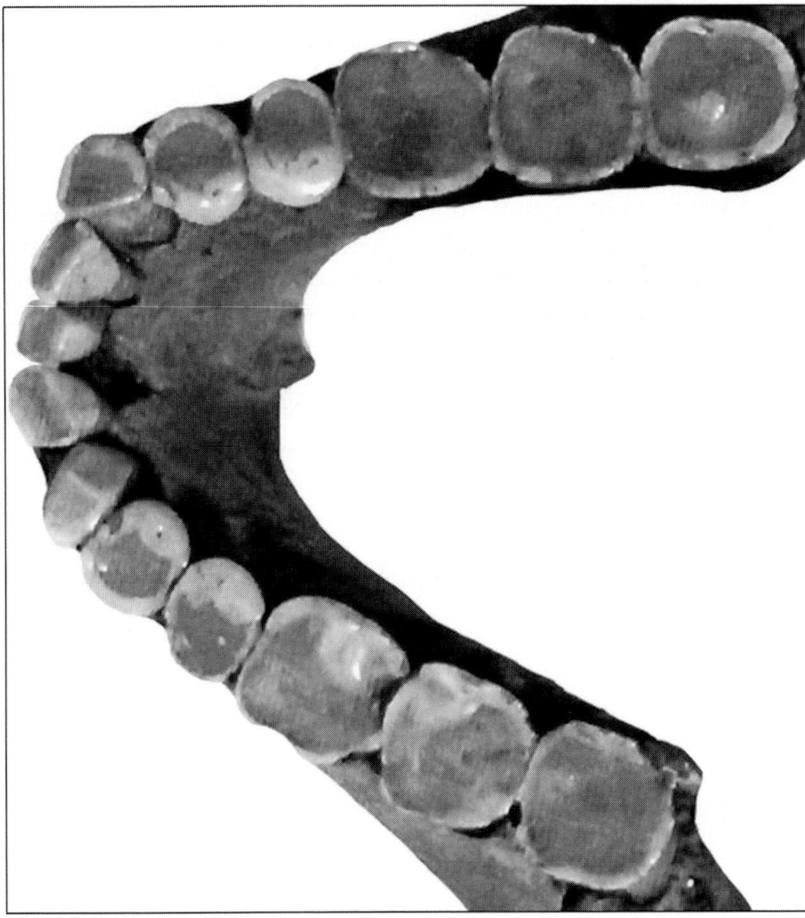

Figure 16.3 Occlusal view of a mandible from Ile de Téviec, a Mesolithic site in France, that demonstrates moderately heavy occlusal attrition to a degree that is typically seen among earlier peoples. Note that most of the enamel has worn away on all teeth, exposing dentine. Not uncommonly, heavier wear than this is seen where the whole crown is missing and the pulp chamber may be covered by a thin layer of secondary dentine, or even exposed prior to gross carious destruction.

There are other problems as well; for instance, how valid is the comparison between mature juvenile and older adult dentitions, regardless of the rigor of the rejection standard? There are also difficulties if dental measurements are used to help identify the sex of children (which is difficult to distinguish in the skeleton), since the method relies on establishing baseline groups of adults whose sex is independently known from pelvic or skull morphology. If their teeth are worn, then no comparison can be made between the baseline group and the less-worn children's teeth. Along the same lines, it is questionable whether it is legitimate to compare a population with one demographic age profile to another that is quite different, since it will not be possible to exclude the effects of wear.

The consequences of reduced sample sizes extend beyond the decreased power of statistical conclusions. The question of variability in tooth size, relative to Late Pleistocene/Early Holocene dental reduction, has never been considered. In most studies, because of small sample sizes, arithmetic means are used to summarize measurements from groups of combined sites, whose remains may range from a single tooth to tens of individual dentitions; this almost certainly gives a false impression of uniformity. Furthermore, comparisons of mean crown size between groups of fossils may be greatly affected by the composition of those groups in terms of ages-at-death of the individuals. There will likely be a differential effect on different tooth types if, for example, incisors are excluded from study at a lesser state of wear than molars. It is therefore possible that some apparent reduction is an artifact of the nature of the assemblages. As such, we sought a measure that would be less affected by all of the problems discussed, and allow us to grapple with the important question of variability.

16.3 Alternative measurements

Conventional crown diameters are arbitrarily chosen maximum dimensions. They are controlled by a complex interaction of genetic and environmental factors (Hillson, 1998) and, based on the discussion so far, may not necessarily be the best record of crown morphology for investigating such phenomena as sexual dimorphism, dental evolution, or the relationships of past populations. There is no reason why other measurements should not be just as good for these purposes, providing they can be recorded reliably. As pointed out by Stojanowski (in press), a number of labor-intensive alternative approaches have been proposed (Biggerstaff, 1969, 1975; Corruccini, 1977a, 1977b, 1978; Corruccini and Potter, 1981; Mayhall, 2000; Morris, 1986).

We decided to take measurements at the base of the crown, along the cement–enamel junction of the cervix. This idea has almost as long of a history as traditional crown diameters (Azouley and Regnault, 1893; Colby, 1996; Falk and Corruccini, 1982; Goose, 1963), but has not often been employed and, where it has, measurements were taken parallel to the usual crown diameters. The buccolingual cervical diameter of the crown is defined as the greatest distance between the buccal and lingual tooth surfaces at the cement–enamel junction. Mesial and distal sides of the crown and root are often concave at the cement–enamel junction, so care is needed when measuring points in the mesiodistal cervical diameter.

Colby (1996) follows the mesiodistal crown diameter description of Tobias (1967), and defines the cervical diameter as the distance between two parallel lines, perpendicular to the mesiodistal axis and tangential to the most mesial and most distal parts of the cement–enamel junction. This means that for teeth *in situ* in the jaw, the sides of the caliper points must be parallel and be as small as 1 mm or so in width to pass between teeth at the cervix. The problem is that it is difficult to obtain points that are thin enough to pass between teeth, yet be stiff enough to not bend when the caliper jaws close. Therefore, we decided to define the mesiodistal cervical diameter differently. Figure 16.4 gives instructions on how the cervical measures should be taken.

We also recognized that conventional calipers are unable to accommodate all requirements of our cervical measures, and that we must, therefore, develop a new instrument to accomplish two different tasks. In the first, points need to be thin enough to pass between teeth in the jaw, but not so pointed that they scratch valuable specimens. After many trials, the best points were found to be 2 mm stainless steel rods, machined to a fine taper with a narrow rounded tip, and finely polished. When tested, it proved impossible to scratch the teeth. The second task that they must accomplish is to take a buccolingual diameter under the main bulge of the cingulum of the crown. This requires the points to be held differently, so that they meet end-to-end. After developing two separate calipers, each carrying out one of the tasks, the authors collaborated with Jim Kondrat of Paleo-Tech Inc. (http://paleo-tech.com) to design an instrument that combines both types of points (Figure 16.5). These new calipers have digital displays that read to 0.01 mm, and allow direct input to the RS232 serial port or PS2 port of a computer; in that way, measurements can be entered directly into an Access (or other) database.

Before using cervical measures in our dental reduction project we conducted a large pilot study using dental remains from a fourteenth-century London site (Hillson *et al.*, 2005). The goals were to determine: (1) the repeatability with which cervical diameters can be measured, as no such study had been published before, and (2) the extent to which they can be related to standard crown diameters. The teeth from this previous study are unworn permanent teeth isolated from their jaws; this resulted in ideal conditions for us to directly compare measures using the two alternative approaches, one of which is affected by wear and the other which is not.

Results of the inter-observer-error portion of this study demonstrate that cervical and diagonal measurements can be recorded as reliably as the usual

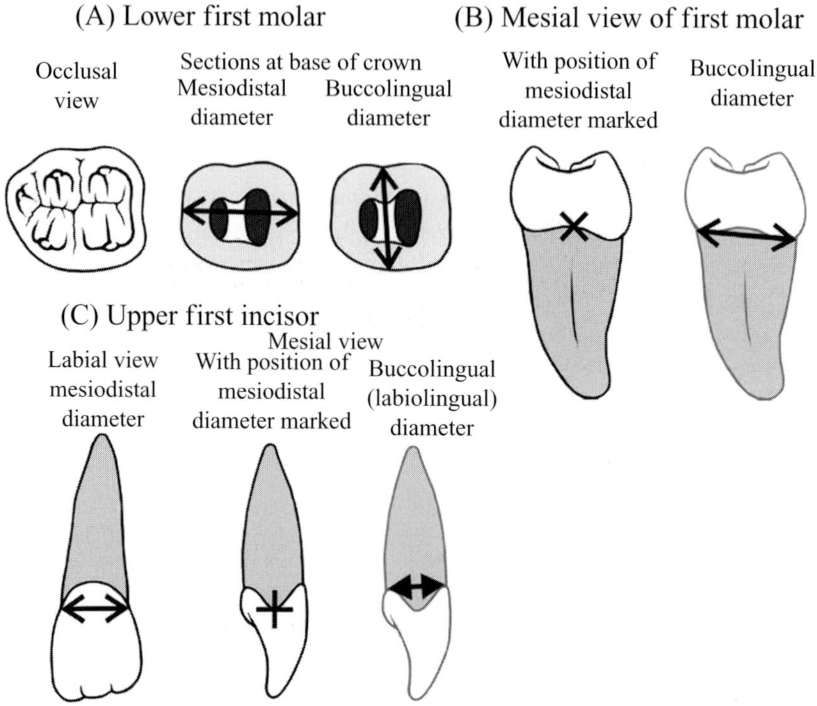

Figure 16.4 Directions on how to take the cervical diameters are given in this figure. The definitions that follow will refer to aspects of the figure. The mesiodistal cervical diameter for incisors and canines is the distance between the most occlusal points of the cement–enamel junction curve on the mesial and distal sides, which make natural measurement landmarks. Since the mesial curve rises more to occlusal than the distal curve, the axis of measurement is not strictly parallel to the occlusal plane of the tooth. C shows this in a labial view of an upper first incisor and it also indicates where a caliper point should be placed in the mesial side. The mesiodistal cervical diameter of premolars and molars cannot be defined using natural landmarks since these are lacking in cheek teeth. The measurement points are therefore defined as midway along the cement–enamel junction on the mesial and distal sides of the crown, as shown in A and B. Buccolingual cervical diameter for incisors, canines, and premolars: in these teeth, the cement–enamel junction makes a single curve apically and outwards to labial/buccal and lingual/palatal. This means that the buccolingual cervical diameter can be defined simply as the maximum measurement at the cement–enamel junction from labial/buccal to lingual/palatal, as illustrated in C. Once again, these landmarks are not necessarily at equal levels, so the axis of measurement may not be parallel to the occlusal plane. Buccolingual cervical diameter for molars: the cement–enamel junction does not have a single outward curve on the buccal and lingual sides of molars. This means that the cervical diameter cannot be defined as the maximum measurement since there would then be at least two maxima. Instead, the measurement is taken on the cement–enamel junction at points midway along the buccal and lingual/palatal sides. In most upper molars, this point is the maximum bulge above the single lingual/palatal root, and there is usually a slight depression midway along the buccal side between the two buccal roots. For lower molars, there is usually a slight depression on both the lingual and buccal sides, between roots, which is where the measurement is taken. This is shown in A and B. Where there is a large enamel extension, the measurement should be taken to one side or the other of it, whichever gives the maximum value.

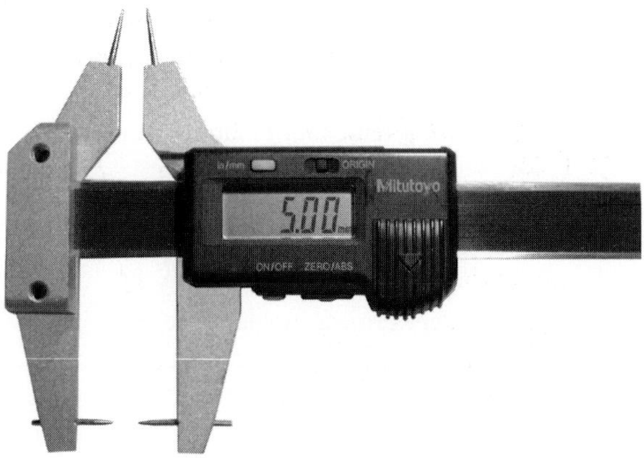

Figure 16.5 Hillson-FitzGerald calipers developed in collaboration with Paleo-Tech, Inc. and used in our dental reduction project.

crown diameters (Hillson *et al.*, 2005). We also found that the buccolingual cervical measurement is strongly correlated with the normal buccolingual crown diameter in all teeth, whereas the mesiodistal cervical measurement is highly correlated with the normal mesiodistal crown diameter in incisors and canines, but less so in premolars and molars (Hillson *et al.*, 2005). Crown areas (robustness index) calculated from maximum diameters are strongly correlated with crown areas from cervical measurements (Hillson *et al.*, 2005). Therefore, it appears to us that, despite the lengthy usage of the more usual maximum crown diameters, the alternatives can be measured just as reliably and record similar information. A recent study by Stojanowski (in press) largely supports our results in this respect.

We hoped that the use of cervical diameters would increase the number of measurements taken in our large study of dental reduction in Late Pleistocene and Holocene hominids and, additionally, increase the veracity of these measurements. Because cervical diameters are not affected by wear until most of the crown is gone, they overcome the handicap that weakens the effectiveness of conventional maximum measures; therefore, we anticipated that they would provide a significant advantage in archaeological populations. This advantage may be less important for buccolingual diameters, but we think that it is crucial for mesiodistal diameters, especially in anterior teeth.

The main downside of using cervical diameters, that we originally foresaw, is the presence of heavy supragingival calculus deposits in teeth where continuous eruption or loss of periodontal tissues would have resulted in moving the gingival attachment down from the crown onto the root. Such deposits might, on occasion, cover the cement–enamel junction. Without removing these deposits, it may not be possible to take cervical measurements; however, we thought that this would be relatively rare in archaeological collections where, if present, calculus frequently falls off during removal of matrix or in storage.

16.4 Methods and materials

The overall objective of the larger project in which we were involved was the detailed examination of dental reduction in the Late Pleistocene and Early Holocene (*c.* 12 0000 to 5000 BP) evolution of both anatomically modern humans and Neandertals (FitzGerald and Hillson, 2002, 2004, 2005; Hillson and FitzGerald, 2003). We made comparisons between regions, periods, and taxa to test the uniformity of the dental reduction phenomenon, and to test the main hypotheses for dental reduction previously put forward. This was done by recording, in all specimens, observations and measurements designed to examine dentition and jaw function, dental pathology, craniofacial development, and general body size and robustness.

For each tooth we recorded up to four measurements, along with 25 other observations (e.g. caries, wear, etc.). For each individual we made as many as 75 additional observations, including the lengths of lower long bones and up to 13 measurements of the mandible. Thus, for an individual with a complete dentition, 1003 variables were recorded. This number necessitated collection of data electronically by, as noted, using calipers that provide input directly to a laptop. In addition, a set of five standard digital photographs were taken of each specimen's cranial elements to investigate, among others, cusp morphology and chewing mechanics. We also did some application programming in Microsoft Access to assist data collection by formatting special forms.

In terms of the narrower methodology relating to tooth measurement, we collected mesiodistal and buccolingual diameters using the definitions discussed above. Every tooth was measured, which means that data were collected on antimeres. In fact, this approach was incorporated into our collection protocol by using the specially programmed Access forms. The result is a program that sorts the display of teeth to be measured so that left and right antimere diameters are displayed adjacent to each other. When two antimeres are measured, the results are immediately compared; in the study, if measurements differed by more than 0.03 mm this fact was flagged. In such cases, the two antimeres were re-measured to ensure that no error was made and that genuine asymmetry existed. Although it was planned to measure the usual maximum diameters, these were recorded only if teeth were not "too worn." We experimented to determine the degree of wear that can be suffered before the maximum crown dimension is lost; Smith's (1984) wear scales were chosen because they are easy to apply and can be quickly assessed. As such, maximum measures are *not* recorded for teeth meeting the following criteria:

Maximum diameter	Tooth type	Smith (1984) wear stage
Mesiodistal	Incisor	≥ 4
Mesiodistal	Canine, premolar, molar	≥ 5
Buccolingual	All	≥ 6

To ensure that worn teeth were not inadvertently measured in our study, we programmed our Access collection form with these criteria, and the input field for maximum diameter measures was blocked from receiving data if wear had been recorded for a particular tooth above defined levels. The investigator, therefore, did not have to make a decision on whether to measure or not.

Data collection concentrated on samples housed in institutions in Europe, Israel, and North America, with the focus on European, Middle Eastern, and North African hominids from the Late Pleistocene and Early Holocene. About 40 institutions were visited.

16.5 Results

A bar graph illustrating the total number of teeth measured, by tooth type, ($n = 6631$) is shown in Figure 16.6. It is apparent that fewer teeth from the upper jaw were measured than from the lower; similarly, more posterior teeth were measured than anterior teeth in both jaws.

Figures 16.7 and 16.8 show bar graphs plotting the number of cervical and maximum measures taken for each tooth type for mesiodistal and buccolingual diameters, respectively. For mesiodistal diameters, more cervical than maximum measures could be made in all tooth types except M2 and M3. Table 16.1 provides a breakdown of Figure 16.7, listing the number of cervical and maximum diameters as figures and percentages of the total for each measurable tooth type. It also shows the differences between cervical and maximum measures. It can be seen that 4046 cervical diameters were measured versus 3704 maximum, a difference of about 5%. It is clear from Table 16.1 that cervical measures performed more consistently than maximum measures. Percentages range around 60–65% of possible measurements in all teeth except the upper and lower M1s and M2s; in the latter four tooth types, percentages are only slightly lower, ranging from 49–56%. On the other hand, maximum diameters

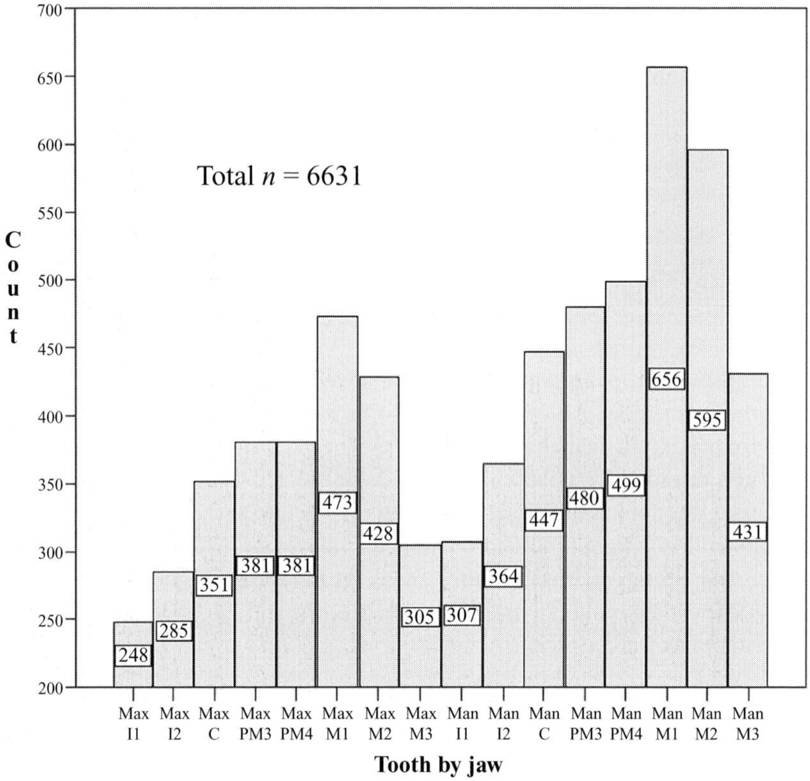

Figure 16.6 Total number of teeth measured by tooth type.

performed poorly for the upper and lower incisors, ranging from about 32–37% of possible measurements. There is also a broad spread in percentages for the remaining tooth types – from 43–75%.

Figure 16.8 and Table 16.2 illustrate the corresponding data for buccolingual diameters. Overall, more buccolingual cervical ($n = 5161$) and maximum ($n = 4717$) diameters were taken than mesiodistal. Moreover, there is a different pattern of effectiveness for buccolingual vs. mesiodistal measurements. More cervical diameters were measured in all teeth except for the upper and lower M3s, where the differences are slight. The % difference between cervical measurable and maximum measurable is also greater at 6.7%. Both cervical and maximum buccolingual diameters performed more consistently, though, again the maximum has a greater range than the cervical (i.e. 57% to 82% for the former against 75% to 84% for the latter).

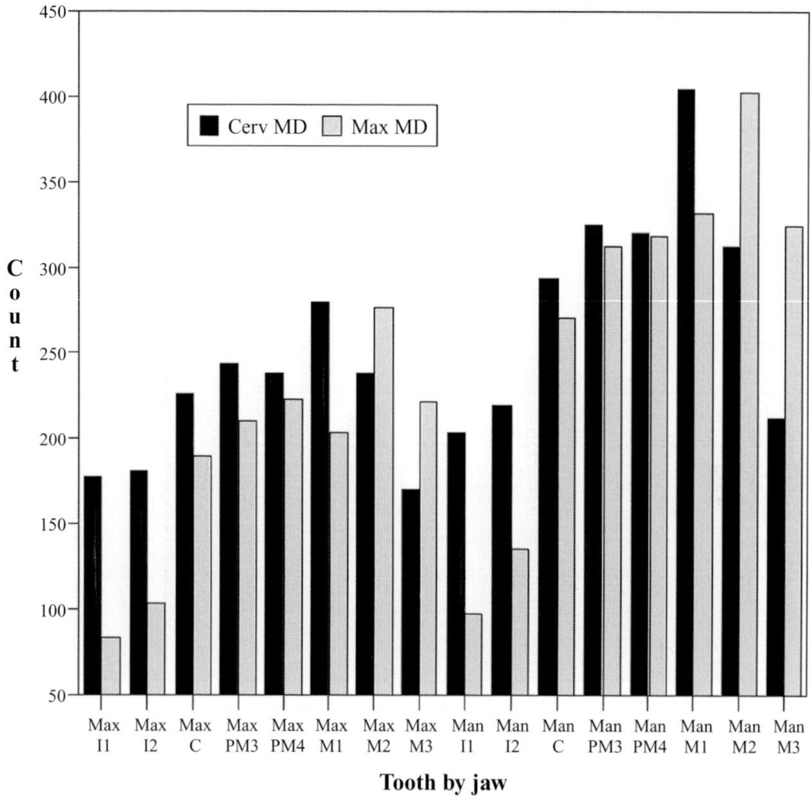

Figure 16.7 Comparison of the frequency of cervical and maximum mesiodistal measures.

Figures 16.9 and 16.10 compare the percentage of teeth measured for mesiodistal and buccolingual cervical and maximum diameters across all teeth, plotted against Smith's (1984) wear stages (0 = no wear; 8 = most severe). Both figures demonstrate the same phenomenon: a greater proportion of maximum than cervical measures were recordable at lesser stages of tooth wear, while at greater wear stages the converse prevails. Indeed, because of the data collection protocol prohibiting the taking of maximum measures above certain Smith (1984) stages, no maximum diameter data are seen at higher levels. The mesiodistal dimension in Figure 16.9 shows this phenomenon more clearly; this diameter is more sensitive to occlusal wear, and Smith's (1984) cut-off stages are lower than for the corresponding buccolingual diameter.

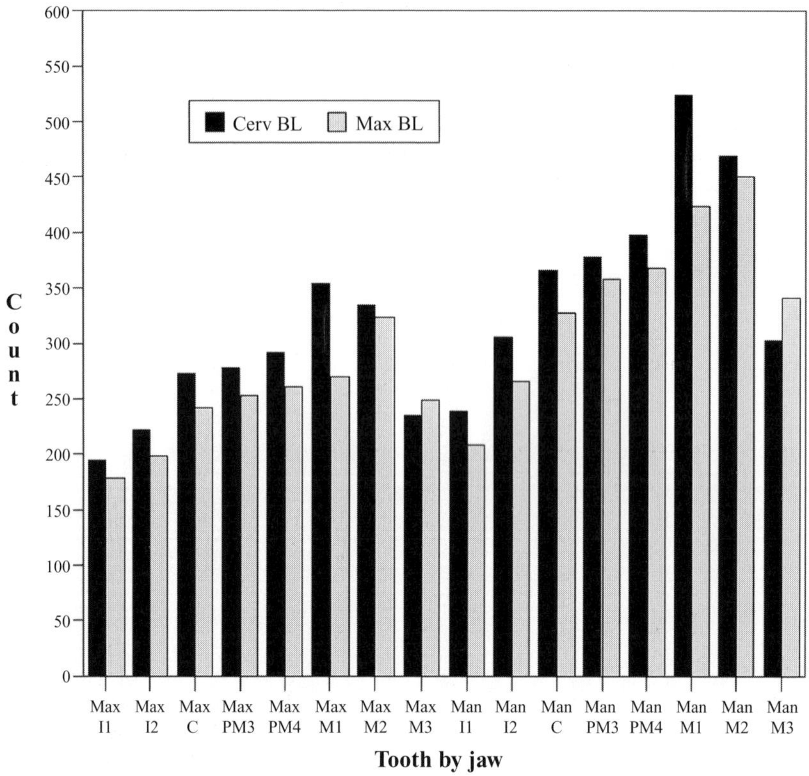

Figure 16.8 Comparison of the frequency of cervical and maximum buccolingual measures.

16.6 Discussion

There is ample evidence from the dental reduction study that cervical measures meet their primary objective of increasing overall sample size. In both mesiodistal and buccolingual diameters, more teeth were measured cervically than maximally. Overall, 5% and 7% are modest improvements, but they are affected by the nature of the dentitions included in the group studied. Because there are many more molars in the study sample than anterior teeth, and because cervical measures are more effective in anterior teeth, these two factors tend to offset one another. A different sample, with a higher proportion of anterior teeth, would show a greater absolute and percentage difference of cervical over maximum diameters.

The impact on maximizing overall sample size of the cervical measures is more apparent in Figures 16.11 and 16.12, which compare the number

Table 16.1 *Mesiodistal cervical and maximum diameters measured by tooth type*

			Mesiodistal diameters					
		Total num. of teeth	Cervical		Maximum		Diff. Cerv-Max	
			N	%	*N*	%	*N*	%
Upper	I1	248	177	71.4	84	33.9	93	37.5
	I2	285	181	63.5	104	36.5	77	27.0
	C	351	226	64.4	190	54.1	36	10.3
	PM3	381	244	64.0	211	55.4	33	8.7
	PM4	381	239	62.7	223	58.5	16	4.2
	M1	473	280	59.2	204	43.1	76	16.1
	M2	428	239	55.8	276	64.5	−37	−8.6
	M3	305	170	55.7	222	72.8	−52	−17.0
Total upper		2852	1756	61.6	1514	53.1	242	8.5
Lower	I1	307	204	66.4	98	31.9	106	34.5
	I2	364	219	60.2	135	37.1	84	23.1
	C	447	294	65.8	270	60.4	24	5.4
	PM3	480	325	67.7	312	65.0	13	2.7
	PM4	499	320	64.1	318	63.7	2	0.4
	M1	656	404	61.6	331	50.5	73	11.1
	M2	595	312	52.4	402	67.6	−90	−15.1
	M3	431	212	49.2	324	75.2	−112	−26.0
Total lower		3779	2290	60.6	2190	58.0	100	2.6
Grand total		6631	4046	61.0	3704	55.9	342	5.2

of diameters (i.e. mesiodistal and buccolingual, respectively) that could be assessed where only one measurement was possible. That is, they identify the teeth where either a cervical- or maximum-only diameter was measured, because some impediment prevented the other diameter from being taken. For example, this impediment may have been excessive wear, which would prevent the recording of a reliable maximum diameter. These two figures show the same patterns as Figures 16.7 and 16.8, which illustrate total diameters in each approach that could be measured, though with the main features more exaggerated. For instance, upper and lower M1s for both diameters, particularly buccolingual, and upper I1s and I2s for both diameters show a significant differential in the number of cervical over maximum measures. This situation is almost certainly due to wear, since these tooth types in most study assemblages have the greatest levels of attrition.

Given what has been said about these four figures, there is an important question that needs answering: why do cervical diameters not outnumber maximum diameters in *every* tooth type? In the case of mesiodistal diameters, more

Table 16.2 *Buccolingual cervical and maximum diameters measured by tooth type*

		Total num. of teeth	Mesiodistal diameters					
			Cervical		Maximum		Diff. Cerv-Max	
			N	%	*N*	%	*N*	%
Upper	I1	248	195	78.6	179	72.2	16	6.5
	I2	285	222	77.9	199	69.8	23	8.1
	C	351	272	77.5	242	68.9	30	8.5
	PM3	381	278	73.0	253	66.4	25	6.6
	PM4	381	292	76.6	260	68.2	32	8.4
	M1	473	354	74.8	270	57.1	84	17.8
	M2	428	334	78.0	323	75.5	11	2.6
	M3	305	235	77.0	249	81.6	−14	−4.6
Total upper		2852	2182	76.5	1975	69.2	207	7.3
Lower	I1	307	239	77.9	208	67.8	31	10.1
	I2	364	305	83.8	266	73.1	39	10.7
	C	447	365	81.7	328	73.4	37	8.3
	PM3	480	377	78.5	358	74.6	19	4.0
	PM4	499	397	79.6	368	73.7	29	5.8
	M1	656	523	79.7	423	64.5	100	15.2
	M2	595	470	79.0	450	75.6	20	3.4
	M3	431	303	70.3	341	79.1	−38	−8.8
Total lower		3779	2979	78.8	2742	72.6	237	6.3
Grand total		6631	5161	77.8	4717	71.1	444	6.7

cervical measures could be made than maximum in all tooth types except for upper and lower M2s and M3s; for buccolingual diameters the exceptions are upper and lower M3s. The answer lies in the difficulties of measuring these diameters in teeth that are still *in situ* within the jaws. These difficulties are greatest in the lower M2 and M3 cervical mesiodistal diameters, in which only 52.4% and 49.2%, respectively, could be measured; these are compared to 67.6% and 75.2% for the maximum diameters (from Table 16.1), though the upper jaws were also difficult to measure.

Figure 16.13 illustrates the problem. In some of the jaws the forward points of the Hillson–FitzGerald calipers could not be inserted, due to insufficient space, to record a mesiodistal measurement. The mandible (or maxilla) may have been too narrow and/or shallow, and the space between the inside edges of the alveolar ridges may not have been sufficient to allow proper placement of the caliper jaws; in mandibles, the ramus might have also blocked access to the molars from the outside. On the whole, cervical buccolingual diameters are easier to take in all teeth, although there are still some upper and lower M3s

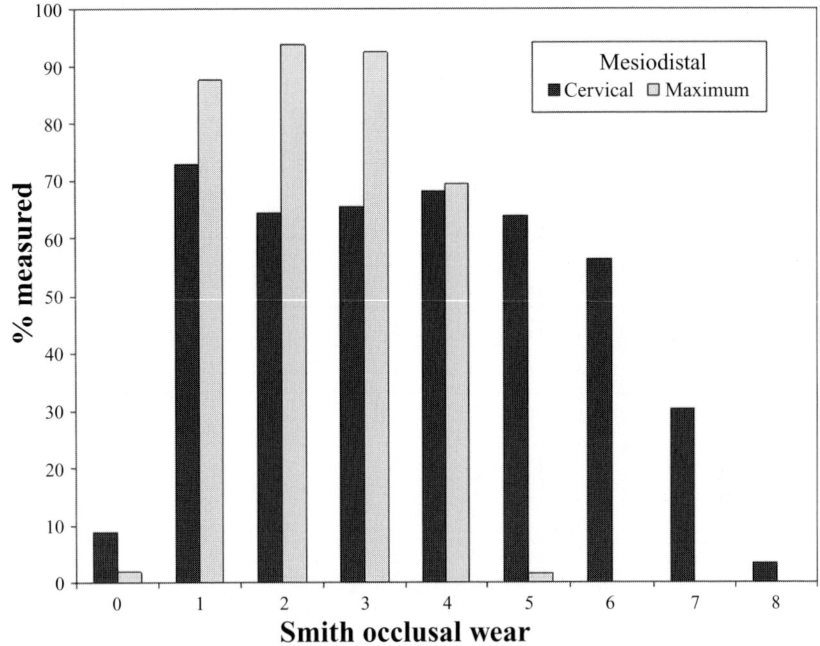

Figure 16.9 This bar graph plots the percentage of mesiodistal cervical and maximum diameters that could be measured in each Smith (1984) wear stage (where 0 represents no wear, and 8 the most severe wear).

that were difficult or impossible to access with the calipers; those that could be measured include 77.0% for upper and 70.3% for lower cervical, vs. 81.6% for upper and 79.1% for lower maximum (again see Table 16.2 and Figure 16.13).

We had anticipated that cervical diameters would be impossible to take when heavy supragingival calculus was present. Stojanowski (in press, p. 3) also identifies several other causes of missing data for what he calls "cervicometrics" that include: "extensive attrition and subsequent root-splitting, root loss, and cervical abrasion with cingulum chipping, cervical caries, inter-proximal grooves, idiosyncratic use-related attrition, [and] malocclusion." We did not record reasons for not taking cervical measures per se, so we cannot statistically examine rejection categories. However, calculus was not a severe problem in our mostly ancient and already frequently measured samples; still, we did encounter some collections with a variety of non-calculus deposits that prevented the recording of cervical diameters (e.g. Figure 16.14).

In any event, the overall increase in sample size largely results from the exclusion of maximum measures at higher levels of attrition. As shown in Figures 16.9 and 16.10, the total number of maximum measures taken for both

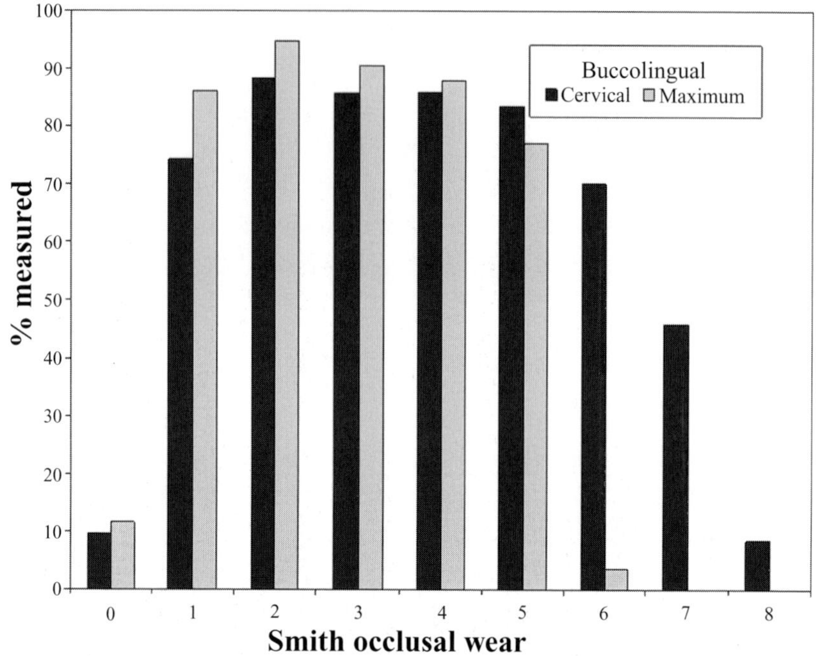

Figure 16.10 This bar graph plots the percentage of buccolingual cervical and maximum diameters that could be measured in each Smith (1984) wear stage (where 0 represents no wear, and 8 the most severe wear).

diameters exceeds cervical measures in Smith (1984) wear stages that are equal to or less than four. For mesiodistal diameters only, a few maximum measures were taken at stage five, and none above this; for the buccolingual only, slightly more cervical measures were taken at stage five than maximum measures, only a few maximums were taken at stage six, and no maximums were taken at levels above this.

The gain of cervical measures at higher wear levels more than offsets the slightly higher maximum measures at low wear levels; the result is a net increase in sample size. Stojanowski (in press) claims that anterior maxillary mesiodistal cervical diameters in his study: (1) demonstrate low correlations between cervical and maximum diameters, (2) are not included in first principal component loadings, indicating that they are not loading for general dental size, and (3) show small left to right side correlations. On these bases he does not feel that they are an appropriate proxy for homologous maximum diameters. The correlations in our study are different (Hillson *et al.*, 2005); since we measured both left and right antimeres, when available, we were also able to establish that these are not significantly different. However, we believe that neither of these

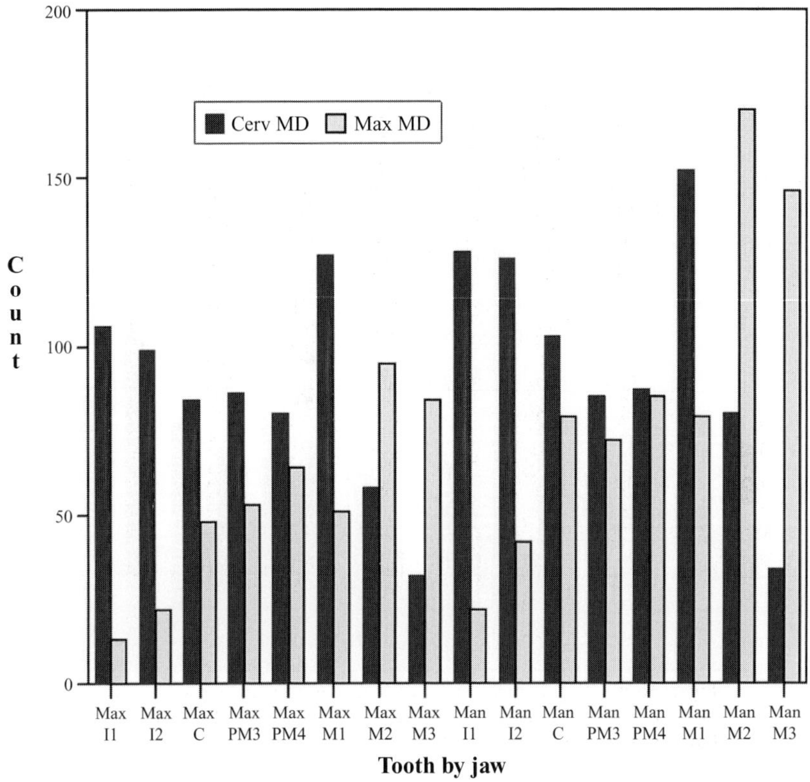

Figure 16.11 Comparison of the frequency of cervical and maximum mesiodistal measures in teeth where it was possible to take only one measurement

points affects the utility of cervical diameters in situations where the maximum measures simply cannot be taken.

All tooth diameter measurements are arbitrary and have been historically selected for reasons that are not strictly related to their information-bearing capability. The most essential characteristic they must possess is measurement repeatability, and if this is established their utility will then depend on the accumulation of a *corpus* of comparative statistics from as many other teeth as possible.

16.7 Conclusions

The use of cervical diameters permitted us to assemble a very robust data set of Late Pleistocene and Early Holocene tooth measurements whose sample size was maximized despite the heavy wear exhibited by most specimens. In this

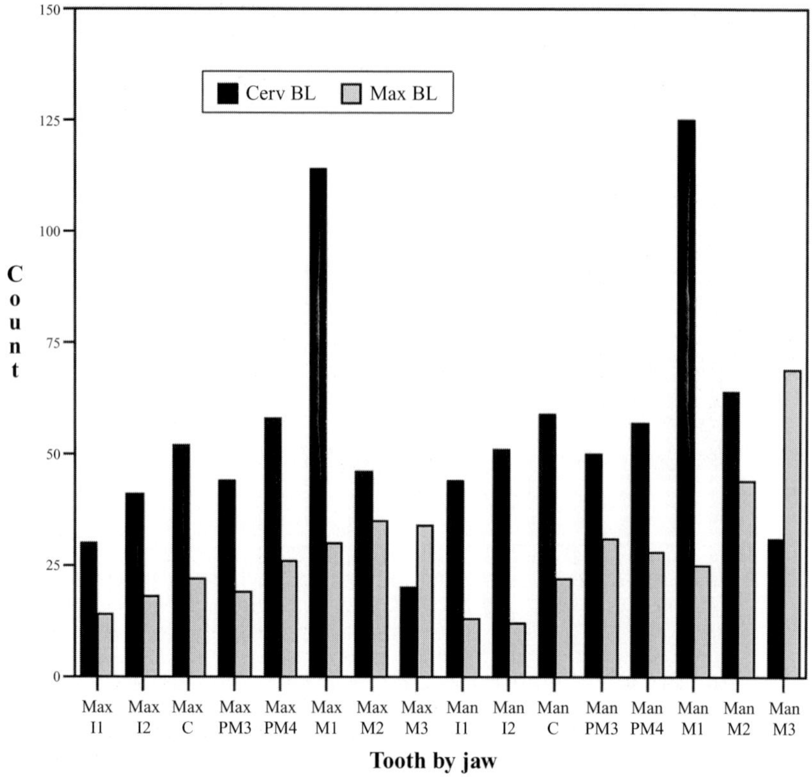

Figure 16.12 Comparison of the frequency of cervical and maximum buccolingual measures in teeth where it was possible to take only one measurement.

respect, cervical diameters meet the objective that we had set for them. However, it is also clear from our results that there are situations where the usual maximum diameters can be taken and the cervical diameters cannot. We therefore make the following recommendations for formulating an odontometric data collection strategy:

(1) Both cervical and the usual maximum diameters should be employed.
(2) A protocol that defines the specific levels of wear at which maximum diameters can be used should be established at the beginning of the study and strictly adhered to throughout.

Acknowledgments

The authors would like to acknowledge the support provided by the Natural Environment Research Council of the UK (Grant GR3/12924). They are also

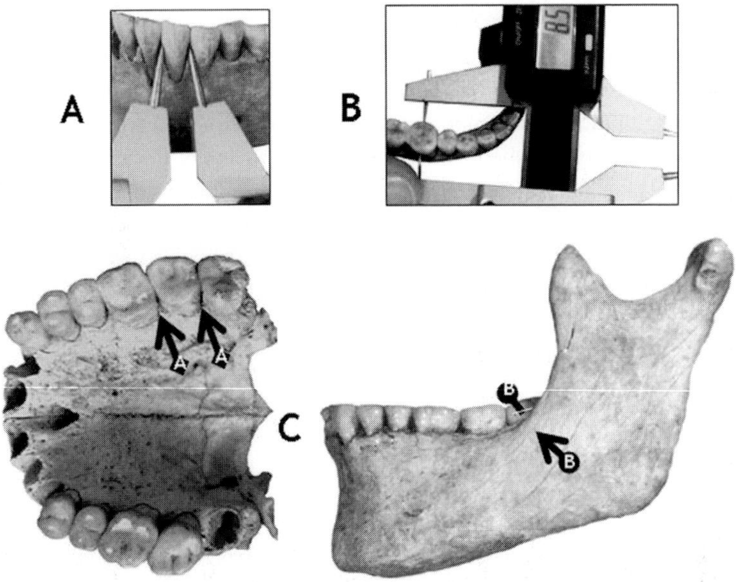

Figure 16.13 This figure illustrates some of the difficulties involved in taking cervical measures toward the back of the jaws. Inset A shows the placement of the forward points of the Hillson–FitzGerald calipers to take the cervical mesiodistal measurement, into the interproximal spaces on either side of an incisor. Inset B shows an occlusal view of the placement of the side-to-side points of the Hillson–FitzGerald calipers to take the cervical buccolingual measurement of a molar. C shows the occlusal view of an upper jaw on the left and the lateral view of a mandible on the right. The arrows labeled A indicate where the points should be inserted between the teeth to measure the mesiodistal diameter of this M2, but if the upper jaws are narrow (or shallow), the space between the inside edges of the alveolar ridges is not sufficient to allow the proper placement of the caliper jaws. The arrows labeled B indicate where points should be placed to take a buccolingual measure of the M3. There is clearly a problem here with the ramus blocking proper access, but in the upper jaw there may also not be enough space to manouver the caliper into place if the maxilla is still *in situ* in the skull and there is a prominent maxillary tuberosity with little retromolar room.

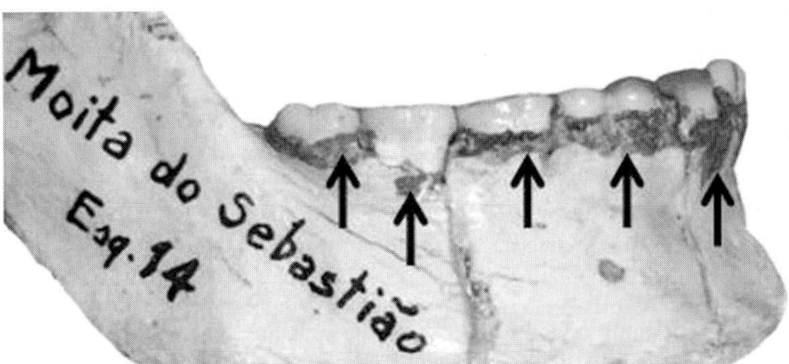

Figure 16.14 This is a mandible from Moita do Sebastião, a Mesolithic shell midden site in Portugal, which shows a particularly severe calcareous deposit that prevented cervical measurements from being taken.

grateful for the assistance of G. Martin (University of Sussex), who designed and built some of the original modifications to the calipers and points, Michael Town (Department of Biochemical Engineering, University College London), for suggesting the penultimate design of the caliper points and for making them, and Jim Kondrat (Paleo-Tech, Inc.), who developed (and now markets) the final design of the calipers. Finally, and most importantly, they owe many thanks to all of the people who have permitted access to original fossil material in their care or who have provided assistance during the three years of data collection in the many museums and institutions visited.

References

Azouley, O. and Regnault, O. (1893). Variation in the form of the teeth. *Bulletins et Memoires de la Societe d'Anthropologie de Paris*, **4**, 266.

Biggerstaff, R. H. (1969). The basal area of posterior tooth crown components: the assessment of within tooth variations of premolars and molars. *American Journal of Physical Anthropology*, **31**, 163–70.

Biggerstaff, R. H. (1975). Cusp size, sexual dimorphism, and heritability of cusp size in twins. *American Journal of Physical Anthropology*, **42**, 127–39.

Brace, C. L. (1964). The probable mutation effect. *The American Naturalist*, **98**, 453–5.

Brace, C. L. (1967). Environment, tooth form, and size in the Pleistocene. *Journal of Dental Research*, **46**, 809–16.

Brace, C. L. (2000). Tooth size differences and the antiquity of cooking (abstract). *American Journal of Physical Anthropology Supplement*, **30**, 110–11.

Brace, C. L., Rosenberg, K. R., and Hunt, K. D. (1987). Gradual change in human tooth size in the Late Pleistocene and Post-Pleistocene. *Evolution*, **41**, 705–20.

Calcagno, J. M. (1989). *Mechanisms of Human Dental Reduction: A Case Study from Post-Pleistocene Nubia*. Lawrence: University of Kansas.

Calcagno, J. M. and Gibson, K. R. (1991). Selective compromise: evolutionary trends and mechanisms in hominid tooth size. In *Advances in Dental Anthropology*, ed. M. A. Kelley and C. S. Larsen. New York: Wiley-Liss, pp. 59–76.

Carlson, D. S. and van Gerven, D. P. (1977). Masticatory function and post-Pleistocene evolution in Nubia. *American Journal of Physical Anthropology*, **46**, 495–506.

Colby, G. R. (1996). Analysis of dental sexual dimorphism in two western Gulf of Mexico precontact populations utilizing cervical measurements (abstract). *American Journal of Physical Anthropology*, Supplement 22, p. 87.

Corruccini, R. S. (1977a). Cartesian coordinate analysis of the hominoid second lower deciduous molar. *Journal of Dental Research*, **56**, 699.

Corruccini, R. S. (1977b). Crown component variation in the hominoid lower second premolar. *Journal of Dental Research*, **56**, 1093–6.

Corruccini, R. S. (1978). Crown component variation in hominoid upper first premolars. *Archives of Oral Biology*, **23**, 491–4.

Corruccini, R. S. and Potter, R. H. (1981). Developmental correlates of crown component asymmetry and occlusal discrepancy. *American Journal of Physical Anthropology*, **55**, 21–31.

Falk, D. and Corruccini, R. S. (1982). Efficacy of cranial versus dental measurements for separating human populations. *American Journal of Physical Anthropology*, **57**, 123–8.

FitzGerald, C. M. and Hillson, S. W. (2002). Dental reduction in Late Pleistocene and Early Holocene hominids (abstract). *American Journal of Physical Anthropology Supplement*, **34**, 70.

FitzGerald, C. M. and Hillson, S. W. (2004). Testing hypotheses for dental reduction in Late Pleistocene and Early Holocene hominids (abstract). *American Journal of Physical Anthropology Supplement*, **38**, 95.

FitzGerald, C. M. and Hillson, S. W. (2005). Dental reduction in Late Pleistocene and Early Holocene hominids: alternative approaches to assessing tooth size (abstract). *American Journal of Physical Anthropology Supplement*, **40**, 102.

Frayer, D. W. (1978). *Evolution of the Dentition in Upper Paleolithic and Mesolithic Europe*. Lawrence: University of Kansas.

Frayer, D. W. (1984). Biological and cultural change in the European Late Pleistocene and Early Holocene. In *The Origin of Modern Humans: A World Survey of the Fossil Evidence*, ed. F. H. Smith and F. Spencer. New York: Alan R. Liss, pp. 211–50.

Goose, D. H. (1963). Dental measurement: an assessment of its value in anthropological studies. In *Dental Anthropology*, ed. D. R. Brothwell. London: Pergamon Press, pp. 125–48.

Hillson, S. W. (1998). Crown diameters, tooth crown development, and environmental factors in growth. In *Human Dental Development, Morphology and Pathology: A Tribute to Albert A. Dahlberg*, ed. J. R. Lukacs. Eugene: University of Oregon, pp. 17–28.

Hillson, S. W. and FitzGerald, C. M. (2003). Tooth size variation and dental reduction in Europe, the Middle East and North Africa between 12 0000 and 5000 BP (abstract). *American Journal of Physical Anthropology Supplement*, **36**, 114.

Hillson, S. W., FitzGerald, C. M., and Flinn, H. (2005). Alternative dental measurements: proposals and relationships with other measurements. *American Journal of Physical Anthropology*, **126**, 413–26.

Kieser, J. A. (1990). *Human Adult Odontometrics*. Cambridge: Cambridge University Press.

Mayhall, J. T. (2000). Dental morphology: techniques and strategies. In *Biological Anthropology of the Human Skeleton*, ed. M. A. Katzenberg and S. R. Saunders. New York: Wiley-Liss, pp. 103–34.

Moorrees, C. F. and Reed, R. B. (1954). Correlations among crown diameters of human teeth. *Archives of Oral Biology*, **9**, 685–97.

Morris, D. H. (1986). Maxillary molar occlusal polygons in five human samples. *American Journal of Physical Anthropology*, **70**, 333–8.

Smith, B. H. (1984). Patterns of molar wear in hunter-gatherers and agriculturalists. *American Journal of Physical Anthropology*, **63**, 39–56.

Stojanowski, C. M. (in press). Comment on “Alternative Dental Measurements” by Hillson *et al. American Journal of Physical Anthropology.*
Tobias, P. V. (1967). *Olduvai Gorge II: The Cranium and Maxillary Dentition of* Australopithecus (Zinjanthropus) boisei. Cambridge: Cambridge University Press.
Wolpoff, M. H. (1969). The effect of mutations under conditions of reduced selection. *Social Biology*, **16**, 11–23.
y’Edynak, G. (1989). Disease and dimensional compensation during Yugoslav dental reduction (abstract). *American Journal of Physical Anthropology*, **78**, 327.
y’Edynak, G. (1992). Dental pathology: a factor in post-Pleistocene Yugoslav dental reduction. In *Culture, Ecology and Dental Anthropology*, ed. J. R. Lukacs. Delhi: Kamla-Raj Enterprises, pp. 133–44.

Endnotes

1. Although some dispute exists over which diameter is to be considered the width and which the length, we follow Wolpoff (1969).

17 *Dental microwear analysis: historical perspectives and new approaches*

PETER S. UNGAR, ROBERT S. SCOTT, JESSICA R. SCOTT, AND MARK TEAFORD

17.1 Introduction

Diet is widely recognized as the single most important parameter underlying behavioral and ecological differences among living animals. Bioarchaeologists and paleontologists reconstruct diets of past peoples and extinct animals for what they can teach us about matters ranging from the health status of individuals to adaptations and evolution of species. Dental microwear analysis is among the most effective ways of inferring diets of past peoples and fossil species. This approach involves the study of microscopic patterns of use-wear on teeth and is applicable to a broad range of species, giving a direct record of what an individual ate during its lifetime.

Researchers have recognized for decades that foods with given material properties leave characteristic patterns of scratches and pits in the molar teeth of humans and other animals. Foods requiring distinct types or levels of ingestive behavior also leave characteristic microscopic wear patterns in incisor teeth. Our understandings of relationships between dental microwear and diet/subsistence is improving with each passing year as new methods of analysis are developed and investigators continue to expand the number and variety of samples examined.

In this chapter we summarize one new method, dental microwear texture analysis, and offer some new data to illustrate the potential of this approach. We also briefly review some of the seminal microwear studies conducted over the past half century that put this and other work into historical context. The field of dental microwear research is growing at an unprecedented rate, and we now have the potential to infer subtle aspects of diet and tooth use, such as within-group variation in subsistence strategies and whether adaptive morphology reflects food preferences or fallback resources. As more microwear researchers join the ranks and our databases expand, it is becoming increasingly apparent that a repeatable method for characterizing and comparing microwear patterns is

Technique and Application in Dental Anthropology ed. Joel D. Irish and Greg C. Nelson
Published by Cambridge University Press.

needed. Microwear texture analysis provides one rapid, objective alternative to traditional approaches that promises to stretch the limits of what teeth can tell us about diet and feeding behaviors.

17.2 A brief history of dental microwear research

17.2.1 Early studies

The first published dental microwear analyses date back more than a half century. These earliest works stemmed from Simpson's (1933) view of teeth as guides for specific types of jaw movements. The angles at which opposing teeth meet in chewing were said to depend on properties of the particular foods eaten. In the 1950s, Butler (1952, ff.) and Mills (1955, ff.) recognized that microscopic scratch orientation on occlusal wear facets could be used to infer directions of jaw movements, and, presumably, diet. This work was followed by Baker *et al.*'s (1959) confirmation that dental microwear on sheep teeth did indeed result from chewing, and that individual features were caused as opal phytoliths in grass blades and exogenous quartz grit from soil scraped across the teeth during mastication.

Dental microwear entered the anthropological literature in 1962, when Dahlberg and Kinzey (1962) reported on modern and bioarchaeological human teeth examined by light microscopy. These authors presaged the idea that microwear variation within and among groups would allow the inference of differences in diet, however little further work was done over the following decade. The first dental microwear analysis of non-human primates was then published by Phillip Walker (1976). He suggested, again based on study using optical light microscopy, that terrestrial cercopithecoids have more striated incisal dentine surfaces than do arboreal Old World monkeys. Walker speculated that feeding substrate, siliceous material in foods eaten, and the mechanical demands of ingestion all affected striation incidence. He also noted diet-related differences, such that folivores had more laterally oriented scratches on their incisal surfaces than did frugivores – presumably related to stripping leaves laterally across the incisors.

17.2.2 Scanning electron microscopy and dental microwear analysis

Researchers soon realized that optical light microscopy had significant limitations for dental microwear research, and hence limited further progress in the field. The two main limitations of conventional optical light microscopy for dental microwear research were its limited depth of field and resolving power. These led to little more than narrow bands in focus, which posed problems for analyses of curved microwear surfaces. Also, magnifications were insufficient to visualize smaller microwear features, which often proved to be sub-micron in diameter. By the late 1970s, several workers had independently adopted the scanning electron microscope (SEM) as the instrument of choice for microwear analysis (Grine, 1977; Rensberger, 1978; Ryan, 1979; Walker *et al.*, 1978). As Ryan (1980a) noted, the SEM has approximately 200 × the resolving power, 100 × the maximal resolution, 100 × the maximum working distance and 10 × the depth of field at a given magnification when compared with conventional optical light microscopy. Thus the SEM allowed researchers to image smaller microwear features for the first time, with whole fields of view in focus, even when surfaces were curved or irregular.

Early SEM based microwear work focused on two areas: (1) determining whether different diets leave different and predictable microwear patterns, and (2) examining dental microwear for clues to diet in early hominins. Rensberger (1978) examined molar microwear in several genera of rodents, defining discrete types of microwear features and relating them to both diet and underlying dental enamel structure. At the same time, Alan Walker and coworkers (Walker *et al.*, 1978) related seasonal differences in diet to molar microwear patterns in hyraxes. They argued that browsing produced pitted surfaces, whereas grazing resulted in striated ones. Soon thereafter, Ryan (1980a, 1981) examined anterior tooth microwear in Old World monkeys and apes. Much like Rensberger (1978), Ryan (1980a, 1981) identified several different types of microwear features, suggesting that the differing incidences of each type reflected different ingestive behaviors, and, by implication, different diets.

Other microwear researchers in the late 1970s and early 1980s focused on the dietary implications of dental microwear in early hominins. Puech and colleagues (Puech, 1979; Puech and Prone, 1979; Puech *et al.*, 1981) used both transmitted light and electron microscopy to compare enamel surfaces of fossil hominins with experimentally produced microwear. These authors examined specimens representing several East African and European fossil hominin species, arguing that microwear surfaces preserved antemortem wear that reflected a range of diets, from grit-laden vegetarian fare, to acidic fruits, to meat. At the same time, Grine (1977, 1981) examined molar enamel microwear in Southern African early hominins, noting that *Paranthropus robustus* molars were dominated by microscopic pits, whereas *Australopithecus africanus* molars tended to have more striated wear facets. He opined in 1981 that heavy pitting on robust australopith molars evinces a diet of small, hard objects, whereas the striations on the gracile australopith molars indicated a diet of softer fruits and immature leaves.

Ryan (1980a) and Alan Walker (1981) applied the comparative method to microwear analysis of early hominins, using apparent associations between dental microwear and diet for living primates (including humans) and other mammals to infer diet from microwear patterns in fossil species. Ryan suggested, for example, that *Australopithecus afarensis* had a mosaic of gorilla- and baboon-like microwear features indicative of use of the incisors to ingest seeds and to strip grit-laden roots and rhizomes. Walker, in contrast, looked to molar microwear, suggesting that *Paranthropus boisei* did not show microwear patterns expected of a specialized grass-seed grazer or of a bone-crushing scavenger; two popular hypotheses at the time. He argued, to the contrary, that *P. boisei* had a microwear pattern similar to those of frugivorous Old World monkeys and apes. Researchers entered the 1980s optimistic about the potential of dental microwear for inferring diet in fossils as observations in living primates were related directly to feeding behaviors observed in the wild.

This optimism was, however, short lived. In fact, a series of papers came out between 1981 and 1983 that forced a complete re-evaluation of dental microwear as a tool for reconstructing diet. First, Covert and Kay (1981) published an experimental study on opossums that suggested no differences in microwear patterns between those fed diets that included plant fiber and those that ate insect chitin. This implied to them that microwear might not even be capable of distinguishing gross diet differences (such as between herbivory and insectivory). Peters (1982) then found that chert fragments and opal phytoliths produced similar microscopic scratches in experimental studies. He thus speculated that silicates within plants and grit on foods could cause similar microwear striations. This, combined with Peters' observation that dicotyledonous seed coats did not score enamel at all, led to further questions about the value of microwear for distinguishing at least some types of diets.

Gordon (1982, 1984, 1988) countered that microwear can be useful for reconstructing diet, but that other factors affecting patterns (such as magnification, tooth position, facet type, and SEM instrumentation settings) must be controlled if researchers were to use this approach to infer feeding behaviors. Indeed, Gordon and Walker (1983) suggested that Covert and Kay's (1981) inability to distinguish opossums by diet was due more to the fact that confounding factors were not taken into account than to limitations inherent to microwear research. Kay and Covert (1983, 1984) rebutted this by reiterating that grit and plant opals can leave similar microwear patterns, and by questioning studies (i.e. Gordon, 1982) on museum collections because of a lack of sufficient dietary control.

17.2.3 Quantitative and comparative analyses

Nevertheless, microwear researchers persevered, with Gordon's analyses setting the precedent for quantitative analyses. Her studies clearly showed the need for standardization of magnification and SEM instrumentation settings as well as control of tooth and even facet type used in analyses (Gordon, 1982, 1984, 1988); truisms that continue to be borne out today (Organ *et al.*, 2006a; see Mahoney, 2006c). Indeed, much of the work that has followed has built upon the techniques that Gordon and Alan Walker pioneered. Teaford and Walker (1984; see also Walker and Teaford, 1989) for example, counted and measured microscopic scratches and pits at a consistent magnification on homologous facets of homologous teeth of a range of anthropoid primates with broadly differing diets. Their results showed that frugivores have more pitting on Phase II molar facets, whereas folivores have more scratches on these surfaces. Further, harder object feeders tend to have higher pit-to-scratch ratios than do soft fruit eaters. Similar studies of other primates have demonstrated that among insectivores, those that specialize on hard beetles have more molar microwear pitting than those that feed on soft moths (Strait, 1991, 1993; see also Crompton *et al.*, 1998). This and other research has determined empirically that microwear patterning does indeed reflect diet.

Much of the primate microwear research that followed focused on documenting differences between samples, and on trying to understand the mechanics of feature formation. Some researchers demonstrated microwear differences between closely related species or sub-species with subtle differences in diet (Daegling and Grine, 1999; King *et al.*, 1999a; Oliveira, 2001; Solounias and Hayek, 1993; Teaford, 1985, 1986, 1993). Others found seasonal and ecological zone differences in microwear within taxa (Merceron *et al.*, 2004a; Teaford and Robinson, 1989). To this point, researchers have documented molar microwear of dozens of primate species representing all higher level taxa within our order (see Rose and Ungar, 1998; Teaford, 2006, 2007; Ungar, 1992, 1998). In fact, microwear studies have now expanded to include fish (Purnell *et al.*, 2006) and mammals of many different orders, from bats (Strait, 1993) to moles (Silcox and Teaford, 2002), pigs to sheep (Mainland, 1998, 2000, 2003, 2006; Ward and Mainland, 1999), antelopes to zebras (Hayek *et al.*, 1991; Solounias and Hayek, 1993; Solounias and Moelleken, 1992a), various marsupials (Robson and Young, 1990; Young *et al.*, 1987a), to large African cats (Van Valkenburgh *et al.*, 1990) and many others. One of the clearest contrasts, for example, has been between grazing and browsing ungulates (Merceron *et al.*, 2005b; Solounias and Moelleken, 1992a, 1992b, 1994) – a contrast that has important implications for reconstructing paleoenvironments (e.g. Merceron and Madelaine, 2006; Merceron and Ungar, 2005; Schubert *et al.*, 2007; Teaford *et al.*, 2007).

Some of the most productive research to date has involved the study of dental microwear and diet in wild primates. Decades of work by Teaford, Glander, and colleagues on mantled howler monkeys at Hacienda La Pacifica in Costa Rica, for example, has revealed much about the relationships between microwear patterning, food properties, and abrasives on and in those foods (Burnell *et al.*, 1994; Pastor *et al.*, 1995; Teaford and Glander, 1991, 1996; Teaford *et al.*, 2006; Ungar *et al.*, 1995). As another example, Nystrom *et al.* (2004) have demonstrated effects of season and grassland phenology on microwear patterning for baboons in the Awash National Park, Ethiopia, where microwear patterns are also influenced by extraneous grit on foods.

While most of this work has been on molar teeth, researchers have also considered incisors, and what their microwear patterns can tell us about ingestive behaviors and tooth use (Kelley, 1990; Ryan, 1981; Teaford, 1983a, 1983b; Ungar, 1990, 1994, 1998). Striation density on anthropoid incisors, for example, has been related to degree of habitual front tooth use in food processing. Further, it has been argued that preferred feature orientation indicates directions that foods are pulled across the front teeth, and that scratch breadth reflects the sizes of abrasive particles that cause dental microwear. As with molar studies, incisor microwear has been examined in other mammals, from Canadian moose (Young and Marty, 1986) to Australian kangaroos (Young *et al.*, 1987b).

17.2.4 Reconstructing diets of past peoples and extinct species

The principal motivation for all of this work is, of course, the inference of diets of past peoples and extinct species; bioarchaeologists and paleontologists have used dental microwear to provide new and important insights into life in the past. Bioarchaeologists have looked to microwear to infer aspects of subsistence and food preparation for a broad range of prehistoric peoples (Bullington, 1991; Danielson and Reinhard, 1998; Fine and Craig, S1981; Gugel *et al.*, 2001; Harmon and Rose, 1988; Hojo, 1989; Minozzi *et al.*, 2003; Molleson and Jones, 1991; Muendel, 1997; Organ *et al.*, 2006b; Reinhard and Danielson, 2005; Ungar and Spencer, 1999).

Much of this work has focused on identifying the transition from gathering and hunting to agricultural subsistence in areas ranging from North America (e.g. Larsen *et al.*, 2001; Rose and Marks, 1985; Schmidt, 2001; Teaford *et al.*, 2001) to Europe (e.g. Borgognini *et al.*, 1989), Africa (e.g. Gambarotta, 1995; Puech *et al.*, 1983b), the Levant (e.g. Mahoney, 2006a, 2006b), and the Indian sub-continent (Lukacs and Pastor, 1988; Pastor, 1993; Pastor and Johnson, 1992). Many have also examined food preparation technology using microwear (e.g. Harmon and Rose, 1988; Molleson *et al.*, 1993; Teaford and Lytle, 1996) and even found evidence for changes in diet from youth to adulthood (e.g. Bullington, 1991; Pérez-Pérez *et al.*, 1994).

Microwear research has focused on the diets of a broad range of fossil forms too, especially primates. Paleontologists have examined dental microwear for primate species representing all higher-order groups, and every epoch for which they are well known, from the Eocene (e.g. Strait, 1991, 1997) and the Oligocene (e.g. Teaford *et al.*, 1996) to the Miocene (e.g. Jacobs, 1981; Kelley, 1986; King, 2001; King *et al.*, 1999a; Leakey *et al.*, 2003; Merceron *et al.*, 2005a; Teaford and Walker, 1984; Ungar, 1996, 1998; Ungar *et al.*, 2004; Walker *et al.*, 1994), Pliocene and Pleistocene (Daegling and Grine, 1994; El Zaatari *et al.*, 2006; Galbany *et al.*, 2005; Godfrey *et al.*, 2004, 2005b; Lucas and Teaford, 1994; Rafferty *et al.*, 2002; Teaford and Leakey, 1992; Ungar and Teaford, 1996). Much of this work has centered on early hominins, from the australopiths and early *Homo* of the Plio-Pleistocene (Grine, 1981, 1986; Grine *et al.*, 2006; Puech, 1986; Puech and Albertini, 1984; Puech *et al.*, 1986; Ryan and Johanson, 1989; Ungar and Grine, 1991; Ungar *et al.*, 2005; Walker, 1981) to more recent members of our own genus (Pérez-Pérez *et al.*, 1999, 2003; Ryan, 1980b). Microwear studies have also been applied to a broad range of other fossil taxa, from Paleozoic conodonts (Purnell, 1995), to Mesozoic dinosaurs (Barrett, 2006; Fiorillo, 1991, 1998; Rybczynski and Vickaryous, 2006; Schubert and Ungar, 2005), mammal-like reptiles (Goswami *et al.*, 2005), and primitive mammals (Biknevicius, 1986; Krause, 1982; O'Leary and Teaford, 1992), to past perissodactyls (e.g. Hayek *et al.*, 1991; Kaiser *et al.*, 2003; MacFadden *et al.*, 1999; Solounias and Semprebon, 2002), artiodactyls (e.g. Dompierre and Churcher, 1996; Franz-Odendaal and Solounias, 2004; Hunter and Fortelius, 1994; Merceron and Madelaine, 2006; Merceron and Ungar, 2005; Merceron *et al.*, 2004a, 2005b; Rivals and Deniaux, 2003; Schubert *et al.*, 2007; Semprebon *et al.*, 2004a; Solounias and Moelleken, 1993; Solounias *et al.*, 1988), rodents (e.g. Gutierrez *et al.*, 1998; Hopley *et al.*, 2006; Lewis *et al.*, 2000), carnivorans (Anyonge, 1996; Van Valkenburgh *et al.*, 1990), proboscideans (Capozza, 2001; Filippi *et al.*, 2001; Green *et al.*, 2005; Palombo *et al.*, 2005), and other groups.

17.2.5 Evolving approaches to characterizing microwear patterns

With all of these researchers documenting microwear for such a dizzying array of living and fossil samples, it would seem at first glance that we are fast approaching the point where comparative studies will allow unprecedented understanding of the ranges of subsistence practices of past peoples, and the adaptive radiations of primates and other mammals. This would be true if only researchers adopted a standard method for quantitative characterization of dental microwear patterns that allows comparisons across studies.

The earliest approaches to dental microwear analysis were largely qualitative, and relied on optical light microscopy. Researchers documented such attributes as microscopic striation presence/absence, density (high or low), and approximate preferred orientation direction if there was one (e.g. Dahlberg and Kinzey, 1962; Walker, 1976). The adoption of the SEM as the instrument of preference quickly led researchers to identify a number of discrete feature types that could be used to describe surfaces in detail. Rensberger (1978), for example, developed a classification of distinctive microwear surface features including polish, striations, furrows, fissures, flaked pits, and pebbly texture. Other terms, such as "microflakes" (Ryan, 1981), crenulations (Puech *et al.*, 1983a), and "compression fractures" (Rose and Marks, 1985) were also commonly used to describe individual microwear features.

It soon became obvious, however, that with larger samples of increasing variety, quantitative characterization of surfaces would be necessary to provide a statistical basis for evaluating probable diets of fossil species and past peoples (Walker, 1981). Several similar approaches emerged, focusing on characterizing average numbers, sizes, shapes, and orientations of individual features. These ranged from counting and measuring scratches and pits on paper photomicrographs using calipers and protractors (Gordon, 1982; Grine, 1986; Maas, 1991; Ryan, 1981; Strait, 1993; Ungar and Grine, 1991) or a digitizing tablet (Pastor, 1993; Solounias *et al.*, 1988; Teaford, 1988a; Teaford and Walker, 1984) to a mouse driven cursor on a computer screen (Ungar, 1995; Ungar *et al.*, 1991). Data on feature lengths, widths and orientations emerged, along with the ubiquitous "pit percentage" – the ratio of pits to scratches on a surface. Pit percentage data proved particularly useful for distinguishing primates by broad diet category; though the length:breadth ratio used to distinguish feature types remained arbitrary (given that that both measures are continuous) and initially inconsistent (e.g. 10:1 versus 4:1, with researchers eventually switching to the 4:1 ratio based on Grine's observation (1986) that it most closely approximated what the human eye would recognize as the boundary between pits and scratches).

While quantification allowed for statistical comparison, this approach was time-consuming and expensive. Preparation of specimens, imaging of surfaces, and identification of features on photomicrographs for a single individual can take hours, and SEM time and supplies can be very expensive (Rose and Ungar, 1998; Solounias and Semprebon, 2002). To this end, Solounias and Semprebon (2002) proposed a return to low-magnification microscopy, where observers classify and tally microwear features by eye while viewing surfaces through a binocular light microscope. A variant of this approach, suggested by Merceron and colleagues (Merceron, 2003a, 2003b; Merceron *et al.*, 2004a, 2004b, 2005a, 2005b), involves a compromise technique combining imaging by light microscopy and measurement of features on a computer screen.

Low-magnification light microscopy certainly offers a rapid and inexpensive approach, and it has gained popularity in recent years (Godfrey *et al.*, 2004, 2005b; Green *et al.*, 2005; Kaiser, 2003; Nelson *et al.*, 2005; Rivals and Semprebon, 2006; Semprebon *et al.*, 2004b; Solounias and Semprebon, 2002). Further, its advocates have demonstrated that the experienced observer can use it to distinguish gross differences in diet. Still, this new low-magnification approach has not magically resolved the original limitations of light microscopy (e.g. depth of field, magnification) that caused microwear researchers to look to the SEM in the 1970s. Given its inherent limitations, even experienced researchers can have difficulty distinguishing some microwear types, such as puncture pits and dentine lakes (Godfrey *et al.*, 2005a; Semprebon *et al.*, 2005). More importantly, it is not possible to resolve the smaller (micron scale) microwear features that dominate wear facets. These are the very features that are often key to finer dietary distinctions and to the differentiation of antemortem microwear from postmortem damage (Teaford, 2006).

The most pressing problem facing both SEM and low-magnification light microscopy studies, however, is measurement error. This leads to low repeatability, and limited accuracy of wear surface characterization. In a recent study by Grine *et al.* (2002) for example, inter-observer error rates using the SEM approaches averaged about 9%. Semprebon *et al.* (2004b) report that their inter-observer absolute error rates are similar to those reported for SEM when using comparable measurement techniques – although no data have been reported for the categorization of features into various sizes. While studies have demonstrated empirically that broad diet differences can be resolved despite measurement error, this is a significant source of variation that likely limits the resolution of microwear both for assessing subtle differences between samples and for describing and assessing within sample variation (Scott *et al.*, 2005).

These high error rates are due to two factors: (1) observer measurement error, and (2) data loss inherent in characterizing 3D surfaces in two dimensions. First, identification of individual features by observers adds subjectivity to the measurement of microwear scratches and pits. A surface visualized by SEM, for example, can have hundreds of features, the boundaries of which are irregular and commonly overlap the borders of others and the edges of the field of view (Rose and Ungar, 1998). Observer error is to be expected, especially given that low correlations between results of investigators are often found when measurement endpoints are difficult to define (Jamison, 1974).

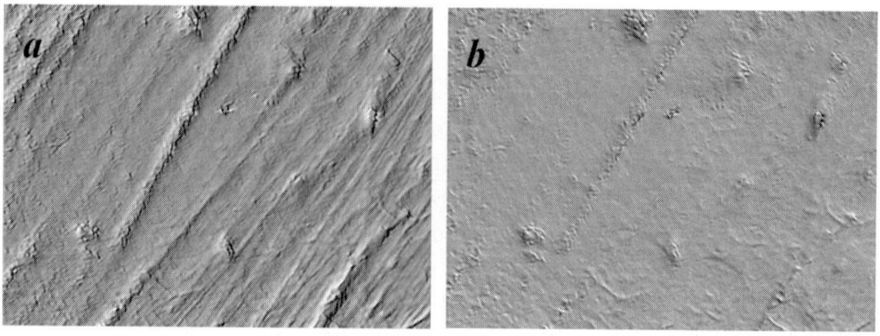

Figure 17.1 Photosimulation of single microwear surface with "pseudo light" oriented perpendicular to the preferred orientation of features (a) and in line with the preferred orientation of features (b).

Various researchers have tried, over the past two decades, to limit measurement error by developing automated surface characterizations. Phillip Walker *et al.* (1987) for example, suggested thresholding of gray levels to isolate features on SEM photomicrographs. Unfortunately, automatic pattern recognition software available 20 years ago was not well-suited to resolving features on SEM photomicrographs given complex variations in gray level across images. Kay (1987) proposed alternatively that Fourier power spectra could be used to characterize whole surfaces. While this would certainly mitigate problems inherent in individual feature identification and measurement, the technique was not broadly adopted, perhaps in part because subsequent study showed that it did not separate taxa as well as did more conventional approaches (Grine and Kay, 1987).

Another important limitation of both SEM and low-magnification light microscopy approaches relates to data loss inherent in the characterization of a 3D surface in two dimensions. Features are identified as "relief" suggested by shadows and decreasing light or electron beam intensity with depth. The image formed for any given surface then depends on the geometric relations of the light or electron source, subject surface plane, and optics or electron collector. Changing the geometry of this system will change the image (Figure 17.1, see also, Gordon, 1988; Pastor, 1993; Solounias and Semprebon, 2002). As Solounias and Semprebon (2002, p. 7) have noted, "while adjusting the manner in which light strikes the cast (i.e. angle of incident light beam and intensity), the visualization of microwear features can vary from none visible to a few or many." Indeed, "the angle of light often needs to be altered slightly to view pits versus scratches" (Solounias and Semprebon, 2002, p. 7). For SEM-based studies, other variables, such as the type of electrons used (e.g. backscattered vs. secondary), voltage, and coating materials and thickness can also affect the resulting image (Gordon, 1988). Even if all of these variables are held constant between studies, 2D characterizations of 3D features are not ideal, as they are inherently incomplete, with the type of data lost depending on decisions made by the observer. In short, we do not know what we are missing in characterizing a 3D surface in 2D.

Researchers have recognized for some time that an instrument capable of measuring a surface in 3D would be a better alternative. Boyde and Fortelius (1991) for example, proposed the use of a confocal reflection microscope. They suggested that resulting elevation data could be used to isolate and identify features by thresholding. This approach was not broadly adopted, however, probably in part because surface analysis software available at the time was of limited value for thresholding these complex surfaces. Other tools, such as the mechanical profilometer and atomic force microscope, have also been suggested as possible tools for microwear analysis (Walker and Hagen, 1994), but these each come with their own limitations related to resolution, work envelope, and depth of field.

17.3 Dental microwear texture analysis

It is against this backdrop that we and our colleagues have developed dental microwear texture analysis (Scott *et al.*, 2005, 2006; Ungar *et al.*, 2003). This approach was designed to solve all three of the major problems inherent to conventional microwear analyses: time and expense, data loss in surface characterization, and observer error in measurement. Dental microwear texture analysis combines white-light confocal microscopy (though other instruments capable of producing a high-resolution point cloud model would also work) with scale-sensitive fractal analysis (SSFA). The result is the quantitative description of whole surfaces at a range of scales. This approach offers a suite of objective, repeatable measures of microwear in 3D that can be compared between groups with differing diets. Further, white-light confocal microscopy is quicker, easier to use, and less costly than SEM, and automated fractal analysis requires *much* less time and effort from individual researchers than does identification and measurement of individual features.

The most important advance is the elimination of observer error in measurement, which allows direct comparisons between studies and the establishment of a large database that researchers can tap for interpretation of their results. Indeed, dental microwear texture analysis is now progressing on a wide range of samples, from bioarchaeological collections to living and fossil primates (including hominins), bovids, and reptiles. Some of this work on living anthropoid primates is summarized here to illustrate how the approach works.

17.3.1 Specimens examined

Here we present dental microwear topography data for eight primate taxa. Data for four of the species are summarized from Scott *et al.* (2006) including two cercopithecoids, *Lophocebus albigena* ($n = 15$) and *Trachypithecus cristatus* ($n = 12$) and two platyrrhines, *Alouatta palliata* ($n = 11$) and *Cebus apella* ($n = 13$). New data on four extant ape taxa, *Gorilla gorilla beringei* ($n = 16$), *G. g. gorilla* ($n = 14$), *Pan troglodytes troglodytes* ($n = 17$), and *Pongo pygmaeus pygmaeus* (including some specimens presented by Merceron *et al.* (2006)) ($n = 15$) are also presented here. High resolution replicas of M_2s were made following conventional procedures. Original specimens were cleaned with acetone-soaked cotton swabs, and vinyl impressions were taken using a polyvinylsiloxane dental impression material. High-resolution epoxy was then poured into the molds and allowed to harden. This procedure results in high-resolution replicas that faithfully reproduce microwear features on the order of a fraction of a micron (see Ungar, 1994 ff. for details).

All individuals examined were wild-shot specimens housed in the Tappen collection at the University of Minnesota (*L. albigena*), the US National Museum of Natural History (*T. cristatus*, *C. apella, A. palliata, G. g. beringei*), the American Museum of Natural History (*G. g. gorilla*), the Cleveland Museum of Natural History (*G. g. gorilla*, *Pa. troglodytes*), and the Bavarian State Collection of Anthropology and Palaeoanatomy in Munich (*Po. pygmaeus*). Specimens were collected in Mukono, Uganda (*L. albigena*); Bahia, Brazil (*C. apella*), Boca del Drago, Panama (*A. palliata*); Cameroon (mostly Ebolwa and Abong Mbong), (*G. g. gorilla, Pa. troglodytes*); the Virunga Mountains of Rwanda (*G. g. beringei*); Skalau, West Kalimantan (*Po. pygmaeus*); and other localities in Indonesia (*T. cristatus*).

These taxa were chosen because of their contrasting diets, and because of differences in microwear demonstrated using conventional microwear analyses (Teaford, 1988a; Teaford and Ungar, 2006). *Cebus apella* and *L. albigena* have diets that include some hard, brittle objects such as palm nuts, bark, and seeds (Chalmers, 1968; Lambert *et al.*, 2004). These can be compared with *A. palliata* and *T. cristatus*, which eat more tough, pliant items such as leaves and stems (Brotoisworo and Dirgayusa, 1991; Estrada, 1984). *Pa. troglodytes* is reported to consume more fruit flesh than *G. gorilla*, which eats more tough, fibrous stems and leaves (Kuroda, 1992; Tutin *et al.*, 1991; Williamson *et al.*, 1990), with *Pongo pygmaeus* intermediate in diet between the two African apes – though the orangutans also consume harder shelled nuts and seeds on occasion (MacKinnon, 1977; Rodman, 1977). The mountain and western lowland gorillas are considered separately here because *G. g. beringei* was reported to more regularly consume tough, fibrous foods than *G. g. gorilla*. As with all such generalizations, however, caveats concerning use of museum samples (Kay and Covert, 1983) and differing methods for the collection of primate feeding data (Doran *et al.*, 2002) apply.

17.3.2 Methods of analysis

Methods developed for microwear texture analysis are described in detail elsewhere (Scott *et al.*, 2006; Ungar *et al.*, 2003). Facet 9 of each specimen was scanned using a Sensofar Plμ white-light scanning confocal microscope (Solarius, Sunnyvale, California) using a 100 × objective. The resulting point cloud had a lateral sampling interval of 0.18 μm and a vertical resolution of 0.005 μm. We collected data for four adjoining fields, sampling an area of 276 × 204 μm. The resulting resolving power exceeds that of typical SEM based microwear images taken at 500 ×, which are usually digitized at 200 dpi yielding a resolution of 0.25 μm per pixel (Grine *et al.*, 2002; Ungar, 1996). Only those surfaces that clearly preserved antemortem microwear (following criteria of Teaford (1988b) and King *et al.* (1999b)) were included in the analysis, and artifacts, such as adherent dust particles, were excluded by thresholding, erase operators and slope-filtering as necessary.

Resulting point clouds were analyzed in Toothfrax and SFrax software (Surfact, www.surfact.com). Scale-sensitive fractal analysis is based on the fact that apparent characteristics of a surface (e.g. length of a profile, area, and volume) vary with scale of observation. Surface textures can appear smooth at coarse scales, but rough at finer ones. Changes in apparent texture at different scales can be examined for profiles across a surface (length-scale analysis), or whole surfaces (area-scale and volume-filling vs. scale analyses). Our research group has to date identified several texture variables of potential value to microwear researchers (Scott *et al.*, 2005, 2006; Ungar *et al.*, 2003). We present data for four of these here: complexity, scale of maximal complexity, anisotropy, and textural fill volume. Values for individual surfaces are reported as medians of the four fields sampled following Scott *et al.* (2006).

It is beyond the scope of this chapter to describe the theoretical underpinnings of these variables in detail, but a brief summary will hopefully convey what they represent. Those interested in more comprehensive descriptions should see Ungar *et al.* (2003) and Scott *et al.* (2006).

*Complexity (*Asfc*)*

Complexity is measured as change in surface roughness at different scales. *Asfc* is basically the slope of the steepest part of curve fit to a plot of measured area over the range of scales at which those measurements are made. The steeper the slope is, the more complex the surface. Pits and scratches of different sizes overlaying one another would present a complex surface.

*Scale of maximum complexity (*Smc*)*

This is the fine scale limit of the steepest part of the curve described for the *Asfc* measure. Surfaces with greater values for *Smc* will tend to have less wear at very fine scales and/or more wear features at coarser scales. For instance, a surface dominated by large pits with an absence of fine scratches might have a high *Smc*.

*Anisotropy (*epLsar*)*

Anisotropy is a measure of orientation concentration of surface roughness. *epLsar* is a measure of differences in lengths of depth profiles sampled across a surface at different orientations at a given scale; in this case a sample interval of 5° and a scale of 1.8 μm (see Scott *et al.*, 2006). Average lengths of profiles and their orientations (treated as vectors) are normalized using the exact proportion method, and the mean vector length is calculated. A surface dominated by scratches all running in the same direction would have a high *epLsar*.

*Textural fill volume (*Tfv*)*

This measure examines summed volumes of square cuboids of a given scale that fill a surface. *Tfv* is computed as the difference in summed volume for very fine cuboids (in this case 2 μm on a side) and larger ones (in this case 10 μm on a side). This removes the structure of the overall surface (e.g. facet curvature), limiting characterization to the microwear features themselves. A surface dominated with more features in the mid-scale range would have a high *Tfv*.

Statistical analyses

Statistical analyses were performed to determine the extent of variation in microwear texture between taxa following Ungar *et al.* (2006). All data were rank-transformed before analysis because unranked microwear data typically violate assumptions associated with parametric statistical tests (Conover and Iman, 1981). Data for the four variables were compared among species using a multivariate analysis of variance model, with taxon as the factor, *Asfc, Smc, epLsar*, and *Tfv* as the dependent variables, and values for each individual as the replicates. This test assesses significance of variation among the taxa in overall microwear surface texture. Single classification ANOVAs for each variable and multiple comparisons tests were used to determine the sources of significant variation. Because these groups were chosen for their dietary (and expected microwear) differences, Fisher's LSD a priori tests were used to compare species. Tukey's HSD *post hoc* tests were also run though, to balance risks of Type I and Type II errors (Cook and Farewell, 1996).

17.3.3 Results and discussion

Results illustrate the efficacy of dental microwear texture analysis. Summary and analytical statistics are presented in Tables 17.1 and 17.2, and examples of microwear in 3D are illustrated in Figure 17.2. Both Wilks' λ and Pillai Trace results indicated significant variation among the taxa in overall microwear texture. Further, the individual ANOVAs for *Asfc, Smc, epLsar*, and *Tfv* all showed significant variation among the taxa.

The multiple comparisons tests suggested unique texture patterns for several taxa. For example, *Alouatta* and *Trachypithecus* both had low *Asfc* values, with significantly less texture complexity than the other taxa. *Alouatta* also had lower *Lsar* values than other taxa, with more anisotropy on average than all except *Trachypithecus* (the latter was also fairly anisotropic, significantly more than at least *Pan*). The howler monkeys also had very low *Tfv* values, significantly lower than all other taxa except *Pongo. Lophocebus* tended to have fairly coarse scales of maximum complexity, with *Smc* values significantly higher in value than *Pan* and marginally higher (defined by a significant difference in the LSD but not the HSD test) than in *Cebus, Pongo*, and *Trachypithecus*. The mangabeys also had a high *Tfv* on average, significantly higher than *Pongo* and *G. g. gorilla*. Finally, *Cebus* had a relatively high average *Asfc*, especially compared with the folivores, but also had marginally more complex microwear than *Lophocebus*, *Pongo*, and *G. g. beringei*.

While a detailed consideration of the biological implications of these results is beyond the scope of this chapter, the data do point to some interesting contrasts. First, the folivorous monkeys, especially *Alouatta*, tend to have less complex microwear than the other primates, with surfaces dominated by fine features with some directionality. More subtle differences are also evident, such that, for example, *Lophocebus* averages somewhat higher *Smc* but lower *Tfv* values than *Cebus*. This suggests that the mangabeys have microwear concentrated at a coarser scale, but show less overall surface complexity than do the capuchins. This may relate to different degrees of exploitation of hard, brittle foods between the two primates (see Scott *et al*., 2006 for discussion); an idea consistent with Lambert *et al*.'s (2004) behavioral observations concerning mangabey dietary preferences and fallback food exploitation.

More remarkable than the differences between taxa, however, is the extreme variability within some groups and the degree of overlap between them. This will come as no surprise to anyone that has spent an extended period of time

Table 17.1 *Descriptive statistics*

Taxon	Statistic	*n*	*Asfc*	*Smc*	*epLsar*	*Tfv*
Alouatta palliata	Median	11	0.315	−0.574	0.006	1351
	Mean		0.360	−0.188	0.006	2610
	SD		0.183	1.050	0.002	3225
	Skewness		0.402	2.653	−0.306	0.853
	Kurtosis		−1.125	7.408	−0.512	−1.021
Cebus apella	Median	13	2.882	−0.574	0.003	9707
	Mean		5.466	−0.178	0.004	9682
	SD		6.304	1.101	0.002	4923
	Skewness		1.624	2.022	0.758	0.746
	Kurtosis		2.294	2.94	−1.053	0.807
Lophocebus albigena	Median	15	1.018	0.886	0.003	11324
	Mean		1.769	0.623	0.004	11388
	SD		1.740	1.064	0.002	3390
	Skewness		2.304	−0.100	1.213	0.193
	Kurtosis		5.637	−1.382	1.343	1.794
Pan troglodytes	Median	17	2.114	−0.821	0.002	9647
	Mean		2.246	−0.522	0.003	9345
	SD		1.523	0.528	0.001	5477
	Skewness		0.917	1.776	0.607	0.173
	Kurtosis		0.175	2.255	−0.125	−1.368
Pongo pygmaeus	Median	15	1.122	−0.569	0.004	6732
	Mean		1.356	−0.379	0.004	6574
	SD		0.947	0.426	0.002	6645
	Skewness		1.078	0.630	0.004	1.135
	Kurtosis		0.947	−1.007	−0.905	0.810
Trachypithecus cristatus	Median	12	0.514	−0.626	0.004	10127
	Mean		0.734	−0.365	0.005	9532
	SD		0.660	0.547	0.003	5687
	Skewness		2.618	1.648	0.826	−0.454
	Kurtosis		7.648	2.176	−0.415	−0.883
G.g. beringei	Median	16	1.182	−0.516	0.004	8662
	Mean		1.711	−0.273	0.004	8686
	SD		1.455	0.695	0.002	6025
	Skewness		2.125	2.165	−0.161	0.035
	Kurtosis		5.211	5.515	−1.012	−0.886
G.g. gorilla	Median	14	1.247	−0.626	0.004	6784
	Mean		1.597	−0.384	0.004	8100
	SD		1.012	0.567	0.002	5703
	Skewness		0.723	1.570	−0.108	1.178
	Kurtosis		−0.65	2.422	−0.11	1.612

Table 17.2 *Statistical Analyses*

A. Multivariate Test Statistics

Wilks' Lambda = 0.417
F-statistic = 3.615
df = 28, 369
P = 0.000

Pillai Trace = 0.720
F-statistic = 3.294
df = 28, 420
P = 0.000

B. Univariate F Tests

Effect	**SS**	**df**	**MS**	***F***	***P***
Asfc	42 294.7	7	6042.1	8.14	0.000
Error	77 937.3	105	742.3		
Smc	16 651.0	7	2378.7	2.411	0.025
Error	103 581.0	105	986.5		
epLsar	162 22.8	7	2317.5	2.34	0.029
Error	104 009.2	105	990.6		
Tfv	24 171.2	7	3453.0	3.776	0.001
Error	96 018.8	105	914.5		

C. Multiple Comparisons Tests
(i) *Asfc* Pairwise comparisons test results

	Alouatta	*Cebus*	*Lophocebus*	*Pan*	*Pongo*	*Trachypithecus*	*G.g. beringei*
Cebus	68.042[a]						
Lophocebus	47.539[a]	−20.503[b]					
Pan	59.684[a]	−8.357	12.145				
Pongo	41.539[a]	−26.503[b]	−6	−18.145			
Trachypithecus	17.356	−50.686[a]	−30.183[b]	−42.328[a]	−24.183[b]		
G.g. beringei	47.21[a]	−20.832[b]	−0.329	−12.474	5.671	29.854[b]	
G.g. gorilla	49.344[a]	−18.698	1.805	−10.34	7.805	31.988[b]	2.134

[a] Tukeys HSD and Fishers LSD $p \leq 0.05$.
[b] Fishers LSD only $p \leq 0.05$.

(cont.)

Table 17.2 (*cont.*)

(ii) *Smc* Pairwise comparisons test results

	Alouatta	*Cebus*	*Lophocebus*	*Pan*	*Pongo*	*Trachypithecus*	*G.g. beringei*
Cebus	−2.958						
Lophocebus	22.006	24.964[b]					
Pan	−22.904	−19.946	−44.91[a]				
Pongo	−2.461	0.497	−24.467	20.443			
Trachypithecus	−2.727	0.231	−24.733	20.176	−0.267		
G.g. beringei	−1.477	1.481	−23.483[b]	21.426	0.983	1.25	
G.g. gorilla	−8.37	−5.412	−30.376[b]	14.534	−5.91	−5.643	−6.893

[a] Tukeys HSD and Fishers LSD $p \leq 0.05$.
[b] Fishers LSD only $p \leq 0.05$.

(iii) *epLsar* Pairwise comparisons test results

	Alouatta	*Cebus*	*Lophocebus*	*Pan*	*Pongo*	*Trachypithecus*	*G.g. beringei*
Cebus	−32.469[b]						
Lophocebus	−30.145[b]	2.323					
Pan	−46.487[a]	−14.018	−16.341				
Pongo	−28.812[b]	3.656	1.333	17.675			
Trachypithecus	−17.379	15.09	12.767	29.108[b]	11.433		
G.g. beringei	−28.483[b]	3.986	1.663	18.004	0.329	−11.104	
G.g. gorilla	−25.117[b]	7.352	5.029	21.37	3.695	−7.738	3.366

[a] Tukeys HSD and Fishers LSD $p \leq 0.05$.
[b] Fishers LSD only $p \leq 0.05$.

(iv) *Tfv* Pairwise comparisons test results

	Alouatta	*Cebus*	*Lophocebus*	*Pan*	*Pongo*	*Trachypithecus*	*G.g. beringei*
Cebus	42.063[a]						
Lophocebus	55.242[a]	13.179					
Pan	40.85[a]	−1.213	−14.392				
Pongo	22.276	−19.787	−32.967[b]	−18.575			
Trachypithecus	42.867[a]	0.804	−12.375	2.017	20.592		
G.g. beringei	36.159[b]	−5.904	−19.083	−4.691	13.883	−6.708	
G.g. gorilla	31.981[b]	−10.082	−23.262[b]	−8.87	9.705	−10.887	−4.179

[a] Tukeys HSD and Fishers LSD $p \leq 0.05$.
[b] Fishers LSD only $p \leq 0.05$.

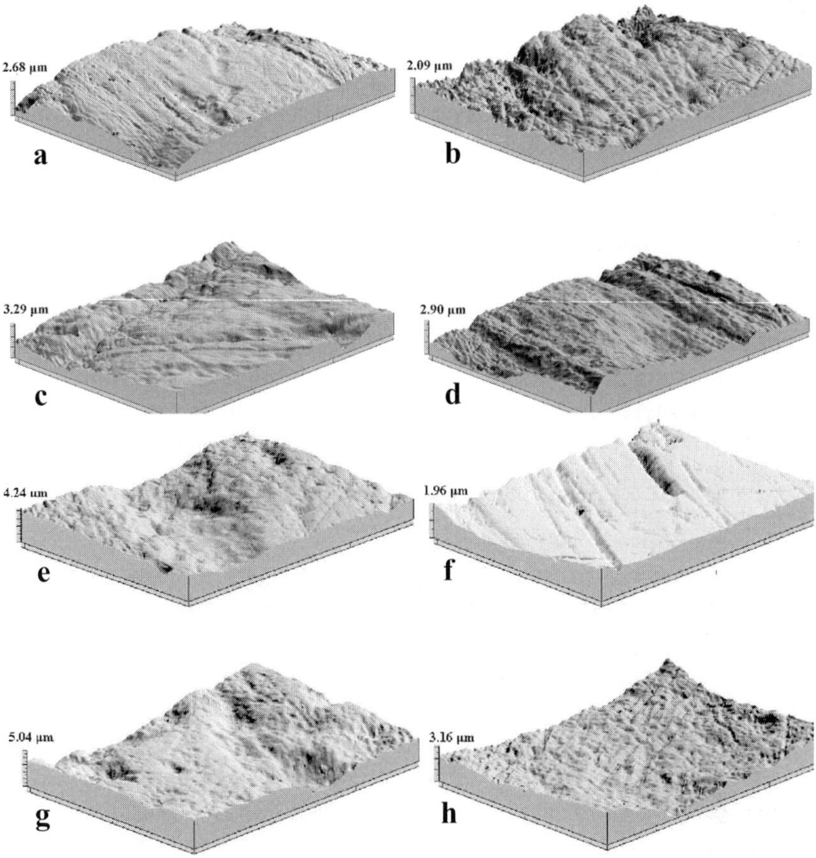

Figure 17.2 3D photosimulations of microwear surfaces from *Pan troglodytes* CMNH-B3537 (a), *Pongo pygmaeus* SAPM198162 (b), *G.g. gorilla* CMNH-B1410 (c), *G.g. beringei* NMNH545027 (d), *Cebus paella* NMNH518289 (e), *Alouatta palliata* NMNH315790 (f), *Lophocebus albigena* UMN238 (g), and *Trachypithecus cristatus* NMNH154723 (h). Each photosimulation is 102 µm by 139 µm with vertical relief noted on the figure.

observing feeding behavior in wild anthropoid primates. Primate diets vary greatly, depending on availability of preferred and fallback resources. The differences between taxa are further obscured by the fact that primates pigeonholed in the popular literature into very different dietary categories will often eat similar foods, e.g. gorillas have been reported to consume 73% of the same species eaten by sympatric chimpanzees at Lopé, Gabon (Tutin and Fernandez, 1985). Thus, the lack of clear differences in central tendencies between chimpanzees and gorillas (and between the sub-species of gorillas for that matter) is not unexpected. Because microwear reflects at most a week of feeding behavior, there would likely be something wrong if these samples did *not* show substantial variability and overlap!

This suggests that perhaps a measure other than central tendency is important for using microwear to understand dietary adaptations and behaviors of primates. Given the relatively short lifespan of individual features, microwear may well give us the opportunity to examine within-species variation in patterns. A few outlier specimens, such as is observed for *Asfc* of *Cebus*, are likely to be more informative of differences in dietary behaviors in many cases (such as fallback food exploitation) than would comparisons of sample means (see Scott *et al.*, 2005 for discussion). The ability to detect subtle differences in within-sample variation may then be a key to realizing the potential of dental microwear analyses. If so, microwear characterizations free from measurement error, such as afforded by texture analysis, may well help unlock the door.

17.4 Conclusions and implications

Researchers have recognized since the 1950s that foods leave characteristic and predictable patterns of microscopic use-wear in teeth, and the field of dental microwear research has come a long way in the past half century. Early studies were brimming with optimism, suggesting that much could be learned by qualitative comparison between the samples of interest and a baseline series of individuals with known diets. Subsequent work demonstrated empirically that microwear patterns do indeed reflect feeding behaviors and the fracture properties of foods; though control over surfaces examined and standardization of data collection protocols is necessary.

The work that has followed has focused on two principal areas: (1) improving comparative baseline series and determining the limits of microwear analysis; and (2) using these baselines to infer aspects of tooth use and diet in past peoples and fossil species. Studies of microwear etiology have involved in vitro experiments, analyses of museum specimens, and investigations of microwear of animals living in the wild. This work has led to new and important insights into relationships between microwear patterns and diet/tooth use. Bioarchaeologists and paleontologists have used these to uncover tantalizing clues about the subsistence practices of early peoples and the diets of fossil species. Today, more researchers than ever before are using dental microwear to infer the diets of a greater and greater range of past peoples and animals.

Nevertheless, it has been argued that conventional dental microwear research has reached a plateau (Ungar *et al.*, 2003). The history of the field shows a feedback loop between research and technological innovation. While there was a 15-year hiatus in microwear studies following initial light-microscopy analyses, the first use of the SEM in such studies in the late 1970s prompted a flurry of activity. Initial quantitative studies sparked another flood of research, and new computer-assisted techniques have facilitated quantification to the point that more researchers are publishing microwear results for a broader range of groups every year. At the same time, workers are trying to identify subtler differences in diet using microwear techniques. Finally, as more work is published, more workers are comparing more data across more studies.

This presents a problem because the lack of standardization in techniques and significant observer measurement error can make comparisons between studies difficult. The most pressing challenge facing the field today is the development of a rapid, objective and repeatable approach to characterizing dental microwear surfaces in 3D.

We propose that dental microwear texture analysis offers one solution. The white-light confocal microscope models surfaces as high-resolution 3D point clouds. The SEM and optical light microscope project a surface on to a 2D plane, with the resulting image and data loss dependent on specimen orientation relative to electron or light source and collector or objective lens. The white-light confocal microscope has the further advantage over SEM in that it is dead easy to operate and uses a white-light source that costs pennies per hour to run.

Scale-sensitive fractal analysis also has several advantages over feature-based microwear characterizations. First, SSFA characterizes whole surfaces, without the need to measure individual features, or to classify them as discrete types. A 4:1 length-to-breadth ratio threshold for distinguishing pits and scratches may, for example, be of value, but it is inherently arbitrary. How many other "types" of features are useful to define given that features vary in length and breadth along a continuum? Further, there is no one-to-one correspondence between an individual feature and a single feeding event. Whole surface analyses can offer more objective and repeatable measures than do ratios of feature "types" or average feature dimensions. In addition, scale-sensitive approaches allow us to look at patterns across a range of scales, without having to decide whether $35\times$ or $500\times$ is more appropriate for distinguishing diets. Finally, because the process is automated, it requires little investment of human effort. That translates to no more weeks of counting and measuring tens of thousands of scratches and pits for the typical SEM-based project! And it provides repeatable, error-free measurements.

The field of dental microwear shows much promise for progress in the future as technology facilitates more repeatable and better characterizations of dental microwear patterning. Approaches such as texture analysis can allow researchers to develop large comparative databases of microwear patterns associated with known diets, be it published diets, or diets directly observed in the field or in the lab. Objective, repeatable measurement facilitates comparisons between studies, with the potential for unprecedented understandings of the ranges of subsistence practices of past peoples, and the adaptive radiations of primates and other mammals. To be sure, more conventional approaches remain valuable for contrasting animals with orthodox diets (e.g. grazing and browsing ungulates). Still, for studies of groups with more catholic proclivities, such as humans and many other primates, error-free measurements of within-sample variation may well afford a deeper understanding of the subtle details of feeding adaptations, such as individual variation in diet, food preferences, and seasonal fallback resource exploitation.

Acknowledgments

We thank Joel Irish and Greg Nelson for inviting us to contribute to this volume. We also thank curators at the American Museum of Natural History, the Bavarian State Collection of Anthropology and Palaeoanatomy, the Cleveland Museum of Natural History, the University of Minnesota Department of Anthropology, and the US National Museum of Natural History for their help and access to specimens in their care. We are grateful to our many colleagues, especially Chris Brown, Fred Grine, Rich Kay, and Alan Walker for many long hours of discussion and debate on the merits of dental microwear study and especially texture analysis. Research described in this chapter was funded in part by grants from the National Science Foundation and the LSB Leakey Foundation.

Appendix 17.1 Raw data

Specimen	Taxon	*Asfc*	*Smc*	*epLsar*	*Tfv*
NMNH315790	*Alouatta palliata*	0.3149	−0.6808	0.0057	0
NMNH315791	*Alouatta palliata*	0.1437	−0.5687	0.0065	7864
NMNH315792	*Alouatta palliata*	0.1961	0.4970	0.0079	0
NMNH315796	*Alouatta palliata*	0.2377	−0.0925	0.0089	0
NMNH315798	*Alouatta palliata*	0.5350	−0.8115	0.0018	1476
NMNH315805	*Alouatta palliata*	0.6797	−0.6563	0.0047	5580
NMNH315806	*Alouatta palliata*	0.3878	−0.5524	0.0046	0
NMNH315818	*Alouatta palliata*	0.1399	−0.8236	0.0037	1351
NMNH315819	*Alouatta palliata*	0.5591	−0.5738	0.0048	4445
NMNH315831	*Alouatta palliata*	0.4911	−0.5739	0.0079	112
NMNH316592	*Alouatta palliata*	0.2779	2.7649	0.0075	7892
NMNH518263	*Cebus apella*	8.3981	−0.5741	0.0025	20885
NMNH518265	*Cebus apella*	21.4166	−0.8076	0.0024	9707
NMNH518266	*Cebus apella*	12.9628	−0.8179	0.0029	13276
NMNH518286	*Cebus apella*	2.3418	−0.6734	0.0014	5994
NMNH518287	*Cebus apella*	2.8818	−0.5566	0.0035	4922

Specimen	Taxon	*Asfc*	*Smc*	*epLsar*	*Tfv*
NMNH518288	*Cebus apella*	1.1142	−0.6767	0.0056	2847
NMNH518289	*Cebus apella*	0.9191	0.1364	0.0059	9186
NMNH518290	*Cebus apella*	10.9773	−0.8225	0.0020	13628
NMNH518293	*Cebus apella*	3.1923	1.9367	0.0033	11114
NMNH518297	*Cebus apella*	4.3825	−0.8234	0.0024	4232
NMNH518303	*Cebus apella*	0.8176	−0.5738	0.0064	6813
NMNH518304	*Cebus apella*	1.1936	−0.5682	0.0024	13377
NMNH518306	*Cebus apella*	0.4576	2.5116	0.0069	9892
NMNH239883	*Gorilla gorilla beringei*	0.5179	−0.2221	0.0030	11988
NMNH395636	*Gorilla gorilla beringei*	0.9680	1.8638	0.0054	11707
NMNH396934	*Gorilla gorilla beringei*	0.5729	−0.6674	0.0050	0
NMNH396935	*Gorilla gorilla beringei*	0.8943	−0.8225	0.0029	0
NMNH396936	*Gorilla gorilla beringei*	6.1242	−0.6787	0.0014	9007
NMNH397351	*Gorilla gorilla beringei*	0.7904	−0.6807	0.0027	13279
NMNH397358	*Gorilla gorilla beringei*	1.8843	−0.4663	0.0021	17732
NMNH545027	*Gorilla gorilla beringei*	0.8764	−0.0263	0.0060	12348
NMNH545028	*Gorilla gorilla beringei*	1.9205	−0.8242	0.0038	19093
NMNH545030	*Gorilla gorilla beringei*	0.5485	−0.4654	0.0010	5845
NMNH545031	*Gorilla gorilla beringei*	3.5846	−0.6800	0.0050	13888
NMNH545032	*Gorilla gorilla beringei*	1.7627	0.4969	0.0033	8316
NMNH545034	*Gorilla gorilla beringei*	1.9730	−0.0256	0.0051	4137
NMNH545035	*Gorilla gorilla beringei*	0.8658	−0.5648	0.0053	226
NMNH545036	*Gorilla gorilla beringei*	1.3969	0.2258	0.0026	4371
NMNH545037	*Gorilla gorilla beringei*	2.6891	−0.8238	0.0039	7043
AMNH167325	*Gorilla gorilla gorilla*	2.0684	−0.6815	0.0025	4468
AMNH167327	*Gorilla gorilla gorilla*	3.4986	−0.8240	0.0035	13568
AMNH167330	*Gorilla gorilla gorilla*	2.0298	−0.8238	0.0008	5928
AMNH167332	*Gorilla gorilla gorilla*	1.7357	−0.5721	0.0047	2250
AMNH167334	*Gorilla gorilla gorilla*	3.1091	−0.8149	0.0027	4287
AMNH167339	*Gorilla gorilla gorilla*	1.3028	−0.8177	0.0055	12715
AMNH200501	*Gorilla gorilla gorilla*	0.9808	−0.6791	0.0038	22304
CMNH-B1075	*Gorilla gorilla gorilla*	0.5549	1.1024	0.0073	7275
CMNH-B1076	*Gorilla gorilla gorilla*	1.1921	0.1817	0.0053	1347
CMNH-B1181	*Gorilla gorilla gorilla*	0.9371	−0.1757	0.0049	8393
CMNH-B1410	*Gorilla gorilla gorilla*	0.8954	0.1324	0.0047	2580
CMNH-B1419	*Gorilla gorilla gorilla*	2.9942	−0.8227	0.0011	12770
CMNH-B1899	*Gorilla gorilla gorilla*	0.2902	−0.0143	0.0049	6293
CMNH-B1908	*Gorilla gorilla gorilla*	0.7708	−0.5695	0.0029	9218
UMN163	*Lophocebus albigena*	0.9802	1.7862	0.0052	14563
UMN165	*Lophocebus albigena*	0.9944	1.5103	0.0053	13995
UMN207	*Lophocebus albigena*	1.0181	1.1181	0.0014	9914
UMN226	*Lophocebus albigena*	2.3968	−0.6754	0.0066	11752
UMN227	*Lophocebus albigena*	6.9706	−0.8242	0.0020	11125
UMN229	*Lophocebus albigena*	0.9952	1.8828	0.0037	12012
UMN235	*Lophocebus albigena*	4.2833	−0.5744	0.0018	19171
UMN236	*Lophocebus albigena*	1.4650	0.8861	0.0027	7754
UMN237	*Lophocebus albigena*	0.5387	−0.3749	0.0024	10457
UMN238	*Lophocebus albigena*	1.9588	0.4703	0.0035	8437

(*cont.*)

Specimen	Taxon	*Asfc*	*Smc*	*epLsar*	*Tfv*
UMN249	*Lophocebus albigena*	1.6396	2.2979	0.0086	12221
UMN251	*Lophocebus albigena*	1.5829	−0.8226	0.0025	11324
UMN257	*Lophocebus albigena*	0.6491	0.9502	0.0039	13619
UMN260	*Lophocebus albigena*	0.8416	1.3336	0.0029	10223
UMN272	*Lophocebus albigena*	0.2163	0.3803	0.0040	4258
CMNH-B1722	*Pan troglodytes*	0.9770	0.1792	0.0017	9846
CMNH-B1903	*Pan troglodytes*	2.6588	−0.8228	0.0034	6956
CMNH-B1956	*Pan troglodytes*	2.3079	−0.8241	0.0007	6593
CMNH-B2027	*Pan troglodytes*	2.3413	−0.8231	0.0020	17174
CMNH-B2033	*Pan troglodytes*	0.5661	0.9080	0.0040	3816
CMNH-B2034	*Pan troglodytes*	4.1740	−0.8234	0.0013	6649
CMNH-B2756	*Pan troglodytes*	2.1137	−0.8233	0.0022	9822
CMNH-B2771	*Pan troglodytes*	0.3947	−0.8209	0.0039	2937
CMNH-B3398	*Pan troglodytes*	1.2423	−0.0113	0.0019	17931
CMNH-B3412	*Pan troglodytes*	2.7852	−0.8231	0.0020	1566
CMNH-B3413	*Pan troglodytes*	1.4836	−0.6788	0.0043	16261
CMNH-B3418	*Pan troglodytes*	0.7073	−0.8240	0.0025	9647
CMNH-B3434	*Pan troglodytes*	5.4613	−0.6781	0.0021	13980
CMNH-B3437	*Pan troglodytes*	5.1744	−0.8186	0.0025	13800
CMNH-B3537	*Pan troglodytes*	0.9769	−0.6806	0.0047	2365
CMNH-B3538	*Pan troglodytes*	2.9140	−0.8236	0.0031	4588
CMNH-B3553	*Pan troglodytes*	1.9077	0.3084	0.0057	14926
SAPM1981103	*Pongo pygameus*	0.3261	0.1303	0.0047	672
SAPM1981106	*Pongo pygameus*	3.6270	−0.8206	0.0010	6941
SAPM1981111	*Pongo pygameus*	0.2401	0.4064	0.0064	1118
SAPM1981113	*Pongo pygameus*	1.1925	−0.5739	0.0026	9396
SAPM1981145	*Pongo pygameus*	1.1219	−0.8234	0.0056	10511
SAPM1981147	*Pongo pygameus*	0.5301	0.2731	0.0037	21746
SAPM198159	*Pongo pygameus*	2.7256	−0.6815	0.0020	8521
SAPM198162	*Pongo pygameus*	0.8175	−0.3806	0.0038	0
SAPM198174	*Pongo pygameus*	2.1927	−0.0794	0.0055	4025
SAPM198178	*Pongo pygameus*	1.8544	−0.8230	0.0051	8060
SAPM198188	*Pongo pygameus*	0.9249	−0.5740	0.0036	336
SAPM198190	*Pongo pygameus*	1.6829	−0.8206	0.0016	899
SAPM198196	*Pongo pygameus*	0.9820	−0.3785	0.0027	18537
SAPM198197	*Pongo pygameus*	1.6077	−0.5693	0.0027	6732
SAPM198199	*Pongo pygameus*	0.5121	0.0279	0.0042	1117
NMNH113071	*Trachypithecus cristatus*	2.6655	−0.8124	0.0028	14858
NMNH113171	*Trachypithecus cristatus*	0.3911	−0.5719	0.0031	16840
NMNH113172	*Trachypithecus cristatus*	0.3742	−0.1447	0.0064	8746
NMNH114515	*Trachypithecus cristatus*	0.3021	−0.6793	0.0101	10082
NMNH115670	*Trachypithecus cristatus*	0.9004	−0.6804	0.0024	895
NMNH115672	*Trachypithecus cristatus*	0.6216	−0.6813	0.0021	3809
NMNH123036	*Trachypithecus cristatus*	0.4469	−0.8228	0.0059	15655
NMNH124711	*Trachypithecus cristatus*	0.4423	−0.4635	0.0073	15063
NMNH144371	*Trachypithecus cristatus*	1.1060	−0.6795	0.0035	10877
NMNH154723	*Trachypithecus cristatus*	0.7514	−0.2217	0.0025	10171
NMNH156305	*Trachypithecus cristatus*	0.2216	0.9511	0.0038	0
NMNH156314	*Trachypithecus cristatus*	0.5812	0.4273	0.0077	7391

References

Anyonge, W. (1996). Microwear on canines and killing behavior in large carnivores: saber function in *Smilodon fatalis*. *Journal of Mammology*, **77**, 1059–67.

Baker, G., Jones, L. H. P., and Wardrop, I. D. (1959). Cause of wear in sheep teeth. *Nature*, **184**, 1583–4.

Barrett, P. M. (2006). Tooth wear and possible jaw action of *Scelidosaurus harrisonii* Owen and a review of feeding mechanisms in other thyreophoran dinosaurs. In *The Armored Dinosaurs*, ed. K. Carpenter. Bloomington: Indiana University Press, pp. 25–52.

Biknevicius, A. R. (1986). Dental function and diet in the Carpolestidae (Primates, Plesiadapiformes). *American Journal of Physical Anthropology*, **71**, 157–71.

Borgognini, T., Della Santina, D., Francalacci, P., and Repetto, E. (1989). Reconstruction of Mesolithic diet using dental microwear and trace element analysis: the case of Grotta dell'Uzzo (Sicily). In *People and Culture in Change*, ed. I. Hershkovitz. Oxford: BAR International Series, pp. 283–320.

Boyde, A. and Fortelius, M. (1991). New confocal LM method for studying local relative microrelief with special references to wear studies. *Scanning*, **13**, 429–30.

Brotoisworo, E. and Dirgayusa, I. W. A. (1991). Ranging and feeding behavior of *Presbytis cristata* in the Pangandaran Nature Reserve, West Java. In *Primatology Today*, ed. A. Ehara, T. Kimura, O. Takenaka, and M. Iwamonto. Amsterdam: Elsevier Science, pp. 115–18.

Bullington, J. (1991). Deciduous dental microwear of prehistoric juveniles from the lower Illinois River Valley. *American Journal of Physical Anthropology*, **84**, 59–73.

Burnell, C. L., Teaford, M. F., and Glander, K. E. (1994). Dental microwear differs by capture site in live-caught Alouatta from Costa Rica. *American Journal of Physical Anthropology*, Supplement 18, 62.

Butler, P. M. (1952). The milk molars of Perissodactyla, with remarks on molar occlusion. *Proceedings of the Zoological Society of London*, **121**, 777–817.

Capozza, M. (2001). Microwear analysis of *Mammuthus meridionalis* (Nesti, 1825) molar from Campo del Conte (Frosinone, Italy). In *The World of Elephants – International Congress, Rome 2001*, pp. 529–33.

Chalmers, N. R. (1968). Group composition, ecology and daily activities of free living mangabeys in Uganda. *Folia Primatologica*, **8**, 247–62.

Conover, W. J. and Iman, R. L. (1981). Rank transformations as a bridge between parametric and nonparametric statistics. *American Statistician*, **35**, 124–9.

Cook, R. J. and Farewell, V. T. (1996). Multiplicity considerations in the design and analysis of clinical trials. *Journal of the Royal Statistical Society, Series A*, **159**, 93–110.

Covert, H. H. and Kay, R. F. (1981). Dental microwear and diet – implications for determining the feeding behaviors of extinct primates, with a comment on the dietary pattern of *Sivapithecus*. *American Journal of Physical Anthropology*, **55**, 331–6.

Crompton, R. H., Savage, R., and Spears, I. R. (1998). The mechanics of food reduction in *Tarsius bancanus*: hard-object feeder, soft-object feeder or both? *Folia Primatologica*, **69**, 41–59.

Daegling, D. J. and Grine, F. E. (1994). Bamboo feeding, dental microwear, and diet of the Pleistocene ape *Gigantopithecus blacki*. *South African Journal of Science*, **90**, 527–32.

Daegling, D. J. and Grine, F. E. (1999). Terrestrial foraging and dental microwear in *Papio ursinus*. *Primates*, **40**, 559–72.

Dahlberg, A. A. and Kinzey, W. (1962). Etude microscopique de l'abrasion et de l'attrition sur la surface des dents. *Bulletin du Groupement International Pour la Recherche Scientifique En Stomatologie*, **5**, 242–51.

Danielson, D. R. and Reinhard, K. J. (1998). Human dental microwear caused by calcium oxalate phytoliths in prehistoric diet of the lower Pecos region, Texas. *American Journal of Physical Anthropology*, **107**, 297–304.

Dompierre, H. and Churcher, C. S. (1996). Premaxillary shape as an indicator of the diet of seven extinct late Cenozoic new world camels. *Journal of Vertebrate Paleontology*, **16**, 141–8.

Doran, D. M., McNeilage, A., Greer, D. *et al.* (2002). Western lowland gorilla diet and resource availability: new evidence, cross-site comparisons, and reflections on indirect sampling methods. *American Journal of Primatology*, **58**, 91–116.

El Zaatari, S., Grine, F. E., Teaford, M. F., and Smith, H. F. (2006). Molar microwear and dietary reconstruction of fossil Cercopithecoidea from the Plio-Pleistocene deposits of South Africa. *Journal of Human Evolution*, **51**, 297–319.

Estrada, A. (1984). Resource use by howler monkeys (*Alouatta palliata*). *International Journal of Primatology*, **5**, 105–31.

Filippi, M. L., Palombo, M. R., Barbieri, M. *et al.* (2001). Isotope and microwear analyses on teeth of late Middle Pleistocene *Elephas antiquus* from the Rome area (La Polledrara, Casal de' Pazzi). In *The World of Elephants – International Congress, Rome 2001*, pp. 534–9.

Fine, D. and Craig, G. T. (1981). Buccal surface wear of human premolar and molar teeth: a potential indicator of dietary and social differentiation. *Journal of Human Evolution*, **10**, 335–44.

Fiorillo, A. (1991). Dental microwear on the teeth of *Camarasaurus* and *Diplodocus*: implications for sauropod paleoecology. In *Fifth Symposium on Mesozoic Terrestrial Ecosystems and Biota*, ed. Z. Kielan-Jaworowska, N. Heintz, and H. Nakrem. Paleontological Museum, University of Oslo, pp. 23–4.

Fiorillo, A. (1998). Dental microwear patterns of the sauropod dinosaurs, *Camarasaurus* and *Diplodocus*: evidence for resource partitioning in the Late Jurassic of North America. *Historical Biology*, **13**, 16.

Franz-Odendaal, T. A. and Solounias, N. (2004). Comparative dietary evaluations of an extinct giraffid (*Sivatherium hendeyi*) (Mammalia, Giraffidae, Sivatheriinae) from Langebaanweg, South Africa (early Pliocene). *Geodiversitas*, **26**, 675–85.

Galbany, J., Moya-Sola, S., and Perez-Perez, A. (2005). Dental microwear variability on buccal tooth enamel surfaces of extant catarrhini and the Miocene fossil *Dryopithecus laietanus* (Hominoidea). *Folia Primatologica*, **76**, 325–41.

Gambarotta, J. P. (1995). Nombre, densité et dimensions des micro-traces d'usure dentaire chez des populations ancienne et actuelles du Nord du Maroc. *Bulletin de la Société d'Anthropologie de Paris*, N. S. O. **7**, 159–76.

Godfrey, L. R., Semprebon, G. M., Jungers, W. L. *et al.* (2004). Dental use wear in extinct lemurs: evidence of diet and niche differentiation. *Journal of Human Evolution*, **47**, 145–69.

Godfrey, L. R., Semprebon, G. M., Jungers, W. L. *et al.* (2005a). Dental use wear in extinct lemurs: evidence of diet and niche differentiation *Journal of Human Evolution*, **49**, 662–3.

Godfrey, L. R., Semprebon, G. M., Schwartz, G. T. *et al.* (2005b). New insights into old lemurs: the trophic adaptations of the Archaeolemuridae. *International Journal of Primatology*, **26**, 825–54.

Gordon, K. D. (1982). A study of microwear on chimpanzee molars: implications for dental microwear analysis. *American Journal of Physical Anthropology*, **59**, 195–215.

Gordon, K. D. (1984). Hominoid dental microwear: complications in the use of microwear analysis to detect diet. *Journal of Dental Research* **63**, 1043–6.

Gordon, K. D. (1988). A review of methodology and quantification in dental microwear analysis. *Scanning Microscopy*, **2**, 1139–47.

Gordon, K. D. and Walker, A. C. (1983). Playing "possum": a microwear experiment. *American Journal of Physical Anthropology*, **60**, 109–12.

Goswami, A., Flynn, J. J., Ranivoharimananac, L., and Wyss, A. R. (2005). Dental microwear in triassic amniotes: implications for paleoecology and masticatory mechanics. *Journal of Vertebrate Paleontology*, **25**, 320–9.

Green, J. L., Semprebon, G. M., and Solounias, N. (2005). Reconstructing the palaeodiet of Florida *Mammut americanum* via low-magnification stereo microscopy. *Palaeogeography, Palaeoclimatology and Palaeoecology*, **223**, 34–48.

Grine, F. E. (1977). Analysis of early hominid deciduous molar wear by scanning electron microscopy: a preliminary report. *Proceedings of the Electron Microscopy, Society of South Africa*, **7**, 157–8.

Grine, F. E. (1981). Trophic differences between "gracile" and "robust" australopithecines: a scanning electron microcope analysis of occlusal events. *South African Journal of Science*, **77**, 203–30.

Grine, F. E. (1986). Dental evidence for dietary differences in *Australopithecus* and *Paranthropus* – a quantitative-analysis of permanent molar microwear. *Journal of Human Evolution*, **15**, 783–822.

Grine, F. E. and Kay, R. F. (1987). Quantitative analysis of occlusal microwear in *Australopithecus* and *Paranthropus*. *Scanning Microscopy*, **1**, 647–56.

Grine, F. E., Ungar, P. S., and Teaford, M. F. (2002). Error rates in dental microwear quantification using scanning electron microscopy. *Scanning*, **24**, 144–53.

Grine, F. E., Ungar, P. S., Teaford, M. F., and El Zaatari, S. (2006). Molar microwear in *Praeanthropus afarensis*: evidence for dietary stasis through time and under diverse paleoecological conditions. *Journal of Human Evolution* (in press).

Gugel, I. L., Grupe, G., and Kunzelmann, K. H. (2001). Simulation of dental microwear: characteristic traces by opal phytoliths give clues to ancient human dietary behavior. *American Journal of Physical Anthropology*, **114**, 124–38.

Gutierrez, M., Lewis, P. J., and Johnson, E. (1998). Evidence of paleoenvironmental change from muskrat dental microwear patterns. *Current Research in the Pleistocene*, **15**, 107–8.

Harmon, A. M. and Rose, J. C. (1988). The role of dental microwear analysis in the reconstruction of prehistoric diet. In *Diet and Subsistence: Current Archaeological Perspectives*, ed. B. V. Kennedy, and G. M. Le Moine. Calgary: Archaeolgoical Association of the University of Calgary, pp. 267–72.

Hayek, L. A. C., Bernor, R. L., Solounias, N., and Steigerwald, P. (1991). Preliminary studies of hipparionine horse diet as measured by tooth microwear. *Annales Zoologici Fennici*, **28**, 187–200.

Hojo, T. (1989). Dietary differences and microwear on the teeth of late stone age and early modern people from western Japan. *Scanning Microscopy*, **3**, 623–8.

Hopley, P. J., Latham, A. G., and Marshall, J. D. (2006). Palaeoenvironments and palaeodiets of mid-Pliocene micromammals from Makapansgat Limeworks, South Africa: a stable isotope and dental microwear approach. *Palaeogeography, Palaeoclimatology, and Palaeoecology*, **233**, 235–51.

Hunter, J. P. and Fortelius, M. (1994). Comparative dental occlusal morphology, facet development, and microwear in two sympatric species of *Listriodo*n (Mammalia, Suidae) from the Middle Miocene of Western Anatolia (Turkey). *Journal of Vertebrate Paleontology*, **14**, 105–26.

Jacobs, L. L. (1981). Miocene lorisid primates from the Pakistan Siwaliks. *Nature*, **289**, 585–7.

Jamison, P. L. (1974). Influence of interobserver measurement error on multivariate population comparisons. *American Journal of Physical Anthropology*, **40**, 141.

Kaiser, T. M. (2003). The dietary regimes of two contemporaneous populations of *Hippotherium primigenium* (Perissodactyla, Equidae) from the Vallesian (Upper Miocene) of Southern Germany. *Palaeogeography, Palaeoclimatology, and Palaeoecology*, **198**, 381–402.

Kaiser, T. M., Bernor, R. L., Franzen, J., Scott, R. S., and Solounias, N. (2003). New interpretations of the systematics and palaeoecology of the Dorn Dürkheim 1 hipparions (Late Miocene, Turolian Age [MN11]), Rheinhessen, Germany. *Senckenbergiana lethaea*, **83**, 103–33.

Kay, R. F. (1987). Analysis of primate dental microwear using image processing techniques. *Scanning Microscopy*, **1**, 657–62.

Kay, R. F. and Covert, H. H. (1983). True grit: a microwear experiment. *American Journal of Physical Anthropology*, **61**, 33–8.

Kay, R. F. and Covert, H. H. (1984). Anatomy and behavior of extinct primates. In *Food Acquisition and Processing in Primates*, ed. D. J. Chivers, B. A. Wood, & A. Bilsborough, pp. 467–508. New York: Plenum Press.

Kelley, J. (1986). *Paleobiology of Miocene hominoids.* Ph.D. Dissertation, Yale University.

Kelley, J. (1990). Incisor microwear and diet in three species of Colobus. *Folia Primatologica*, **55**, 73–84.

King, T. (2001). Dental microwear and diet in Eurasian Miocene catarrhines. In *Phylogeny of the Neogene Hominoid Primates in Europe*, ed. L. de Bonis, G. D. Koufos, and P. Andrews. Cambridge: Cambridge University Press, pp. 102–17.

King, T., Aiello, L. C., and Andrews, P. (1999a). Dental microwear of *Griphopithecus alpani*. *Journal of Human Evolution*, **36**, 3–31.

King, T., Andrews, P., and Boz, B. (1999b). Effect of taphonomic processes on dental microwear. *American Journal of Physical Anthropology*, **108**, 359–73.

Krause, D. W. (1982). Jaw movement, dental function, and diet in the Paleocene multituberculate *Ptilodus*. *Paleobiology*, **8**, 265–81.

Kuroda, S. (1992). Ecological interspecies relationships between gorillas and chimpanzees in the Ndoki-Nouabale Reserve, Northern Congo. In *Topics in Primatology, Volume 2, Behavior, Ecology and Conservation.*, ed. N. Itoigawa, Y. Sugiyama, G. P. Sackett, and R. K. R. Thompson. Tokyo: University of Tokyo Press, pp. 385–94.

Lambert, J. E., Chapman, C. A., Wrangham, R. W., and Conklin-Brittain, N. L. (2004). Hardness of cercopithecine foods: implications for the critical function of enamel thickness in exploiting fallback foods. *American Journal of Physical Anthropology*, **125**, 363–8.

Larsen, C. S., Griffen, M. C., Hutchinson, D. L. *et al.* (2001). Frontiers of contact: bioarchaeology of Spanish Florida. *Journal of World Prehistory*, **15**, 69–123.

Leakey, M. G., Teaford, M. F., and Ward, C. V. (2003). Cercopithecidae from Lothagam. In *Lothagam*, ed. M. G. Leakey and J. Harris. New York: Columbia University Press, pp. 130–77.

Lewis, P. J., Gutierrez, M., and Johnson, E. (2000). *Ondatra zibethicus* (Arvicolinae, Rodentia) dental microwear patterns as a potential tool for palaeoenvironmental reconstruction. *Journal of Archaeological Science*, **27**, 789–98.

Lucas, P. W. and Teaford, M. F. (1994). Functional morphology of colobine teeth. In *Colobine Monkeys: Their Ecology, Behaviour and Evolution*, ed. A. G. Davies and J. F. Oates. Cambridge: Cambridge University Press, pp. 173–203.

Lukacs, J. R. and Pastor, R. F. (1988). Activity-induced patterns of dental abrasion in prehistoric Pakistan: evidence from Mehrgarh and Harappa. *American Journal of Physical Anthropology*, **76**, 377–98.

Maas, M. C. (1991). Enamel structure and microwear: an experimental study of the response of enamel to shearing force. *American Journal of Physical Anthropology*, **85**, 31–49.

MacFadden, B. J., Solounias, N., and Cerling, T. E. (1999). Ancient diets, ecology, and extinction of 5-million-year-old horses from Florida. *Science*, **283**, 824–7.

MacKinnon, J. (1977). A comparative ecology of Asian Apes. *Primates*, **18**, 747–72.

Mahoney, P. (2006a). Brief communication: intertooth and intrafacet dental microwear variation in an archaeological sample of modern humans from the Jordan Valley. *American Journal of Physical Anthropology*, **129**, 39–44.

Mahoney, P. (2006b). Dental microwear from Natufian hunter-gatherers and Early Neolithic farmers: comparisons within and between samples. *American Journal of Physical Anthropology*, **130**, 308–19.

Mahoney, P. (2006c). Microwear and morphology: functional relationships between human dental microwear and the mandible. *Journal of Human Evolution*, **50**, 452–9.

Mainland, I. L. (1998). Dental microwear and diet in domestic sheep (*Ovis aries*) and goats (*Capra hircus*): distinguishing grazing and fodder-fed ovicaprids using a quantitative analytical approach. *Journal of Archaeological Science*, **25**, 1259–71.

Mainland, I. L. (2000). A dental microwear study of seaweed-eating and grazing sheep from Orkney. *International Journal of Osteoarchaeology* **10**, 93–107.

Mainland, I. L. (2003). Dental microwear in grazing and browsing Gotland sheep (*Ovis aries*) and its implications for dietary reconstruction. *Journal of Archaeological Science*, **30**, 1513–27.

Mainland, I. L. (2006). Pastures lost? A dental microwear study of ovicaprine diet and management in Norse Greenland. *Journal of Archaeological Science*, **33**, 238–52.

Merceron, G. (2003a). *Dental microwear analysis of primates and ungulates from the late Miocene of eastern Mediterranean: paleobiological and paleoenvironmental implications.* Ph.D. Thesis University of Poitiers, France.

Merceron, G. (2003b). Une nouvelle méthodologie pour la quantification de la micro-usure dentaire: application à l'hominoïde fossile *Ouranopithecus macedoniensis* (Miocène, Grèce). *Bulletin et Mémoires de la Société d'Anthropologie de Paris*, **15**, 300–1.

Merceron, G., Blondel, C., Brunet, M. *et al.* (2004a). The Late Miocene paleoenvironment of Afghanistan as inferred from dental microwear in artiodactyls. *Palaeogeography, Palaeoclimatology, and Palaeoecology*, **207**, 143–63.

Merceron, G., Blondel, C., de Bonis, L., Koufos, G. D., and Viriot, L. (2005a). A new method of dental microwear analysis: application to extant primates and *Ouranopithecus macedoniensis* (Late Miocene of Greece). *Palaios*, **20**, 551–61.

Merceron, G., Bonis, L. D., Viriot, L., and Blondel, C. (2005b). Dental microwear of fossil bovids from northern Greece: paleoenvironmental conditions in the eastern Mediterranean during the Messinian. *Palaeogeography, Palaeoclimatology, and Palaeoecology*, **217**, 173–85.

Merceron, G. and Madelaine, S. (2006). Molar microwear pattern and palaeoecology of ungulates from La Berbie (Dordogne, France): environment of Neanderthals and modern human populations of the Middle/Upper Palaeolithic. *Boreas*, **35**, 272–8.

Merceron, G., Taylor, S., Scott, R., Chaimanee, Y., and Jaeger, J. J. (2006). Dietary characterization of the hominoid *Khoratpithecus* (Miocene of Thailand): evidence from dental topographic and microwear texture analyses. *Naturwissenschaften*, **93**, 329–33.

Merceron, G. and Ungar, P. (2005). Dental microwear and palaeoecology of bovids from the Early Pliocene of Langebaanweg, Western Cape province, South Africa. *South African Journal of Science*, **101**, 365–70.

Merceron, G., Viriot, L., and Blondel, C. (2004b). Tooth microwear pattern in roe deer (*Capreolus capreolus*, L.) from Chize (Western France) and relation to food composition. *Small Ruminant Research*, **53**, 125–32.

Mills, J. R. E. (1955). Ideal dental occlusion in primates. *Dental Practice*, **6**, 47–51.

Minozzi, S., Manzi, G., Ricci, F., di Lernia, S., and Tarli, S. M. B. (2003). Nonalimentary tooth use in prehistory: an example from early Holocene in Central Sahara (Uan Muhuggiag, Tadrart Acacus, Libya). *American Journal of Physical Anthropology*, **120**, 225–32.

Molleson, T. and Jones, K. (1991). Dental evidence for dietary change at Abu Hureyra. *Journal of Archaeological Science*, **18**, 525–39.

Molleson, T., Jones, K., and Jones, S. (1993). Dietary change and the effects of food preparation on microwear patterns in the Late Neolithic of Abu Hureyra, Northern Syria. *Journal of Human Evolution*, **24**, 455–68.

Muendel, M. G. (1997). *Dental microwear analysis of Averbuch: a dietary reconstruction of a Mississippian culture*. Ph.D. Thesis, University of Tennessee.

Nelson, S., Badgley, C., and Zakem, E. (2005). Microwear in modern squirrels in relation to diet. *Palaeontologia Electronica*, **8**, Art. No. 14A.

Nystrom, P., Phillips-Conroy, J. E., and Jolly, C. J. (2004). Dental microwear in anubis and hybrid baboons (*Papio hamadryas, sensu lato*) living in Awash National Park, Ethiopia. *American Journal of Physical Anthropology*, **125**, 279–91.

O'Leary, M. and Teaford, M. F. (1992). Dental microwear and diet of Mesonychids. *Journal of Vertebrate Paleontology*, **12**, 45A.

Oliveira, E. V. (2001). Micro-desgaste dentário em alguns Dasypodidae (Mammalia, Xenarthra). *Acta Biologica Leopoldensia*, **23**, 83–91.

Organ, J. M., Ruff, C. B., Teaford, M. F., and Nisbett, R. A. (2006a). Do mandibular cross-sectional properties and dental microwear give similar dietary signals? *American Journal of Physical Anthropology*, **130**, 501–7.

Organ, J. M., Teaford, M. F., and Larsen, C. S. (2006b). Dietary inferences from dental occlusal microwear at Mission San Luis de Apalachee. *American Journal of Physical Anthropology*, **128**, 801–11.

Palombo, M. R., Filippi, M. L., Iacumin, P. *et al.* (2005). Coupling tooth microwear and stable isotope analyses for palaeodiet reconstruction: the case study of late Middle Pleistocene *Elephas (Palaeoloxodon) antiquus* teeth from Central Italy (Rome area). *Quaternary International*, **126–8**, 153–70.

Pastor, R. F. (1993). *Dental microwear among prehistoric inhabitants of the Indian subcontinent: a quantitative and comparative analysis*. Ph.D. Thesis, University of Oregon.

Pastor, R. F. and Johnson, T. L. (1992). Dental microwear and attrition. In *Human Skeletal Remains from Mahadaha: A Gangetic Mesolithic Site*, ed. K. A. R. Kennedy. Ithaca: Cornell University, pp. 271–304.

Pastor, R. F., Teaford, M. F., and Glander, K. E. (1995). Method for collecting and analyzing airborne abrasive particles from neotropical forests. *American Journal of Physical Anthropology*, Suppl. 20, 168.

Pérez-Pérez, A., Bermudez de Castro, J. M., and Arsuaga, J. L. (1999). Nonocclusal dental microwear analysis of 300 000-year-old *Homo heidelbergensis* teeth from Sima de los Huesos (Sierra de Atapuerca, Spain). *American Journal of Physical Anthropology*, **108**, 433–57.

Pérez-Pérez, A., Espurz, V., Bermudez de Castro, J. M., de Lumley, M. A., and Turbon, D. (2003). Non-occlusal dental microwear variability in a sample of Middle and Late Pleistocene human populations from Europe and the Near East. *Journal of Human Evolution*, **44**, 497–513.

Pérez-Pérez, A., Lalueza, C., and Turbon, D. (1994). Intraindividual and intragroup variability of buccal tooth striation pattern. *American Journal of Physical Anthropology*, **94**, 175–87.

Peters, C. R. (1982). Electron-optical microscopic study of incipient dental microdamage from experimental seed and bone crushing. *American Journal of Physical Anthropology*, **57**, 283–301.

Puech, P. F. (1979). Diet of early man – evidence from abrasion of teeth and tools. *Current Anthropology*, **20**, 590–2.

Puech, P. F. (1986). *Australopithecus afarensis* Garusi-1, variability and specialization of early hominids in their masticatory apparatus. *Comptes Rendus de l'Academie des Sciences Serie II*, **303**, 1819.

Puech, P. F. and Albertini, H. (1984). Dental microwear and mechanisms in early hominids from Laetoli and Hadar. *American Journal of Physical Anthropology*, **65**, 87–91.

Puech, P. F., Albertini, H., and Serratrice, C. (1983a). Tooth microwear and dietary patterns in early hominids from Laetoli, Hadar and Olduvai. *Journal of Human Evolution*, **12**, 721–9.

Puech, P. F., Cianfarani, F., and Roth, H. (1986). Reconstruction of the maxillary dental arcade of Garusi Hominid 1. *Journal of Human Evolution*, **15**, 325–32.

Puech, P. F. and Prone, A. (1979). Mechanical process of dental wearing down by abrasion, reproduced by experimentation and applied to fossil man and his paleoecological surroundings. *Comptes Rendus Hebdomadaires des Seances de l'Academie des Sciences Serie D*, **289**, 895.

Puech, P. F., Prone, A., and Albertini, H. (1981). Mechanical process of dental surface alteration by non-abrasive and non-adhesive friction, reproduced by experimentation and applied to the diet of early man. *Comptes Rendus de l'Academie des Sciences Serie II*, **293**, 729–34.

Puech, P. F., Serratrice, C., and Leek, F. F. (1983b). Tooth wear as observed in ancient Egyptian skulls. *Journal of Human Evolution*, **12**, 617–29.

Purnell, M. A. (1995). Microwear on conodont elements and macrophagy in the first vertebrates. *Nature*, **374**, 798–800.

Purnell, M. A., Hart, P. J. B., Baines, D. C., and Bell, M. A. (2006). Quantitative analysis of dental microwear in threespine stickleback: a new approach to analysis of trophic ecology in aquatic vertebrates. *Journal of Animal Ecology*, **75**, 967–77.

Rafferty, K. L., Teaford, M. F., and Jungers, W. L. (2002). Molar microwear of subfossil lemurs: improving the resolution of dietary inferences. *Journal of Human Evolution*, **43**, 645–57.

Reinhard, K. J. and Danielson, D. R. (2005). Pervasiveness of phytoliths in prehistoric southwestern diet and implications for regional and temporal trends for dental microwear. *Journal of Archaeological Science*, **32**, 981–8.

Rensberger, J. M. (1978). Scanning electron microscopy, of wear and occlusal events in some small herbivores. In *Development, Function, and Evolution of Teeth*, ed. P. M. Butler and K. A. Joysey. New York: Academic Press, pp. 415–38.

Rivals, F. and Deniaux, B. (2003). Dental microwear analysis for investigating the diet of an argali population (*Ovis ammon antiqua*) of mid-Pleistocene age, Caune de l'Arago cave, eastern Pyrenees, France. *Palaeogeography, Palaeoclimatology, and Palaeoecology*, **193**, 443–55.

Rivals, F. and Semprebon, G. M. (2006). A comparison of the dietary habits of a large sample of the Pleistocene pronghorn *Stockoceros onusrosagris* from the Papago

Springs Cave in Arizona to the modern *Antilocapra americana*. *Journal of Vertebrate Paleontology*, **26**, 495–500.

Robson, S. K. and Young, W. G. (1990). A comparison of tooth microwear between an extinct marsupial predator, the Tasmanian tiger *Thylacinus cynocephalus* (Thylacinidae) and an extant scavenger, the Tasmanian devil *Sarcophilus harrisii* (Dasyuridae, Marsupialia). *Australian Journal of Zoology*, **37**, 575–89.

Rodman, P. S. (1977). Feeding behaviour of orangutans of the Kutai Nature Reserve, East Kalimantan. In *Primate Ecology: Studies of Feeding and Ranging Behaviour in Lemurs, Monkeys and Apes*, ed. T. H. Clutton Brock. London: Academic Press, pp. 383–413.

Rose, J. C. and Ungar, P. S. (1998). Gross wear and dental microwear in historical perspective. In *Dental Anthropology: Fundamentals, Limits, Prospects*, ed. K. W. Alt, F. W. Rosing, and M. Teschler-Nicola. Stuttgart: Gustav-Fischer, pp. 349–86.

Rose, J. V. and Marks, M. K. (1985). Bioarcheology of the Alexander Site. In *The Alexander Site*, ed. Arkansas Archeological Survey. Fayetteville, AR: Arkansas Archeological Survey, pp. 76–98.

Ryan, A. S. (1979). Wear striation direction on primate teeth – scanning electron microscope examination. *American Journal of Physical Anthropology*, **50**, 155–67.

Ryan, A. S. (1980a). *Anterior dental microwear in hominid evolution: comparisons with human and nonhuman primates.* Ph.D. Thesis, University of Michigan.

Ryan, A. S. (1980b). Anterior dental microwear in Neanderthals. *American Journal of Physical Anthropology*, **52**, 274.

Ryan, A. S. (1981). Anterior dental microwear and its relationhips to diet and feeding behavior in three African primates (*Pan troglodytes troglodytes, Gorilla gorilla gorilla*, and *Papio hamadryas*). *Primates*, **22**, 533–50.

Ryan, A. S. and Johanson, D. C. (1989). Anterior dental microwear in *Australopithecus afarensis*: comparisons with human and nonhuman primates. *Journal of Human Evolution*, **18**, 235–68.

Rybczynski, N. and Vickaryous, M. K. (2006). Evidence of complex jaw movement in the Late Cretaceous ankylosaurid *Euoplocephalus tutus* (Dinosauria: Thyreophora). In *The Armored Dinosaurs*, ed. K. Carpenter. Bloomington: Indiana University Press, pp. 299–317.

Schmidt, C. W. (2001). Dental microwear evidence for a dietary shift between two nonmaize-reliant prehistoric human populations from Indiana. *American Journal of Physical Anthropology*, **114**, 139–45.

Schubert, B. and Ungar, P. S. (2005). Wear facets and enamel spalling in tyrannosaurid dinosaurs. *Acta Palaeontologica Polonica*, **50**, 93–9.

Schubert, B., Ungar, P. S., Sponheimer, M., and Reed, K. E. (2007). Microwear evidence for Plio-Pleistocene bovid diets from Makapansgat Limeworks Cave, South Africa. *Palaeogeography, Palaeoclimatololgy, and Palaeoecology,* **241**, 301–19.

Scott, R. S., Ungar, P. S., Bergstrom, T. S. *et al.* (2006). Dental microwear texture analysis: technical considerations. *Journal of Human Evolution*, **51**, 339–49.

Scott, R. S., Ungar, P. S., Bergstrom, T. S., Brown, C. A., Grine, F. E., Teaford, M. F., and Walker, A. (2005). Dental microwear texture analysis reflects diets of living primates and fossil hominins. *Nature*, **436**, 693–5.

Semprebon, G., Janis, C., and Solounias, N. (2004a). The diets of the dromomerycidae (Mammalia: Artiodactyla) and their response to Miocene vegetational change. *Journal of Vertebrate Paleontology*, **24**, 427–44.

Semprebon, G. M., Godfrey, L. R., Solounias, N., Sutherland, M. R., and Jungers, W. L. (2004b). Can low-magnification stereo microscopy reveal diet? *Journal of Human Evolution*, **47**, 115–44.

Semprebon, G. M., Godfrey, L. R., Solounias, N., Sutherland, M. R., and Jungers, W. L. (2005). [Erratum] Can low-magnification stereo microscopy reveal diet? *Journal of Human Evolution*, **49**, 662–3.

Silcox, M. T. and Teaford, M. F. (2002). The diet of worms: an analysis of mole dental microwear. *Journal of Mammology*, **83**, 804–14.

Simpson, G. G., (1933). Paleobiology of Jurassic mammals. *Paleobiologica*, **5**, 127–58.

Solounias, N. and Hayek, L. A. C. (1993). New methods of tooth microwear analysis and application to dietary determination of two extinct antelopes. *Journal of Zoology*, **229**, 421–45.

Solounias, N. and Moelleken, S. M. C. (1992a). Dietary adaptations of two goat ancestors and evolutionary considerations. *Geobios*, **25**, 797–809.

Solounias, N. and Moelleken, S. M. C. (1992b). Tooth microwear analysis of *Eotragus sansaniensis* (Mammalia: Ruminantia), one of the oldest known bovids. *Journal of Vertebrate Paleontology*, **12**, 113–21.

Solounias, N. and Moelleken, S. M. C. (1993). Tooth microwear and premaxillary shape of an archaic antelope. *Lethaia*, **26**, 261–8.

Solounias, N. and Moelleken, S. M. C. (1994). Dietary differences between two archaic ruminant species from Sansan, France. *Historical Biology*, **7**, 203–20.

Solounias, N. and Semprebon, G. (2002). Advances in the reconstruction of ungulate ecomorphology with application to early fossil equids. *American Museum Novitiates* (3366) 1–49.

Solounias, N., Teaford, M., and Walker, A. (1988). Interpreting the diet of extinct ruminants: the case of a non-browsing giraffid. *Paleobiology*, **14**, 287–300.

Strait, S. G. (1991). *Dietary reconstruction in small-bodied fossil primates.* Ph.D. Thesis, State University of New York at Stony Brook.

Strait, S. G. (1993). Molar microwear in extant small-bodied faunivorous mammals: an analysis of feature density and pit frequency. *American Journal of Physical Anthropology*, **92**, 63–79.

Strait, S. G. (1997). Tooth use and the physical properties of food. *Evolutionary Anthropology*, **5**, 199–211.

Teaford, M. F. (1983a). Differences in molar wear gradient between adult macaques and langurs. *International Journal of Primatology*, **4**, 427–44.

Teaford, M. F. (1983b). The morphology and wear of the lingual notch in macaques and langurs. *American Journal of Physical Anthropology*, **60**, 7–14.

Teaford, M. F. (1985). Molar microwear and diet in the genus *Cebus. American Journal of Physical Anthropology*, **66**, 363–70.

Teaford, M. F. (1986). Dental microwear and diet in two species of *Colobus*. In *Proceedings of the Tenth Annual International Primatological Conference. Volume 2: Primate Ecology and Conservation*, ed. J. G. Else and P. Lee. Cambridge: Cambridge University, pp. 63–6.

Teaford, M. F. (1988a). A review of dental microwear and diet in modern mammals. *Scanning Microscopy*, **2**, 1149–66.

Teaford, M. F. (1988b). Scanning electron microscope diagnosis of wear patterns versus artifacts on fossil teeth. *Scanning Microscopy*, **2**, 1167–75.

Teaford, M. F. (1993). Dental microwear and diet in extant and extinct *Theropithecus*: preliminary analyses. In *Theropithecus: The Life and Death of a Primate Genus*, ed. N. G. Jablonski. Cambridge: Cambridge University, pp. 331–49.

Teaford, M. F. (2006). What do we know and not know about dental microwear and diet? In *Evolution of the Human Diet: The Known, the Unknown, and the Unknowable*, ed. P. S. Ungar. New York: Oxford University Press, 106–31.

Teaford, M. F. (2007). Dental microwear and paleoanthropology: cautions and possibilities. In *Dental Perspectives on Human Evolution*, ed. S. Bailey and J. J. Hublin, Springer, in press.

Teaford, M. F. and Glander, K. E. (1991). Dental microwear in live, wild-trapped *Alouatta palliata* from Costa Rica. *American Journal of Physical Anthropology*, **85**, 313–19.

Teaford, M. F. and Glander, K. E. (1996). Dental microwear and diet in a wild population of mantled howling monkeys (*Alouatta palliata*). In *Adaptive Radiations of Neotropical Primates*, ed. M. A. Norconk, A. L. Rosenberger, and P. A. Garber. New York: Plenum Press, pp. 433–49.

Teaford, M. F., Larsen, C. S., Pastor, R. F., and Noble, V. E. (2001). Dental microwear and diet in La Florida. In *Bioarchaeology of La Florida*, ed. C. S. Larsen. Gainesville: University of Florida, pp. 82–112.

Teaford, M. F. and Leakey, M. G. (1992). Dental microwear and diet in Plio Pleistocene cercopithecoids from Kenya. *American Journal of Physical Anthropology*, Suppl. 14, 160.

Teaford, M. F., Lucas, P. W., Ungar, P. S., and Glander, K. E. (2006). Mechanical defenses in leaves eaten by Costa Rican *Alouatta palliata. American Journal of Physical Anthropology*, **129**, 99–104.

Teaford, M. F. and Lytle, J. D. (1996). Brief communication: diet-induced changes in rates of human tooth microwear: a case study involving stone-ground maize. *American Journal of Physical Anthropology*, **100**, 143–7.

Teaford, M. F., Maas, M. C., and Simons, E. L. (1996). Dental microwear and microstructure in early Oligocene primates from the Fayum, Egypt: implications for diet. *American Journal of Physical Anthropology*, **101**, 527–43.

Teaford, M. F. and Robinson, J. G. (1989). Seasonal or ecological differences in diet and molar microwear in *Cebus nigrivittatus. American Journal of Physical Anthropology*, **80**, 391–401.

Teaford, M. F. and Ungar, P. S. (2006). Dental adaptations of African apes. In *Handbook of Paleoanthropology. Volume 1: Principles, Methods, and Approaches*, ed. W. Kenke, W. Rothe, and I. Tattersall. Heidelberg: Springer Verlag, in press.

Teaford, M. F., Ungar, P. S., and Grine, F. E. (2007). Dental microwear and hominin paleoecology. In *Early Hominin Paleoecology*, ed. M. Sponheimer, P. Ungar, K. Reed, and J. Lee-Thorp. Boulder: University of Colorado Press, in press.

Teaford, M. F. and Walker, A. (1984). Quantitative differences in dental microwear between primate species with different diets and a comment on the presumed diet of *Sivapithecus*. *American Journal of Physical Anthropology*, **64**, 191–200.

Tutin, C. E. G. and Fernandez, M. (1985). Foods consumed by sympatric populations of *Gorilla g. gorilla* and *Pan t. troglodytes* in Gabon: some preliminary data. *International Journal of Primatology*, **6**, 27–43.

Tutin, C. E. G., Williamson, E. A., Rogers, M. E., and Fernandez, M. (1991). A case study of a plant-animal relationship – Cola-Lizae and lowland gorillas in the Lope Reserve, Gabon. *Journal of Tropical Ecology*, **7**, 181–99.

Ungar, P. S. (1990). Incisor microwear and feeding behavior in *Alouatta seniculus* and *Cebus olivaceus*. *American Journal of Primatology*, **20**, 43–50.

Ungar, P. S. (1992). Dental evidence for diet in primates. *Anthropolologiai Közlemények*, **34**, 141–55.

Ungar, P. S. (1994). Incisor microwear of Sumatran anthropoid primates. *American Journal of Physical Anthropology*, **94**, 339–63.

Ungar, P. S. (1995). A semiautomated image analysis procedure for the quantification of dental microwear. 2. *Scanning*, **17**, 57–9.

Ungar, P. S. (1996). Dental microwear of European Miocene catarrhines: evidence for diets and tooth use. *Journal of Human Evolution*, **31**, 335–66.

Ungar, P. S. (1998). Dental allometry, morphology, and wear as evidence for diet in fossil primates. *Evolutionary Anthropology*, **6**, 205–17.

Ungar, P. S., Brown, C. A., Bergstrom, T. S., and Walker, A. (2003). Quantification of dental microwear by tandem scanning confocal microscopy, and scale sensitive fractal analyses. *Scanning*, **25**, 185–93.

Ungar, P. S. and Grine, F. E. (1991). Incisor size and wear in *Australopithecus africanus* and *Paranthropus robustus*. *Journal of Human Evolution*, **20**, 313–40.

Ungar, P. S., Grine, F. E., and Teaford, M. F. (2006). Diet in early *Homo*: a review of the evidence and a new model of adaptive versatility. *Annual Review of Anthropology*, **35**, in press.

Ungar, P. S., Grine, F. E., Teaford, M. F., and El Zaatari, S. (2005). Dental microwear and diets of African early *Homo*. *Journal of Human Evolution*, **50**, 78–95.

Ungar, P. S., Simon, J. C., and Cooper, J. W. (1991). A Semiautomated Image Analysis Procedure for the Quantification of Dental Microwear. *Scanning*, **13**, 31–6.

Ungar, P. S. and Spencer, M. A. (1999). Incisor microwear, diet, and tooth use in three Amerindian populations. *American Journal of Physical Anthropology*, **109**, 387–96.

Ungar, P. S., and Teaford, M. F. (1996). Preliminary examination of non-occlusal dental microwear in anthropoids: implications for the study of fossil primates. *American Journal of Physical Anthropology*, **100**, 101–13.

Ungar, P. S., Teaford, M. F., Glander, K. E., and Pastor, R. F. (1995). Dust accumulation in the canopy: a potential cause of dental microwear in primates. *American Journal of Physical Anthropology*, **97**, 93–9.

Ungar, P. S., Teaford, M. F., and Kay, R. F. (2004). Molar microwear and shearing crest development in Miocene catarrhines. *Anthropologie* (Brno), **42**, 21–35.
Van Valkenburgh, B., Teaford, M. F., and Walker, A. (1990). Molar microwear and diet in large carnivores: inferences concerning diet in the sabretooth cat, *Smilodon fatalis*. *Journal of Zoology*, **222**, 319–40.
Walker, A. (1981). Diet and teeth. Dietary hypotheses and human evolution. *Philosophical Transactions of the Royal Society London B, Biological Science*, **292**, 57–64.
Walker, A., Hoeck, H. N., and Perez, L. (1978). Microwear of mammalian teeth as an indicator of diet. *Science*, **201**, 908–10.
Walker, A. and Teaford, M. (1989). Inferences from quantitative analysis of dental microwear. *Folia Primatologica*, **53**, 177–89.
Walker, A., Teaford, M. F., and Ungar, P. S. (1994). Enamel microwear differences between species of *Proconsul* from the early Miocene of Kenya. *American Journal of Physical Anthropology*, Suppl. **18**, 202–3.
Walker, P. L. (1976). Wear striations on the incisors of cercopithecoid monkeys as an index of diet and habitat preference. *American Journal of Physical Anthropology*, **45**, 299–308.
Walker, P. L., Bernstein, S. A., and Gordon, K. D. (1987). An image processing system for the quantitative analysis of dental microwear. *American Journal of Physical Anthropology*, **72**, 267.
Walker, P. L. and Hagen, E. H. (1994). A topographical approach to dental microwear analysis. *American Journal of Physical Anthropology*, Suppl. 18, 203.
Ward, J. and Mainland, I. L. (1999). Microwear in modern rooting and stall fed pigs: the potential of dental microwear analysis for exploring pig diet and management in the past. *Environmental Archaeology*, **4**, 25–32.
Williamson, E. A., Tutin, C. E. G., Rogers, M. E., and Fernandez, M. (1990). Composition of the diet of lowland gorillas at Lope in Gabon. *American Journal of Primatology*, **21**, 265–77.
Young, W. G. and Marty, T. M. (1986). Wear and microwear on the teeth of a moose (*Alces alces*) population in Manitoba, Canada. *Canadian Journal of Zoology*, **64**, 2467–79.
Young, W. G., Robson, S. K., and Jupp, R. (1987a). Microwear on the molar teeth of the Koala *Phascolarctos cinereus*. *Journal of Dental Research* **66**, 828.
Young, W. G., Stephens, M., and Juff, R. (1987b). Tooth wear and enamel structure in the mandibular incisors of six species of kangaroo (Marsupiala: Macropodinae). *Delivered at the De Vis Symposium*, Queensland Museum, Australia.

18 *Virtual dentitions: touching the hidden evidence*

ROBERTO MACCHIARELLI, LUCA BONDIOLI
AND ARNAUD MAZURIER

18.1 Introduction

Recent advances in dental developmental biology, quantitative genetics, and micro-anatomy (e.g. Dean, 2000, 2006; Hlusko, 2004; Hlusko *et al.*, 2004; Jernvall, 2000; Jernvall and Jung, 2000; Mitsiadis and Smith, 2006; Olejniczak *et al.*, 2004; Pereira *et al.*, 2006; Smith T. M., 2006; Smith T. M. *et al.*, 2006a; Thesleff *et al.*, 2001) have made clear that a critical amount of structural data is preserved in primate dental tissues. Such data can be used to reconstruct/assess evolutionary pathways and phylogenetic relationships, adaptive strategies, growth rates and developmental timing, and age- and sex-related variation patterns in fossil taxa; they may even be used to tentatively outline aspects of their life-history, including fluctuating health conditions and seasonally related individual–environment dynamic relationships recorded during growth (Beynon *et al.*, 1998; Chaimanee *et al.*, 2006; Dean and Leakey, 2004; Dean *et al.*, 2001; FitzGerald *et al.*, 2006; Guatelli-Steinberg *et al.*, 2005; Kelley and Smith, 2003; Lacruz *et al.*, 2006; Macchiarelli *et al.*, 2006; Marivaux *et al.*, 2006a; Ramirez-Rozzi and Bermúdez de Castro, 2004; Schwartz *et al.*, 2003; Smith P. *et al.*, 2006; Smith T. M. *et al.*, 2005a, 2006b; Sponheimer *et al.*, 2006). Nonetheless, a significant portion of this valuable paleobiological archive is hidden deep within the crown and root(s). Since it is not possible or, in the case of scarce fossils, desirable to section every specimen, non-invasive analytical approaches can be used in addition to histomorphometry. Such approaches can facilitate extraction, "cleaning," and decoding of the usually noisy endo-microstructural signature at the most appropriate resolution. Accordingly, beyond the "classic" study topics and investigative strategies, three major research trends have characterized dental (paleo)anthropology during the last two decades: (1) a shift in focus from outer to inner tooth morphology, (2) the related development of advanced, sharper non-destructive analytical tools,

Technique and Application in Dental Anthropology ed. Joel D. Irish and Greg C. Nelson
Published by Cambridge University Press.

and (3) integration of the third dimension in structural visualization and quantitative analysis (Macchiarelli, in press).

Standard 2D radiography has been a common tool to allow non-invasive access to inner dental morphology (see Harris and Hicks, 1998; Harris *et al.*, 2001; rev. in Olejniczak and Grine, 2006), and was widely used to comparatively describe the fossil record (e.g. Molnar *et al.*, 1993; Nagatoshi, 1990; Zilberman and Smith, 1992; Zilberman *et al.*, 1992). As a whole, this approach is qualitatively and quantitatively informative, comprehensive, and, when assisted by advanced digital image processing techniques, likely represents the most practical solution to quickly and "easily" document fossil specimens. However, a critical evaluation of its accuracy discourages extensive utilization in dental paleoanthropology, at least in quantitative measurements of enamel thickness (Grine *et al.*, 2001).

From the late 1980s until recently, medical computed tomography (CT), often integrated by stereolithographic reconstruction, constituted the most effective technology to explore inner structural variation at the millimetric scale, and to help visualize dental elements and tissues in 3D (e.g. Alt and Buitrago-Téllez, 2004). In principle, because specimens are imaged in multiple directions, computed tomography overcomes the problem of parallax distortion and structure superimposition typical of plain film radiography (Spoor *et al.*, 2000). The development of computer-aided segmentation methods has also granted access to otherwise unobservable features and volumes in fossil specimens. Besides its pioneering applications in dental paleoanthropology (Conroy, 1991; Conroy and Vannier, 1987; Conroy *et al.*, 1995; Macho and Thackeray, 1992; Schwartz *et al.*, 1998), a number of methodological studies were developed to test the degree of reliability of CT-based quantitative estimates (e.g. Grine, 1991; Spoor *et al.*, 1993, 2000). Of course, the major constraint in such dental investigations is the limited spatial resolution.

Recently, substantial technological improvements in the rheological sciences and reverse engineering allowed the realization of a more powerful and accurate tool for the non-invasive exploration, high-resolution imaging, and detailed assessment of linear, surface, and volumetric variables in tooth-sized objects; this tool, microfocal X-ray computed tomography (or microtomography), is fostering new research perspectives and quickly affecting our traditional habits and thinking in dental paleoanthropology.

18.2 X-ray computed microtomography (μCT)

X-ray computed microtomography (mCT, or XMT, or CMT, or μCT) operates at microscopic-level resolutions. Relative to medical CTs, industrial and laboratory μCTs actually provide much higher spatial resolution – on the order of a few to about 200 μm (Mees *et al.*, 2003). Because of this and its versatility, microtomography is highly recommended for non-destructive paleobiological studies dealing with virtual exploration and 2D to 3D quantitative analyses of the finest structural variation in mineralized (or remineralized) tissues – most notably teeth (Ketcham and Carlson, 2001; Mazurier *et al.*, 2006; Rossi *et al.*, 2004; Tafforeau *et al.*, 2006).

In principle, a microtomographic examination comprises the recording of a variable number (depending on the resolution needed) of X-ray projections in a specimen from different angles. The projections are formed on a detector by the X-ray beam passing through the object, where the differences in X-ray attenuation are proportional to its topographic density variation (Davis and Wong, 1996). According to the acquisition geometry of the system, unlike a medical CT, the object is rotated through 180 or 360 angular degrees to complete the scan. From these projections, a 3D volumetric digital representation is reconstructed with the help of stochastic (for cone/fan shaped X-ray beams) or exact (for parallel X-ray beans) algorithms (Feldkamp *et al.*, 1984). The size of a volume element, called a voxel (i.e. 3D equivalent of a pixel), is commonly used as a measure of the system's resolution power. The value of a voxel represents the X-ray linear attenuation coefficient of the corresponding volume in the specimen; this variable is intimately related to the mineral composition and density of the material within each specific volume unit (Salvo *et al.*, 2003).

Under some general conditions and specific technical constraints, all available laboratory microtomographic equipment can reproduce the external morphology of a specimen to a satisfactory degree. However, in the case of highly mineralized tissues, the ability to delineate the general external shape of the "container," and the subtle site-specifically varied structure of the "content" strongly depends on: (1) the individual characteristics of the equipment, (2) the calibrated set-up of the record, and (3) the diagenetic history of the sample, which can slightly vary topographically (Mees *et al.*, 2003). Indeed, system resolution is, by itself, not an adequate parameter to assure quality results; the geometry of the cone X-ray beam, its energy spectrum, the sample size and its distance from the beam, the efficiency of the detector, focal spot size, beam intensity and power, angular positions, and integration time are all additional key parameters.

Currently available medical microtomographers (e.g. Scarfe *et al.*, 2006) are normally of limited use in dental paleoanthropology; they do not reach appropriate resolutions to discriminate among mineralized tissues, and are specifically designed for low-dose radiation to limit patient exposure. Conversely, thanks to their varied micrometric (or nanometric) focal-spot size and flexible setting possibilities, industrial μCT equipments for rheological analyses grant a wide range of technical solutions. However, because they mostly utilize X-ray tubes that produce cone-shaped polychromatic beams, they rely upon stochastic algorithms for the reconstructions, with errors increasing as a function of the distance from the central plane (normal to the rotation axis). They are also prone to produce beam hardening artifacts, i.e. "noisy" effects that invariably occur when the effective energy is shifted to a higher value as X-rays pass through the target (Salvo *et al.*, 2003); they can be only partially reduced by pre-filtering of the beam and digital post-processing of the images (Ketcham and Carlson, 2001).

In paleobiological research, the major limit of laboratory μCT equipment is that they can usually accommodate only small objects, not exceeding a few centimeters in diameter. Moreover, although individual primate teeth fit the μCT camera space, the power that theoretically represents the most appropriate solution/compromise for high resolution documentation of fragile specimens on site, does not necessarily assure an optimal contrast between mineralized tissues and matrix; thus, reliable quantification of their relative proportions is prevented (Mazurier *et al.*, 2006).

An "ideal" system for imaging remineralized fossils uses a parallel, monochromatic, high photon flux beam with continuous energy spectrum, and should be equipped with a relatively large sample holder and powerful detector. These requirements are currently met only by the latest generation synchrotrons optimized for hard X-ray (e.g. Ito *et al.*, 2003; Kunz, 2001; Salomé *et al.*, 1999; Salvo *et al.*, 2003). In fact, synchrotron radiation-based microtomography (SR-μCT) assures the best imaging; it involves very low signal/noise ratio, the theoretical absence of beam hardening artifacts (thanks to the beam monochromaticity), and allows the use of exact back-projection algorithms (thanks to the parallel beam geometry) for 3D reconstructions.

The nature of the detector also heavily influences the quality of the results. Conventional image detectors consist of a digital camera coupled with a device that converts X-rays into visible light. The system processes the input signal at various stages, starting from conversion of input X-ray photons into light, conversion of light into electrical signals and, finally, conversion of electrical signal strength into digital form. At each stage of the process some electronic "noise" is usually introduced (via X-ray crosstalk, optical crosstalk, optical scatter); as a result, the signal is almost invariably corrupted and the image quality affected at different degrees. Accordingly, a new generation of detection systems has been specifically designed to assure an almost optimal signal/noise ratio (e.g. Bravin *et al.*, 2003).

At present, the highest μCT resolutions are on the order of 0.15 μm (for synchrotron X-ray tomographic microscopy, see Donoghue *et al.* 2006). Theoretically, higher resolutions allow finer detail recovery but, at least in routine dental paleoanthropological research, this parameter should be carefully tuned to grant the best compromise between (paleo)biological question(s) posed by the investigator(s) and final data size to be post-processed electronically and manually. Of course, depending on continuous technological enhancements, this "optimal" compromise necessarily tends to shift, allowing sharper noninvasive questions to be answered at an ever higher resolution.

In principle, high resolutions are essential for extracting the finest structural information, and to minimize the partial volume effect (i.e. the averaging of different densities within a voxel) typical of medical CT scanners (Spoor *et al.*, 2000); yet, the fact that virtual volume size grows with the cube of the resolution has to be considered when planning for large-scale records. For example, the virtual volume of a modern human molar crown scanned at 50 μm isometric voxel resolution with an 8 bits representation, occupies about 4 Mb; the same specimen scanned at 10 μm reaches 500 Mb. In addition, because the relative difference in density between enamel and dentine directly impacts the discriminating ability of any X-ray-based radiographic technique, it should be carefully considered that spatial resolution, beam geometry, and detector quality of the μCT equipment are not the only factors influencing the acquisition results in fossil specimens (Mazurier *et al.*, 2006).

Following microtomographic acquisition, the most critical analytical step is the identification and separation of different structural components (mineralized tissues and "empty" spaces) by means of segmentation, i.e. the process of identifying and classifying data in a digitally sampled representation (Russ, 2002). In principle, and by definition, there is no univocal technical solution to this problem when dealing with the fossil record; the most effective segmentation algorithms are usually obtained by running various combinations of components and methods. Parameters of these components are tuned for the characteristics of the image modality used as input and the features of the anatomical structure to be segmented. Interestingly, after the pioneering contribution by Spoor and co-workers (1993), little effort has been devoted to address this critical subject in the paleoanthropological literature (Prossinger *et al.*, 2003; Zollikofer and Ponce de León, 2005). In the case of fossil teeth, time-consuming (and operator-dependent) slice-by-slice manual segmentation is frequently the only feasible solution. A review on manual and semi-automatic segmentation procedures is available at the National Library of Medicine Insight Segmentation and Registration Toolkit web site (www.itk.org).

After segmentation, the final 3D rendering of a sample represents the basic record for the high resolution non-invasive visualization and quantitative assessment of its linear, surface, and volumetric features and, in the case of a tooth, its subtle structural characterization in terms of relative tissue proportions. Accordingly, a new era for dental paleoanthropology is just beginning.

18.3 Virtual fossil dentitions

Several methodological studies of modern/recent dental samples have tested the reliability of microtomography as an advanced, non-destructive, analytical tool capable of producing continuous high-resolution slices (serial imaging) to reveal enamel, dentine, and the pulp chamber (e.g. Amano *et al.*, 2006; Avishai *et al.*, 2004; Dowker *et al.*, 2006; Gantt *et al.*, 2006; Kono, 2004; Olejniczak *et al.*, in press; Peters *et al.*, 2000; Rhodes *et al.*, 1999). Further, some papers focused on key technical problems concerning acquisition protocols and imaging, including section position, congruence between cross sectional and volumetric estimates, intra- and inter-observer error, and accuracy of the μCT-based virtual record with respect to physical sections on reference teeth (e.g. Kono, 2004; Olejniczak and Grine, 2006; Olejniczak *et al.*, 2006a; Suwa and Kono, 2005; for a test on microtomographic vs. histological bony sections, see Fajardo *et al.*, 2002; Müller *et al.*, 1998).

On the whole, the tests performed to date are encouraging, and disclose exciting new perspectives for the finest 2D to 3D structural analysis of the dental fossil record; they assure a reliable investigative shift from the external "hard" evidence to its hidden "virtual" imaging (Macchiarelli and Bondioli, 2005). A growing number of researchers have successfully used microtomography to deal with qualitative and quantitative inner characteristics of archaeological and fossil teeth, including those of non-primate mammals (Brunet *et al.*, 2005; Chaimanee *et al.*, 2006; Coppa *et al.*, 2006; Lihoreau *et al.*, 2006; Macchiarelli *et al.*, 2004, 2006, in press; Marivaux *et al.*, 2006a,b; Mazurier and Macchiarelli, 2005; Mazurier *et al.*, 2006; McErlain *et al.*, 2004; Olejniczak and Grine, 2005; Olejniczak *et al.*, 2006b; Rossi *et al.*, 2004; Smith P. *et al.*, 2006; Smith T. M. *et al.*, 2006b; Tafforeau *et al.*, 2006).

During the last few years we have had the opportunity to detail a variety of fossil specimens by means of several different X-ray (SR)μCT scan systems; these include those at the Department of Physics of the University of Bologna, the Centre de Microtomographie of the University of Poitiers, the Bundesanstalt für Materialforschung und -prüfung (BAM) of Berlin, and the medical Beamline ID 17 of the European Synchrotron Radiation Facility (ESRF) of Grenoble (Coppa *et al.*, 2006; Macchiarelli *et al.*, 2004, 2006, in press; Mazurier and Macchiarelli, 2005; Mazurier *et al.*, 2005, 2006; Olejniczak *et al.*, 2006b; Rook *et al.*, 2004; Rossi *et al.*, 2004; Volpato *et al.*, 2006).

To illustrate both the potential and limitations of research in the growing field of virtual dental paleoanthropology, we will present and briefly discuss three case studies from our hominoid (*Ouranopithecus macedoniensis*) and hominid (*Australopithecus* cf. *A. afarensis*, and Neandertals) studies. Before proceeding, however, it first should be noted that, in addition to variation in "transparency," brightness, and contrast, images of these specimens can be rendered in a wide range of false and, as desired, vibrant colors to delineate the specific feature(s) under study. Such was the case for the following, original images. Unfortunately, because all figures in this volume are required to be black and white and/or half tones, the specimen images had to be modified accordingly. References to the original colors can be found in the figure captions, so the reader can at least use his/her imagination.

18.3.1 **Ouranopithecus macedoniensis *(RPl-83)***

Ouranopithecus is a Late Miocene (Vallesian, MN 10) large-bodied ape from Macedonia (Axios Valley), Greece; it is known from cranial and mandibular remains and, mostly, a large sample of permanent teeth. Recently, the mandibular remains of a young individual bearing a partial mixed dentition was recovered from the *c.* 9.3 Ma site of Ravin de la Pluie (RPl) (Koufos and de Bonis, 2004). The individual was likely a male whose age at death was estimated at 3.5–6 years. The remains are represented by two fragments: RPl-82 (left corpus) and RPl-83 (right corpus).

A virtual reconstruction of the larger RPl-83 fragment is shown in Figure 18.1. The microtomographic acquisition was performed at the BAM using 50 μm spatial resolution. With respect to the specimen's original description, based on its external appearance and radiographic and tomographic record (Koufos and de Bonis, 2004), the μCT-based lingual (Figure 18.1e) and buccal (Figure 18.1f) 3D projections in semi-transparency clarify the position of the residual crown fragment, corresponding to the permanent right central incisor, and distinctly visualize both lateral incisors. In addition, and of greater importance, this high-resolution record permits a subtle quantitative assessment of the degree (pattern) of relative crown and root maturation between the preserved deciduous (drc-, drm1, drm2) and permanent teeth (RI1, RI2, LI2, RC-, RP3, RP4, RM1); this life-history variable is still unknown for this hominoid and may be relevant in refining its status (see Koufos and de Bonis, 2005; Smith T. M. *et al.*, 2005a).

The histological analysis of parallel sections of an isolated lower third molar (RPl-641) shows that *Ouranopithecus* has the thickest relative and absolute enamel of any Miocene great ape yet reported (Smith T. M. *et al.*, 2005a; see also Andrews and Martin, 1991); this variable is commonly counted among diagnostic features for taxonomic and phylogenetic assessment, and as a proxy for dietary adaptations and paleoenvironmental reconstructions. For details on extant and fossil hominoids see, among others, Beynon *et al.* (1998), Chaimanee *et al.* (2006), Dean (2000), Gantt *et al.* (2006), Kelley and Smith (2003), Kono

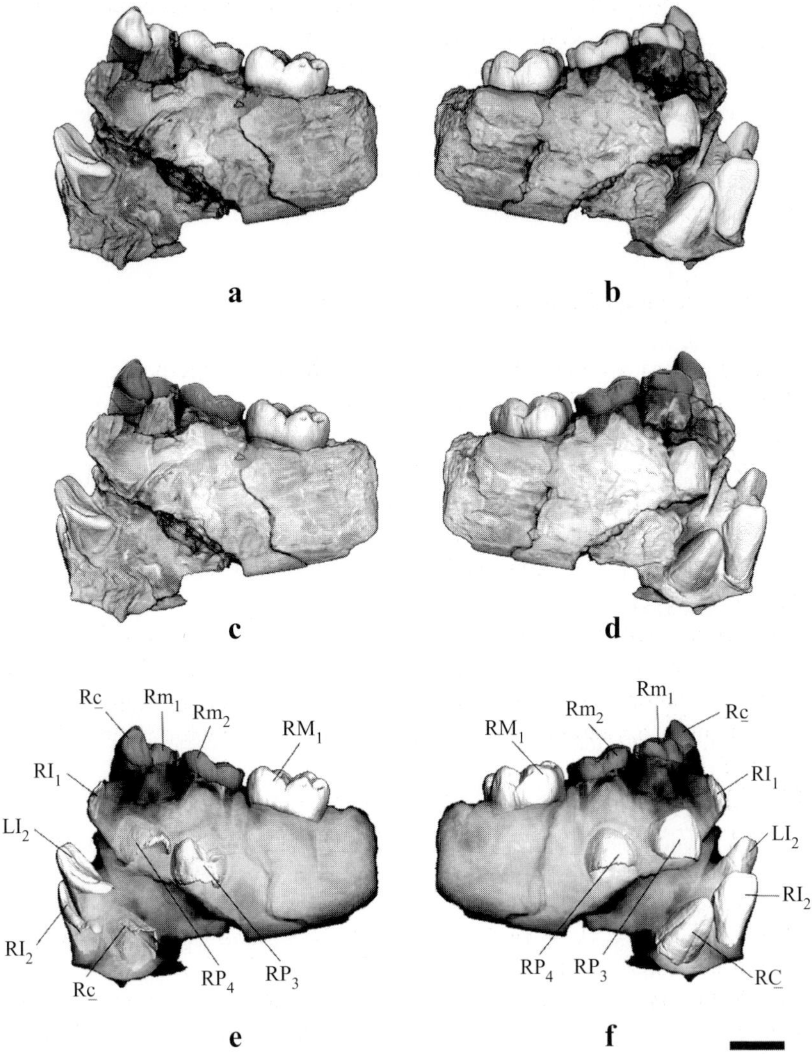

Figure 18.1 μCT-based 3D virtual reconstruction of the right portion of a juvenile *Ouranopithecus* mandible (RPl-83). a: lingual aspect; b: buccal aspect; c, d: same views as a and b with deciduous elements rendered in dark gray (originally purple (see text for explanation of false colors)) and permanent in light gray (originally cyan); e, f: same views with volume rendered in semi-transparency. Scale bar is 1 cm.

(2004), Martin (1985), Martin *et al.* (2003), Schwartz (2000), Schwartz *et al.* (2003), and Smith T. M. *et al.* (2003, 2005a,b); for a recent review on extant humans see Smith T. M. *et al.* (2006a).

A virtual view of the topographic-related variation in enamel thickness on the permanent first molar (M1) and deciduous second molar (m2) of the RPl-83 juvenile *Ouranopithecus* specimen is rendered in Figure 18.2; patterns for *Homo*, *Pan*, and *Gorilla* are also shown for comparative purposes. This visualization technique reveals a significant contrast in the relative volume of occlusal basin enamel between permanent and deciduous crowns that characterizes the fossil compared to extant apes; it also illustrates the overall trans-taxon variation. With respect to conventional methods, the topographic rendering of this feature also allows qualitative and quantitative assessment not only of the cuspal-related occlusal variation, but of likely subtle taxon-specific differences in enamel thickness among the crown walls; the latter is still a poorly explored functional variable that is of potentially great interest in dental paleoanthropology (Kono, 2004; Kono *et al.*, 2002; Schwartz, 2000).

18.3.2 **Australopithecus** ***cf.*** **A. afarensis** ***(GLL 33)***

The shift from a qualitative to quantitative assessment of enamel–dentine junction (EDJ) shape and its topographic relationship with respect to the enamel surface in primate teeth is a complex methodological matter that is receiving growing attention; this matter is of special evolutionary significance in the comparative analysis of extinct taxa (Begun *et al.*, 1997; Dean, 2000, 2006; Heizmann and Begun, 2001; Macchiarelli *et al.*, 2006; Olejniczak *et al.*, 2004; Smith T. M. *et al.*, 2006a). As the EDJ begins to be set earlier in development than enamel or dentine deposition, its shape may be indicative of species-level affiliation (rev. in Smith T. M. *et al.*, 2006a). Accordingly, a major contribution for the 3D modeling of its complex shape in fossil specimens can be expected from non-invasive high-resolution microtomographic imaging (Macchiarelli *et al.*, 2006).

GLL 33 is an isolated lower right third molar from an early Pliocene australopithecine (cf. *A. afarensis*) from Galili, Somali Region, Ethiopia. Although worn and weathered, the crown is nearly complete and exhibits seven cusps (including a *tuberculum intermedium* between the metaconid and entoconid); however, most of the mesial root is absent (Macchiarelli *et al.*, 2004). Its microtomographic record (30 and 60 μm spatial resolution) was again imaged at the BAM (original digitized volume data is available in Weber *et al.*, 2004).

Following surface virtual models, where the enamel was rendered transparent, a 3D rendering of this highly mineralized tooth is shown in Figure 18.3.

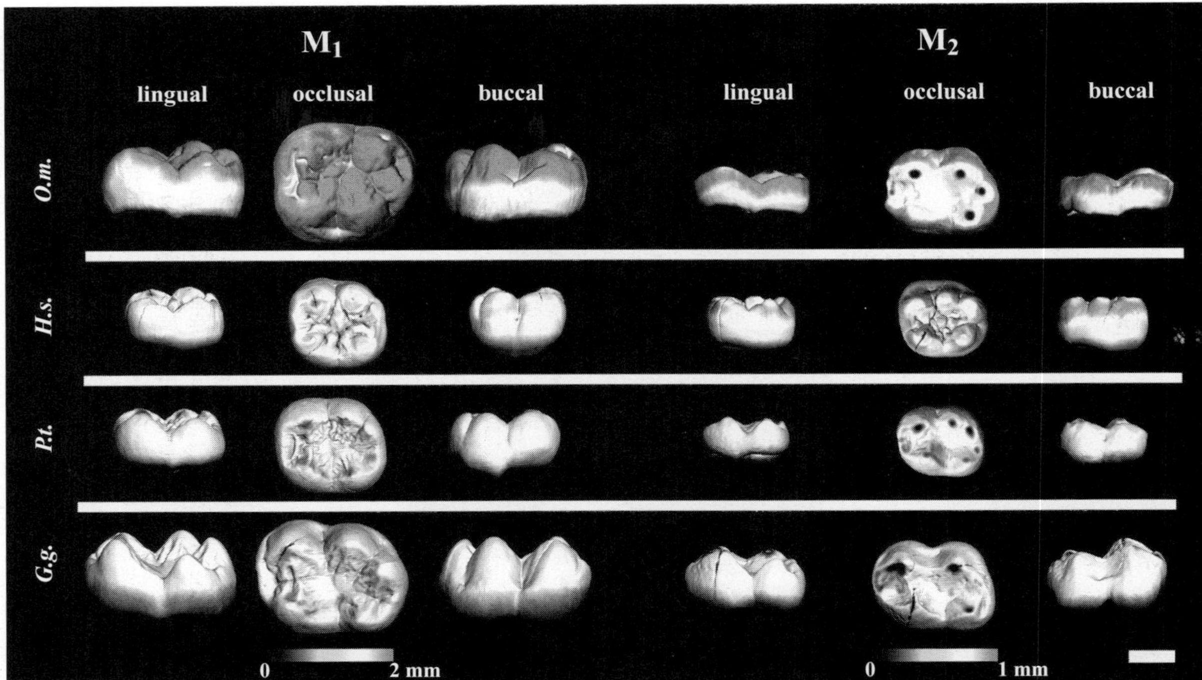

Figure 18.2 μCT-based comparative enamel thickness variation digitally measured on a lower permanent first molar (M_1) and deciduous second molar (m_2) in *Ouranopithecus* (*O.m.*), *Homo* (*H.s.*), *Pan* (*P.t.*), and *Gorilla* (*G.g.*). Crowns shown in lingual, occlusal, and buccal views. The topographic variation in enamel thickness across each crown is represented by light gray (i.e., thin) through dark gray (thick) (originally rendered by blue (thin) to red (thick)). Isolated black spots (originally blue) on occlusal surfaces correspond to cuspal dental wear. The unworn *Ouranopithecus* M_1 has a total enamel volume of 572 mm^3 (vs. 345 in *Gorilla*, 213 in *Homo*, and 210 in *Pan*). The maximum radial thickness measured on the *Ouranopithecus* m_2 is 1.32 mm (vs. 1.12 in *Homo*, 0.75 in *Gorilla*, and 0.74 in *Pan*). Scale bar is 5 mm.

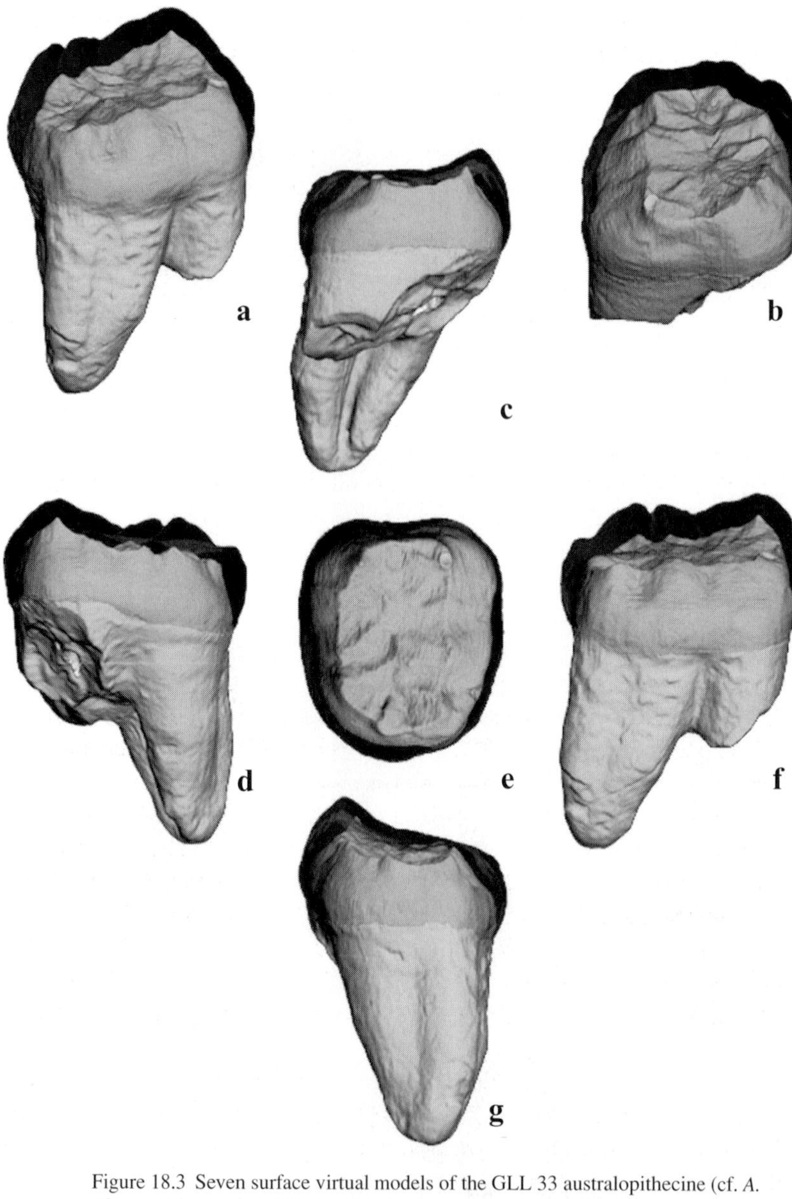

Figure 18.3 Seven surface virtual models of the GLL 33 australopithecine (cf. *A. afarensis*) lower right M3 showing the topography of the enamel-dentine junction. (a): slightly oblique buccal view; (b): oblique mesial view; (c): mesial view; (d): lingual view; (e): occlusal view; (f): buccal view; (g): distal view. Images not to scale.

Despite the fact that dentine usually exhibits a structurally simpler shape than the surface enamel and that, in principle, there does not appear to be a predictive relationship between dentine and enamel topographies (Olejniczak *et al.*, 2004), a good degree of morphological resemblance characterizes this specimen; the dentine shape is quite rough and displays a complex pattern of occlusal ridges and grooves (see Figure 18.3 a,b,e). Nonetheless, the faintly developed mesial trigonid crest, for example, that connects the protoconid and metaconid, is not as developed as it appears on the surface; similarly, the dentine signature of the enamel anterior fovea is barely noticeable.

Compared to an average modern human M_3 from our digital record, the surface area of the GLL 33 EDJ is about 2.4 times larger (333 vs. 141 mm^2) and, mostly, the volume of its coronal dentine – which includes the pulp contained within the enamel cap – is nearly four times larger (663 vs. 171 mm^3). In this early australopithecine, the dentine horn tips are low (see Figure 18.3c,d,g) and, despite the additive effect of functional crown wear and weathering/erosion, the enamel is relatively thick, especially at the cuspal level.

18.3.3 Neandertals

Recent use of microtomography (μCT and SR-μCT) on Neandertal deciduous and permanent teeth is providing fresh quantitative elements to the classic debate about their "unique condition" relative to anatomically modern humans, in terms of structural morphology and growth and developmental patterns. Important advances concern Neandertal prenatal dental growth trajectories, timing of molar crown and root completion, relative proportions of dental tissues, comparative topographies of the EDJ and of the outer enamel surface, and enamel thickness variation (Bayle *et al.*, 2007; Macchiarelli *et al.*, 2006, in press; Mazurier and Macchiarelli, 2005; Olejniczak and Grine, 2005; Olejniczak *et al.*, 2006b; Smith P. *et al.*, 2006; for fossil 'modern' teeth, see Smith T. M. *et al.*, 2006b). However, most of these analyses have dealt with isolated teeth (though see Bayle *et al.*, 2007).

A virtual reconstruction of the Regourdou 1 Neandertal mandible from Montignac-sur-Vézère, France (OIS 4) is presented in Figure 18.4. The image is based on a high-resolution synchrotron radiation microtomographic record (SR-μCT) performed with the beamline ID 17 at the ESRF (45.5 μm spatial resolution). The specimen is from the partial skeleton of a young adult of indeterminate sex (Vandermeersch and Trinkaus, 1995); it contains a complete well-preserved dentition, though with notable occlusal wear on many crowns. Relative to the variation reported for most Neandertals, odontometric

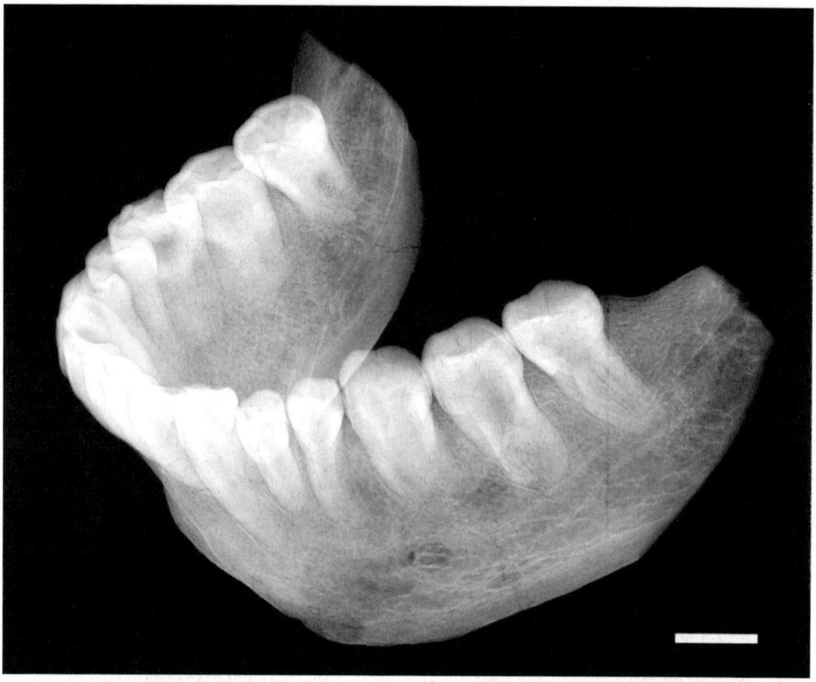

Figure 18.4 SR-μCT-based 3D virtual reconstruction (volume rendered as transparent) of the Regourdou 1 adult Neandertal mandible (antero-lateral oblique view). Scale bar is 1 cm.

study (Maureille *et al.*, 2001) revealed relatively modest crown size, including a reduced LP_3, in this individual.

The 3D digital projection allows a qualitative appreciation of the dental root extension and orientation, the position and shape of the multiple dental and mandibular foramina, and the site-specific textural organization and degree of anisotropy of the trabecular network. With reference to the molars, characteristic Neandertal features include thin occlusal enamel, large anterior foveae with mid-trigonid crests, small occlusal areas relative to maximum contours of the crowns, a lack of cervical constriction, and taurodontism (per Smith P. *et al.*, 2006; see also Macchiarelli *et al.*, 2006; Olejniczak and Grine, 2005; Olejniczak *et al.*, 2006b). Nonetheless, for most endostructural dental features, the extent of variation in Neandertals remains poorly known; no high-resolution quantitative volumetric estimates have been reported so far (though see Macchiarelli *et al.*, 2006; Olejniczak and Grine, 2005; for modern deciduous molars see Amano *et al.*, 2006).

In Figure 18.5, tissue proportions of the Regourdou 1 molars are compared to those in a modern human of similar age at death; to facilitate this comparison,

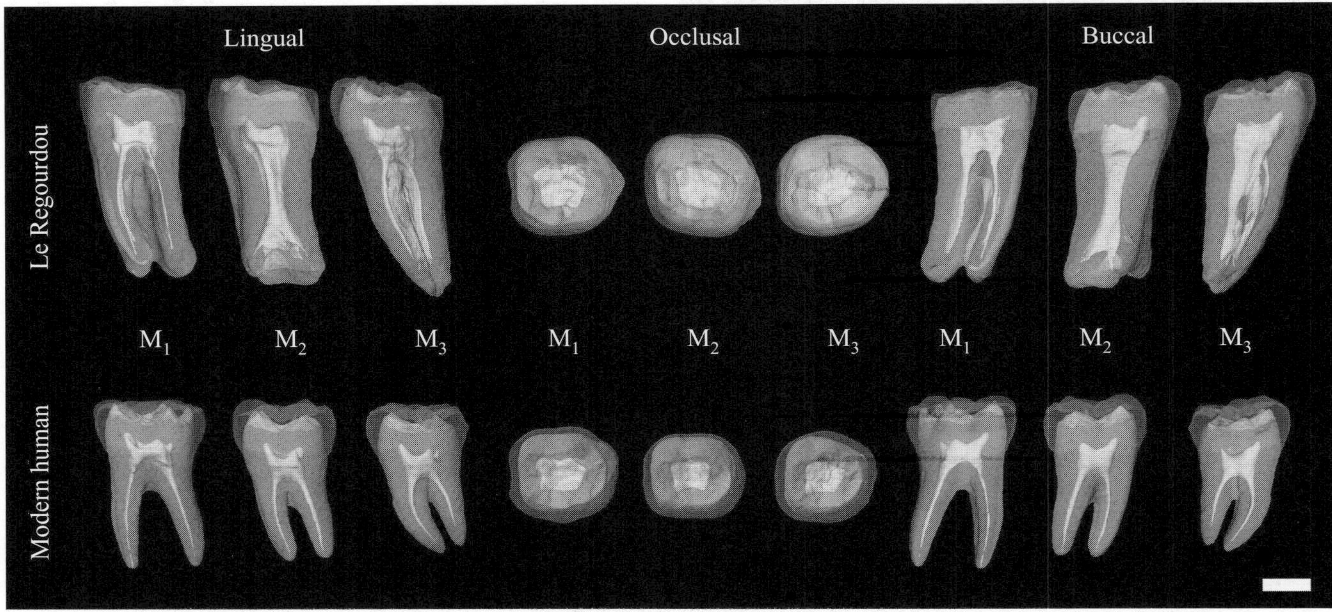

Figure 18.5 Regourdou 1 Neandertal right lower molars (upper row) compared to molars from a modern human for their relative tissue proportions. The enamel caps are transparent; pulp chambers are "virtually" filled and rendered in light gray (originally violet). In lingual, occlusal, and buccal views, respectively. Scale bar is 5 mm.

the enamel was rendered transparent while the pulp chambers were virtually "filled." The fossil pulp cavities exhibit varying sizes and shapes; volumes range from 66 to 104 mm^3 for the first and second molar, respectively (vs. 28–35 mm^3 in the modern specimen's M_3 and M_1). Accordingly, only the Regourdou M_2 can be defined as taurodont, i.e. showing a relative expansion – in both the vertical and transverse diameters – of the pulp chamber, associated with apical root bifurcation. In fact, the volumetric proportion between the pulp components measured above and below the pulp chamber floor bifurcation (as defined in Macchiarelli *et al.*, 2004) is close to 50% only in this tooth (i.e. proportional expansion in M_2 of the lower component which is absolutely smaller in the Regourdou M_1 and M_3, as well as all modern molars). However, even when scaled with respect to total tooth volume (% ratio), all three Neandertal molars have larger cavities relative to the modern condition (M_1: 5.4 vs. 4.3; M_2: 7.2 vs. 4.0; M_3: 6.9 vs. 4.1).

In sum, a 3D quantification of relative dental tissue proportions can be crucial in advanced paleoanthropological studies; such quantification is particularly important when dealing with the functional interpretation and assessment of the evolutionary polarity of structural dental features, such as enamel thickness (e.g. Huber *et al.*, 2007; Olejniczak *et al.*, 2006b).

18.4 Conclusion

Scarce and fragmentary fossils usually constitute the only paleobiological evidence testifying to the life and death of our ancient relatives and ancestors. The appropriate exploitation of this unique heritage for research and educational purposes is crucial for understanding key aspects of our own history, and for modeling possible future scenarios. Nonetheless, accessibility to the original record is deeply affected by its intrinsic uniqueness, fragility, and geographic dispersal. Moreover, even though such specimens may be characterized by a high mineral content, their frequent handling for direct observation, measurement, reproduction, casting, and display, can be risky.

In response to the potentially conflicting requirements of curation vs. study of osteodental fossil collections, a new generation of analytical tools is capable, for the first time, of non-invasive manipulation and extraction. High-resolution reproduction, both virtual and solid, and precise morphometric data collection can be made in any specimen without risk of damage (for ongoing applications to the Neandertal fossil record, see Macchiarelli *et al.*, 2005; Semal *et al.*, 2005). In this way, it is likely that "virtual reality" will play a major role in dental paleoanthropology by permitting new and privileged access to the "hidden evidence."

Acknowledgments

We are deeply indebted to the editors of this volume for their kind invitation, patience, competence, and extraordinary help in enhancing the quality of our work. This contribution is based on the microtomographic record of modern and fossil specimens realized during the past few years at the Bundesanstalt für Materialforschung und -prüfung (BAM) of Berlin, the ESRF beamline ID 17 of Grenoble, the Department of Physics at the University of Bologna, and the Centre de Microtomographie (CdMT) at the University of Poitiers. For their technical and scientific collaboration, we acknowledge A. Bergeret, A. Bravin, F. Casali, B. Illerhaus, C. Nemoz, M. Rossi, P. Sardini, P. Tafforeau, V. Volpato, and G. W. Weber. For having granted access to the fossil specimens discussed in this paper, we are deeply indebted to L. de Bonis, F. Couturas, G. Koufos, G. Marchesseau, V. Merlin-Anglade, H. Seidler, and G. W. Weber. Research was supported by the French CNRS, the EU TNT Project, the ESRF, the University of Poitiers, the GDR 2152 (to R. M.), and the Région Poitou-Charentes (to A. M.). Image elaborations realized by means of AMIRA v4.0 package (Mercury Computer Systems, Inc.).

References

Alt, K. W. and Buitrago-Téllez, C. H. (2004). Dental paleoradiology: applications in paleoanthropology and paleopathology. *Journal of the Canadian Association of Radiologists*, **55**, 258–63.

Amano, M., Agematsu, H., Abe, S. *et al.* (2006). Three-dimensional analysis of pulp chambers in maxillary second deciduous molars. *Journal of Dentistry*, **34**, 503–8.

Andrews, P. and Martin, L. (1991). Hominoid dietary evolution. *Philosophical Transactions of the Royal Society of London, Series B*, **334**, 199–209.

Avishai, G., Müller, R., Gabet, Y. *et al.* (2004). New approach to quantifying developmental variation in the dentition using serial microtomographic imaging. *Microscopy Research and Technique*, **65**, 263–9.

Bayle, P., Braga, J., Mazurier, A., Radovčic, J., and Macchiarelli, R. (2007). Dental developmental patterns in Neandertals: a high-resolution 3D analysis. *American Journal of Physical Anthropology*, Suppl. 41, 70 (abstract).

Begun, D., Ward, C. V., and Rose, M. D. (1997). Events in hominoid evolution. In *Function, Phylogeny, and Fossils: Miocene Hominoid Evolution and Adaptation*, ed. D. Begun, C. V. Ward, and M. D. Rose. New York: Plenum Press, pp. 389–415.

Beynon, A. D., Dean, M. C., Leakey, M. G., Reid, D. J., and Walker, A. (1998). Comparative dental development and microstructure of Proconsul teeth from Rusinga Island, Kenya. *Journal of Human Evolution*, **35**, 163–209.

Bravin, A., Fielder, S., Coan, P. *et al.* (2003). Comparison between a position sensitive germanium detector and a taper optics CCD "FRELON" camera for diffraction enhanced imaging. *Nuclear Instruments and Methods in Physics Research A*, **510**, 35–40.

Brunet, M., Guy, F., Pilbeam, D. *et al.* (2005). New material of the earliest hominid from the Upper Miocene of Chad. *Nature*, **434**, 752–5.

Chaimanee, Y., Yamee, C., Tian, P. *et al.* (2006). *Khoratpithecus piriyai*, a Late Miocene hominoid of Thailand. *American Journal of Physical Anthropology*, **131**, 311–23.

Conroy, G. C. (1991). Enamel thickness in South African australopithecines: noninvasive evaluation by computed tomography. *Palaeontologica Africana*, **28**, 53–9.

Conroy, G. C. and Vannier, M. H. (1987). Dental development of the Taung skull from computerized tomography. *Nature*, **329**, 625–7.

Conroy, G. C., Lichtman, J. W., and Martin, L. B. (1995). Some observations on enamel thickness and enamel prism packing in the Miocene hominoid *Otavipithecus namibiensis*. *American Journal of Physical Anthropology*, **98**, 595–600.

Coppa, A., Bondioli, L., Cucina, A. *et al.* (2006). Early Neolithic dentistry. *Nature*, **440**, 755–6.

Davis, G. R. and Wong, F. S. L. (1996). X-ray microtomography of bones and teeth. *Physiological Measurement*, **17**, 121–46.

Dean, M. C. (2000). Progress in understanding hominoid dental development. *Journal of Anatomy*, **197**, 77–101.

Dean, M. C. (2006). Tooth microstructure tracks the pace of human life-history evolution. *Proceedings of the Royal Society*, **B273**, 2799–808.

Dean, M. C. and Leakey, M. G. (2004). Enamel and dentine development and the life history profile of *Victoriapithecus macinnesi* from Maboko Island, Kenya. *Annals of Anatomy*, **186**, 405–12.

Dean, M. C., Leakey, M. G., Reid, D. *et al.* (2001). Growth processes in teeth distinguish modern humans from *Homo erectus* and earlier hominins. *Nature*, **414**, 628–31.

Donoghue, P. C. J., Bengtson, S., Dong, X. *et al.* (2006). Synchrotron X-ray tomographic microscopy of fossil embryos. *Nature*, **442**, 680–3.

Dowker, S. E. P., Elliott, J. C., Davis, G. R., Wilson, R. M., and Cloetens, P. (2006). Three-dimensional study of human dental fissure enamel by synchrotron X-ray microtomography. *European Journal of Oral Sciences*, **114** (Suppl. 1), 353–9.

Fajardo, R. J., Ryan, T. M., and Kappelman, J. (2002). Assessing the accuracy of high-resolution X-ray computed tomography of primate trabecular bone by comparisons with histological sections. *American Journal of Physical Anthropology*, **118**, 1–10.

Feldkamp, L. A., Davis, L. C., and Kress, J. W. (1984). Practical cone-beam algorithm. *Journal of the Optical Society of America*, **1**, 612–19.

FitzGerald, C., Saunders, S., Bondioli, L., and Macchiarelli, R. (2006). Health of infants in an Imperial Roman skeletal sample: perspective from dental microstructure. *American Journal of Physical Anthropology*, **130**, 179–89.

Gantt, D. G., Kappleman, J., Ketcham, R. A., Alder, M. E., and Deahl, T. H. (2006). Three-dimensional reconstruction of enamel thickness and volume in humans and hominoids. *European Journal of Oral Sciences*, **114** (Suppl. 1), 360–4.

Grine, F. E. (1991). Computed tomography and the measurement of enamel thickness in extant hominoids: implications for its paleontological application. *Palaeontologica Africana*, **28**, 61–9.

Grine, F. E., Stevens, N. J., and Jungers, W. J. (2001). An evaluation of dental radiograph accuracy in the measurement of enamel thickness. *Archives of Oral Biology*, **46**, 1117–25.

Guatelli-Steinberg, D., Reid, D. J., Bishop, T. A., and Larsen, C. S. (2005). Anterior tooth growth periods in Neandertals were comparable to those of modern humans. *Proceedings of the National Academy of Sciences USA*, **102**, 14197–202.

Harris, E. F. and Hicks, J. D. (1998). A radiographic assessment of enamel thickness in human maxillary incisors. *Archives of Oral Biology*, **10**, 825–31.

Harris, E. F., Hicks, J. D., and Barcroft, B. D. (2001). Tissue contributions to sex and race: differences in tooth crown size of deciduous molars. *American Journal of Physical Anthropology*, **115**, 223–37.

Heizmann, E. P. J. and Begun, D. (2001). The oldest Eurasian hominoid. *Journal of Human Evolution*, **41**, 463–81.

Hlusko, L. J. (2004). Integrating the genotype and phenotype in hominid paleontology. *Proceedings of the National Academy of Sciences USA*, **101**, 2653–7.

Hlusko, L. J., Suwa, G., Kono, R. T. and Mahaney, M. C. (2004). Genetics and the evolution of primate enamel thickness: a baboon model. *American Journal of Physical Anthropology*, **124**, 223–33.

Huber, C. D., Bookstein, F. L., and Weber, G. W. (2007). Tooth shape and enamel thickness variation in primate teeth: an approach using topographic thickness maps. *American Journal of Physical Anthropology*, Suppl. 41, 132 (abstract).

Ito, M., Ejiri, S., Jinnai, H., Kono, J. *et al.* (2003). Bone structure and mineralization demonstrated using synchrotron radiation computed tomography (SR-CT) in animal models: preliminary findings. *Journal of Bone and Mineral Metabolism*, **21**, 287–93.

Jernvall, J. (2000). Linking development with generation of novelty in mammalian teeth. *Proceedings of the National Academy of Sciences USA*, **97**, 2641–5.

Jernvall, J. and Jung, H.-S. (2000). Genotype, phenotype, and developmental biology of molar tooth characters. *Yearbook of Physical Anthropology*, **43**, 171–90.

Kelley, J. and Smith, T. M. (2003). Age at first molar emergence in early Miocene *Afropithecus turkanensis* and life-history evolution in the Hominoidea. *Journal of Human Evolution*, **44**, 307–29.

Ketcham, K. A. and Carlson, W. D. (2001). Acquisition, optimization and interpretation of X-ray computed tomographic imagery: applications to the geosciences. *Computers and Geosciences*, **27**, 381–400.

Kono, R. (2004). Molar enamel thickness and distribution patterns in extant great apes and humans: new insights based on a 3-dimensional whole crown perspective. *Anthropological Science*, **112**, 121–46.

Kono, R. T., Suwa, G., and Tanijiri, T. (2002). A three-dimensional analysis of enamel distribution patterns in human permanent first molars. *Archives of Oral Biology*, **47**, 867–75.

Koufos, G. D. and de Bonis, L. (2004). The deciduous lower dentition of *Ouranopithecus macedoniensis* (Primates, Hominoidea) from the Late Miocene deposits of Macedonia, Greece. *Journal of Human Evolution*, **46**, 699–718.

Koufos, G. D. and de Bonis, L. (2005). The Late Miocene hominoids Ouranopithecus and Graecopithecus. Implications about their relationships and taxonomy. *Annales de Paléontologie*, **91**, 227–40.

Kunz, C. (2001). Synchrotron radiation: third generation sources. *Journal of Physics: Condensed Matter*, **13**, 7499–510.

Lacruz, R. S., Ramirez-Rozzi, F., and Bromage, T. G. (2006). Variation in enamel development of South African fossil hominids. *Journal of Human Evolution*, **51**, 580–90.

Lihoreau, F., Boisserie, J.-R., Viriot, L. *et al.* (2006). Anthracothere dental anatomy reveals a late Miocene Chado-Libyan bioprovince. *Proceedings of the National Academy of Sciences USA*, **23**, 8763–7.

Macchiarelli, R. (in press). Dental microstructure and life history: introduction. In *Dental Perspectives on Human Evolution: State of the Art Research in Dental Paleoanthropology*, ed. S. E. Bailey and J.-J. Hublin. Dordrecht: Springer.

Macchiarelli, R. and Bondioli, L. (2005). Virtual dentitions: touching the hidden evidence. *American Journal of Physical Anthropology*, Suppl. 39, 177 (abstract).

Macchiarelli, R., Bondioli, L., Falk, D. *et al.* (2004). Early Pliocene hominid tooth from Galili, Somali Region, Ethiopia. *Collegium Antropologicum*, **28**, 65–76.

Macchiarelli, R., Radovčic, J., Semal, P., and Weniger, G. C. (2005). A "virtual reality" for the Neanderthal fossil record: "The Neanderthal Tools" project. *Bullettin et Mémoires de la Société d'Anthropologie de Paris*, **17**, 278 (abstract).

Macchiarelli, R., Bondioli, L., Debénath, A. *et al.* (2006). How Neanderthal molar teeth grew. *Nature*, **444**, 748–51.

Macchiarelli, R., Mazurier, A., and Volpato V. (in press). L'apport des nouvelles technologies à l'étude des Néandertaliens. In *Les Néandertaliens*, ed. B. Vandermeersch. Paris: Comité des Travaux Historiques et Scientifiques (CTHS).

Macho, G. A. and Thackeray, J. F. (1992). Computed-tomography and enamel thickness of maxillary molars of Plio-Pleistocene hominids from Sterkfontein, Swartkrans, and Kromdraai (South Africa): an exploratory study. *American Journal of Physical Anthropology*, **89**, 133–43.

Marivaux, L., Chaimanee, Y., Tafforeau, P., and Jaeger, J.-J. (2006a). New strepsirrhine primate from the Late Eocene of Peninsular Thailand (Krabi Basin). *American Journal of Physical Anthropology*, **130**, 425–34.

Marivaux, L., Bocat, L., Chaimanee, Y. *et al.* (2006b). Cynocephalid dermopterans from the Palaeogene of South Asia (Thailand, Myanmar and Pakistan): systematic, evolutionary and palaeobiogeographic implications. *Zoologica Scripta*, **35**, 395–420.

Martin, L. (1985). Significance of enamel thickness in hominoid evolution. *Nature*, **314**, 260–3.

Martin, L., Olejniczak, A. J., and Maas, M. C. (2003). Enamel thickness and microstructure in pithecine primates, with comments on dietary adaptations of the Middle Miocene hominoid Kenyapithecus. *Journal of Human Evolution*, **45**, 351–67.

Maureille, B., Rougier, H., Houet, F., and Vandermeersch, B. (2001). Les dents inférieures du néandertalien Regourdou 1 (site de Regourdou, commune de Montignac, Dordogne): analyses métriques et comparatives. *Paléo*, **13**, 183–200.

Mazurier, A. and Macchiarelli, R. (2005). Anterior deciduous dentition in Neanderthals: topographic variation in enamel thickness and inner structural morphology. *Bulletin et Mémoires de la Société d'Anthropologie de Paris*, **17**, 280 (abstract).

Mazurier, A., Bondioli, L., Bravin, A., Nemoz, C., and Macchiarelli R. (2005). High-resolution (3D SR-μCT-based) structural analysis of the primate proximal tibia: evidence for locomotion-related topographic variation. *American Journal of Physical Anthropology*, Suppl. 39, 147 (abstract).

Mazurier, A., Volpato, V., and Macchiarelli, R. (2006). Improved noninvasive microstructural analysis of fossil tissues by means of SR-microtomography. *Applied Physics A, Materials Science and Processing*, **83**, 229–33.

McErlain, D. D., Chhem, R. K., Bohay, R. N., and Holdsworth, D. W. (2004). Micro-computed tomography of a 500-year-old tooth: technical note. *Journal of the Canadian Association of Radiologists*, **55**, 242–5.

Mees, F., Swennen, R., van Geet, M., and Jacobs, P., eds. (2003). *Applications of X-ray Computed Tomography in the Geosciences*. Geological Society, Spec. Publ. 215. London: Geological Society.

Mitsiadis, T. A. and Smith, M. M. (2006). How do genes make teeth to order through development? *Journal of Experimental Zoology Part B: Molecular and Developmental Evolution*, **306 B**, 177–82.

Molnar, S., Hildebolt, C., Molnar, I. M., Radovcic, J., and Gravier, M. (1993). Hominid enamel thickness: I, the Krapina Neandertals. *American Journal of Physical Anthropology*, **92**, 131–8.

Müller, R., van Campenhout, H., van Damme, B. *et al.* (1998). Morphometric analysis of human bone biopsies: a quantitative structural comparison of histological sections and micro-computed tomography. *Bone*, **23**, 59–66.

Nagatoshi, K. (1990). Molar enamel thickness in European Miocene and extant Hominoidea. *International Journal of Primatology*, **11**, 283–95.

Olejniczak, A. J. and Grine, F. E. (2005). High-resolution measurement of Neanderthal tooth enamel thickness by micro-focal computed tomography. *South African Journal of Science*, **101**, 219–20.

Olejniczak, A. J. and Grine, F. E. (2006). Assessment of the accuracy of dental enamel thickness measurements using microfocal X-ray computed tomography. *Anatomical Record*, **288 A**, 263–75.

Olejniczak, A. J., Grine, F. E., and Martin, L. B. (in press). Micro-computed tomography of the primate post-canine dentition. Methodological aspects of three-dimensional data collection. In *Dental Perspectives on Human Evolution: State of the Art Research in Dental Paleoanthropology*, ed. S. E. Bailey and J.-J. Hublin. Dordrecht: Springer.

Olejniczak, A. J., Martin, L. B., and Ulhaas, L. (2004). Quantification of dentine shape in anthropoid primates. *Annals of Anatomy*, **186**, 479–85.

Olejniczak, A. J., Smith, T. M., Tafforeau, P., Temming, H. and Hublin, J.-J. (2006a). A comparison of microtomographic systems for the analysis of dental tissues. *American Journal of Physical Anthropology*, Suppl. 42, 140–41 (abstract).

Olejniczak, A. J., Smith, T. M., Macchiarelli, R. *et al.* (2006b). Enamel volume and thickness in Neanderthal molars: a microtomographic investigation. *Terra Nostra*, **2**, 128–9 (abstract).

Pereira, T. V., Salzano, F. M., Mostowska, A. *et al.* (2006). Natural selection and molecular evolution in primate PAX9 gene, a major determinant of tooth development. *Proceedings of the National Academy of Sciences USA*, **103**, 5676–81.

Peters, O. A., Laib, A., Rüegsegger, P. and Barbakow, F. (2000). Three-dimensional analysis of root canal geometry by high-resolution computed tomography. *Journal of Dental Research*, **79**, 1405–9.

Prossinger, H., Seidler, H., Wicke, L. *et al.* (2003). Electronic removal of encrustations inside the Steinheim cranium reveals paranasal sinus features and deformations, and provides a revised endocranial volume estimate. *Anatomical Record*, **273 B**, 132–44.

Ramirez Rozzi, F. and Bermúdez de Castro, J. M. (2004). Surprisingly rapid growth in Neanderthals. *Nature*, **428**, 936–9.

Rhodes, J. S., Pitt-Ford, T. R., Lynch, J. A., Liepins, P. J., and Curtis, R. V. (1999). Micro-computed tomography: a new tool for experimental endodontology. *International Endodontology Journal*, **32**, 165–70.

Rook, L., Bondioli, L., Casali, F. *et al.* (2004). The bony labyrinth of *Oreopithecus bambolii*. *Journal of Human Evolution*, **46**, 345–52.

Rossi, M., Casali, F., Romani, D. *et al.* (2004). Micro-CTscan in paleobiology: application to the study of dental tissues. *Nuclear Instruments and Methods in Physics Research B*, **213**, 747–50.

Russ, J. C. (2002). *The Image Processing Handbook, 4th Edn*. Boca Raton: CRC Press.

Salomé, M., Peyrin, F., Cloetens, P. *et al.* (1999). A synchrotron radiation microtomography system for the analysis of trabecular bone samples. *Medical Physics*, **26**, 2194–204.

Salvo, L., Cloetens, P., Maire, E. *et al.* (2003). X-ray microtomography: an attractive characterisation technique materials science. *Nuclear Instruments and Methods in Physics Research B*, **200**, 273–86.

Scarfe, W. C., Farman, A. G., and Sukovic, P. (2006). Clinical applications of cone-beam computed tomography in dental practice. *Journal of the Canadian Dental Association*, **72**, 75–80.

Schwartz, G. T. (2000). Taxonomic and functional aspects of the patterning of enamel thickness distribution in extant large-bodied hominoids. *American Journal of Physical Anthropology*, **111**, 221–44.

Schwartz, G. T., Liu, W., and Zheng, L. (2003). Preliminary investigation of dental microstructure in the Yuanmou hominoid (*Lufengpithecus hudienensis*), Yunnan Province, China. *Journal of Human Evolution*, **44**, 189–202.

Schwartz, G. T., Thackeray, J. F., Reid, C., and Van Reenan, J. F. (1998). Enamel thickness and the topography of the enamel–dentine junction in South African Plio-Pleistocene hominids with special reference to the Carabelli trait. *Journal of Human Evolution*, **35**, 523–42.

Semal, P., Toussaint, M., Maureille, B. *et al.* (2005). Numérisation des restes humains néandertaliens belges. Préservation patrimoniale et exploitation scientifique. *Notae Praehistoricae*, **25**, 25–38.

Smith, P., Müller, R., Gabet, Y., and Avishai, G. (2006). Computerized reconstruction of prenatal growth trajectories in the dentition: implications for the taxonomic status of Neandertals. *Terra Nostra*, **2**, 60–3.

Smith, T. M. (2006). Experimental determination of the periodicity of incremental features in enamel. *Journal of Anatomy*, **208**, 99–113.

Smith, T. M., Martin, L. B., and Leakey, M. G. (2003). Enamel thickness, microstructure and development in *Afropithecus turkanensis*. *Journal of Human Evolution*, **44**, 283–306.

Smith, T. M., Martin, L. B., Reid, D. J., de Bonis, L., and Koufous, G. D. (2005a). An examination of dental development in *Graecopithecus freybergi* (*Ouranopithecus macedoniensis*). *Journal of Human Evolution*, **46**, 551–77.

Smith, T. M., Olejniczak, A. J., Martin, L. B., and Reid, D. J. (2005b). Variation in hominoid molar enamel thickness. *Journal of Human Evolution*, **48**, 575–92.

Smith, T. M., Olejniczak, A. J., Reid, D. J., Ferrell, R. J. and Hublin, J.-J. (2006a). Modern human molar enamel thickness and enamel-dentine junction shape. *Archives of Oral Biology*, **51**, 974–95.

Smith, T. M., Olejniczak, A. J., Tafforeau, P. *et al.* (2006b). Molar crown thickness, volume, and development in South African Middle Stone Age humans. *South African Journal of Science*, **102**, 1–5.

Sponheimer, M., Passey, B. H., de Ruiter, D. J. *et al.* (2006). Isotopic evidence for dietary variability in the early hominin *Paranthropus robustus*. *Science*, **314**, 980–2.

Spoor, C. F., Zonneveld, F. W., and Macho, G. A. (1993). Linear measurements of cortical bone and dental enamel by computed tomography: applications and problems. *American Journal of Physical Anthropology*, **91**, 469–84.

Spoor, F., Jeffery N., and Zonneveld, F. (2000). Imaging skeletal growth and evolution. In *Development, Growth and Evolution: Implications for the Study of the Hominid Skeleton*, ed. P. O'Higgins and M. Cohn. London: Academic Press, pp. 123–61.

Suwa, G. and Kono, R. T. (2005). A micro-CT based study of linear enamel thickness in the mesial cusp section of human molars: reevaluation of methodology and assessment of within-tooth, serial, and individual variation. *Anthropological Science*, **113**, 273–89.

Tafforeau, P., Boistel, R., Boller, E. *et al.* (2006). Applications of X-ray synchrotron microtomography for non-destructive 3D studies of paleontological specimens. *Applied Physics A, Materials Science and Processing*, **83**, 195–202.

Thesleff, I., Keranen, S., and Jernvall, J. (2001). Enamel knots as signalling centers linking tooth morphogenesis and odontoblast differentiation. *Advances in Dental Research*, **15**, 14–18.

Vandermeersch, B. and Trinkaus, E. (1995). The postcranial remains of the Regourdou 1 Neandertal: the shoulder and arm remains. *Journal of Human Evolution*, **28**, 439–76.

Volpato, V., Couture, C., Vandermeersch, B., and Macchiarelli, R. (2006). Endostructural characterisation of the Regourdou 1 Neandertal proximal arm: bilateral asymmetry and handedness. *Terra Nostra*, **2**, 140–1 (abstract).

Weber, G. W., Seidler, H., Woldearagay, K. *et al.* (2004). *GLL 33. 3rd Lower Molar, Australopithecus cf. A. afarensis*. Digital Archive of Fossil Hominoids, 6. Vienna-Addis Ababa: Institute of Anthropology and ARCCH (CD-ROM, ISBN 3–9501135–5-X).

Zilberman, U. and Smith, P. (1992). A comparison of tooth structure in Neanderthals and early *Homo sapiens sapiens*: a radiographic study. *Journal of Anatomy*, **180**, 387–93.

Zilberman, U., Skinner, M., and Smith, P. (1992). Tooth components of mandibular deciduous molars of *Homo sapiens sapiens* and *Homo sapiens neanderthalensis*: a radiographic study. *American Journal of Physical Anthropology*, **87**, 255–62.

Zollikofer, C. P. E. and Ponce de León, M. S. (2005). *Virtual Reconstruction: A Primer in Computer-Assisted Paleontology and Biomedicine*. Hoboken, NJ: Wiley-Interscience.

Index